DNA DAMAGE
AND REPAIR IN
HUMAN TISSUES

BASIC LIFE SCIENCES

Ernest H. Y. Chu, Series Editor

The University of Michigan Medical School
Ann Arbor, Michigan

Alexander Hollaender, Founding Editor

A Continuation Order Plan is available for this series. A continuation order will bring delivery
of each new volume immediately upon publication. Volumes are billed only upon actual
shipment. For further information please contact the publisher.

DNA DAMAGE AND REPAIR IN HUMAN TISSUES

Edited by

**Betsy M. Sutherland and
Avril D. Woodhead**

Brookhaven National Laboratory
Upton, New York

PLENUM PRESS • NEW YORK AND LONDON

Library of Congress Cataloging-in-Publication Data

Brookhaven Symposium in Biology (36th : 1989 : Brookhaven National
Laboratory)
    DNA damage and repair in human tissues / edited by Betsy M.
Sutherland and Avril D. Woodhead.
        p.   cm. -- (Basic life sciences ; v. 53)
    "Proceedings of Brookhaven Symposium in Biology no. 36, on DNA
damage and repair in human tissues, held October 1-4, 1989, in
Brookhaven National Laboratory, Upton, New York"--T.p. verso.
    Includes bibliographical references.
    Includes index.
    ISBN-13: 978-1-4612-7903-7   e-ISBN-13: 978-1-4613-0637-5
    DOI: 10.1007/978-1-4613-0637-5
    1. DNA damage--Congresses.   2. DNA repair--Congressses.
3. Mutagenicity testing--Congresses.   4. Human cell culture-
-Congresses.   I. Title.   II. Series.
    [DNLM: 1. DNA Damage--congresses.   2. DNA Repair--congresses.   W3
BA255 v. 53 / QU 58 B872 1989d]
QH465.A1B76   1989
616'.042--dc20
DNLM/DLC
for Library of Congress   90-7499
                                                           CIP

Proceedings of Brookhaven Symposium in Biology No. 36, on
DNA Damage and Repair in Human Tissues. held October 1-4, 1989,
at Brookhaven National Laboratory, Upton, New York

© 1990 Plenum Press, New York
Softcover reprint of the hardcover 1st edition 1990
A Division of Plenum Publishing Corporation
233 Spring Street, New York, N.Y. 10013

PREFACE

Physical and chemical agents in the environment damage the DNA of humans, and pose a major threat to human health today, and to the genetic integrity of human populations. Although studies on isolated DNA *in vitro*, on prokaryotes, on mammalian cells in culture, and on laboratory animals have provided essential background information, it is now possible to study DNA damage and repair in human tissues directly. New techniques of high sensitivity, especially those not requiring radioactive labeling have made possible quantitation of DNA damage and repair, as well as detection of residual, unrepaired DNA lesions.

In recent years, several investigators have taken up the challenge of studying damage and repair responses in humans, and we have chosen that work as the special focus of this Symposium. Major advances in understanding damage and responses in human skin, in blood cells and in human internal organs indicate three major themes. First, DNA damage levels in human tissues depend not only on the initial exposures, but also on the capapacity of that tissue for repair of the specific lesion type. Second, repair in human tissues may differ quantitatively and qualitatively from that in human cells in culture. Third, both the initial damage levels and the repair responses of humans vary over a wide range: variability is a signal characteristic of human populations!

The Symposium Committee, Symposium Coordinator, and Biology Department Business Manager thank first, the sponsors without whose generous support the meeting would not have been possible: Allergan Pharmaceuticals, Inc.; Bristol-Meyers Company; Department of Energy; Estee Lauder Inc.; Food and Drug Administration; Herbert Laboratories; Johnson & Johnson; The Proctor & Gamble Company; Risk Science Institute; and Westwood Pharmaceuticals. We also thank Ms. Kathy Folkers for outstanding work in manuscript processing; Ms. Folkers and Ms. Jean Frejka for assistance during the meeting; Ms. Judi Calace for her patience in manuscript photocopying, and all the staff of the Biology Department and Brookhaven National Laboratory who made the meeting proceed smoothly. We especially thank the many contributors who presented their exciting and, in many cases, unpublished data at the meeting, and to all the speakers who wrote their contributions for the volume promptly to allow for its early publication.

The Symposium Committee
Betsy M. Sutherland, Chair
Steven M. D'Ambrosio
Richard W. Gange
Richard B. Setlow
John C. Sutherland
Avril D. Woodhead
Symposium Coordinator
Helen Z. Kondratuk
Business Manager, Biology Department
Deborah M. Maresca

CONTENTS

DNA LESION MEASUREMENT IN HUMAN TISSUES

DAMAGE AND REPAIR IN SKIN

MEASUREMENT OF DNA ADDUCTS BY IMMUNOASSAYS

Miriam C. Poirier [1], Ainsley Weston [2], Shalina Gupta-Burt [1] and
Eddie Reed [3]

[1] Laboratory of Cellular Carcinogenesis and Tumor Promotion, and
[2] Laboratory of Human Carcinogenesis, Division of Cancer Etiology
[3] Medicine Branch, Division of Cancer Treatment

National Cancer Institute, National Institutes of Health,
Bethesda, MD, 20892

INTRODUCTION

The ability to monitor for chemical carcinogen-DNA adducts in human
tissues provides an indication that human exposure has occurred. Such data
may eventually demonstrate the dose received and/or allow the prediction of
cancer risk. At the present time evidence that the occurrence of certain
adducts is associated with specific chemical exposures is accumulating, and
multiple methods are being validated to confirm these observations.

Among the earliest techniques that made these studies possible are
immunoassays established with antisera elicited against either individual
carcinogen-DNA adducts or carcinogen-modified DNA samples (Poirier, 1984).
The antisera generated are usually specific for adducts of a particular
chemical class, and are not specific for unmodified DNA samples or normal
nucleotides; they have been employed in radioimmunoassays (RIA) and enzyme-
linked immunosorbent assays (ELISA) to measure adducts in the f.mtomole
range, that is approximately 1 adduct in 10^7 normal nucleotides. The
immunoassays are sufficiently sensitive to monitor human tissues for
evidence of exposure, but are not without difficulties since their high
degree of sensitivity is accompanied by high variability. In addition,
cross-reactivities and other properties of the antisera may limit the
capabilities of specific assays. Technical difficulties notwithstanding,
there has been an impressive advancement in this field during the past
several years, as more and more Laboratories are using immunoassays or
combining the use of adduct-specific antisera with other techniques to
determine DNA adducts in humans.

This article will focus on some technical aspects of carcinogen-DNA-
adduct immunoassay development, including characteristics of antisera
raised against DNA adducts and modified DNA samples, and measures which can
be taken to increase immunoassay sensitivity. In addition, an example of
an application of these methods for determination of DNA adducts in humans
will be described; that is, studies designed to measure cisplatin-DNA
adducts in peripheral white blood cell DNA and tissue DNA of patients
undergoing platinum-drug based chemotherapy.

DNA Damage and Repair in Human Tissues
Edited by B. M. Sutherland and A. D. Woodhead
Plenum Press, New York, 1990

Specificities of Antisera Elicited Against Carcinogen-DNA Adducts and Carcinogen-Modified DNA Samples

In order to elicit either polyclonal or monoclonal antisera it is necessary to couple the adduct hapten or modified DNA to a protein carrier. Adduct haptens are generally bonded covalently (10-25 molecules of hapten per molecule of protein) (Erlanger, 1980) while modified DNA samples (containing at least 1 adduct in 100 bases) are mixed with a methylated protein creating an electrostatic coupling, which is stable due to the polymeric nature of DNA (Stollar, 1980). Rabbits injected with a DNA-adduct immunogen usually respond well to repeated injections and late boosting. In contrast, a modified DNA immunogen, even if double stranded, may elicit undesirable anti-DNA antisera if the rabbits are injected many times. New antisera can be characterized by immunoassay; the most common of these are RIA (Zettner, 1973; Butler, 1980) and ELISA (Engvall, 1980), the former requiring a high specific-activity radiolabeled version of the immunogen, and the latter requiring some rather sophisticated equipment for washing and reading microtiter plates (Fig. 1, - - and —). Competitive immunoassays can be used to test for cross-reactivity with unmodified DNA samples, normal nucleotides, the carcinogen alone and other adducts of the

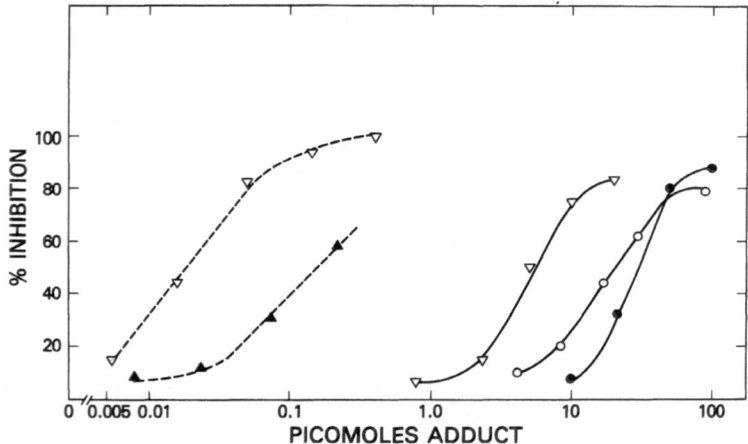

Fig. 1. Immunoassay curves established with a rabbit antiserum elicited against DNA modified with the anti-7,8 diol-9,10 epoxide of benzo(a)pyrene such that the only adduct was trans-(7R)-N²-{ 10 (7β,8α,9α-trihydroxy-7,8,9,10-tetrahydrobenzo[a]pyrene)-yl} - deoxyguanosine (BPdG)(Poirier et al., 1980). For RIA (——) the tracer was ³H-BPdG, and for ELISA (- - -) wells were coated with denatured BPdG-DNA modified to 1% (30 pmoles/ug DNA, the original immunogen). Competition curves for RIA are: the immunogen DNA as native (0) and denatured (▽), and the individual BPdG adduct (●). Competition curves for ELISA are: the denatured immunogen (▼), and a denatured BPdG-DNA modified at 4.5 fmol/ug DNA (Santella et al., 1988)(▲).

same carcinogen as well as adducts and DNA samples modified with carcinogens of the same or different chemical classes (Fig. 1 and 2).

When an antiserum has been elicited against an individual adduct there will often be cross-reactivity for structurally-similar adducts of the same compound (Müller and Rajewsky, 1981; Groopman et al., 1984) or of other compounds in the same chemical class (Poirier, 1981; Santella, 1988). The practical implication of this is that human samples might be expected to contain a mixture of adducts from compounds of the same chemical class and therefore the numbers obtained when samples are quantified against one standard adduct may not be precise. Antisera raised against an individual adduct often recognize that adduct in a modified DNA to a lesser extent than the adduct alone (Poirier, 1981; Poirier and Connor, 1982). Therefore, it is usual to hydrolyze a biological DNA sample in order to measure all of the adducts present. In addition, an anti-adduct antiserum frequently has specificity for ribo-adducts of the same compound. Thus, removal of RNA during the preparation of biological DNA samples ensures exclusive measurement of DNA adducts (Poirier, 1981).

An antiserum elicited against a chemically-modified DNA often has little (Poirier et al., 1980) or no (Reed et al., 1990) cross reactivity for the individual DNA adduct (Fig. 1, ●——●). In this case, biological samples are generally assayed as native or denatured. Such an antiserum may recognize denatured modified DNA better than native modified DNA (Fig. 1, 0 and ▽) even though the immunogen was native (Poirier et al., 1980). Recognition of DNA samples modified with compounds of the same chemical class is frequent. For example, an antiserum raised against DNA modified with benzo(a)pyrene-7,8diol-9,10epoxide is also specific for DNAs modified with a number of polycyclic aromatic hydrocarbon-diol epoxides (Fig. 2; Weston, et al., 1989), and an antiserum raised against cisplatin-DNA recognized DNA samples modified with a number of cisplatin analogs (Lippard et al., 1983). Thus, in practice, results obtained with human samples, in which quantitation is against a specific modified-DNA standard, are not necessarily precise because of the possibility that each DNA sample is composed of a mixture of DNA adducts recognized by that antiserum. In addition, the extent of DNA modification may influence the antibody recognition (Van Schooten et al., 1987; Santella et al., 1988). To be sufficiently immunogenic a modified DNA must have adducts in the range of one adduct in 100 bases; this type of DNA sample is conformationally very different from a biological sample modified in the range of one adduct in 10^6 bases. An antiserum raised against a highly-modified DNA immunogen may not recognize all of the adducts in a DNA modified at a significantly lower level and the resulting inaccuracy will yield an underestimation of the biological samples when they are quantified against a highly-modified DNA standard curve (Van Schooten et al., 1987; Santella et al., 1988; Poirier et al., 1988). If the discrepancy between antibody recognition of high and low modified DNA samples is only several fold it may be possible to obtain accurate values by using a low-modified standard curve (see Fig. 1, ELISA curves). However, in validating the assay it is advisable to check the absolute adduct quantitation by another method, such as a radiolabeled carcinogen (Santella et al., 1988).

Factors Influencing the Sensitivities of RIAs and ELISAs for DNA Adduct Measurements in Humans

In general, the sensitivity of an RIA rests upon the affinity of the antiserum (ideally above 10^8 liters/mole) and the specific activity of the tracer (>6 Ci/mmole). For measurement of human DNA adducts the amount of DNA that can be put into one RIA tube is an important factor which must be determined for each assay. In the case of an anti-DNA adduct antiserum, hydrolysis of the DNA sample is required for quantitative determination,

and a significant increase in sensitivity can be obtained by chromato-
graphing the hydrolysate and assaying the appropriate column fractions for
adduct without the interfering normal nucleosides (Müller and Rajewsky et
al., 1981; Plooy et al., 1985). The sensitivity of an RIA can be augmented
somewhat through the use of sequential saturation (non-equilibrium)
conditions (Zettner and Duly, 1974), in which the tracer is given a short
time to compete after the antiserum and non-radiolabeled inhibitor have
reached equilibrium. Often an RIA will not be as sensitive as an ELISA
(see Fig. 1), but that may depend on the antiserum in question (Poirier,
1990).

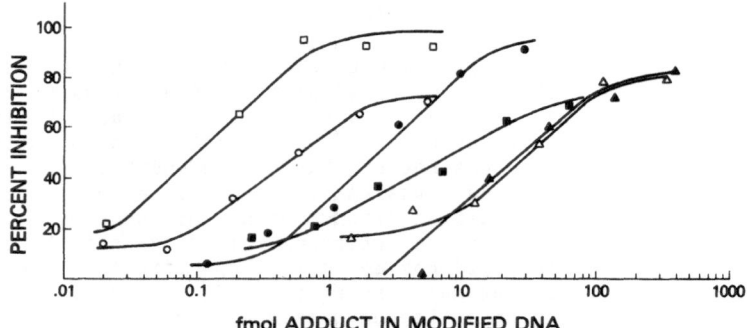

Fig. 2.   Competitive ELISA with the same conditions as Fig. 1 (- - -) in
           which the standard immunogen BPdG-DNA is competed as denatured
           (0). Other curves are denatured DNA samples modified in the
           range of 0.1-1.0% with the diol-epoxides of : chrysene (□),
           benzo[k]fluoranthene (Δ), dibenz[a,c]anthracene (▲) and the bay
           region (0) and non-bay region (■) benz[a,c]anthracenes. This
           ELISA demonstrated that the antiserum has specificity for all of
           the above modified DNA samples.

     For ELISAs the amount of DNA which will not alter the standard curve
provides the limit of sensitivity, and can be in the range of 35-50 ug of
native or denatured DNA per well (Poirier, 1990). Hydrolytic enzymes
generally inhibit ELISA reactions and must be removed before assay; if this
is done chromatographically and the appropriate fractions assayed an
impressive increase in sensitivity can be achieved (Plooy et al., 1985).
The sensitivity of an ELISA can also be augmented by the choice of enzyme
substrate. For example, a 10 fold increase in the sensitivity of the
benzo(a)pyrene-DNA standard curve was obtained by using methyl-
umbelliferyl-phosphate as compared to p-nitro-phenylphosphate. The former
compound gives a fluorescent product with a much more intense signal than
the colorimetric end-point of the latter (Santella et al., 1988).

APPLICATION OF IMMUNOASSAYS FOR THE DETERMINATION OF DNA ADDUCTS IN TISSUE
AND BLOOD CELL DNA OF CANCER PATIENTS

The earliest attempts to measure DNA adducts in human tissues
comprised studies in which lung tumor and surrounding lung tissue were
examined for evidence of polycyclic aromatic hydrocarbon-DNA adduct
formation (Perera et al., 1982) using an ELISA (Fig. 1, - - -)
established with the anti-BPdG-DNA antiserum (Poirier et al., 1980). Even
though a small percentage of the samples were positive in the ELISA, the
investigation encountered serious problems. It was not possible to document
the dose of hydrocarbon received from smoking and other sources even though
extensive questionnaires were administered. In addition, there was no
correlation between the heaviest smokers and the individuals with the
highest adduct levels, and there was a great deal of uncertainty concerning
the choice of a proper control. In an attempt to overcome these
difficulties and validate the use of ELISAs to determine DNA adducts in
human samples, antiserum was elicited against the DNA-damaging
chemotherapeutic agent cisplatin (Fig. 3). The immunogen in these studies
was calf thymus DNA modified to approximately 4 adducts per 100 nucleotides
with cisplatin (Poirier et al.,1982). Our intention was to determine DNA
adducts in a human cohort in which the exact exposure dosage was known, and
this approach had the additional advantage that it would be possible to
obtain truly unexposed controls.

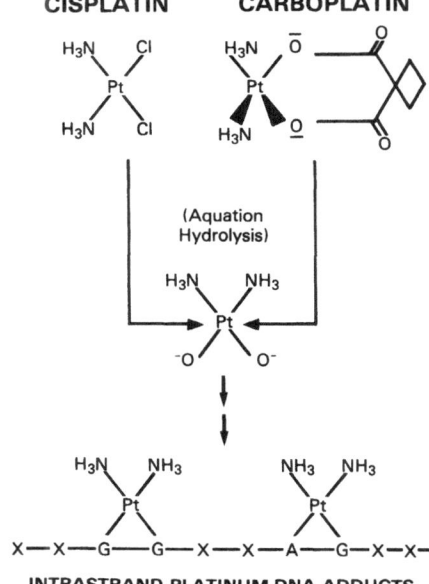

Fig. 3.   Structures of cisplatin and carboplatin (CBDCA), and their major
           intrastrand adducts with DNA.

Cisplatin is a highly effective chemotherapeutic agent (Calvert, 1986; Einhorn et al., 1985) currently in use for a variety of human cancers, and responsible for extensive cures (approximately 90%) in individuals with testicular cancer. This compound, and other cis-reacting analogs such as carboplatin (CBDCA, Fig. 3), bind to DNA at the N7 positions of adjacent deoxyguanosines or a deoxyadenosine and a deoxyguanosine (5'-3') in the same DNA strand. Although interstrand DNA adducts are also formed, the intrastrand bidentate adducts comprise the major fraction of platinum bound to DNA (Plooy et al., 1985) and were the major epitopes recognized by the antiserum elicited against cisplatin-modified DNA (Poirier et al., 1982). In early studies this antiserum was shown to be specific for the highly-modified immunogen DNA, DNA from cultured cells exposed to cisplatin and nucleated blood cell DNA from a patient receiving cisplatin chemotherapy (Fig. 4). In addition, the antiserum was not specific for unmodified calf thymus DNA or DNA from a patient receiving non-platinum-based chemotherapy (Fig. 4). These initial studies suggested that monitoring of human tissues for DNA adducts of platinum drugs would be possible.

Cisplatin-DNA Adducts in Human Tissues Obtained at Autopsy

A variety of tissues were obtained from eight individuals autopsied at the NIH clinical center; the cohort comprised one female with breast cancer, one male with diffuse histiocytic lymphoma and six females with ovarian cancer. These patients ranged in age from 35 to 75 years and had received cumulative platinum drug doses between 700 and 9210 mg/m² of body surface area. Four of the patients with the highest cumulative drug doses

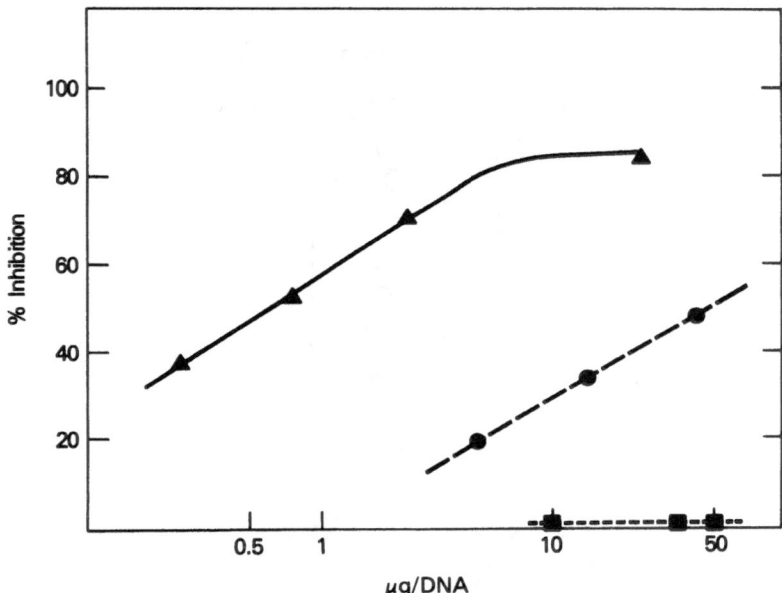

Fig. 4.   Competitive ELISA with anti-cisplatin-DNA antiserum. Immunogen cisplatin-DNA was coated on wells and competed against: (▲) DNA from mouse keratinocytes exposed to 20 u molar cisplatin; (●) DNA from blood of a patient who received 40 mg/m² of body surface area of cisplatin; (■) unmodified calf thymus DNA and a DNA sample from a patient who did not receive platinum drugs.

had achieved remissions of 4-7 months duration prior to events which lead to their final demise, and 6 of the patients had received their most recent therapy between 2 and 15 months before they were evaluated for adducts. Ovarian tumor tissue was obtained on 4 of the 8 individuals, and other tissues included bone marrow, lymph node, spleen, kidney, liver, peripheral nerve and brain. Cisplatin-DNA adducts, determined by ELISA (Table 1), were found in all of these tissues, although not all tissues were present for each individual, and not all tissues of one individual contained adducts.

The results show that cisplatin-DNA adducts accumulate in a wide variety of human tissues, including tissues that are target sites for cisplatin toxicity such as kidney, peripheral nerve, brain and tumor. Adduct levels in tumor were found to be similar to those in other tissues of the same individual. The highly-persistent nature of the intrastrand bidentate adduct was demonstrated in these experiments since at least three of the individuals were autopsied 12-15 months after receiving their last therapy. In a previous study (Poirier et al., 1987) adducts were determined in kidney, liver and spleen from four individuals; one of these individuals had survived 22 months since the last therapy, and adducts were still measurable in the kidney DNA. It is possible that the chemotherapeutic efficacy, as well as the toxic effects of the platinum drugs are related to the widespread adduct distribution and the high degree of persistence observed here. These compounds are rodent carcinogens (Leopold et al.,1979; Barnhart and Bowden, 1985), and may eventually cause second tumors in cancer patients cured of their original malignancies.

Table 1. ELISA Determination of Platinum-DNA Adducts (attomoles of adduct/ ug of DNA) in Multiple Human Tissues Obtained at Autopsy

	Patient Number							
TISSUE	1	2	3	4	5	6	7	8
Tumor	-*	-	106	58	-	176	73	-
Bone Marrow	-	0	100	77	-	-	45	36
Lymph Node	0	143	-	0	-	-	-	-
Spleen	88	343	74	-	141	-	283	113
Kidney	-	511	66	50	-	315	122	184
Liver	-	457	10	45	211	342	96	78
Peripheral Nerve	-	0	-	0	-	62	0	315
Brain - White	-	143	122	62	-	-	-	833
Brain - Grey	-	306	100	112	-	-	-	456

The ELISA lower limit of sensitivity was 25 attomol/ug DNA and is designated by "0". *Specimen not available.

Cisplatin-DNA Adducts in Human Nucleated Blood Cell DNA

Since it is rarely possible to obtain biopsy materials of malignancies or normal tissues from living patients, we investigated the possibility that DNA adducts measured in nucleated blood cell DNA might vary with dose, be indicative of DNA adducts in the tumor, and reflect or predict disease response. For these studies DNA was prepared from 35-45 ml of blood taken from ovarian or testicular cancer patients at the NIH clinical center. Patients were given 5 days of cisplatin infusion and samples were drawn on the morning of day 6. Frequently samples were obtained from the same individual on multiple monthly cycles of therapy since the drug was usually given during one week, and this was followed by three drug-free weeks to comprise one cycle of treatment (Reed et al., 1986). ELISA results are shown in Fig. 5. Adduct levels in 27 positive samples were plotted as a function of cycle of treatment and the dose-related increase in adducts had a linear regression correlation coefficient of 0.79. Six samples obtained from untreated individuals were clearly negative for adduct formation (Fig. 5). What is not shown in Fig. 5 is that in any large group of samples approximately 40% of samples from treated individuals do not contain measurable adducts. However, those which are positive exhibit a dose response suggesting that adducts accumulate during monthly exposures. Since it is known that most nucleated blood cells have a relatively short life-span, it is assumed that this accumulation over weeks of time reflects

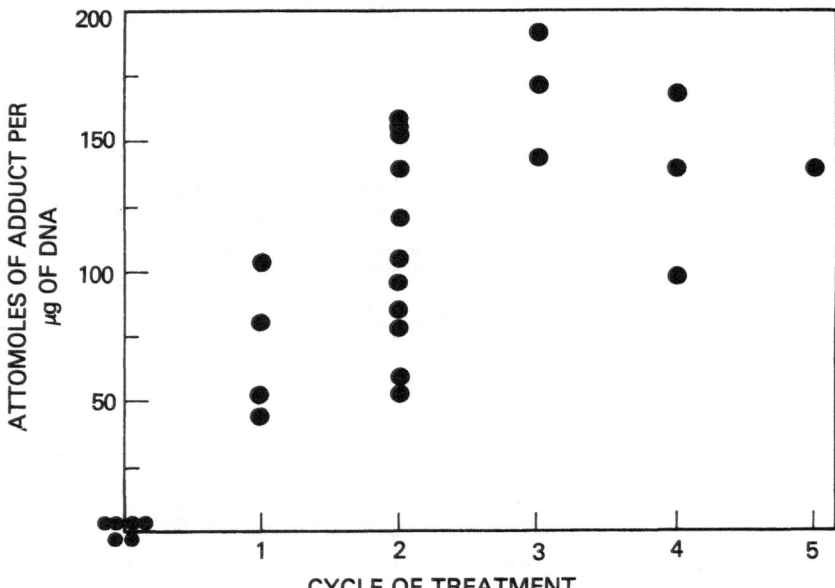

Fig. 5.   Accumulation of cisplatin-DNA adducts in nucleated blood cell DNA of previously-untreated ovarian and testicular cancer patients during monthly cycles of cisplatin-based therapy. Six individuals had samples taken before treatment, serving as unexposed controls.

adduct formation which begins in the granulocyte precursor cells and continues to damage these cells with continuing cisplatin exposure.

The relationship between blood cell DNA adduct formation and disease response was addressed in 55 ovarian and 17 testicular cancer patients treated at the NIH Clinical Center (Reed et al., 1987). The ovarian patients comprised four treatment groups, two on combination chemotherapy and two receiving high-dose, single agent therapy of either cisplatin or carboplatin (Fig. 3). The testicular cancer patients all had metastatic "poor prognosis" disseminated disease and were given one of two combination protocols. Disease response was obtained from the medical records and was categorized as: complete response (CR), or total absence of visible disease; partial response (PR), or greater than 50% tumor reduction; and, no response (NR), or less than 50% tumor reduction. When blood samples were assayed by ELISA and plotted as a function of disease response (Fig. 6) there were many samples from non-responders which did not contain measurable adducts. Conversely, the median adduct level for the CRs was the highest of all three groups (Fig. 6), and decreased significantly with the poorer responses in a statistically significant trend (Reed et al., 1987). Thus, it appears that when a large group of samples is analyzed high adduct levels in blood cell DNA can correlate with a favorable disease response. This is presumably related to the fact that adduct levels in blood cell DNA also reflect adduct levels in the tumor.

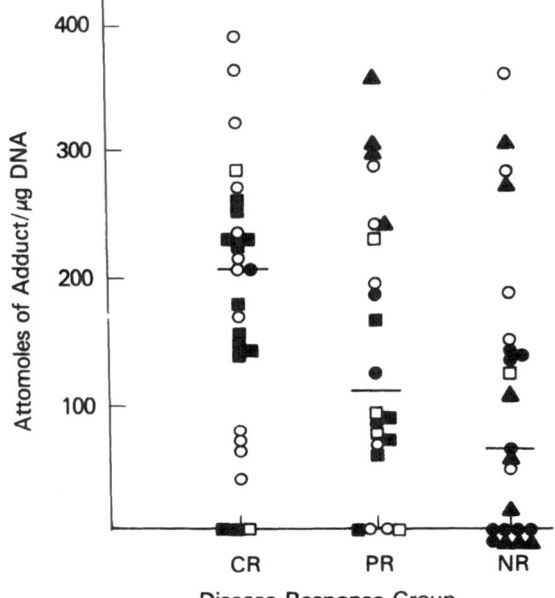

Fig. 6.   Cisplatin-DNA adduct levels in blood cell DNA from 72 testicular and ovarian cancer patients plotted as a function of response to therapy. See text for definitions of complete response (CR), partial response (PR) and no response (NR). Median adduct levels for the group are designated by the solid bars.

CONCLUSIONS

These studies demonstrate the successful utilization of DNA adduct-specific antisera for determination of chemicals bound to DNA in human tissue by immunoassay. Currently, immunoassays provide incontrovertible evidence of human exposure. Data generated by these assays may help elucidate the mechanisms by which DNA binding drugs are clinically active, and may provide information useful in the molecular epidemiology of cancer.

REFERENCES

Barnhart, K. M. and Bowden, G. T., 1985, Cisplatin as an initiating agent in two-stage mouse skin carcinogenesis, Cancer Lett., 29:101.

Butler, J. E., 1980, Antibody-antigen and antibody-hapten reactions, in: "Enzyme-Immunoassay", E. T. Maggio, ed., CRC Press, Inc., Boca Raton, p 6.

Calvert, A. H., 1986, Clinical application of platinum metal complexes, in: "Biochemical Mechanisms of Platinum Antitumor Drugs", D. C. H. McBrien and T. F. Slater, eds., IRL Press, Oxford, p 307.

Einhorn, L. H., Donohue, J. P., Peckham, M. J., Williams, S. D., and Loehrer, P. J., 1985, Cancer of the testes, in: "Cancer - Principles and Practice of Oncology", V. T. DeVita, S. Hellman, and S. A. Rosenberg, eds., Lippincott, Philadelphia, p 979.

Engvall, E., 1980, Enzyme immunoassay ELISA and EMIT, Methods in Enzymology, 70:419.

Erlanger, B. F., 1980, The preparation of antigenic hapten-carrier conjugates: A survey, Methods in Enzymology, 70:85.

Groopman, J. D., Trudel, L. J., Donahue, P. R., Marshak-Rothstein, A., and Wogan, G. N., 1984, High-affinity monoclonal antibodies for aflatoxins and their application to solid-phase immunoassays, Proc. Natl. Acad. Sci. USA, 81:7728.

Leopold, W. R., Miller, E. C., and Miller, J. A., 1979, Carcinogenicity of antitumor cis-platinum(II) coordination complexes in the mouse and rat, Cancer Res., 39:913.

Lippard, S. J., Ushay, H. M., Merkel, C. M., and Poirier, M. C., 1983, Use of antibodies to probe the stereochemistry of antitumor platinum drug binding to deoxyribonucleic acid, Biochemistry, 22:5165.

Müller, R. and Rajewsky, M. F., 1981, Antibodies specific for DNA components structurally modified by chemical carcinogens, J. Cancer Res. Clin. Oncol., 102:99.

Perera, F. P., Poirier, M. C., Yuspa, S. H., Nakayama, J., Jaretzki, A., Curnen, M. M., Knowles, D. M., and Weinstein, I. B., 1982, A pilot project in molecular cancer epidemiology: Determination of benzo[a]pyrene-DNA adducts in animal and human tissues by immunoassays, Carcinogenesis, 3:1405.

Plooy, A. C. M., Fichtinger-Schepman, A. M. J., Schutte, H. H., van Dijk, M., and Lohman, P. H. M., 1985, The quantitative detection of various Pt-DNA-adducts in Chinese hamster ovary cells treated with cisplatin: application of immunochemical techniques, Carcinogenesis, 6:561.

Poirier, M. C., Santella, R., Weinstein, I. B., Grunberger, D., and Yuspa, S. H., 1980, Quantitation of benzo(a)pyrene-deoxyguanosine adducts by radioimmunoassay, Cancer Research, 40:412.

Poirier, M. C., 1981, Antibodies to carcinogen-DNA adducts, JNCI, 67:515.

Poirier, M. C. and Connor, R. J., 1982, Radioimmunoassay for 2-acetylamino-fluorene-DNA adducts, Methods in Enzymology, 84:607.

Poirier, M. C., Lippard, S. J., Zwelling, L. A., Ushay, H. M., Kerrigan, D., Thill, C. C., Santella, R. M., Grunberger, D., and Yuspa, S. H., 1982, Antibodies elicited against cis-diamminedichloroplatinum(II)-modified DNA are specific for cis-diamminedichloroplatinum(II)-DNA adducts formed in vivo and in vitro, Proc. Natl. Acad. Sci. USA, 9:6443.

Poirier, M. C., 1984, The use of carcinogen-DNA adduct antisera for
     quantitation and localization of genomic damage in animal models and
     the human population, Environ. Mutagen., 6:879.
Poirier, M. C., Reed, E., Ozols, R. F., Fasy, T., and Yuspa, S. H., 1987,
     DNA adducts of cisplatin in nucleated peripheral blood cells and
     tissues of cancer patients, Prog. Exp. Tumor Res., 31:104.
Poirier, M. C., Egorin, M. J., Fichtinger-Schepman, A. M. J., and Reed, E.,
     1988, DNA adducts of cisplatin and carboplatin in tissues of human
     cancer patients, in: "Methods for Detecting Damaging Agents in
     Humans: Applications in Cancer Epidemiology and Prevention", H.
     Bartsch, K. Hemminki, and I. K. O'Neill, eds., International Agency
     for Research on Cancer Scientific Publication No. 89, Lyon, p 313.
Poirier, M. C., 1990, Development of immunoassays for the detection of
     carcinogen-DNA adducts, in: "Monitoring Human Exposure to
     Carcinogens: Analytical, Epidemiological and Ethical Considerations"
     P. L. Skipper, F. Koshier, and J. D. Groopman, eds., Telford Press,
     Caldwell, in press.
Reed, E., Ostchega, Y., Steinberg, S. M., Yuspa, S. H., Young, R. C.,
     Ozols, R. F., and Poirier, M. C., 1990, An evaluation of platinum-DNA
     adduct levels relative to known prognostic variables in a cohort of
     ovarian cancer patients, Carcinogenesis, in press.
Reed, E., Ozols, R. F., Tarone, R., Yuspa, S. H., and Poirier, M. C., 1987,
     Platinum-DNA adducts in leukocyte DNA correlate with disease response
     in ovarian cancer patients receiving platinum-based chemotherapy,
     Proc. Natl. Acad. Sci. USA, 84:5024.
Reed, E., Yuspa, S. H., Zwelling, L. A., Ozols, R. F., and Poirier, M. C.,
     1986, Quantitation of cis-diamminedichloroplatinum(II) (Cisplatin)-
     DNA intrastrand adducts in testicular and ovarian cancer patients
     receiving cisplatin chemotherapy. J. Clin. Invest., 77:545.
Santella, R. M., 1988, Application of new techniques for the detection of
     carcinogen adducts to human population monitoring, Mutation Research,
     205:271.
Santella, R. M., Weston, A., Perera, F. P., Trivers, G. T., Harris, C. C.,
     Young, T. L., Nguyen, D., Lee, B. M., and Poirier, M. C., 1988,
     Interlaboratory comparison of antisera and immunoassays for
     benzo[a]pyrene-diol-epoxide-I-modified DNA, Carcinogenesis, 9:1265.
Stollar, B. D., 1980, The experimental induction of antibodies to nucleic
     acids, Methods in Enzymology, 70:70.
Van Schooten, F. J., Kriek, E., Steenwinkel, M. S. T., Noteborn, H. P. J.
     M., Hillebrand, M. J. X., and Leeuwen, F. E. V., 1987, The binding
     efficiency of polyclonal and monoclonal antibodies to DNA modified
     with benzo[a]pyrene diol epoxide is dependent on the level of
     modification. Implications for quantitation of benzo[a]pyrene-DNA
     adducts in vivo, Carcinogenesis, 8:1263.
Weston, A., Manchester, D. K., Poirier, M. C., Choi, J.-S., Trivers, G.E.,
     Mann, D. L., and Harris, C. C., 1989, Derivative fluorescence
     spectral analysis of polycyclic aromatic hydrocarbon-DNA adducts in
     human placenta, Chem. Res. Toxicol., 2:104.
Zettner, A., 1973, Principles of competitive binding assays (saturation
     analyses). I. Equilibrium techniques, Clin. Chem., 19:699.
Zettner, A. and Duly, P. E., 1974, Principles of competitive binding assays
     (saturation analyses). II. Sequential saturation, Clin. Chem., 20:5.

DETECTION OF HUMAN DNA ADDUCTS

BY ^{32}P-POSTLABELING

Kurt Randerath and Erika Randerath

Division of Toxicology, Department of Pharmacology
Baylor College of Medicine
Houston, Texas 77030, USA

INTRODUCTION

Humans are exposed to a wide variety of genotoxic and tumor-promoting agents in their environment. These may occur as individual carcinogens such as certain aromatic amines or hydrocarbons in occupational settings, or as incompletely defined complex mixtures such as cigarette smoke. The important role of tumor promoters in multistage carcinogenesis of experimental animals and humans (Pitot, 1986) is documented by many lines of evidence, but no practical end-point has been developed for the biomonitoring of human exposure to tumor promoters. On the other hand, most known human carcinogens are tumor initiators, and fortunately, a number of sensitive assays have been developed over the past 10-15 years to measure the formation of covalent addition products (adducts) of DNA, a key event in tumor initiation. Some of the assays, such as ^{32}P-postlabeling, allow one to monitor activities of unidentified carcinogens and carcinogen mixtures at the target site (DNA), a feature that is particularly important for assessing human carcinogen exposure. Assays for DNA adducts are currently acquiring an increasingly significant role in the identification of environmental carcinogens and in the estimation of their role played in the causation of human cancer. This article reviews the current status of the ^{32}P-postlabeling assay and its application to human exposures.

THE ^{32}P-POSTLABELING ASSAY

Basic Methodology

The ^{32}P-postlabeling assay for nucleic acid adducts represents an extension of earlier radiolabeling procedures with tritium (E. Randerath et al., 1972; K. Randerath et al., 1980) or [125]I (K. Randerath, 1981) for measuring the normal and modified base content of RNA. These assays entail the initial enzymatic hydrolysis of the RNA or DNA preparation under test to monomers (nucleosides or nucleotides) or dimers. The hydrolysis products are subsequently radiolabeled by chemical or enzymatic reactions and the labeled derivatives are chromatographically separated and quantified by scintillation counting. The ^{32}P-postlabeling assay for DNA adducts has been reviewed recently

DNA Damage and Repair in Human Tissues
Edited by B. M. Sutherland and A. D. Woodhead
Plenum Press, New York, 1990

(K. Randerath et al., 1984a, 1985; Reddy and Randerath, 1987; Watson, 1987; Hemminki and Randerath, 1987; Gupta and Randerath, 1988), and a number of reviews and books have dealt with the general aspects and measurement of carcinogen exposure (Miller and Miller, 1981; Hemminki, 1983; Kriek et al., 1984; Berlin et al., 1984; Wogan and Gorelick, 1985; Farmer et al., 1987; Bartsch et al., 1988).

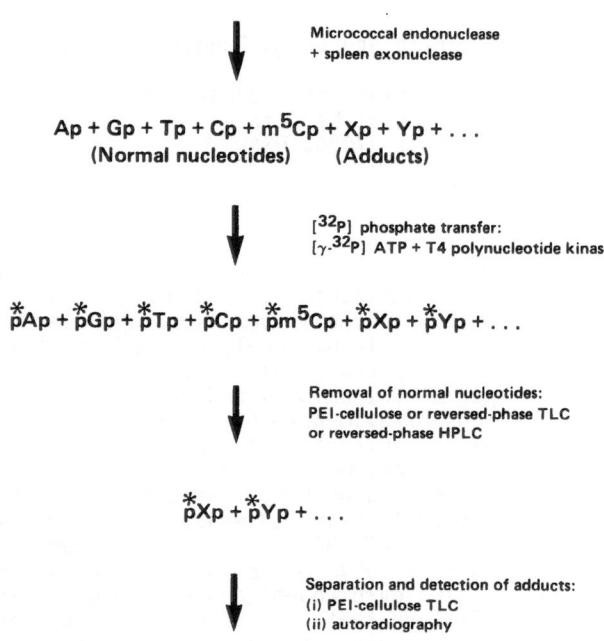

Fig. 1   The basic ^{32}P-postlabeling assay for DNA adducts involves 4 steps: Digestion of DNA to 3'-monophosphate nucleotides, ^{32}P-labeling of digestion products, removal of ^{32}P-labeled non-adduct components, and TLC mapping of ^{32}P-postlabeled adducts. Asterisks indicate ^{32}P-label.

Standard Nucleoside Bisphosphate Assay

In this procedure (K. Randerath et al., 1981; Reddy et al., 1981; Gupta et al., 1982), microgram amounts of DNA are exhaustively digested to deoxyribonucleoside 3'-monophosphates, which are then quantitatively ^{32}P-labeled in the presence of T4 polynucleotide kinase and a molar excess of [γ-^{32}P]ATP (spec. act., ~200 Ci/mmol) (Fig. 1). The ^{32}P-labeled nucleotides are resolved by polyethyleneimine (PEI)-cellulose anion-exchange TLC, first to separate the adducts from the excess of normal DNA nucleotides and then to resolve the adducts from each other (Gupta et al., 1982; K. Randerath et al., 1984a, 1984b, 1985; Reddy et al., 1984). Electrolyte solutions containing 6 - 8.5 M urea have been found particularly useful as chromatographic solvents (Gupta et al., 1982; Reddy et al., 1984). ^{32}P-labeled TLC fractions ("spots") are located on X-ray film by screen-intensified autoradiography and if desired, quantitated by scintillation counting of excised fractions (Gupta et al., 1982; Gupta and Randerath, 1988).

This procedure is applicable to DNA containing individual bulky-aromatic adducts at a minimum level of 1 adduct in 3×10^7 DNA nucleotides and allows reproducible quantitations if adduct levels are in the range of 1 in 10^4 to 5×10^6 nucleotides, as frequently observed in model studies employing cultured cells or experimental animals.

Intensification Version of Assay

This procedure (E. Randerath et al., 1985) is related to the standard assay in that the normal DNA 3'-nucleotides in the original DNA hydrolysate are not removed before ^{32}P-labeling. In contrast to the standard assay, however, a limiting amount of [γ-^{32}P]ATP is added rather than an excess over normal nucleotides. Under such conditions, many bulky or aromatic adducts are labeled at a higher rate than the normal nucleotides. This results in a considerably enhanced sensitivity of adduct detection, particularly if carrier-free [γ-^{32}P]ATP (spec. act., 4000 - 6000 Ci/mmol) is used for labeling. Before this procedure can be applied to adduct quantitation, "intensification factors" (IF's) need to be determined which reflect the variable labeling rates for individual adducts (E. Randerath et al., 1985; Gupta and Randerath, 1988).

The procedure is suitable for DNA samples containing adducts at 10 - 100 times lower levels as compared with the standard assay, provided the adducts are labeled preferentially over the normal nucleotides. The sensitivity of this procedure obviously depends on the magnitude of the intensification factors. This technique has been employed in both animal (E. Randerath et al., 1985, 1986; Schurdak and Randerath 1985, 1989; Schurdak et al., 1987a, 1987b; Schut et al., 1988) and human (Everson et al., 1986) studies. The intensification assay affords reproducible quantitative results for levels of individual aromatic adducts in the range of 1 in 10^5 to 10^8 DNA nucleotides. Since the procedure is technically simpler and requires less DNA than assays involving 3'-monophosphate adduct enrichment, it is superior to other ^{32}P-postlabeling techniques if the adducts are preferentially labeled and their levels are sufficient.

Nuclease P1 Enrichment

This procedure involves the selective enzymatic enrichment of 3'-nucleotide adducts prior to ^{32}P-labeling by 3'-dephosphorylation of normal nucleotides to nucleosides which do not serve as substrates for polynucleotide-kinase labeling (Fig. 2) (Reddy and Randerath, 1986, 1987). The remaining adducts are ^{32}P-labeled with an excess of carrier-free [γ-^{32}P]ATP (4000 - 6000 Ci/mmol), resulting in a sensitivity of detection down to 1 adduct in 10^{10} nucleotides. If this extreme sensitivity is not required (which is often the case), ATP of lower specific activity is used. (ATP of lower specific activity is prepared by diluting carrier-free ^{32}P-labeled ATP with unlabeled ADP-free ATP or by employing a mixture of non-radioactive inorganic phosphate and [^{32}P]phosphate for ATP synthesis.)

Nuclease P1-enhanced ^{32}P-postlabeling has become a standard method for the analysis of human DNA samples for covalent lesions (see APPLICATIONS TO HUMAN DNA) and for the detection and measurement of I-compounds, i.e. putative endogenous DNA modifications in tissues of untreated animals (K. Randerath et al., 1986a, 1988a, 1988b, 1989a; Li et al., 1989). While the method is applicable to a large number of bulky/aromatic DNA adducts, the 3'-monophosphate adducts of arylamines bound to the C8 position of guanine undergo significant dephosphorylation by nuclease P1, resulting in incomplete recoveries (Reddy and Randerath, 1986; K. Randerath et al., 1988a; Gupta and Earley, 1988; Gallagher et al., 1989). In this case, a procedure which does not involve enrichment or which employs another enrichment technique is substituted.

BISPHOSPHATE VERSION OF ASSAY

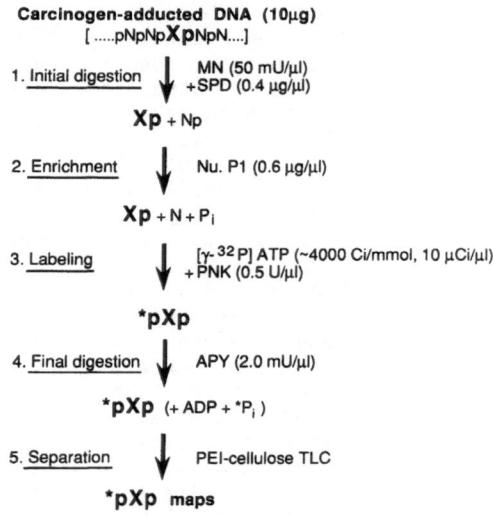

Fig. 2   Nuclease P1 enhancement of the ^{32}P-postlabeling assay entails the removal of normal DNA nucleotides by enzymatic enrichment before ^{32}P-labeling of adducted nucleotides with carrier-free [γ-^{32}P]ATP.

Butanol Enrichment

This procedure entails adduct purification by extraction into n-butanol (Gupta, 1985) rather than by enzymatic enrichment. Similar sensitivity is achieved as in the nuclease P1 procedure (Gupta, 1985; Gupta and Randerath, 1988; Gupta and Earley, 1988) but more time and effort are required. For the reasons outlined in the preceding paragraph, it is superior to enzymatic enrichment as a means to purify certain aromatic-amine adducts. On the other hand, certain adducts are recovered better by enzymatic enrichment (Gupta and Earley, 1988).

HPLC Enrichment

Dunn and San (1988) have described HPLC enrichment of aromatic adducts. Normal and adducted 3'-nucleotides in digests of benzo(a)pyrene-modified DNA were injected onto a reversed-phase HPLC column and normal nucleotides were eluted with 5% methanol, 95% 1 M ammonium formate, pH 3.5. The adducted nucleotides were then recovered from the column by methanol-gradient elution. The collected adduct fractions were dried and then subjected to ^{32}P-postlabeling using carrier-free [γ-^{32}P]ATP. Results were similar to those obtained with nuclease P1 enrichment. This procedure appears applicable to bulky 3'-nucleotide adducts which undergo significant dephosphorylation by nuclease P1.

The procedures outlined so far all take advantage of the marked physicochemical, chromatographic, and biochemical differences between non-polar, bulky/aromatic DNA adducts and normal nucleotides. On the other hand, adduct derivatives of low-molecular weight carcinogens often closely resemble the normal nucleotides in their physicochemical and biochemical properties, so that different procedures need to be applied for their analysis. ^{32}P-labeling of "small" adducts is readily accomplished (K. Randerath et al., 1981), and levels of 1 adduct in 10^4 to 10^5 DNA nucleotides can be measured without enrichment (Reddy et al, 1984); however, more sensitive detection requires adduct purification prior to labeling. Several laboratories have developed techniques for the analysis of small alkyl and etheno adducts (Dietrich et al., 1987; Wilson et al., 1988; Watson and Crane, 1989). This involved reversed-phase HPLC purification to isolate specific 3'-monophosphate adducts of interest, ^{32}P-postlabeling of these adducts, and ^{32}P-adduct separation by HPLC or TLC. A limit of detection of 1 adduct in 10^7 to 10^8 nucleotides was achieved; this level of sensitivity often should be sufficient for monitoring human and animal exposures giving rise to "small" adducts. This area needs further development so that a greater range as well as complex mixtures of polar adducts become amenable to ^{32}P-analysis. Generally applicable procedures for the efficient separation of normal nucleotides from "small" adducts are still lacking.

Nucleoside Monophosphate Version of Assay

This recently developed technique (K. Randerath et al., 1989b) represents a major departure from the conventional postlabeling assay in that the DNA is hydrolysed by a mixture of nuclease P1 and prostatic acid phosphatase rather than micrococcal nuclease and spleen phosphodiesterase. This leads to the generation of different ^{32}P-postlabeled adducts. As shown in Fig. 3, non-polar bulky/aromatic adducts are released from DNA as dinucleotides (XpN) while normal nucleotides are converted to nucleosides (N). The internucleotide linkage on the 3'-side of bulky adducts, X, resists attack by nuclease P1 so that the adducts are excised from DNA in the form of 5'-phosphorylated dinucleotides, pXpN, in contrast to normal nucleotides which are obtained as mononucleotides, pN. In the presence of prostatic acid phosphatase, these products are 5'-dephosphorylated yielding adducted dinucleotides, XpN, which are subsequently ^{32}P-labeled (step 2). (Normal nucleosides, N, are not substrates for labeling). The 5'-^{32}P-labeled products, *pXpN, are mapped as such, or further digested by snake venom phosphodiesterase (step 3) and mapped in 5'-monophosphate, *pX, form (step 4). This scheme does not entail separate adduct enrichment for maximal sensitivity since normal nucleotides are inactivated by enzymatic conversion to nucleosides during the initial DNA hydrolysis.

Overall, this assay is simpler and less time-consuming than the bisphosphate assay. Recoveries of certain polycyclic aromatic adducts appear to be somewhat higher as ^{32}P-labeled pXpN and pX as compared with pXp derivatives. With recent applications of ^{32}P-postlabeling to chemically uncharacterized adducts (Schurdak and Randerath, 1985; Liehr et al., 1986), to DNA lesions elicited by exposures to complex mixtures (E. Randerath et al., 1988, 1989a; Schoket et al., 1988), and to putative indigenous adducts (I-compounds) (K. Randerath et al., 1986a, 1989a), the monophosphate assay allows one to validate the results of the bisphosphate procedure. An important feature of the monophosphate procedure is the quantitative conversion of *pXpN adducts to *pX adducts by venom phosphodiesterase (Fig. 3): This reaction provides evidence that ^{32}P-labeled extra spots actually represent modified DNA derivatives, not non-specific background labeling (K. Randerath et al., 1989b). While the monophosphate assay has not yet been extensively applied in actual adduct analyses, the assay complements other analytical techniques and will improve our ability to detect and measure DNA adducts from diverse sources.

Summary of Properties of ^{32}P-Postlabeling Assay

Work in several laboratories over the past 5-8 years has established the following features of the ^{32}P-postlabeling assay:

(i) The assay can be applied to most chemical carcinogens; even putative non-genotoxic carcinogens may be detected by their

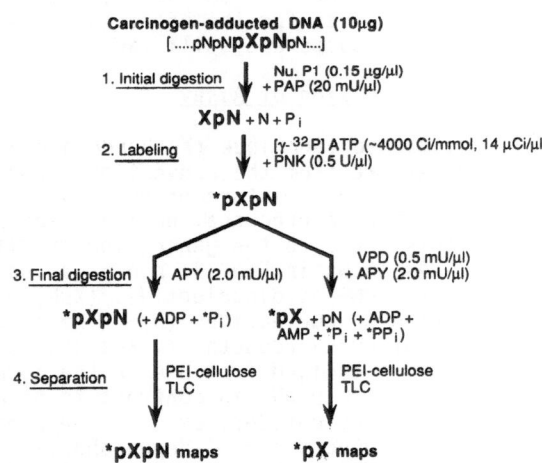

Fig. 3   In the dinucleotide/monophosphate version of the ^{32}P-postlabeling assay bulky/aromatic adducts are first converted to dinucleotides (XpN) by DNA digestion using nuclease P1 and prostatic acid phosphatase. The adducted dinucleotides are subsequently ^{32}P-labeled (*pXpN) and mapped as such or, alternatively, digested to 5'-monophosphates (*pX) by snake venom phosphodiesterase and then mapped. This procedure does not involve a separate adduct-enrichment step.

effects on I-compounds (K. Randerath et al., 1988b; Li et al., 1989; E. Randerath et al., 1989b).

    (ii) The assay is extremely sensitive down to 1 adduct in 10^8 to 10^{10} nucleotides; this sensitivity is achieved with adduct enrichment (bisphosphate version) or without a separate enrichment step (dinucleotide/monophosphate version).

    (iii) Adducts can be quantitated.

    (iv) Radiolabeled carcinogens or anti-adduct antibodies are not required.

    (v) The assay may be used in the screening of chemicals for genotoxic activity.

    (vi) Adducts can be assayed in somatic and germ cells in the intact animal (or human) or in cultured cells.

    (vii) Adduct persistence may be quantified by ^{32}P-postlabeling.

    (viii) Effects of modulators of adduct formation may be investigated.

    (ix) The assay can be used in model systems to correlate DNA adduction with biological effects, e.g., in studies of mechanisms of carcinogenesis.

    (x) Endogenous sources of DNA adduction can be detected and studied by ^{32}P-postlabeling.

    (xi) The assay has become a major tool for monitoring exposures to complex mixtures in animals and humans; its use in human studies will be reviewed in the following sections.

APPLICATIONS TO HUMAN DNA

Importance of Carcinogen-Exposure Monitoring in Man

The majority of chemicals causing human cancer has not been identified, but there is evidence, mostly from epidemiology, that certain human cancers are caused by chemicals in tobacco smoke and by natural and synthetic chemicals of environmental, occupational, medicinal, and dietary origin. At the level of the individual cancer victim (with the major exception of heavy smokers), however, the causative agent(s) have been difficult or often impossible to identify because many cases of cancer appear to arise in humans which have not been demonstrably exposed to unusual levels of known carcinogens. While some of these cancers may be "spontaneous", i.e. be due to endogenous (hereditary, hormonal, etc.) mechanisms, many are probably contingent on as yet poorly characterized chemical exposures. DNA adducts (and protein adducts as their surrogates) represent "fingerprints" of such exposures at the biologically relevant target site; it is hoped, therefore, that the detection, measurement, and characterization of such adducts by modern sensitive and specific methods will eventually lead to the identification of many of the causative chemicals and thus contribute significantly to the prevention of human cancer.

Wogan and Gorelick (1985), Garner (1985), Farmer et al. (1987), and Hemminki and Randerath (1987) have reviewed and discussed in depth the rationale and currently available methods of exposure monitoring by means of DNA and protein adduct measurements.

DNA Damage in Cigarette Smokers

Cigarette smoke-induced, presumably aromatic DNA adducts were initially detected in both mice (K. Randerath et al., 1986b; E. Randerath et al., 1986) and humans (E. Randerath et al., 1986; Everson et al., 1986, 1988) by the intensification version of the ^{32}P-postlabeling assay. Application of the nuclease P1-enhanced version of

the ^{32}P-postlabeling assay (Reddy and Randerath, 1986) allowed much
lower levels of smoking-related DNA adducts to be detected. Results
obtained by this procedure in human and mouse tissues (Fig. 4) (Everson
et al., 1986; E. Randerath et al., 1988) provided evidence for the
presence of DNA adducts. Cigarette smoke-related ^{32}P-labeled material
occupied two extensive diagonal radioactive zones (DRZ 1 and DRZ 2) on
the autoradiographic maps. These results presumably indicate the
presence in the DNA samples of numerous, only partially resolved
aromatic DNA adducts of varying polarities (E. Randerath et al., 1988),
in accord with the presence in cigarette smoke of a large number of
polycyclic aromatic compounds encompassing known as well as unidentified
tumor initiators/carcinogens (Hoffmann et al., 1976, 1987; U.S.
Department of Health and Human Services, 1982; International Agency for
Research on Cancer, 1985). The adducts detected by ^{32}P-postlabeling
thus appear to provide a valid dosimeter for initiator/carcinogen
exposure. The similar patterns of DNA lesions in human and mouse
tissues (Fig. 4), which was also demonstrated for individual smoking-
associated adducts (Everson et al., 1986; E. Randerath et al., 1986),
suggest common characteristics of tobacco-associated carcinogen
activation and adduct formation in different mammalian species. These
results are encouraging in that adduct patterns and levels are
comparable in humans and experimental models.

As shown in Fig. 5, smoking-associated, presumably aromatic DNA
adducts occur in a dose- and time-dependent manner in surgical specimens
of lung, bronchus, and larynx from smokers with cancer of these organs
(E. Randerath et al., 1989a). The available dose-response data best fit
a power curve, $Y = aX^b$, especially if two outlying values from heavy
alcohol users were omitted. Similar results were obtained when exposure
was measured in packs per day. Alcohol abuse appeared to lower the
levels of smoking-associated DNA adducts in heavy smokers, but this
needs further investigation. After cessation of smoking, DNA levels

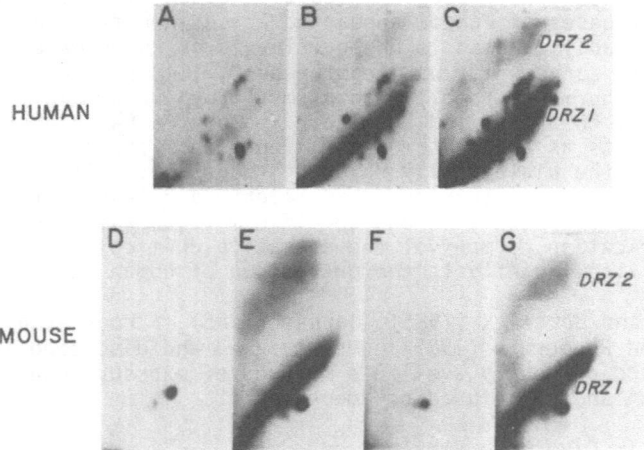

Fig. 4   DNA adduct patterns from smoker's lung (panels B and C)
           resemble those from mouse lung (panel E) and heart (panel G)
           after topical application of cigarette "tar". Panels A, D,
           and F are from unexposed controls. The nuclease P1-enhanced
           version of ^{32}P-postlabeling was used.

declined only slowly: Smoking-associated DNA adducts were still
measurable after 10 or 14 years in ex-smokers with previous heavy
exposure (E. Randerath et al., 1989a). Thus, smoking-induced DNA
lesions persist in human tissues similarly to adducts elicited by
authentic aromatic carcinogens in animals where DNA adduct
concentrations, after an initial decline after carcinogen exposure,
remain stabilized at low levels for extended periods of time (K.
Randerath et al., 1984b; E. Randerath et al., 1985). The extent of DNA
damage in lung and larynx reflects cancer risk and mortality, which
increase with the number of cigarettes smoked and the duration of
smoking (U.S. Department of Health and Human services, 1982; IARC,
1985). Similarly, the persistence of smoking-associated DNA adducts is
in accord with the slow decline of lung and larynx cancer risk and
mortality after cessation of smoking (U.S. Department of Health and
Human Services, 1982; IARC, 1985). These results demonstrate,
therefore, that smoking-associated DNA adducts in major target organs of
human carcinogenesis, as assayed by ^{32}P-postlabeling, provide a valid
dosimeter for initiator/carcinogen exposure. Correlations of aromatic
DNA adduct levels in human lung with cigarette smoking were also
established independently by Phillips et al. (1988a).

Studies of human placental DNA by the intensification version of
the assay have detected a total of 7 different adducts in 53 specimens
(Everson et al., 1986, 1988). The detection of these specific adducts
was facilitated by their preferential labeling in the presence of a
limiting amount of ATP. Three adducts were found almost exclusively in

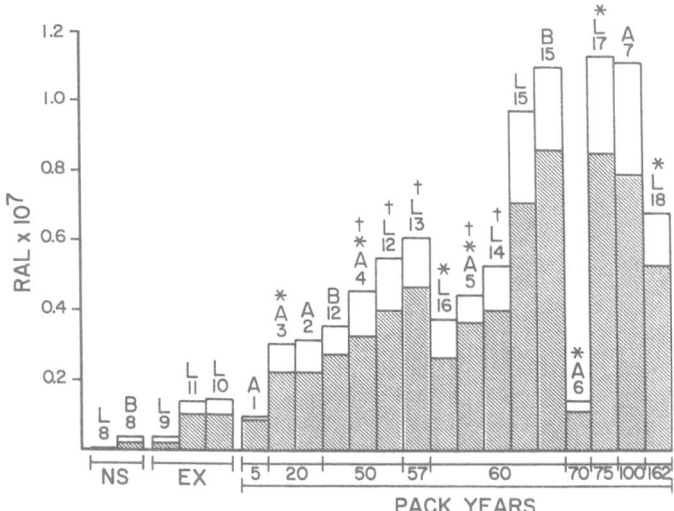

Fig. 5   Levels of smoking-associated DNA adducts (Fig. 4), expressed as
          RAL x 10^7 values, depend on the smoking exposure measured in
          pack years (packs per day x years smoked). RAL values were
          calculated from the radioactivity of DRZ 1 (hatched areas) and
          DRZ 2 (white areas). Specimens investigated were lung (L),
          bronchus (B), and aryepiglottic fold (A). NS, non-smoker;
          EX, ex-smoker; S, smoker; *, heavy alcohol user; +, patient
          quit smoking 12 - 42 days prior to surgery. For details about
          patients (numbers above stacked bars), consult E. Randerath et
          al. (1989a). A relative adduct labeling (RAL) value of 1 x
          10^{-7} corresponds to 1 adduct in 10^7 DNA nucleotides.

smokers, and positive dose-response relationships were established (Everson et al., 1988). One adduct appeared to relate to amounts of caffeine consumption in smokers. Interestingly, levels of smoking-related placental adducts were inversely associated with the birthweight of offspring (Everson et al., 1988). Statistical correlations were strengthened when in addition to questionnaire information, chemical blood data for cotinine (a nicotine metabolite), thiocyanate, and carboxyhemoglobin were considered (Everson et al., 1988).

The tissue distribution of smoking-associated DNA adducts in autopsy samples from heavy smokers (E. Randerath et al., 1989a; see Fig. 6) was found to parallel that seen in mice treated dermally with CSC (E. Randerath et al., 1988), i.e. adduct levels in lung and heart DNA of both species were high (Fig. 7, panels g, h, l, and m), in contrast to considerably lower levels in other human and mouse tissues such as kidney, liver, and spleen. These similarities further suggest that the mouse provides a suitable model system for studying DNA damage and mechanisms of smoking-associated carcinogenesis.

Our results imply that tobacco-related DNA lesions in target organs of carcinogenesis, such as lung and larynx, play a key role in cancer induction in these tissues. In addition, the DNA lesions detected by ^{32}P-postlabeling may conceivably be involved in non-neoplastic lung and heart pathology, such as chronic obstructive lung disease and cardiomyopathy, in line with recent reports that DNA adducts induced by the carcinogenic food pyrolysis product, aminomethyl(α)carboline, are associated with degenerative tissue alterations (Takayama et al, 1985; Yamashita et al., 1986).

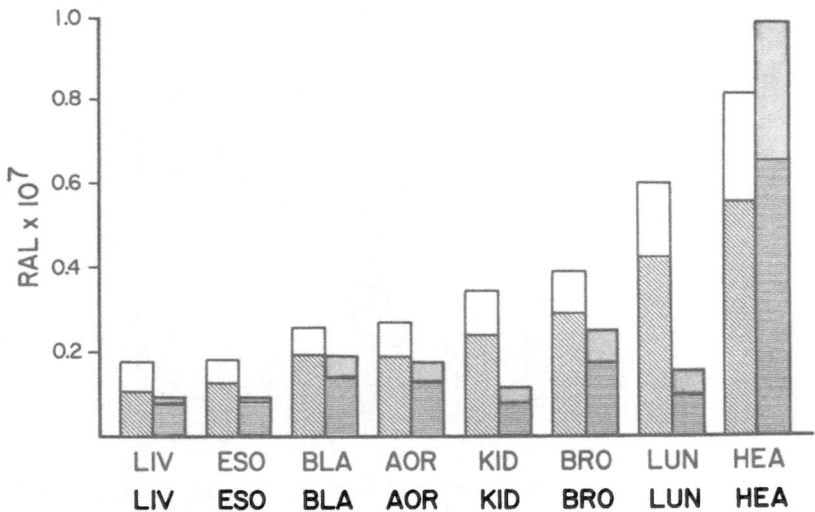

Fig. 6   Levels of smoking-associated DNA adducts are tissue-dependent. Post-mortem tissues of two smokers were liver (LIV), esophagus (ESO), bladder (BLA), ascending aorta (AOR), kidney (KID), bronchus (BRO), lung (LUN), and heart (HEA). The low lung adduct level of the second smoker was presumably due to advanced adult respiratory distress syndrome. For additional details, consult legend to Fig. 5 and E. Randerath et al (1989a).

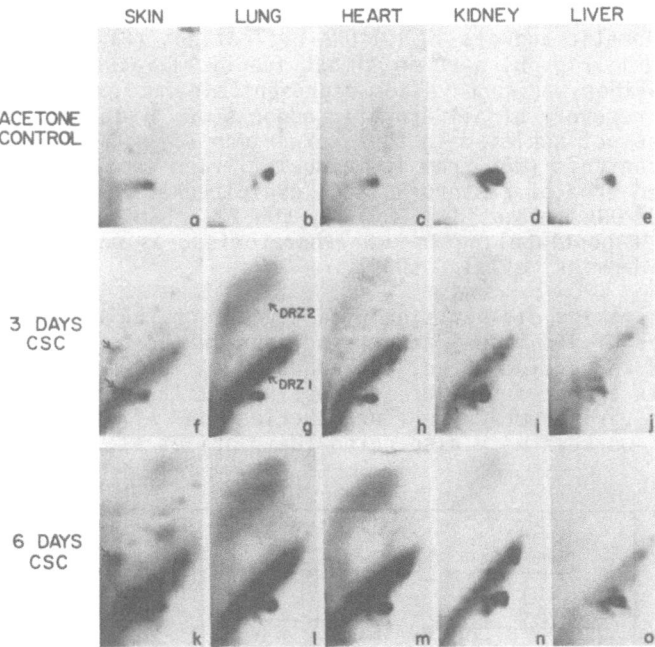

```
        SKIN      LUNG     HEART    KIDNEY    LIVER
```

ACETONE
CONTROL

                  a   b   c   d   e

3 DAYS
CSC
                       DRZ2

                       DRZ1

                  f   g   h   i   j

6 DAYS
CSC

                  k   l   m   n   o

Fig. 7. Various organs of mice treated topically with cigarette "tar"
         display typical cigarette smoke-associated DNA adducts that
         increase with exposure time (panels f - o). Panels a - e are
         from unexposed control tissues. The nuclease P1-enhanced
         version of ^{32}P-postlabeling was used.

Coke Oven Workers

Aromatic compounds, such as polycyclic aromatic hydrocarbons (PAH),
are ubiquitous environmental contaminants emitted mainly as a
consequence of human activity (World Health Organization, 1987). They
are thought to contribute to the incidence of some occupational cancers
and be associated with global variations of cancer occurrence (World
Health Organization, 1987; Doll and Peto, 1981). Some work processes
involve high exposures to PAH, such as chimney sweeping, roofing,
aluminum or coke production, and iron founding, leading to elevated
cancer risks in these occupations (IARC, 1984, 1987). As first
suggested by the results on smokers' DNA, the ^{32}P-postlabeling assay
appears well suited to search for and measure DNA adducts elicited by
additional environmental and occupational exposures in humans. Thus
far, DNA specimens of coke oven workers (Hemminki et al., 1989), foundry
workers (Hemminki et al., 1988; Phillips et al., 1988b), and pregnant
women exposed to residential wood combustion smoke (Reddy et al., 1987)
have been examined.

In a recent study by Hemminki et al. (1989), DNA adducts were
analyzed in coded white blood cell (WBC) samples of coke workers from
four factories in Silesia, a highly industrialized area of Poland, and
compared with controls (Fig. 8). In addition to ^{32}P-postlabeling
including nuclease P1 enrichment, the DNA samples were analyzed by
immunoassay (competitive ELISA) for PAH-DNA adducts. Mean adduct levels
by ^{32}P-postlabeling in the coke workers' WBC-DNA samples were 4.4,

23

presumably aromatic adducts in 10^8 DNA nucleotides (Fig. 8), while local controls (CON 1, Fig. 8) gave an almost identical value of 4.5 adducts in 10^8 nucleotides. (These values represent minimum estimates because quantitative recovery of all aromatic adducts in ^{32}P-labeled form presumably was not achieved in these experiments.) On the other hand, countryside controls (WBC from individuals living in a non-industrialized area of Eastern Poland) exhibited a low value of 0.84 adducts in 10^8 DNA nucleotides (Fig. 8, CON 2). Similar results were obtained by ^{32}P-postlabeling in two laboratories, as well as by immunoassay (Hemminki et al., 1989).

Age and smoking did not significantly affect the results obtained. The identities of individual adducts present in these DNA samples (Fig. 8) still need to be elucidated, but adduct profiles among workers and local controls appeared similar, suggesting similar exposures. Mean adduct levels varied among the four cokeries, and effects of job categories of workers were also noted (Hemminki et al., 1989).

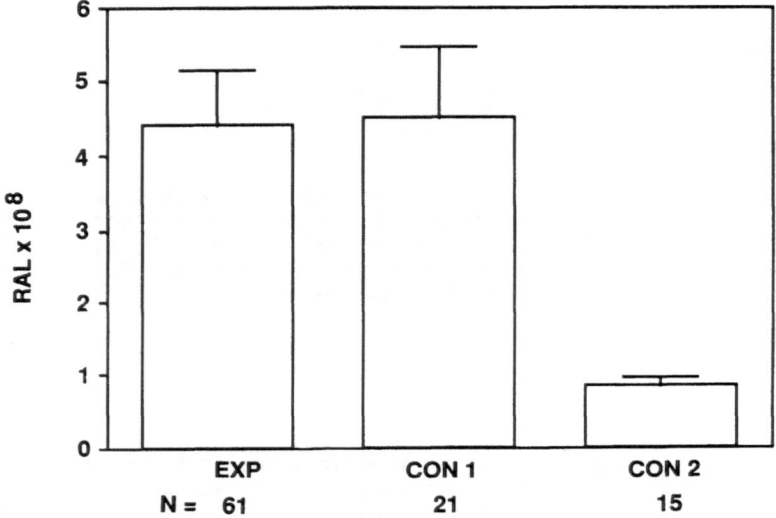

Fig. 8 Adduct levels in WBC of coke workers (Hemminki et al., 1989). EXP, exposed workers; CON 1, local controls; CON 2, countryside controls. For details, consult text.

An intriguing result was the difference between the two control populations (CON 1 and CON 2, Fig. 8). Mean adduct levels of the Polish countryside controls were similar to those of the controls of a Finnish foundry worker study (Perera et al., 1988). Another intriguing aspect related to the dose-response relationships among workers from different job categories and between workers and local controls: Ambient air levels of PAH which differed by a factor of about 10 within the factory (battery versus non-battery sites) and between the cokery and adjacent residential areas were not reflected by the adduct levels measured. It is possible that routes of exposure other than inhalation, such as skin absorption and ingestion, may play a significant role. A comparison with the countryside controls indicated a clear association of the WBC-DNA adducts with environmental pollution, however. It is also clear from these results that the ^{32}P-postlabeling assay can be used as a dosimeter of human exposure to carcinogenic compounds in the occupational setting.

24

Iron Foundry Workers

Iron-founding processes have been reviewed in relation to cancer by IARC (1984). PAH are formed during thermal decomposition of the organic ingredients of the mold material, and the levels of PAH formed are dependent on the types of molds used (IARC, 1984). Levels of PAH are known to differ extensively by workplace within the foundry (IARC, 1984; Schimberg et al., 1980).

For analyzing DNA adducts in WBC of foundry workers and unexposed controls, the nuclease P1-enhanced ^{32}P-postlabeling assay was used (Hemminki et al., 1988; Phillips et al., 1988b; M.V. Reddy, K. Hemminki, and K. Randerath, manuscript in preparation). Benzo(a)pyrene (BP) levels in the workplace atmosphere were used as guidelines to designate the exposure as high (>0.2 μg BP/m^3), medium (0.05 - 0.2 μg BP/m^3), and low (<0.05 μg BP/m^3). Adducts in individual samples were scored for statistical evaluation from 0 - 3, where 0 is <5.0, 1 is 5.0 -10, 2 is 10 - 20, and 3 is >20 adducts in 10^8 DNA nucleotides, as estimated by ^{32}P-postlabeling (Reddy and Randerath, 1986). The mean scores were 2.4, 1.7, 0.7, and 0.2 adducts/10^8 nucleotides in high, medium, low, and control populations, respectively (Fig. 9), the differences between each group being statistically significant. Adduct scores varied by job description in agreement with industrial hygienic measurements of atmospheric PAH levels (K. Hemminki, K. Randerath, and M.V. Reddy, unpublished results).

These data showed a high correlation between the estimated exposure to PAH in an iron foundry and the levels of aromatic DNA adducts in WBC.

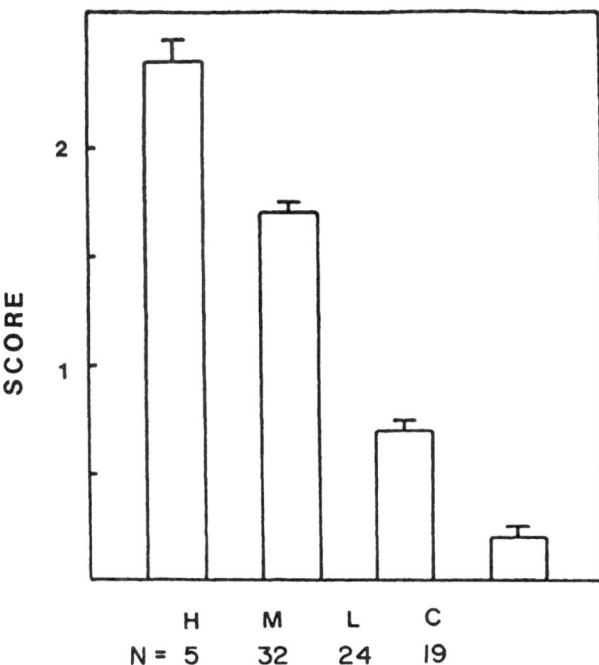

Fig. 9   Adduct levels in WBC of iron foundry workers (Hemminki et al., 1988). H, M, L = high, medium, low exposure group. C, unexposed controls. For definition of adduct scores and other details, consult text.

A similar result was obtained by immunoassay conducted with an antibody raised against BP-modified DNA (Perera et al., 1988), but it is not yet clear whether the same adducts were being measured by the two analytical techniques. Also, adduct profiles between foundry workers and coke workers have yet to be compared. These studies reinforce the notion that the ^{32}P-postlabeling assay represents a sensitive dosimeter of human exposure to genotoxicants in the environment and the workplace.

Persons Exposed to Residential Wood Combustion Smoke

Residential wood combustion (RWC), which is being increasingly used in the United States as a heating source, is of health concern because emissions from RWC contain carcinogenic aromatic hydrocarbons and other toxic compounds such as CO, aldehydes, and phenols (Cooper, 1980). To assess health risk, the possible formation of polycyclic aromatic DNA adducts in placentas and WBC of non-smoking women exposed to RWC smoke during pregnancy was measured by the nuclease P1-enhanced ^{32}P-postlabeling assay (Reddy et al., 1987). Examination of DNA samples from 12 exposed specimens (8 WBC, 4 placentas) and 13 unexposed controls (8 WBC, 5 placentas) showed no exposure-related adducts. All placental DNA maps exhibited one major (47±10%) and 12 minor extra spots, however, that were not seen on the WBC-DNA maps. On the other hand, WBC-DNA showed four very weak spots that were absent in placental DNA. The results suggested that RWC smoke does not elicit detectable levels of aromatic adducts in human placenta and WBC, and that placental and WBC-DNA contain covalent modifications of unknown origin. These DNA derivatives may be caused by ingestion or inhalation of, or skin contact with, low levels of environmental genotoxicants or may arise from endogenous electrophiles, i.e. represent I-compounds (as defined in K. Randerath et al., 1986a, 1989a).

CONCLUSIONS AND FUTURE PROSPECTS

Due to its versatility and sensitivity, ^{32}P-postlabeling has become a major method in the detection and measurement of DNA lesions induced by genotoxic chemicals. It complements other existing methods such as anti-body-based and spectroscopic assays for DNA adducts in many cases; in others, it is the only method currently available. For example, no other method exists for the detection of adducts formed by reaction of DNA with endogenous electrophiles (I-compounds, certain estrogen-induced adducts, etc.). ^{32}P-postlabeling certainly has not as yet attained its full potential: Further developments are expected in the area of "small" adducts, and ^{32}P-postlabeling can perhaps be adapted, also, to the analysis of oxygen free-radical induced genetic damage. Procedures for the identification of individual ^{32}P-postlabeled adducts, especially in human samples, need to be worked out. It may be hoped that ^{32}P-postlabeling, in its existing form and through future developments, will play an important role in the biomonitoring and risk assessment of human chemical-carcinogen exposure and contribute to our understanding of human carcinogenesis.

Acknowledgements

Work in our laboratory on the ^{32}P-postlabeling assay reviewed in this article was supported by grants from the USPHS (CA 25590, CA 32157, CA 43263) awarded by the National Cancer Institute and by a Du Pont Environmental and Occupational Health Grant. Our collaborators, especially Drs. R.B. Everson, R.C. Gupta, K. Hemminki, D. Li, L.-J.W. Lu, D.H. Phillips, and M.V. Reddy, have made many important contributions to the development and application of the assay. We also express our gratitude to Drs. R.B. Everson, K. Hemminki, R.H. Miller, and H.A. Dunsford for providing human tissue samples. T.A. Avitts and K.L. Putman provided expert technical help in ^{32}P-postlabeling assays of human DNA samples.

REFERENCES

Bartsch, H., Hemminki, K. and O'Neill, I.K. eds., 1988, Methods for Detecting DNA Damaging Agents in Humans: Applications in Cancer Epidemiology and Prevention. IARC Scientific Publication No. 89. International Agency for Research on Cancer, Lyon, France.

Berlin, A., Draper, M., Hemminki, K. and Vainio, H. eds., 1984, Monitoring Human Exposure to Carcinogenic and Mutagenic Agents. IARC Scientific Publication No. 59. International Agency for Research on Cancer, Lyon, France.

Cooper, J.A., 1980, Environmental impact of residential wood combustion emissions and its implications, J. Air Pollution Control Assoc. 30: 855.

Dietrich, M.W., Hopkins, W.E., Asbury, K.J. and Ridley, W.P. 1987, Liquid chromatographic characterization of the deoxyribonucleoside 5'-phosphates and deoxyribonucleoside 3', 5'-bisphosphates obtained by ^{32}P-postlabeling of DNA, Chromatographia 24: 545.

Doll, R. and Peto, R., 1981, The causes of cancer: quantitative estimates of avoidable risks of cancer in the United States today, J. Natl. Cancer Inst. 66: 1191.

Dunn, B.P. and San, R.H.C., 1988, HPLC enrichment of hydrophobic DNA-carcinogen adducts for enhanced sensitivity of ^{32}P-postlabeling analysis, Carcinogenesis 9: 1055.

Everson, R.B., Randerath, E., Avitts, T.A., Schut, H.A.J. and Randerath, K., 1986, Preliminary investigations of tissue specificity, species specificity, and strategies for identifying chemicals causing DNA adducts in human placenta, Prog. Exp. Tumor Res. 31: 86.

Everson, R.B., Randerath, E., Santella R.M., Avitts, T.A., Weinstein, I.B. and Randerath, K., 1988, Quantitative associations between DNA damage in human placenta and maternal smoking and birth weight, J. Natl. Cancer Inst. 80: 567.

Farmer, P.B., Neumann, H.-G. and Henschler, D., 1987, Estimation of exposure of man to substances reacting covalently with macromolecules, Arch. Toxicol. 60: 251.

Gallagher, J.E., Jackson, M.A. George, M.H., Lewtas, J. and Robertson, J.G.C., 1989, Differences in detection of DNA adducts in the ^{32}P-postlabeling assay after either 1-butanol extraction or nuclease P1 treatment, Cancer Lett. 45: 7.

Garner, R.C., 1985, Assessment of carcinogen exposure in man, Carcinogenesis 6: 1071.

Gupta, R.C., 1985, Enhanced sensitivity of ^{32}P-postlabeling analysis of aromatic carcinogen DNA adducts, Cancer Res. 45: 5656.

Gupta, R.C. and Earley, K., 1988, ^{32}P-adduct assay: comparative recoveries of structurally diverse DNA adducts in the various enhancement procedures, Carcinogenesis 9: 1687.

Gupta, R.C. and Randerath, K. 1988, Analysis of DNA adducts by ^{32}P-labeling and thin-layer chromatography. In DNA Repair, A Laboratory Manual of Research Procedures, vol. 3 (eds. E.C. Friedberg and P.C. Hanawalt), pp. 399-418. Marcel Dekker, Inc., New York.

Gupta, R.C., Reddy, M.V. and Randerath, K., 1982, ^{32}P-Postlabeling analysis of nonradioactive aromatic carcinogen-DNA adducts, Carcinogenesis 3: 1081.

Hemminki, K., 1983, Nucleic acid adducts of chemical carcinogens and mutagens, Arch. Toxicol. 52: 249.

Hemminki, K., Grzybowska, E., Chorazy, M., Twardowska-Saucha, K., Scroczynski, J.W., Putman, K.L., Randerath, K., Phillips, D.H., Hewer, A., Santella, R.M. and Perera, F.P., 1989, DNA adducts in humans related to occupational and environmental exposure to aromatic compounds. In IARC Scientific Publications, in press, International Agency for Research on Cancer, Lyon, France.

Hemminki, K., Perera, F.P., Phillips, D.H., Randerath K., Reddy, M.V. and Santella, R.M., 1988, Aromatic DNA adducts in white blood cells of foundry workers. In IARC Scientific Publications No. 89, pp. 190-95. International Agency for Research on Cancer, Lyon.

Hemminki, K. and Randerath, K., 1987, Detection of genetic interaction of chemicals by biochemical methods: Determination of DNA and protein adducts, in: "Mechanisms of Cell Injury: Implications for Human Health" ed. B.A. Fowler, pp.209-27. J. Wiley and Sons, New York.

Hoffmann, D., Schmeltz, I., Hecht, S.S. and Wynder, E.L., 1976, Chemical studies on tobacco smoke. XXXIX. On the identification of carcinogens, tumor promoters, and cocarcinogens in tobacco smoke. In DHEW Publication (NIH) - 76-1221, Smoking and Health. Vol. 1: Modifying the Risk for the Smoker, pp. 125-46. United States Department of Health, Education, and Welfare, Rockville, MD.

Hoffmann, D., Wynder, E.L., Hecht, S.S., Brunnemann, K.D., Lavoie, E.J. and Haley, N.J., 1987, Chemical carcinogens in tobacco. In Cancer Risks. Strategies for Elimination (ed.P.Bannasch), pp. 101-13. Springer Verlag, New York.

IARC, 1984, IARC Monographs on the Evaluation of Carcinogenic Risks of Chemicals to Humans. Vol. 34, pt. 3. Polynuclear Aromatic Compounds. International Agency for Research on Cancer, Lyon, France.

IARC, 1985, IARC Monographs on the Evaluation of the Carcinogenic Risk of Chemicals to Humans. Vol. 38. Tobacco Smoking.

International Agency for Research on Cancer, Lyon, France.

IARC, 1987, _IARC Monographs on the Evaluation of Carcinogenic Risks to Humans._ _Vol. 1-42, Suppl. 7._ _Overall Evaluations of Carcinogenicity:_ _An Updating of IARC Monographs._ International Agency for Research on Cancer, Lyon, France.

Kriek, E., den Engelse, L., Scherer, E. and Westra, G., 1984, Formation of DNA modifications by chemical carcinogens. Identification, localization and quantification, _Biochim. Biophys. Acta_ 738: 181.

Li, D., Chandar, N., Lombardi, B. and Randerath, K., 1989, Reduced accumulation of I-compounds in liver DNA of rats fed a choline-devoid diet, _Carcinogenesis_ 10: 605.

Liehr, J.G., Avitts, T.A., Randerath, E. and Randerath, K., 1986, Estrogen-induced endogenous DNA adduction: Possible mechanism of hormonal cancer, _Proc. Natl. Acad. Sci. U.S.A._ 83: 5301.

Miller, E.C. and Miller, J.A., 1981, Searches for ultimate chemical carcinogens and their reactions with cellular macromolecules, _Cancer_ 47: 2327.

Perera, F.P., Hemminki, K., Young, T.L., Santella, R.M., Bremer, D. and Kelly, G., 1988, Detection of polycyclic aromatic hydrocarbon-DNA adducts in white blood cells of foundry workers, _Cancer Res._ 48: 2288.

Phillips, D.H., Hemminki, K., Alhonen, A., Hewer, A. and Grover, P.L., 1988b, Monitoring occupational exposure to carcinogens: Detection by ^{32}P-postlabelling of aromatic DNA adducts in white blood cells from iron foundry workers, _Mutat. Res._ 204: 531.

Phillips, D.H., Hewer, A., Martin, C.N., Garner, R.C. and King M.M., 1988a, Correlation of DNA adduct levels in human lung with cigarette smoking, _Nature (Lond.)_ 336: 790.

Pitot, H.C., 1986, _Fundamentals of Oncology,_ 3rd ed. Marcel Dekker, New York.

Randerath, E., Agrawal, H.P., Weaver, J.A., Bordelon, C.B. and Randerath, K., 1985, ^{32}P-Postlabeling analysis of DNA adducts persisting for up to 42 weeks in the skin, epidermis and dermis of mice treated topically with 7,12-dimethylbenz(a)anthracene, _Carcinogenesis_ 6: 1117.

Randerath, E., Avitts, T.A., Reddy, M.V., Miller, R.H., Everson, R.B. and Randerath, K., 1986, Comparative ^{32}P-analysis of cigarette smoke induced DNA damage in human tissues and mouse skin, _Cancer Res._ 46: 5869.

Randerath, E., Miller, R.H., Mittal, D., Avitts, T.A., Dunsford, H.A. and Randerath, K., 1989a, Covalent DNA damage in tissues of cigarette smokers as determined by ^{32}P-postlabeling assay, _J. Natl. Cancer Inst._ 81: 341.

Randerath, E., Mittal, D. and Randerath, K., 1988, Tissue distribution of covalent DNA damage in mice treated dermally with cigarette "tar": Preference for lung and heart DNA, Carcinogenesis 9: 75.

Randerath, E., Randerath, K., Reddy, R., Rao, M.S. and Reddy, J. K., 1989b, Rat liver DNA alterations induced by the peroxisome proliferate ciprofibrate, Proc. Am. Assoc. Cancer Res. 30: 146.

Randerath, E., Yu, C.-T. and Randerath, K., 1972, Base analysis of ribopolynucleotides by chemical tritium labeling: A methodological study with model nucleosides and purified tRNA species, Anal. Biochem. 4: 172.

Randerath, K., 1981, 3-([3-^{125}I]Iodo-4-hydroxyphenyl)propionyl carbohydrazide, a new radioiodination reagent for ultrasensitive detection and determination of periodate-oxidized nucleoside derivatives and other carbonyl compounds, Anal. Biochem. 115: 391.

Randerath, K., Gupta, R.C. and Randerath, E., 1980, ^{3}H and ^{32}P derivative methods for base composition and sequence analysis of RNA. In Methods in Enzymology, Vol. 65, Part I, Nucleic Acids, pp. 638-80. Academic Press, New York.

Randerath, K., Haglund, R.E., Phillips, D.H. and Reddy, M.V., 1984b, ^{32}P-Postlabeling analysis of DNA adducts formed in the livers of animals treated with safrole, estragole and other naturally-occurring alkenylbenzenes. I. Adult female CD-1 mice, Carcinogenesis 5: 1613.

Randerath, K., Liehr, J.G., Gladek, A. and Randerath, E., 1989a, Age-dependent covalent DNA alterations (I-compounds) in rodent tissues: Species, tissue and sex specificities, Mutat. Res. 219: 121.

Randerath, K., Lu, L.-J.W. and Li, D., 1988a, A comparison between different types of covalent DNA modifications (I-compounds, persistent carcinogen adducts and 5-methylcytosine) in regenerating rat liver, Carcinogenesis 9: 1843.

Randerath, K., Putman, K.L., Randerath, E., Mason, G., Kelley, M. and Safe, S., 1988b, Organ-specific effects of long term feeding of 2,3,7,8-tetrachlorodibenzo-p-dioxin and 1,2,3,7,8-pentachlorodibenzo-p-dioxin on I-compounds in hepatic and renal DNA of female Sprague-Dawley rats, Carcinogenesis 9: 2285.

Randerath, K., Randerath, E., Agrawal, H.P., Gupta, R.C., Schurdak, M.E. and Reddy, M.V., 1985, Postlabeling methods for carcinogen-DNA adduct analysis, Environ. Health Persp. 62: 57.

Randerath, K., Randerath, E., Agrawal, H.P. and Reddy, M.V., (1984a). Biochemical (postlabeling) methods for analysis of carcinogen-DNA adducts, in: Monitoring Human Exposure to Carcinogenic and Mutagenic Agents, IARC Scientific Publications No. 59, pp. 217-31, International Agency for Research on Cancer, Lyon, France.

Randerath, K., Randerath, E., Danna, T.F., van Golen, K.L. and Putman, K.L., 1989b, A new sensitive ^{32}P-postlabeling assay

based on the specific enzymatic conversion of bulky DNA
lesions to radiolabeled dinucleotides and nucleoside 5'-
monophosphates, Carcinogenesis, 10: 1231.

Randerath, K., Reddy, M.V., Avitts, T.A., Miller, R.H., Everson,
R.B. and Randerath, E., 1986, ^{32}P-Postlabeling test for
smoking-related DNA adducts in animal and human tissues. In
Mechanisms in Tobacco Carcinogenesis, Banbury Report 23 (eds.
D. Hoffmann and C.C. Harris), pp. 85-98. Cold Spring Harbor
Laboratory, Cold Spring Harbor, NY.

Randerath, K., Reddy, M.V. and Disher, R.M., 1986a, Age- and
tissue-related DNA modifications in untreated rats:
Detection by ^{32}P-postlabeling assay and possible significance
for spontaneous tumor induction and aging, Carcinogenesis 7:
1615.

Randerath, K., Reddy, M.V. and Gupta, R.C., 1981, ^{32}P-Labeling
test for DNA damage, Proc. Natl. Acad. Sci. U.S.A. 78: 6126.

Reddy, M.V., Gupta, R.C., Randerath, E. and Randerath, K., 1984,
[32]P-Postlabeling test for covalent DNA binding of chemicals
in vivo: Application to a variety of aromatic carcinogens
and methylating agents, Carcinogenesis 5: 231.

Reddy, M.V., Gupta, R.C. and Randerath K., 1981, ^{32}P-Base analysis
of DNA, Anal. Biochem. 117: 271.

Reddy, M.V., Kenny, P.C. and Randerath, K., 1987, ^{32}P-Assay of DNA
adducts in white blood cells (WBC) and placentas of pregnant
women exposed to residential wood combustion (RWC) smoke,
Proc. Am. Assoc. Cancer Res. 26: 97.

Reddy, M.V. and Randerath, K., 1986, Nuclease P1-mediated
enhancement of sensitivity of ^{32}P-postlabeling test for
structurally diverse DNA adducts, Carcinogenesis 7: 1543.

Reddy, M.V. and Randerath, K., 1987, ^{32}P-Postlabeling assay for
carcinogen-DNA adducts: Nuclease P1-mediated enhancement of
its sensitivity and applications, Environ. Health Persp. 76:
41.

Schimberg, R.W., Pfäffli, P. and Tossavainen, A., 1980, Polycyclic
aromatic hydrocarbons in foundries, J. Toxicol. Environ.
Health 6: 1187.

Schoket, B., Hewer, A., Grover, P.L. and Phillips, D.H., 1988,
Formation of DNA adducts in human skin maintained in short-
term organ culture and treated with coal-tar, creosote or
bitumen, Int. J. Cancer 42: 622.

Schurdak, M.E. and Randerath, K., 1985, Tissue-specific DNA adduct
formation in mice treated with the environmental carcinogen,
7H-dibenzo(c,g)carbazole, Carcinogenesis 6: 1271.

Schurdak, M.E. and Randerath, K., 1989, Effects of route of
administration on tissue distribution of DNA adducts in mice:
Comparison of 7H-dibenzo(c,g)carbazole, benzo(a)pyrene, and
2-acetylaminofluorene, Cancer Res. 49: 2633.

Schurdak, M.E., Stong, D.B., Warshawsky, D. and Randerath, K., 1987a, ^{32}P-postlabeling analysis of DNA adduction in mice by synthetic metabolites of the environmental carcinogen, 7H-dibenzo(c,g)carbazole: chromatographic evidence for 3-hydroxy-7H-dibenzo(c,g)carbazole being a proximate geno-toxicant in liver but not skin, <u>Carcinogenesis</u> 8: 591.

Schurdak, M.E., Stong, D.B., Warshawsky, D. and Randerath, K., 1987b, N-methylation reduces the DNA-binding activity of 7H-dibenzo(c,g)carbazole ~300-fold in liver but only ~2-fold in skin: possible correlation with carcinogenic activity, <u>Carcinogenesis</u> 8: 1405.

Schut, H.A.J., Putman, K.L. and Randerath, K., 1988, DNA adduct formation of the carcinogen 2-amino-3-methylimidazo[4,5-f]quinoline (IQ) in target tissue of the F-344 rat, <u>Cancer Lett.</u> 41: 345.

Takayama, S., Nakatsura, Y., Ohgakij, H., Sato, S. and Sugimura, T., 1985, Atrophy of salivary glands and pancreas of rats fed on diet with aminomethyl-α-carboline, <u>Proc. Japan Acad., Ser. B</u> 61: 277.

United States Department of Health and Human Services, 1982, <u>The Health Consequences of Smoking: Cancer. A Report of the Surgeon General.</u> Rockville, MD.

Watson, W.P., 1987, Post-radiolabeling for detecting DNA damage, <u>Mutagenesis</u> 2: 319.

Watson, W.P. and Crane, A.E., 1989, HPLC-^{32}P-postlabelling analysis of 1,N^6-ethenodeoxyadenosine and 3,N^4-ethenodeoxycytidine, <u>Mutagenesis</u> 4: 75.

Wilson, V.L., Basu, A.K., Essigmann, J.M., Smith, R.A. and Harris, C.C., 1988, O^6-Alkyldeoxyguanosine detection by ^{32}P-postlabeling and nucleotide chromatographic analysis, <u>Cancer Res.</u> 48: 2156.

Wogan, G.N. and Gorelick, N.J., 1985, Chemical and biochemical dosimetry of exposure to genotoxic chemicals, <u>Environ. Health Perspect.</u> 62: 5.

World Health Organization, 1987, <u>Air Quality Guidelines of Europe.</u> WHO, Copenhagen.

Yamashita, K., Takayama, S., Nagao, M., Sato, S. and Sugimura T., 1986, Amino-methyl-α-carboline induced DNA modification in rat salivary glands and pancreas detected by ^{32}P-postlabeling method, <u>Proc. Japan Acad., Ser. B</u> 62: 45.

IMMUNOLOGIC METHODS FOR THE DETECTION OF CARCINOGEN ADDUCTS IN HUMANS

Regina M. Santella, Xiao Yen Yang, Ling Ling Hsieh, Tie Lan Young, Xiao Qing Lu, Marina Stefanidis and Frederica P. Perera

Cancer Center and Division of Environmental Science, School of Public Health, Columbia University, New York, NY 10032

INTRODUCTION

Immunologic methods are now available for the sensitive detection and quantitation of carcinogen-DNA adducts. Monoclonal and polyclonal antibodies have been developed against a number of specific adducts as well as against UV-damaged DNA (Poirier, 1981; Santella, 1988). Antibodies can be developed against either the carcinogen adduct covalently coupled to carrier protein or the modified DNA electrostatically complexed to methylated bovine serum albumin. These antibodies can be used in highly sensitive competitive enzyme-linked immunosorbent assays (ELISA) with color- or fluorescence-endpoint detection. Since femtomole (10^{-15}) sensitivities are readily attainable, DNA adduct levels in the range of $1/10^8$ nucleotides can be measured. With monoadduct-specific antibodies, higher sensitivities may be obtainable if large amounts of DNA are available and the adduct is isolated by various chromatographic procedures before quantitation in the ELISA. Table 1 lists the monoclonal antibodies recognizing carcinogen-DNA adducts which we have developed to date. Several of these antibodies, including those recognizing aflatoxin, benzo(a)pyrene diol epoxide and 8-methoxypsoralen-DNA adducts, have been applied to adduct detection in humans.

DETECTION OF 8-METHOXYPSORALEN-DNA ADDUCTS

The combination of 8-methoxypsoralen (8-MOP) and UVA light (320–400 nm), termed PUVA, is used clinically in the treatment of psoriasis, a hyperproliferative disease of the skin. It has also been used extracorporeally as a cytoreductive treatment in the leukemic phase of cutaneous T-cell lymphoma (CTCL). We have utilized these patient populations as model systems for the development and validation of methods to measure carcinogen-DNA adducts since high, well-defined exposures are administered and unexposed controls readily identified.

8-MOP photoreacts primarily with thymine forming both monoadducts and interstrand cross-linked adducts. We have developed antibodies whose primary specificity is for the monoadduct, but which also react with crosslinks (Santella et al., 1985). These antibodies do not crossreact with nonmodified DNA or free 8-MOP. For quantitation of adducts in biological samples, a highly sensitive competitive ELISA was

DNA Damage and Repair in Human Tissues
Edited by B. M. Sutherland and A. D. Woodhead
Plenum Press, New York, 1990

Table 1. Monoclonal Antibodies Recognizing Carcinogen-DNA Adducts

---

Acetylaminofluorene-DNA   Yang and Santella, 1987
Aflatoxin-DNA   Hsieh et al., 1988
4-Aminobiphenyl-guanosine   unpublished*
Aminopyrene-DNA   Hsieh et al., 1985
Benzo(a)pyrene diol epoxide-DNA   Santella et, al., 1984
Benzo(a)pyrene diol epoxide-guanosine Santella et al., 1984
Ethenoadenine   Young and Santella, 1988
Ethenocytidine   Young and Santella, 1988
7-(Hydroxyethyl)guanosine   unpublished*
8-Methoxypsoralen-DNA   Santella et al., 1985
8-Oxoguanosine   unpublished*
Trimethylangelicine-DNA   Miolo et al., 1989
*Work carried out in our laboratory

---

established for antibody 8G1 utilizing alkaline phosphatase-labeled
second antibodies. When p-nitrophenyl phosphate is utilized as the
substrate for measurement of enzyme activity, 50% inhibition is at 17
fmol (Fig. 1). Sensitivity can be further increased by the use of 4-
methylumbelliferyl phosphate, a substrate which becomes fluorescent
after phosphate cleavage (50% inhibition at 4 fmol). With this level of
sensitivity, adducts could easily be measured in white blood cell DNA of
CTCL patients treated by oral administration of 8-MOP, followed by
extracorporeal photopheresis. All patients (n=10) had detectable levels
of adducts ranging from 0.1-15/10^7 nucleotides (Santella et al., 1988).
These high levels result from the in vitro irradiation of the white
blood cells in the photopheresis apparatus. In contrast, no adducts
were detectable in white blood cell DNA from psoriasis patients treated
by oral administration of 8-MOP and skin irradiation (Yang et al.,
1989). It has been estimated that lymphocytes are exposed to
approximately 1-5% of the skin surface dose of UVA (Kraemer and
Weinstein, 1977). Prolonged treatment results in skin pigmentation and
may decrease the effective UVA dose. Therefore, it is not surprising
that adduct levels in lymphocytes were below the detectable level of
$1/10^8$.

Antibodies recognizing PAH-DNA adducts have been found in the sera
of humans and it has been suggested that the presence of these
antibodies can serve as a marker of exposure to PAHs (Harris et al.,

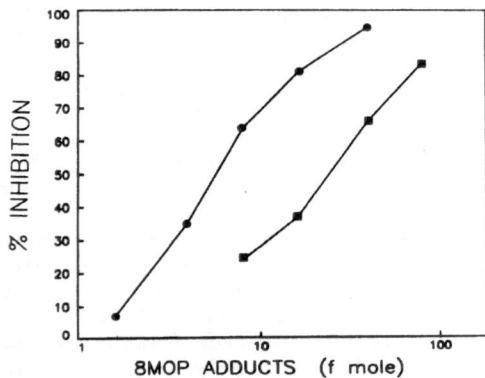

Fig. 1.   Competitive inhibition of monoclonal antibody 8G1 binding to 8-
          MOP-DNA using color (■) or fluorescence (●) endpoint detection.

Table 2. Immunofluorescence staining and 8-MOP DNA adduct levels in human keratinocytes.

Dose 8-MOP (ug/ml)	Relative Immuno- fluorescence staining	8-MOP-DNA adducts/ 10^6 nucleotides	
		^{3}H	ELISA
0	--	-	-
0.25	+		3.0
0.5	++	76	128
2.5	+++	340	340

1985). For this reason, we investigated whether patients treated with PUVA had detectable levels of circulating anti 8-MOP-DNA antibodies in their sera. Neither psoriasis patients with long term exposure (n=5) nor CTCL patients (n=20) demonstrated significant serum titers against 8-MOP-DNA (unpublished).

We have also utilized the 8-MOP-DNA specific antibodies in indirect immunofluorescence studies to visualize adducts in cells and tissues. Human keratinocytes treated with 8-MOP and UVA were fixed with ethanol then treated with RNase A to eliminate potential crossreactivity with RNA adducts. They were then treated with proteinase K to release proteins from the DNA to enhance antibody binding. This was followed by treatment with 4N HCl to denature the DNA and further increase sensitivity. Staining with adduct specific antibody was followed by fluorescein-conjugated secondary antisera. Adducts could be visualized in keratinocytes treated with as little as 0.25 ug/ml 8-MOP and 12 J/cm^2 UVA (Yang et al., 1987) (Fig. 2a). Control cells treated with vehicle alone were negative (Fig. 2b). Additional controls, consisting of 8-MOP treated cells stained with nonspecific antiserum or with specific antiserum preabsorbed with 8-MOP-DNA, were negative. Treatment of cells with DNase before staining also gave negative results. Quantitation of adducts by competitive ELISA on DNA isolated from the treated cells indicated that the limit of sensitivity of the immunofluorescence method

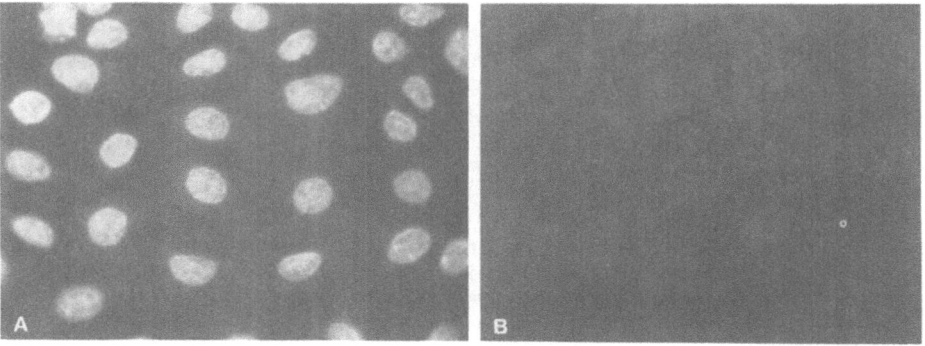

Fig. 2. Immunofluorescence staining of human keratinocytes treated with 0.25 ug/ml 8-MOP and 12 J/cm^2 UVA (a) and untreated control cells (b). Sections were stained with antibody 9D8 (1:10) and goat anti-mouse IgG antisera conjugated with fluorescein (1:10).

is about 3 adducts/10^6 nucleotides (Table 2). Thus, the immunofluorescence method is not as sensitive as the ELISA on isolated DNA, which can detect adduct levels as low as $1/10^8$. Also shown in Table 2 is the comparison of adduct quantitation by ELISA compared to that determined by measurement of bound radioactivity. These types of studies are important in the validation of an ELISA for quantitation of adducts in biological samples.

The immunofluorescence procedure was also utilized to visualize adducts in the skin of animals treated ip with 8-MOP followed by skin irradiation (Yang et al., 1987). More recently, we have observed adducts in skin biopsies from a volunteer who had 8-MOP topically applied, a punch biopsy removed and irradiated, as well as in biopsies from psoriasis patients treated by oral administration and skin irradiation before biopsy (Yang et al., 1989). Figure 3a shows the specific nuclear staining visible in the stratified squamous epithelium of the epidermis in the biopsy of the volunteer. A similar biopsy stained with non-specific antiserum was negative (Figure 3b). Other controls, including treatment of the section with DNase or preabsorption of the antiserum with 8-MOP-DNA before use, were also negative.

The 8-MOP-DNA antibodies have also been used for flow cytometric analysis of adducts formed in human keratinocytes during different stages of the cell cycle (Yang et al. 1988). Treated keratinocytes were stained with adduct specific antibody followed by fluorescein-labeled second antibodies for adduct detection and with propidium iodide for simultaneous determination of DNA content. The sensitivity of the method was determined by quantitation of adduct levels in DNA isolated from treated cells by ELISA. Current sensitivity is limited to detection of adduct levels around $1/10^5$. Using this technique, two separate cell populations with a DNA content indicative of cells in G_1 but with different levels of fluorescein labeling were observed in 8-MOP treated keratinocytes. Pretreatment of cells with aphidicolin decreased the number of cells in S phase and only one fluorescein staining G_1 population was observed. Since it is difficult to distinguish late-G_1

a   b

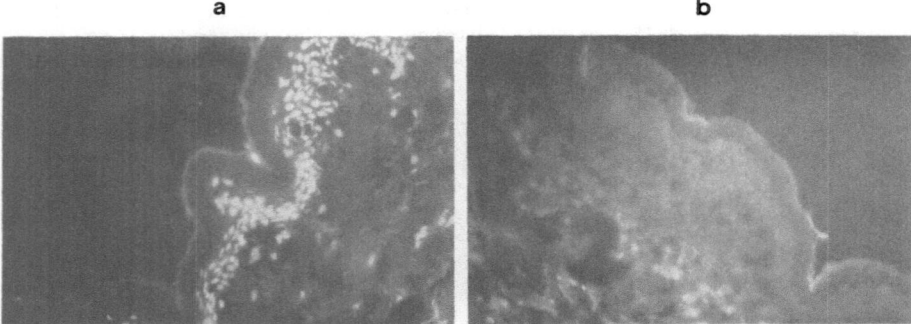

Fig. 3. Indirect immunofluorescence staining of a human skin biopsy from volunteer treated topically with 8-MOP (30 ul 0.1% solution /4 cm^2) and biopsied 30 min later. The biopsy was irradiated with with 22 J/cm^2. Sections were stained with antibody 9D8 (1:10) and goat anti-mouse IgG antisera conjugated with fluorescein (1:10). a, biopsy stained with specific antiserum; b, biopsy stained with no-specific antiserum. From Yang et al. 1989.

cells from those in early S, the "G₁" population with the higher fluorescein staining may be early S-phase cells. Partial unwinding of the DNA during cell replication could result in increased accessibility to the DNA and higher levels of adduct formation. These studies demonstrate the applicability of adduct specific antibodies to various studies on basic mechanisms of chemical carcinogenesis.

DETECTION OF POLYCYCLIC AROMATIC HYDROCARBON-DNA ADDUCTS

Antibodies developed against benzo(a)pyrene diol epoxide modified DNA (BPDE-I-DNA) have been used to quantitate adducts in biological samples obtained from humans with occupational or environmental exposure to polycyclic aromatic hydrocarbons (PAH). These antibodies crossreact with structurally related diol epoxide adducts of several other polycyclic aromatic hydrocarbons including chrysene and benz(a)anthracene (Santella et al., 1987). Figure 4 shows competitive ELISA curves for polyclonal antibody #29. This antibody recognizes DNA modified by chrysene-1,2-diol-3,4-epoxide more efficiently (50% inhibition at 18 fmol) than it recognizes BPDE-I-DNA (50% inhibition at 30 fmol). Also shown in Fig. 4 is antibody reactivity with DNA modified by benz(a)anthracene-8,9-diol-10,11-epoxide (50% inhibition at 42 fmol) and by 3,4-diol-1,2-epoxide (50% inhibition at 114 fmol). Since humans are exposed to BP in complex mixtures containing a number of other PAHs, these results indicate that multiple adducts may be detected by the ELISA. The identity of the adducts cannot be determined and thus absolute quantitation of adducts is not possible. However, since a number of PAHs in addition to BP are carcinogenic, the ELISA provides a biologically relevant general index of DNA binding by this class of compounds. Measured values are expressed as femtomole equivalents of BP adducts which would cause a similar inhibition in the assay. Similar results have been found with monoclonal antibody 5D11 developed against BPDE-I-DNA (Santella et al., 1987).

We have also recently determined that this antibody detects adducts more efficiently in highly modified DNA (1.2 adducts/100 nucleotides) than in low modified DNA (1.5/10⁵) (Santella et al., 1988). This efficiency also varied with the type of ELISA used. With the color endpoint ELISA there was a 2.5 fold difference between the high and low

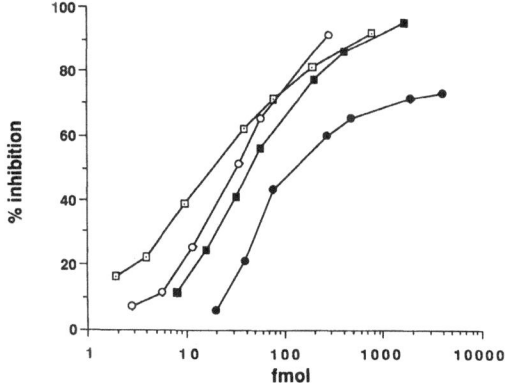

Fig. 4. Competitive inhibition of anti BPDE-I-DNA antibody #29 binding to BPDE-I-DNA. The competitors are chrysene-1,2-diol-3,4-oxide-DNA (□), BPDE-I-DNA (○), benz(a)anthracene-8,9-diol-10,11-oxide-DNA (■) and benz(a)anthracene-3,4-diol-1,2-oxide (●).

modified DNA samples but with the fluorescence endpoint ELISA the difference was 10 fold (Figure 5). The antigen used for antibody development was highly modified DNA. Clustering of adducts or some unique determinents present on highly modified DNA may be responsible for the higher sensitivity with these samples. Utilization of highly modified DNA in the standard curve in our original studies resulted in an underestimation of adduct levels. In contrast, antibodies recognizing 8-MOP-DNA have similar crossreactivity with adducts in high and low modified DNA (Yang et al., 1987). These results demonstrate the importance of thorough characterization of antisera before application to human samples and the utilization of appropriate standards for analyzing biological samples.

Antibodies recognizing PAH-DNA adducts have been used in several studies to quantitate adducts levels in humans. In collaboration with K. Hemminki, Institute of Occupational Health, Finland, adduct levels were measured in white blood cell DNA from foundry workers and controls (Perera et al., 1988). Workers were classified into high, medium, or low exposure to BP based on air monitoring data and an industrial hygenist's evaluation of the job description. Mean adduct levels for high exposed workers (>0.2 ug BP/m^3) were 5/10^7 nucleotides, for medium exposed (0.05-0.2 ug/m^3) 2.1/10^7, and for low exposed (<0.05 ug/m^3) 0.80/10^7. Controls, not occupationally exposed to PAHs, had a mean adduct level of 0.22/10^7. Adducts in these samples were also analyzed by two other laboratories by ^{32}P postlabeling (Phillips et al., 1988). While adduct levels were lower in the postlabeling assay, there was a good correlation between the immunoassay and postlabeling data.

In contrast to these results, several studies on adducts in smokers and nonsmokers have not detected significant differences between these populations. Mean adduct levels in placental DNA of smokers were 1.9/10^7 and in nonsmokers 1.2/10^7 (Everson et al., 1988; Everson et al., 1986). White blood cell DNA adducts were lower than in placenta but also were not significantly different in smokers (0.15/10^7) compared to nonsmokers (0.12/10^7) (Perera et al., 1987). These results probably reflect the ubiquitous exposure of the general population to PAHs from a number of sources including air pollution and, more importantly, diet. Recently we have also found a seasonal effect on adduct levels with

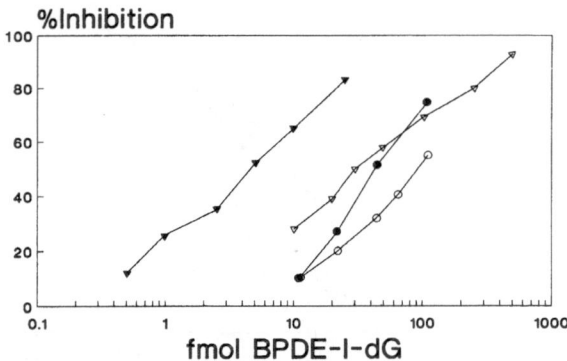

Fig. 5. Competitive inhibition of polyclonal antibody #29 binding to BPDE-I-DNA. The competitors were high modified DNA (1.2 adducts/100 nucleotides,▽) and low modified DNA (1.5 adducts/10^5,○) with color endpoint detection and high modified DNA (▼) and low modified DNA (●) with fluorescence endpoint detection.

blood samples collected during the late summer and early fall showing higher levels than those collected during the other two seasons (Perera et al., 1989) (Figure 6) This seasonal effect is consistent with observations of a peak in aryl hydrocabon hydroxylase (AHH) inducibility during this period (Paigen et al., 1981). The data in Figure 6 are from sample collected throughout the year. Repeat measurements on the same individual during the year should provide further information about the relationship of adduct formation and season.

Serum antibodies against PAH–diol expoxide–DNA adducts have been detected in individuals with various exposures to PAHs (Harris et al., 1985, Weston et al., 1987). The presence of such antisera may indicate adduct formation in vivo and may be useful as an alternate marker of exposure to PAHs. To test this hypothesis, we screened the sera of the Finnish foundry workers, roofers, and controls by noncompetitive ELISA on plates coated with calf thymus DNA and BPDE-I-DNA. Criteria for positive titer, defined by Harris et al., 1985, was an absorbance value for the modified DNA greater than two standard deviations above that for the control, unmodified DNA. Two of the four foundry workers with high exposure to PAHs demonstrated significant titer, 5/7 with medium exposure and 4/4 with low exposure. For controls, not occupationally exposed to PAHs, 6/10 sera showed positive titer. With the samples obtained from roofers only 4/12 were positive, while 6/12 age, sex and smoking matched controls were positive. Thus, no significant difference was seen between the number of samples with positive titer in the sera of control individuals compared to those with high occupational exposure. These results are in contrast to the large differences in white blood cell DNA adduct levels seen in these same populations.

DETECTION OF AFLATOXIN–DNA ADDUCTS

Epidemiological studies have demonstrated a strong association between exposure to aflatoxin B_1 (AFB$_1$), a potent liver carcinogen, and human liver cancer incidence in Africa and Southeast Asia (Busby and Wogan, 1984). The major adduct of AFB$_1$ at the N7 position of guanine is an unstable and either depurinates or imidazole ring-opens (Wogan, 1976). The ring opened AFB$_1$-FAPy adducts are stable, accumulate in DNA and may play an important role in hepatocarcinogenesis (Croy and Wogan, 1981). We have developed monoclonal antibodies recognize AFB$_1$-FAPy adducts with a limit of sensitivity of 5/10^7 (Hsieh et al., 1988). No crossreactivity is seen with free AFB$_1$ or AFB$_1$-protein adducts. These antibodies have been used to detect adducts in tissues obtained from

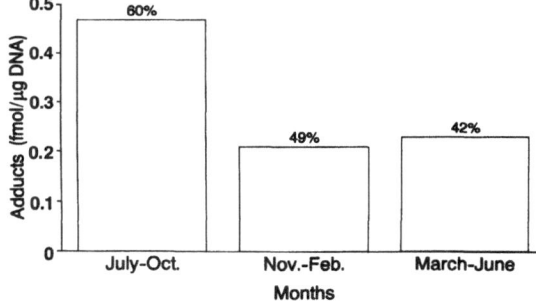

Fig. 6. Seasonal variation in PAH–DNA adducts in white blood cell DNA. Values shown are the means for positive samples; numbers above the bars are percentage of positive samples.

Table 3. Levels of AFB$_1$-FAPY Adducts in Human Liver

Patient	Tumor	Adjacent-normal
	adducts/10^6 nucleotides	
1	3.5	ND*
2	3.2	ND
3	1.2	ND
4	3.4	1.7
5	1.2	1.2
6	1.8	ND
7	–	ND
8	–	ND
9	1.3	NA

*ND, non detectable
NA, not assayed

liver cancer patients from Taiwan. Adducts were detectable in 2 of 8 adjacent-normal tissues and 7 of 7 tumor tissues (Table 3). The difference between tumor and nontumor tissue may not be significant because of the small number of samples but will be further investigated in ongoing studies. In addition, because of the high adduct levels present in some samples we have recently begun to utilize fluorescence methods to confirm adduct levels quantitated by ELISA. Initial studies with in vitro modified DNA indicate that the fluorescence method can readily detect adducts down to a level of 1/10^7. We are also developing immunoaffinity techniques to further increase this sensitivity by isolation of DNA fragments enriched in adduct before fluorescence measurement.

DETERMINATION OF MULTIPLE ADDUCTS

Human exposure to environmental carcinogens usually occurs in the form of complex mixtures. To monitor exposure to these mixtures, we would ideally like to perfom multiple ELISAs on DNA samples from the same individual to determine all adducts present on DNA. To circumuent the limited availability of peripheral blood cell DNA, we have initially tested whether two different DNA adducts can be measured in a DNA sample with specific antibodies recognizing the individual adducts. DNA modified in vitro with BPDE-I was subsequently modified with 8-methoxypsoralen and UVA light. A mixture of the antibodies recognizing both adducts, each at the appropriate final dilution for the ELISA, was then made. The competitive ELISA was carried out on serial dilutions of the mixed DNAs and mixed antibodies. This competitive mixture was first added to plates coated with BPDE-I-DNA and after a 90 min incubation transferred to plates coated with 8-MOP-DNA. Each plate was then incubated with the appropriate alkaline phosphatase conjugate as in the standard assay. These assays were compared to the standard assay for both antibodies (Fig. 7) and indicate that when BPDE-I-DNA is analyzed alone or in the presence of 8-MOP-DNA similar 50% inhibition values result. Similarly, for 8-MOP-DNA, no difference is seen when analyzed alone or in the presence of BPDE-I-DNA. These results suggest that it may be possible to make a cocktail of antisera to specific DNA adducts and, by sequential transfer to plates coated with the appropriate antigen, quantitate a number of different DNA adducts. Since the adducts are not destroyed by incubation with antibodies in the ELISA, DNA can be recovered from the competitive mixture on the microwell plate and repurified with phenol/chloroform extraction. The DNA can then be utilized for additional analysis by alternate methods such as postlabeling or fluorescence.

DISCUSSION

These studies demonstrate that immunologic methods have sufficient sensitivity to monitor human exposure to environmental carcinogens. Immunoassays also have the advantage of ease of application to large number of samples making them ideal for epidemiologic studies. However, human samples frequently have adducts levels near the limits of sensitivity of these assay. In addition, because competitive ELISAs measure general inhibition of antibody binding to plates, artifacts can sometimes interfer with quantitation. For these reasons, it is advantageous to use other methods to confirm adducts levels determined by ELISA. Unfortunately, alternate methods, with the required sensitivity, are sometimes not available. The studies discussed above on PAH adducts in foundry workers are examples of this approach. While the postlabeling assay may not be measuring the same adducts as the ELISA, and the values were somewhat lower than the those determined by ELISA, the correlation of both assays with exposure level and with each other provides support for the accuracy of the determinations. Similarly, for aflatoxin-DNA adducts we are attempting to utilize fluorescence measurements to confirm immunoassay data.

The current immunofluorescence method is limited to the detection of adduct levels around $1/10^6$ nucleotides. Computer – assisted video microscopy systems or the use of biotin-streptavidin staining should further increase sensitivity. It may then be possible to utilize these methods for adduct detection in human samples from occupational or environmental exposures. Since adducts can in theory be visualized in single cells, the small amount of material obtained at biopsy could be utilized.

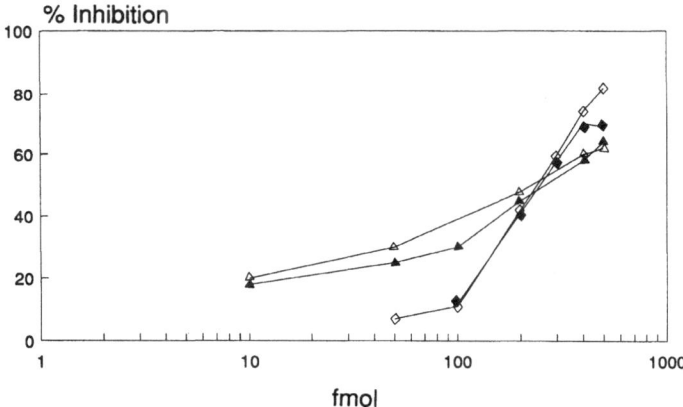

Fig. 7. Multiple adduct analysis by competitive ELISA. The competitors were BPDE-I-DNA in the standard assay with antibody #29 (△) and 8-MOP-DNA in the standard assay with antibody 8G1 (◇). For the multiple adduct assay, DNA modified by BPDE-I and 8-MOP was mixed with antisera #29 and 8G1 and sequentially incubated on plates coated with BPDE-I-DNA (▲) and 8-MOP-DNA (◆).

While methods for the determination of DNA adducts in humans provides information about the biologically effective dose of a carcinogen, information about the relationship of these measurements to risk is unknown. Future epidemiologic studies are needed to provide this information.

ACKNOWLEDGEMENTS

Studies on placental DNA adducts, in smokers and nonsmokers were carried out in collaboration with R. Everson. Studies on 8-MOP treated patients were carried out in collaboration with F. Gasparro and V. DeLeo. The cooperation of S-W Hsu and D-S Chen in the collection of samples from cancer patients in Taiwan is also greatfully acknowledged. This work was supported by grants ESO3881 and CA21111 and by a grant from the Lucille P. Markey Charitable Trust.

REFERENCES

Busby, W. F., and Wogan, G. N., 1984, Aflatoxins. in: "Chemical Carcinogens". Searle, C. D., ed., ACS, Washington, DC.

Croy, R. G., and Wogan, G. N., 1981, Temporal patterns of covalent DNA adducts in rat liver after single and multiple doses of aflatoxin B. Cancer Res., 41: 197.

Everson, R. B., Randerath, E., Santella, R. M., Cefalo, R. C., Avitts, T. A., and Randerath, K., 1986, Detection of smoking-related covalent DNA adducts in human placenta. Science, 231: 54.

Everson, R. B., Randerath, E., Santella, R. M., Avitts, T. A., Weinstein, I. B., and Randerath, K., 1988, Quantitative associations between DNA damage in human placenta and maternal smoking and birth weight. J. Natl. Cancer Inst., 80, 567.

Harris, C. C., Vahakangas, K., Newman, J. M., Trivers, G. E., Shamsuddin, A., Sinopoli, N., Mann, D. L., and Wright, W. E. 1985, Detection of benzo[a]pyrene diol epoxide-DNA adducts in peripheral blood lymphocytes and antibodies to the adducts in serum from coke oven workers. Proc. Natl. Acad. Sci. USA, 82: 6672.

Hsieh, L. L., Hsu, S. W., Chen, D. S., and Santella, R. M., 1988, Immunological detection of aflatoxin Bl-DNA adducts formed in vivo. Cancer Res., 48: 6328.

Hsieh, L. L., Jeffrey, A. M., and Santella, R. M., 1985, Monoclonal antibodies to l-aminopyrene-DNA. Carcinogenesis, 6: 1289

Kraemer, K. H., and Weinstein, G. D., 1977, Decreased thymidine incorporation in circulating leucocytes after treatment of psoriasis with psoralen and long-wave ultraviolet light. J. Invest. Dermatol., 69: 211.

Miolo, G., Stefanidis, M., Santella, R. M., Acqua, F., and Gasparro, F., 1989, 6,4,4'-Trimethylangelecin photoadduct formation in DNA: production and characterization of a specific monoclonal antibody. Photochem. Photobiol., 3: 101.

Paigen, B., Ward, E., Reilly, A., Houten, L., Gurtoo, H. L., Minowada, J., Steenland, K., Havens, M. B., and Satori, P., 1981, Season bariation of aryl hydrocarbon hydroxylase activity in human lymphocytes. Cancer Res., 41: 2757.

Perera, F. P., Hemminiki, K., Young, T. L., Santella, R. M., Brenner, D., and Kelly, G., 1988, Detection of polycyclic aromatic hydrocarbon-DNA adducts in white blood cells of foundry workers. Cancer Res., 48: 2288.

Perera, F. P., Santella, R. M., Brenner, D., Poirier, M. C., Munshi, A.

A., Fischman, H. K., and VanRyzin, J., 1987, DNA adducts, protein adducts and SCE in cigarette smokers and nonsmokers. J. Natl. Cancer Inst., 79: 449.

Perera. F. P., Mayer, Jl, Jaretzki, A., Hearne, S., Brenner, D., Young, T. L., Fishman, H. K., Fishman, H. K., Grimes, M., Grantham, S., Tang, M. X., Tsai, W. Y., Santella, R. M., 1989, Comparison of DNA adducts and sister chromatid exchange in lung cancer cases and controls. Cancer Research, 49: 4446.

Phillips, D. H., Hemminki, K., Alhonen, A., Hewer, A., and Grover, P. L., 1988, Monitoring occupational exposure to carcinogens: detection by 32P-postlabelling of aromatic DNA adducts in white blood cells from iron foundry workers. Mutation Res., 204: 531.

Poirier, M. C., 1981, Antibodies to carcinogen-DNA adducts. J. Natl. Cancer Inst., 67: 515.

Santella, R. M., 1988, Application of new techniques for the detection of carcinogen adducts to human population monitoring. Mutation Res., 205: 271.

Santella, R. M., Dharmaraja, N., Gasparro, F. P., and Edelson, R. L., 1985, Monoclonal antibodies to DNA modified by 8-methoxypsoralen and ultraviolet A light. Nucleic Acids Res., 13: 2533.

Santella, R. M., Gasparo, F. P., and Hsieh, L. L., 1987, Quantitation of carcinogen-DNA adducts with monoclonal antibodies. Prog. Exper. Tumor Res., 31: 63.

Santella, R. M., Lin, C. D., Cleveland, W. L., and Weinstein, I. B., 1984, Monoclonal antibodies to DNA modified by a benzo[a]pyrene diol epoxide. Carcinogenesis, 5: 373.

Santella, R. M., Weston, A., Perera, F. P., Trivers, G. T., Harris, C. C., Young, T. L., Nguyen, D., Lee, B. M. and Poirier, M. C., 1988, Interlaboratory comparison of antisera and immunoassays for benzo(a)pyrene-diol-epoxide--I-modified DNA. Carcinogenesis, 9: 1265.

Santella, R. M., Yang, X. Y., DeLeo, V. A., and Gasparro, F. P., 1988, Detection and quantification of 8-methoxypsoralen-DNA adducts, in: Bartsch, H., Hemminki, K., and O'Neil, I.K. ed.," Methods for Detecting DNA Damaging Agents in Human: Applications in Cancer Epidemiology and Prevention". IARC, Lyon.

Weston, A., Trivers, G., Vahakangas, K., Newman, M., and Rowe, M., 1987, Detection of carcinogen-DNA adducts in human cells and Antibodies to These Adducts in Human Sera. Prog. Exper. Tumor Res., 31: 76.

Wogan, G. N., 1976, Aflatoxins and their relationship to hepatocellular carcinoma, in: "Hepatocellular Carcinoma, " Okuda, K. and Peters, R.L., ed., John Wiley and Sons, New York.

Yang, X. Y., DeLeo, V., and Santella, R. M., 1987, Immunological detection and visualization of 8-methoxypsoralen-DNA photoadducts. Cancer Res.., 47: 2451.

Yang, X. Y., Delohery, T., and Santella, R. M., 1988, Flow cytometric analysis of 8-methoxypsoralen-DNA photoadducts in human keratinocytes. Cancer Res., 48: 7013.

Yang, X. Y., Gasparro, F. P., DeLeo, V. A., and Santella, R. M., 1989, 8-Methoxypsoralen-DNA adducts in patients treated with 8-methoxypsoralen and ultraviolet A light. J. Invest. Dermatol., 92: 59.

Yang, X. Y., and Santella, R. M., 1987, Development of monoclonal antibodies to acetylaminofluorene modified DNA and poly(dG-dC)-poly(dG-dC)., in: Carcinogenic and Mutagenic Responses to Aromatic Amines and Nitroarenes., King. C. M., Romano, L. J., and Schuetzle, D., ed., Elsevier, New York.

43

Yang, T. L., and Santella, R. M., 1988, Development of techniques
   to monitor for exposure to vinyl chloride: monoclonal
   antibodies to ethenoadenosine and ethenocytine.
   Carcinogenesis, 9: 5892.

LESION MEASUREMENT IN NON-RADIOACTIVE DNA

BY QUANTITATIVE GEL ELECTROPHORESIS

John C. Sutherland, Chun Zhang Chen, Ann Emrick,
Haim Hacham, Denise C. Monteleone, Eldred
Ribeiro, John Trunk and Betsy M. Sutherland

Biology Department
Brookhaven National Laboratory
Upton, New York 11973, USA

INTRODUCTION

The important role of DNA damage and repair in homeostasis has been clearly demonstrated by studies involving isolated DNA, procaryotic cells and eukaryotic cells growing in culture. The information obtainable from these model systems, while extremely valuable, can never replace the need for data from intact higher organisms. The gel electrophoresis method developed during the past ten years in our laboratories makes possible the quantitation of UV induced pyrimidine dimers, gamma ray induced single- and double-strand breaks and many other types of lesions in nanogram quantities of DNA. The DNA does not have to be labeled with radionuclides or of a particular conformation, thus facilitating the use of the method in measuring damage levels and repair rates in the DNA of intact organisms -- including man.

The gel method can quantitate any lesion in DNA that either is, or can be converted to a single- or double-strand break. The formation of a strand break produces two shorter DNA molecules for each molecule that existed before the treatment that produced the break. Determining the number of breaks, and hence the number of lesions, becomes a matter of comparing the average lengths of molecules in samples differing only in lesion-induced breaks. This requires that we determine the distribution of mass of DNA on a gel as a function of its distance of migration and also the dispersion function (the relationship between molecular length and distance of migration) in the gel electrophoresis system.

The distribution of DNA mass in a gel is determined by staining with a fluorophore such as ethidium bromide and recording the intensity of ethidium fluorescence from a uniformly UV irradiated gel. We have replaced photographic recording of ethidium fluorescence by an electronic imaging

DNA Damage and Repair in Human Tissues
Edited by B. M. Sutherland and A. D. Woodhead
Plenum Press, New York, 1990

system which is more accurate and much faster. The
sensitivity of the method has been further increased by
electrophoresis procedures that separate longer DNA molecules
by temporal modulation of the strength of the electric field
or its direction relative to the gel, and by the use of a
second generation electronic imaging system with improved
photometric performance.

DEVELOPMENT OF THE GEL ELECTROPHORESIS METHOD FOR
QUANTITATION OF LESIONS IN UNLABELED HETEROGENEOUS DNA

Our gel electrophoresis method for the quantitation of
DNA damage is the conceptual descendant of methods in which
DNA of different lengths are separated by centrifugation.
The theoretical and practical aspects of this method were
reviewed by Lett (1981). While methods based on
centrifugation were important in many studies of DNA damage
and repair, they are labor intensive, usually require that
the DNA be prelabeled with a radionuclide and provide limited
spatial resolution of the material in the centrifuge tube,
and hence, have limited sensitivity compared to gel
electrophoresis. By separating the population of DNA
molecules as some known function of their length, one can
compute the number of **molecules** per unit mass of DNA. The
number of strand breaks per unit mass (or length) of DNA
induced by some treatment is the difference between the
number of molecules per unit mass for two samples, only one
of which has received the treatment. In the case of UV-
induced pyrimidine dimers, strand breaks are induced by
treatment with an endonuclease that produces a single-strand
scission adjacent to a dimer and has no other site of action.
Setlow's group and subsequent work at Brookhaven used the
UV-specific endonuclease from <u>Micrococcus</u> <u>luteus</u> (Carrier and
Setlow, 1970), but endonuclease V from bacteriophage T4 has
equivalent properties (see the review by Seawell et al.,
1981). Both the endonuclease treated sample and a control
sample that received the same UV exposure but was not treated
with endonuclease are exposed to high pH to separate the DNA
strands. These samples are then subjected to electrophoresis
in an alkaline agarose gel to separate the single-stranded
DNA molecules as a function of their length. The preparation
of UV-irradiated DNA in the determination of pyrimidine
dimers is shown schematically in Fig. 1. A schematic diagram
of the appearance of a typical gel post electrophoresis is
shown in Fig. 2 and a photograph of the image of an actual
gel is shown in Fig. 3. The integrated profiles of the lanes
of the gel shown in Fig. 3 containing endonuclease-treated
DNA samples are shown in Fig. 4.

<u>Qualitative Observation of Pyrimidine Dimer Production and
Repair in Lower Eukaryotes</u>

Richard Setlow and his colleagues pioneered the use of
gel electrophoresis to study the effects of 254 nm UV on the
DNA of cells from three species of fish, <u>Prionace glauca</u>
(Woodhead et al., 1978), <u>Poecilia</u> <u>formosa</u> (Achey et al.,
1989) and <u>Anoptichthys</u> <u>jordani</u> (Woodhead and Achey, 1979),and
a tapeworm, <u>Hymenolepis</u> <u>diminuta</u> (Woodhead and Achey, 1981).
While they did not attempt to determine absolute molecular
lengths of their DNA samples, they demonstrated both the

DNA (in cells)

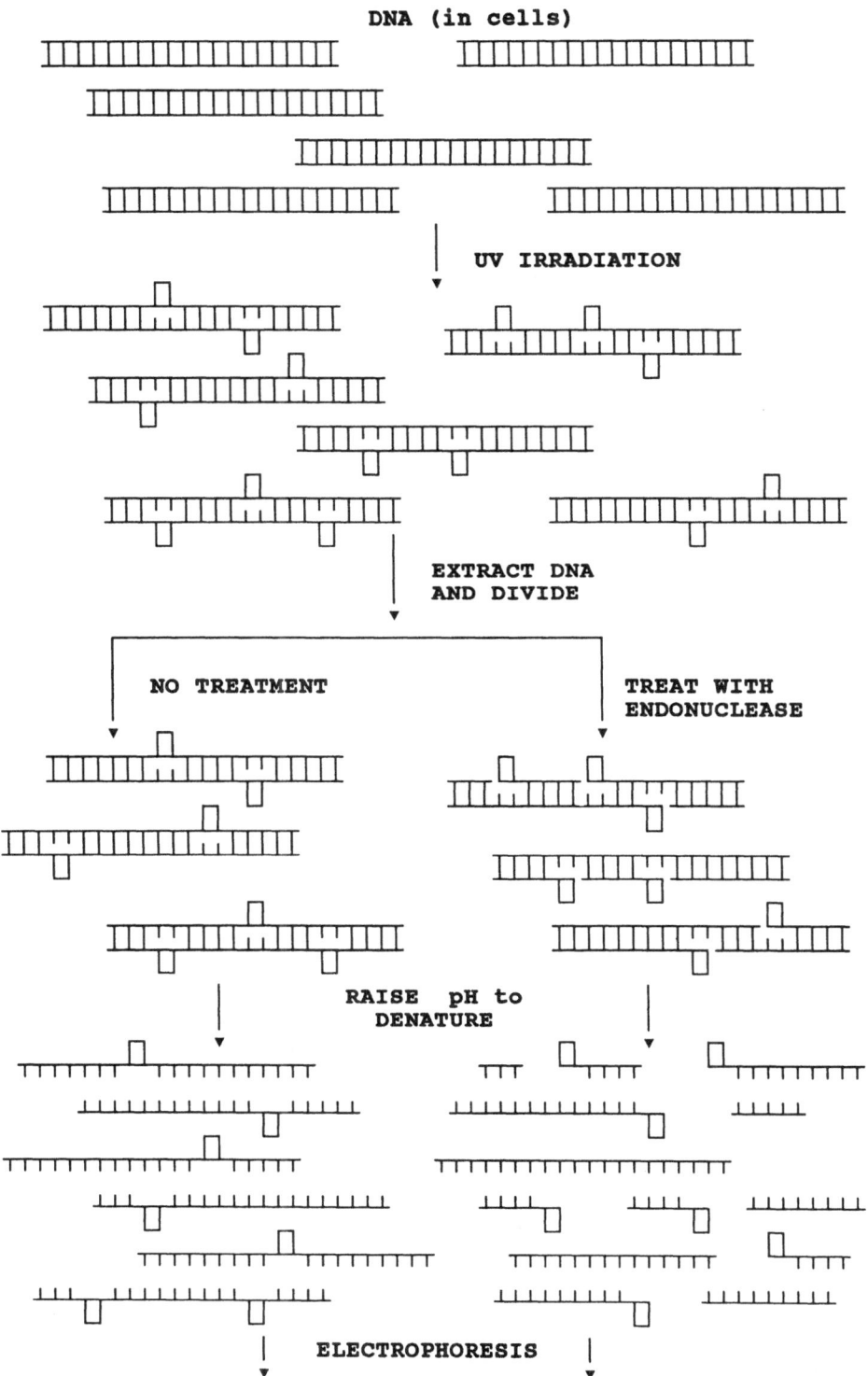

Fig. 1. Diagram of the gel method applied to the measurement
of pyrimidine dimers formed in DNA by UV radiation.

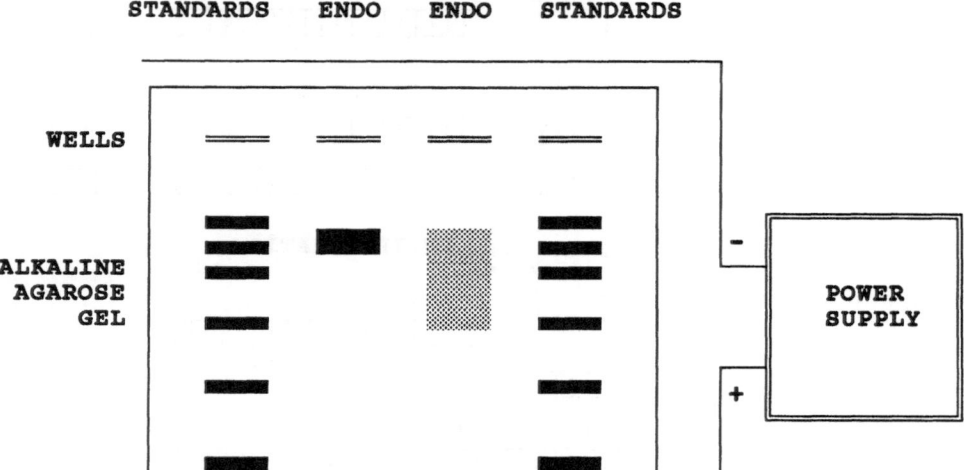

Fig. 2. Schematic diagram of the distribution of DNA on a gel after electrophoresis. The two outside lanes contain molecular length standards that are used to determine the dispersion function of the electrophoresis system, while the two center lanes contain samples of UV-irradiated DNA prepared as outlined in Fig. 1.

formation of pyrimidine dimers and their subsequent repair by photoreactivation. Setlow and his colleagues resorted to gel electrophoresis because of the difficulty of labeling the DNA of higher organisms with radionuclides and the need to use less DNA.

Quantitation of Dimers by the Gel Method and Its Application to Pyrimidine Formation in the DNA of Cells of UV-Irradiated Human Skin

Betsy Sutherland and her associates adopted the gel method for similar reasons. Since they studied the formation and repair of pyrimidine dimers in the DNA from cells in human skin UV-irradiated in situ (Sutherland et al., 1980), the ability to work with small quantities of DNA was critical. In addition, prelabeling of the target DNA with radionuclides was proscribed for ethical as well as technical reasons. Sutherland and her colleagues made a quantum advance by introducing **quantitation** of lesions to the gel method (Sutherland et al., 1980; Sutherland and Shih, 1983).

The first procedure for quantifying the frequency of lesions using the gel electrophoresis method was based on: photographing the ethidium bromide stained gel to obtain the distribution of DNA in each lane, scanning each lane of the photographic negative with a densitometer and determining the median position of the densitometric profile using a "cut and weigh" procedure. By definition, one half of the DNA in a lane migrates further than the median migration distance.

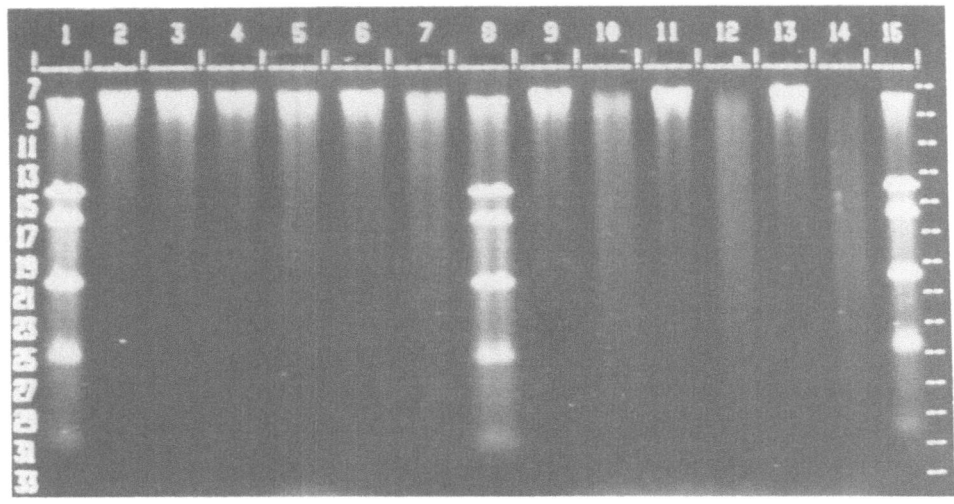

Fig. 3. Photograph of a video monitor showing the distribution of ethidium bromide fluorescence from an alkaline agarose gel, as recorded by our electronic imaging system. Lanes 1, 8 and 15 contain a mixture of DNA molecules of known lengths from bacteriophage (T4, 170 kb; lambda, 48.5 kb; T7, 40 kb and the fragments produced by a terminal digestion of T7 DNA with the restriction endonuclease Bgl I: 22.5, 13.5, and 4 kb respectively) that are used to determine the dispersion function of the electrophoresis system. The other lanes contain samples of DNA from human cells that received increasing doses of 254 nm UV radiation: lanes 2 and 3, 0 J/m^2; lanes 4 and 5, 0.2 J/m^2; lanes 6 and 7, 0.5 J/m^2; lanes 9 and 10, 1.0 J/m^2; lanes 11 and 12, 2 J/m^2; lanes 13 and 14, 3 J/m^2. In each pair of samples that received the same dose, the one in the higher numbered lane was treated with the pyrimidine dimer specific endonuclease prior to electrophoresis and the sample in the lower numbered lane was not treated with endonuclease.

The location on the negative of a series of bands containing DNA molecules of known length was used to construct a plot of molecular length versus distance of migration (i. e. the "dispersion function of the electrophoresis system). This empirical curve was used to determine the molecular length of DNA corresponding to the median distance of migration. The critical link to the determination of lesion frequency is that for a suitably heterogeneous population of DNA molecules, the number average length equals 60% of the median length (Veatch and Okada, 1969). The number of single-strand breaks per unit length of DNA, η, is the difference between the reciprocal of the number average length of a DNA sample that has been treated with a pyrimidine dimer specific endonuclease, $N^{-1}(+endo)$, minus the reciprocal of the number average length of a sample that has not been treated, $N^{-1}(-endo)$, (Lett, 1981,

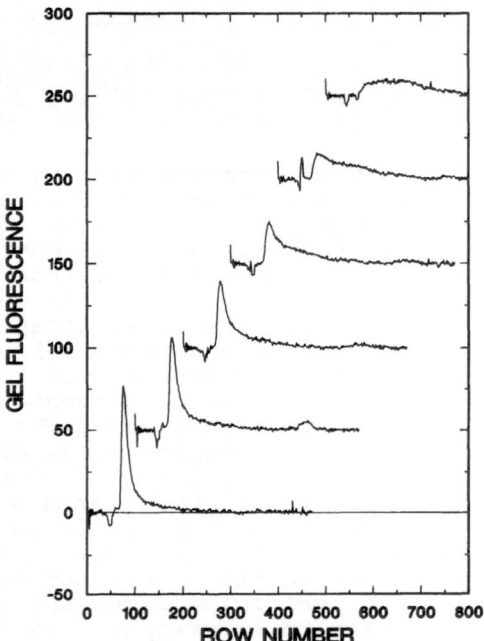

Fig. 4. Integrated lane profiles of the lanes in Fig. 3
containing endonuclease-treated DNAs. As the UV dose
increases, the average length of the DNA decreases
and the shorter molecules migrate further during
electrophoresis. Each profile is offset 100 rows to
the right and 50 units vertically relative to the
previous trace.

50

Freeman et al., 1986). The frequency of endonuclease sites and hence dimers is calculated from the equation:

$$\eta - N^{-1}(+endo) - N^{-1}(-endo) \qquad Eqn. \ 1$$

The units of η are sites per kilobase or sites per megabase. Hence, η is also referred to as the "frequency" of endonuclease sensitive sites.

Computerized Analysis and Improved Accuracy

The introduction of quantitation to the gel assay by Sutherland et al. (1980) was a critical milestone in the development of the method. However, the procedure used to obtain the number average lengths was extremely tedious and required the use of several approximations. One way to make the measurement of dimers faster and less labor intensive was to obtain the optical density profile of each lane in digital form so that the calculation of the median distance of migration could be performed by a computer. Thus, we developed a computer controlled scanner and programs to perform this function (Sutherland et al., 1984). After the program to compute the median distance of migration of the DNA in each lane was working, we wrote a program to construct the DNA-length vs distance-of-migration function. We chose the empirical "offset hyperbolic" relationship reported by Southern (1979). However, we modified the equation describing this function to give physically meaningful names to two of the constants (Freeman et al., 1986). Our version of the offset hyperbolic dispersion function is:

$$L(x) - \frac{C}{x - x_\infty} - \frac{C}{x_0 - x_\infty} \qquad Eqn. \ 2$$

where $L(x)$ is the length of the DNA molecules migrating to position x on the gel, C is the "gel constant" for the particular electrophoresis system and x_0 and x_∞ are the distances of migration of molecules of "zero" and "infinite" length, respectively. For static field gel electrophoresis, x_∞ corresponds to some finite distance of migration (McDonnell et al., 1977) due to the process of reptation (Lerman, and Frisch, 1982; Lumpkin and Zimm, 1982). At the other extreme, x_0 corresponds to the motion of very short molecules that are not retarded by the sieving effect of the gel. The values of C, x_0, and x_∞ are obtained from the observed distances of migration of a set of length standards of known length using the least-squares procedure of Schaffer and Sederoff (1981). For brevity, and by analogy with the function of optical instruments that separate a broad spectrum of light into its individual components, we call $L(x)$ the "dispersion function" of the electrophoresis system (Sutherland et al., 1988).

Once we could determine $L(x)$, we realized that we could use the experimental distribution of the mass of DNA down a lane, $\Phi(x)$, to compute the number average lengths, N, directly, hence avoiding the approximation introduced by the use of the median length of the population, that is:

$$N^{-1} = \frac{\int \frac{\Phi(x) \times dx}{L(x)}}{\int \Phi(x) \times dx} \qquad \textit{Eqn. 3}$$

We choose to write Eqn. 3 in terms of the reciprocal of **N** because this is the quantity directly related to the frequency of lesions, i. e. Eqn. 1. The integral in the denominator of Eqn. 3 is just the total mass of DNA in the lane and, hence, the computation of lesion frequency from Eqn. 1 is independent of the quantity of DNA in both the treated and untreated samples. Actually, the parameter that we measure is not the distribution of mass in each lane but rather the distribution of fluorescence which is proportional to the quantity of DNA at each position down the lane. Since the same constant appears in the integrals of both numerator and denominator of Eqn. 3, the value of N^{-1} is independent of this factor.

Photographic Recording of Gel Fluorescence

While testing the gel scanner, we discovered that the integrated optical density of a band of a photographic negative is not exactly proportional to the quantity of DNA in the band. This results from the fact that the optical density of a developed photographic negative is not simply proportional to the total number of photons incident upon it during an exposure. Rather, the optical density of a negative is a sigmoidal function of the logarithm of the incident light (see e. g. Ditchburn, 1965). The central portion of the film response function is essentially a straight line. Pulleyblank et al. (1977), Prunell et al. (1977), and Prunell (1980) described procedures to convert optical density to a parameter proportional to ethidium bromide fluorescence from a gel. They used optical density data recorded on chart paper and hence, their methods were quite laborious, but when the optical density data are recorded by a computer, the conversion is swift and transparent to the user (Sutherland et al., 1984).

Two other precautions are necessary when photography is used in quantitative studies to record fluorescence from a gel. Since gel fluorescence is a nonlinear function of optical density and the distribution of DNA across the width of a lane is not uniform, it is imperative that the conversion be performed on the optical density recorded at each point on the gel, before any averaging or summation across the lane (Sutherland et al., 1984). In addition, the actual film function depends on several factors, including the duration of the exposure. That is, for exposures lasting more than a few seconds, there is a failure of "time-intensity reciprocity". Ribeiro et al. (1989) have recently investigated this problem in detail and demonstrated that it can be overcome by including a calibration procedure as part of the recording and analysis of each photographic image. Their procedure also extends the range of optical densities that can be converted accurately to values of gel fluorescence by including nonlinear portions of the film function.

Enhanced Sensitivity by Separation of Longer DNA Molecules

The lowest frequency of dimers or other lesions that can be measured is limited by the length of the longest DNA molecules that the electrophoresis system can separate since a lesion is not detected if the product molecules migrate to the same position on the gel as their precursor. In static-field gel electrophoresis, DNA molecules longer than about 100 kilobases -- the maximum length is influenced by a variety of experimental parameters including the agarose content of the gel and the strength of the electric field -- migrate together, independent of their exact length, due to the process of reptation (Lerman and Frisch, 1982; Lumpkin and Zimm, 1982). The length-limited sensitivity of the gel method is the maximum length of molecules that can be resolved divided by the fractional difference between the number average lengths of two samples that can be detected reliably. Thus, if the number average lengths of molecules in the range of 100 kb can be determined reliably to within 10 %, then the length limited sensitivity of the method is one dimer per megabase ($10^5/0.1 = 10^6$). In practice, we found that with static-field alkaline gel electrophoresis and photographic imaging of fluorescence, dimer frequencies of three per megabase were readily achievable (Freeman et al., 1986).

Schwartz and Cantor (1984) discovered that periodically switching the direction of the electric field with respect to the gel overcomes the effects of reptation and makes possible the separation of **very** long DNA molecules. They believed (incorrectly) that the separation process depended on the presence of gradients in the electric field and, indeed, initially called the technique "pulsed field **gradient** gel electrophoresis". The field gradients resulted in curved lanes in their gels. Identical samples placed in different wells moved different distances. Thus, while the method of Schwartz and Cantor represented an important breakthrough in electrophoresis technology, their implementation was unsuitable for our quantitative method.

Unidirectional Pulsed Field Gel Electrophoresis. We developed another approach to separating longer DNA molecules in which the electric current through a standard electrophoresis cell is switched on for a short time, typically 0.1 to 0.3 sec and then turned off for a longer time, typically 10 sec (Sutherland et al., 1987b; Sutherland et al., 1988). In the case of single-stranded DNA in alkaline agarose gels, the limit of separation is increased to above 300 kb, far lower than achievable with the method of Schwartz and Cantor but sufficient to increase significantly the length-limited sensitivity of lesion detection. However, the lanes are straight, so quantitative analysis is possible! An additional benefit is that for alkaline gels the same function used for static-field gel electrophoresis (i. e. Eqn. 2) describes the dispersion function, thus eliminating the need for additional analysis software. The apparatus costs only slightly more than that required for static-field gel electrophoresis and heating of the gel by the electric current is never a problem because the time-average power is very low.

The mechanism by which longer DNA molecules are separated appears to be different from that in the method of Schwartz and Cantor. In their case, the field is on for a sufficiently long time that all of the longer molecules have been extruded into an extended linear conformation by the action of the electric field forcing them into the porous gel and, hence, are moving through the gel at the same speed by the process of reptation. Separation based on length is achieved because when the direction of the field is switched, longer molecules require more time to reorganize and begin reptating in the new direction (see e. g. Deutsch, 1987, 1988). In contrast, in our method the "random coil" resting molecules presumably do not have adequate time to change conformation and the long interpulse period permits them to relax completely. Thus, molecules that are forced into a linear conformation and move by reptation in the presence of a static field retain a globular conformation and are separated by the sieving action of the gel. In support of this hypothesis we found that the least squares fitting procedure for the gel dispersion function (Eqn. 2) puts x_{∞} near the edge of the well. That is, very long molecules do not enter the gel at all. We call the technique **unidirectional** pulsed field gel electrophoresis to distinguish it from the method described by Cantor and Schwartz.

Lesion Quantitation Using Alternating Field Direction Gel Electrophoresis. The ability of the Schwartz-Cantor method to separate very long DNA molecules prompted other workers to develop variations in which the lanes run straight and the mobilities of samples are independent of the lane in which they run (Carle et al., 1986; Chu et al., 1986; Gardiner et al., 1986; Serwer, 1987; Southern et al., 1987; Bancroft and Wolk, 1988; Clark et al., 1988). Most applications involve the analysis of discrete bands, but the same techniques can be applied to the analysis of heterogeneous populations, as required in the quantitation of DNA lesions.

The procedure for the analysis of DNA lesions must be modified when using alternating field direction gel electrophoresis. First, the dispersion functions for these systems for molecules longer than 100 kb or kbp are clearly not hyperbolic. Indeed, over a wide range of lengths, they are linear. Thus, we have modified the analysis software to include generation of dispersion functions by spline function and polynomial fitting of sets of length standards. For double stranded DNA on native gels, ladders of concatonated DNA from bacteriophage lambda can be used as length standards up to about 1.5 Mbp and chromosomal DNAs from Saccharomyces cerevisiae and Schizosaccharomyces pombe to greater than 5 Mbp, however, the lengths of the chromosomal DNAs from the latter are much less certain. Long single-stranded length standards are far more difficult to obtain. Our best results to date have been with the DNA from bacteriophage G, which is about 780 kb in length. In order to obtain DNA molecules this long, it is necessary to embed cells in agarose plugs which are then treated to remove other cellular components.

Since the longest chromosomal DNA from <u>Schizo</u>
<u>saccharomyces</u> <u>pombe</u>, which is longer than 5 Mbp, has
been resolved, the length-limited sensitivity should
approach, and perhaps exceed, one lesion in 50 million base
pairs or about 60 lesions per human genome! Our experience
to date indicates that such high sensitivities cannot yet be
achieved because for very long double stranded DNAs, not all
of the sample placed in a well will enter the gel, thus
precluding the standard analysis described above. For
single-stranded DNAs, the lack of length standards longer
than about 1 Mb will limit the sensitivity to roughly one
lesion per 10 Mb. However, this sensitivity can be increased
by more accurate procedures for determining number average
lengths.

Electronic Imaging System for Quantification of Fluorescence from Ethidium Bromide Stained Gels

The limitations inherent in the use of photographic
imaging of the distribution of fluorescence from gels
prompted us to investigate other approaches. We wanted an
imaging system that: responds linearly to the intensity of
light from the source, provides adequate spatial resolution,
has photometric sensitivity comparable to or exceeding that
of photography and produces the image in digital form
immediately suitable for quantitative analysis and archival
storage.

<u>First generation electronic imaging system.</u> The first
system we built for electronic imaging of gel fluorescence is
based on an industrial TV camera that employs a charged
coupled device (CCD) to detect incident light (Sutherland et
al., 1987a). A schematic diagram of this system is shown in
Fig. 5. A CCD is an integrated circuit (chip) containing a
rectangular array of image sensors. The CCD in our first
imaging system has about 200,000 individual light detectors,
but special "scientific" CCDs are available with more than 4
million individual detectors. The signal from a CCD is a
linear function of the light that exposed it, thus greatly
simplifying the processing of image data compared to
photography. The sensitivity of this electronic imaging
system is greater than that of the Polaroid type 55 film used
previously (Freeman et al., 1986) and hence exposure times
are reduced. Detection of fluorescence from many gels is,
however, far too weak to yield a good image in the standard
(1/30 sec) exposure of a TV camera. Thus, we modified the
camera and frame-grabber (the device that digitizes, stores
and displays the voltage output from the camera) and built
additional timing logic to permit the camera system -- under
computer control -- to record images for extended periods.
The functional limit on the exposure period is the
accumulation of thermally generated charge in the CCD. The
rate of buildup of the thermal "background" is a function of
temperature. Thus, we cool the CCD detector to less than
30°C. Operating at this temperature, the CCD detector
saturates in about 15 min, hence, exposures of up to 1 min
are not greatly influenced by thermal background. At room
temperature, the CCD saturates in less than a second.

The camera can be operated in either the extended
exposure mode, described above, or at the normal TV rate.

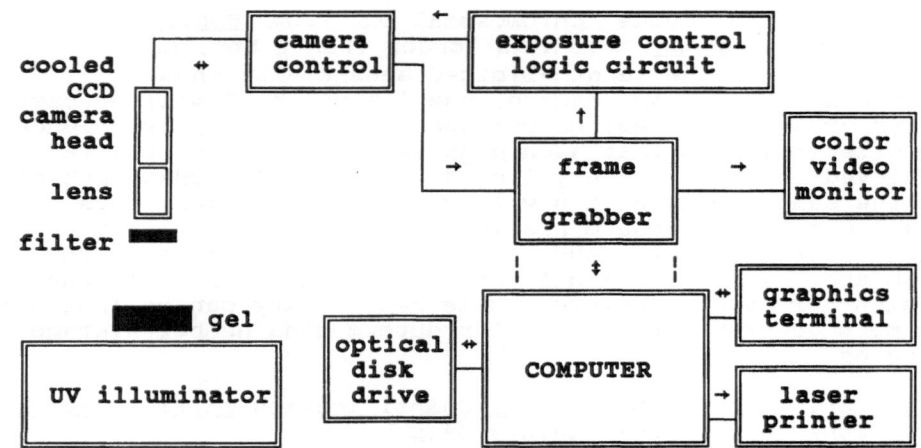

Fig. 5. Schematic diagram of the electronic imaging system
described by Sutherland et al. (1987a). The gel is
placed upon a UV illuminator constructed to provide
uniform illumination of the entire gel. Ethidium
bromide fluorescence is detected by an electronic
camera with a charge-coupler device, CCD, detector.
The signal from the camera is digitized by a "frame-
grabber" which is installed in a computer. In order
to record weak fluorescence from gels, the camera and
frame-grabber were modified and a control logic
circuit was added to permit exposures longer than the
0.33 msec. of a conventional TV camera. In addition,
the camera sense head, which contains the CCD, is
cooled to less than 30°C, to permit exposures that
can last up to one minute without excessive "dark
current" that otherwise would saturate the image.
The image recorded by the camera is displayed, either
in black and white or in pseudocolor, on a monitor
attached to the frame-grabber. The system is
controlled and the images of gel fluorescence
analyzed from a graphics monitor connected to the
computer. The camera can also be run at normal video
rates and the "real time" image stream displayed on
the color monitor to facilitate the focusing of the
lens system and the proper alignment of gels. The
arrows indicate the direction of flow of control
signals and data between the several components.

In both modes, the analog voltage signal from the camera is
digitized by the frame-grabber and displayed on a color
monitor. The ability to operate at the standard TV rate is
extremely useful in aligning the gel (using visible light)
prior to recording the image of ethidium fluorescence.
However, the rapid rate of digitization limits the
photometric resolution of the system to 256 intensity levels
(8 bits). Images can be displayed either in black and white
or the different intensity levels can be color coded to aid
in distinguishing smaller variations in intensity and in
alerting the operator to camera saturation. Pseudocolor
images from the gel imaging system have been published

elsewhere (Sutherland et al., 1987a; Chen and Sutherland, 1989). Digital images are archived on an optical disk. The operator controls the camera system and analyzes data extracted from images from a graphics terminal. Images of gels suitable for storing in laboratory notebooks are produced either with a video printer (not shown in Fig. 5) or on a laser printer, which is also used for plotting data extracted from digital images (Fig. 4 is an example) and printing reports of analyzed data. In addition to the above improvements is accuracy resulting from a linear response to incident light, the electronic imaging system greatly reduces the time required to analyze a gel and hence increases laboratory productivity. In addition, more complicated types of data analysis, e. g. background subtraction based on interpolation between areas between lanes that do not contain DNA and summing over the width of the lane at each position, are possible on a routine basis.

Second generation electronic imaging system. We have constructed another imaging system based on a slow readout or "scientific" CCD camera. These cameras offer several improvements in performance compared to systems based on TV type CCD cameras. The slower readout rate permits digitization to 12 or 14 bits (4096 and 16384 intensity levels, respectively). They are designed to operate at lower temperatures, and hence permit longer exposure times. Finally, some of these cameras can be equipped with CCDs containing many more individual detectors or "pixels" compared to TV type CCD cameras, but at a steeply higher price. The TV based imaging system, however, has the edge in ease of operation, since it can be operated at the normal video rate of 30 frames/sec. This feature, which is not available with a scientific CCD based system, is convenient for focusing the cameras lens and aligning gels. Sutherland (1990) discussed the properties and merits of both types of CCD systems plus laser scanners in which a light beam is swept over the surface of the gel and the resulting fluorescence is recorded with a photomultiplier.

APPLICATIONS

The gel method can be used to detect and quantify any lesion or class of lesions in DNA that either is a single- or double-strand break or which can be converted to a single- or double-strand break, either chemically or enzymatically. The theory of analysis of the data are basically similar for the various types of lesions. The important experimental differences are in the type of gel, native for double-strand breaks and denaturing, typically alkaline, for single-strand breaks, and also in the agent used, if necessary, to convert the lesion into a break.

Pyrimidine Dimers

Pyrimidine dimers are, by far, the most extensively studied UV-induced lesion in DNA and also the lesion to which the gel method has been most often applied. In just over a decade since the first qualitative (Woodhead et al. , 1978) and quantitative (Sutherland et al., 1980) observations, the method has evolved rapidly in sophistication and has been applied to problems ranging from demonstrating the harmful effects of the artificial lights used in "sun tanning parlors" (Freeman et al., 1987) to the prediction of increases in UV-induced skin cancers resulting from depletion of stratospheric ozone (Freeman et al., 1989). We forsee numerous future applications of the method, particularly in studies of the repair of dimers in UV-irradiated human skin (Sutherland et al., 1980; Freeman, 1988).

Other DNA lesions

Chen and Sutherland (1989) used the gel method to quantify the frequency of gamma-ray induced single- and double-strand breaks in DNA irradiated in situ. The potential exists for increasing the sensitivity of the method, especially for the biologically more important double-strand breaks, so that accurate measurements can be made for biologically relevant doses for DNA irradiated in vivo. This improvement in sensitivity would be based on the analysis of longer DNA molecules, since the length limited sensitivity of the gel method is inversely proportional to the number average length of the population of **unnicked** molecules. Alternating-field direction gel electrophoresis can separate molecules 100 times longer than those used by Chen and Sutherland (1989), but, as noted above, it has not yet been possible to get all of the molecules from an irradiated organism to enter the gel.

Most endonucleases involved in DNA repair, in contrast to the dimer specific enzymes from M. luteus and phage T4, form single-strand breaks near a spectrum of lesions, not just one type. They can, therefore, be used to monitor the formation and repair of all lesions in the class. Experiments of this sort have been reported using assays based on centrifugal separations and radionuclide labeled DNA, but could also be pursued in men and other organisms that are difficult to label using the gel method.

ACKNOWLEDGMENTS

Research supported by the Office of Health and Environmental Research, U.S.D.O.E, and by grants from the NIH (GM-40936 to JCS and CA-23096 to BMS).

REFERENCES

Achey, P. M., Woodhead, A. D. and Setlow, R. B., 1979, Photoreactivation of pyrimidine dimers from thyroid cells of the teleost, Poecilia formosa, Photochem. Photobiol., 29:305-310.
Bancroft, I. and Wolk, C. P., 1988, Pulsed homogeneous field gel electrophoresis (PHOGE), Nucleic Acids Res., 16:7405-7418.
Carle, G. F., Frank, M. and Olson, M. V., 1986, Electrophoretic separations of large DNA molecules by periodic inversion of the electric field, Science, 232:65-68.
Carrier, W. L. and Setlow, R. B., 1970. Endonuclease from Micrococcus luteus which has activity towards ultraviolet irradiated deoxyribonucleic acid:

purification and properties, <u>J. Bact.</u>, 102:178-186.

Chen C-Z. and Sutherland. J. C., 1989, Gel electrophoresis method for quantitation of gamma ray induced single- and double-stranded breaks in DNA in vitro, <u>Electrophoresis</u>, 10:316-326.

Chu, G., Vollrath, D. and Davis, R. W., 1986, Separation of large DNA molecules by contour-clamped homogeneous electric fields, <u>Science,</u> 234:1582-1585.

Clark, S. M., Lai, E., Birren, B. W. and Hood, L., 1988, A novel instrument for separating large DNA molecules with pulsed homogeneous electric fields, <u>Science</u>, 241:1203-1205.

Deutsch, J. M., 1987, Dynamics of pulsed-field electrophoresis, <u>Physical Review Letters</u>, 59:1255-1258.

Deutsch, J. M., 1988, Theoretical studies of DNA during gel electrophoresis, <u>Science</u>, 240:922-924.

Ditchburn, R. W., 1965, <u>Light</u>, vols 1, John Wiley, New York.

Freeman, S. E., Blackett, A. D., Monteleone, D. C., Setlow, R. B., Sutherland, B. M., and Sutherland, J. C., 1986, Quantitation of radiation-, chemical- or enzyme-induced single strand breaks in nonradioactive DNA by alkaline gel electrophoresis: application to pyrimidine dimers, <u>Analyt. Biochem.</u>, 158:119-129.

Freeman, S. E., Sutherland, J. C., Sutherland, B. M., Gange, R. W., and Matzinger, E. A., 1987, Production of pyrimidine dimers in DNA of human skin exposed in situ to UVA radiation, <u>J. Invest. Dermatol.</u>, 88:430-433.

Freeman, S. E., 1988, Variations in excision repair of UVB-induced pyrimidine dimers in DNA of human skin In Situ, <u>J. Invest. Dermatol.</u>, 90:814-817.

Freeman, S. E., Hacham, H., Gange, R. W., Maytum, D., Sutherland, J. C., and Sutherland, B. M., 1989, Wavelength dependence of pyrimidine dimer formation in DNA of human skin irradiated in situ, <u>Proc. Nat. Acad. Sci. U.S.</u>, 86:5605-5609.

Gardiner, K., Laas, W., Patterson, D., 1986, Fractionation of large mammalian DNA restriction fragments using vertical pulsed-field gradient gel electrophoresis, <u>Somatic Cell and Molecular Genetics</u>, 12:185-195.

Lerman, L. S. and Frisch, H. L., 1982, Why does the electrophoretic mobility of DNA vary with the length of the molecule?, <u>Biopolymers</u>, 21:995-997.

Lett, J. T., 1981, Measurement of single-strand breaks by sedimentation in alkaline sucrose gradients, <u>In</u>, "DNA Repair, A Laboratory Manual of Research Procedures 1, part B", E. C. Friedberg, and P. C. Hanawalt, eds., Marcel Dekker, Inc. New York.

Lumpkin, O. J. and Zimm, B. H., 1982, Mobility of DNA in gel electrophoresis, <u>Biopolymers</u>, 21:2315-2316.

McDonnell, M. W., Simon, M. N. and Studier, F. W., 1977, Analysis of restriction fragments of T7 DNA and determination of molecular weights by electrophoresis in neutral and alkaline gels, <u>J. Mol. Biol.</u>, 110:119-146.

Prunell, A., Strauss, F. and Leblanc, B., 1977, Photographic quantitation of DNA in gel electrophoresis, <u>Analyt. Biochem.</u>, 78:57-65.

Prunell, A., 1980,. A Photographic method to quantitate DNA in gel electrophoresis, <u>Methods in Enzymology</u>, 65:353-358.

Pulleyblank, D. E., Shure, M. and Vinograd, J., 1977, The quantitation of fluorescence by photography, <u>Nucleic Acids Res.</u>, 4:1409-1418.

Ribeiro, E., Larcom, L. L. and Miller, D. P., 1989, Quantitative fluorescence of DNA intercalated ethidium bromide of agarose gels, Analyt. Biochem., **181**:197-208.

Schaffer, H. E. and Sederoff, R. R., 1981, Improved estimation of DNA fragment lengths from agarose gels, Analyt. Biochem., 115:113-122.

Schwartz, D. C. and Cantor, C. R., 1984, Separation of yeast chromosome-sized DNAs by pulsed field gradient gel electrophoresis, Cell, 37:67-75.

Seawell, P. C., Friedberg, E. C., Ganesan, A. K., and Hanawalt, P. C., 1981, Purification of endonuclease V of bacteriophage T4. in, "DNA Repair, A Laboratory Manual of Research Procedures 1, part B". E. C. Friedberg and P. C. Hanawalt, eds, Marcel Dekker, Inc. New York.

Serwer, P., 1987, Gel electrophoresis with discontinuous rotation of the gel: an alternative to gel electrophoresis with changing direction of the electric field, Electrophoresis, 8:301-304.

Southern, E. M., 1979, Measurement of DNA length by gel electrophoresis, Analyt. Biochem., 100:319-323.

Southern, E. M., Anand, R., Brown, W. R. A., and Fletcher, D. S., 1987, A model for the separation of Large DNA molecules by crossed field Electrophoresis, Nucleic Acids Res., 15:5925-5943.

Sutherland, B. M., Harbor, L. C. and Kochevar, I. E., 1980, Pyrimidine dimer formation and repair in human skin, Cancer Res., 40:3181-3185.

Sutherland, B. M. and Shih, A. G., 1983, Quantitation of pyrimidine dimer content of nonradioactive deoxyribonucleic acid by electrophoresis in alkaline agarose gels, Biochem., 22:745-749.

Sutherland, J. C., Monteleone, D. C., Trunk, J. and Ciarrocchi, G., 1984, Two dimensional, computer-controlled film scanner: quantitation of fluorescence from ethidium bromide-stained DNA gels, Analyt. Biochem., 139:390-399.

Sutherland, J. C., Lin, B.; Monteleone, D. C., Mugavero, J., Sutherland, B. M., and Trunk, J. 1987a, Electronic imaging system for direct and rapid quantitation of fluorescence from electrophoretic gels: application to ethidium bromide-Stained DNA, Analyt. Biochem., 163:446-457.

Sutherland, J. C., Monteleone, D. C., Mugavero, J. H., and Trunk, J., 1987b, Undirectional pulsed-field electrophoresis of single- and double-stranded DNA in agarose gels: analytical expressions relating mobility and molecular length and their application in the measurement of strand breaks, Analyt. Biochem., 162:511-520.

Sutherland, J. C., Bergman, A. M., Chen, C-Z., Monteleone, D. C., Trunk, J., and Sutherland, B. M., 1988, Measurement of DNA damage using gel electrophoresis and electronic imaging, in: "Electrophoresis '88", C. Schafer-Nielsen, ed., VCH Verlagsgesellschaft, Weinheim.

Sutherland, J. C., 1990, Electronic imaging systems for quantitative electrophoresis of DNA. in: "Non-invasive Techniques in Biology and Medicine", San Francisco Press. (in the press).

Veatch, W. and Okada, S., 1969, Radiation induced breaks in cultured mammalian cells, Biophys. J., 9:330-346.

Woodhead, A. D., Achey, P., Setlow, R. B. and Grist, E.,
   1978, Photoenzymatic repair of ultraviolet-irradiated
   DNA in the cells of a shark, _Prionace glauca_, _Comp._
   Biochem. Physiol., 60B,205-208.
Woodhead, A. D. and Achey, P., 1979, Photoreactivating enzyme
   in the blind cave fish, _Anoptichthys jordani_, _Comp._
   Biochem. Physiol., 63B:73-76.
Woodhead, A. D. and Achey, P., 1981, Photoreactivating enzyme
   activity in the rat tapeworm, _Hymenolepis diminuta_, _J._
   Parasitol., 67:386-371.

FLUORESCENCE DETECTION OF LESIONS IN DNA

Ainsley Weston[1], Elise D. Bowman[1], David K. Manchester[2] and
Curtis C. Harris[1,3]

[1]Laboratory of Human Carcinogenesis, Division of Cancer
Etiology, National Cancer Institute, NIH, Bethesda, MD
20892

[2]Department of Pediatrics, The Children's Hospital,
Denver, CO 80218

[3]To whom correspondence should be addressed

INTRODUCTION

Polycyclic aromatic compounds are commonly encountered environmental contaminants (Anonymous, 1972). Many of these chemicals present
hazards to humans through diet, occupation and life-style (World Health
Organization, 1973; 1983). Metabolism and activation of chemicals that
reach target-organs lead to the formation of carcinogen-DNA adducts,
which are recognized as human cancer risk factors (Doll and Peto, 1981).

During the last ten years a variety of sensitive methods have been
developed to measure carcinogen-DNA adducts for human cancer risk
assessment. These include enzyme immunoassays (Hsu et al., 1980; Poirier
et al., 1980; Harris et al., 1982; Santella et al., 1988; Perera et al.,
1989), ^{32}P-nucleotide postlabeling (Randerath et al., 1981; 1986; 1989;
Gupta et al., 1982; Foiles et al., 1989), electrochemical detection
(Floyd et al., 1986a; 1986b), gas chromatography/mass spectrometry
(Manchester et al., 1988; Weston et al., 1989a) and fluorescence spectroscopy (Herron and Shank, 1980; Shugart et al., 1983; Vahakangas et
al., 1988; Jankowiak et al., 1988). Each of these methods has its own
advantages and disadvantages and corroborative end-point analyses are of
considerable value (Weston et al., 1987a; Harris et al., 1987a). This
report deals primarily with synchronous fluorescence spectroscopy as a
means to measure potentially carcinogenic lesions in human DNA and gas
chromatography/mass spectroscopy as a means of corroborative analysis.
With special reference to fluorescence assays, three techniques are
currently being developed: fluorescence line narrowing spectroscopy
(Jankowiak et al., 1988), synchronous fluorescence spectroscopy
(Vo-Dinh, 1982; 1985) and fixed wavelength fluorescence detection
combined with high performance liquid chromatography (Herron and Shank,
1980). These latter two methods have proved useful in measuring
carcinogen-DNA adducts in humans, whereas the sensitivity of fluorescence line narrowing spectroscopy requires improvement before it can
effectively be applied to analysis of human samples. Herron and Shenk

DNA Damage and Repair in Human Tissues
Edited by B. M. Sutherland and A. D. Woodhead
Plenum Press, New York, 1990

63

(1980) showed that methylation of DNA could be detected in human liver following dimethylnitrosamine poisoning using fixed wavelength fluorescence detection and high performance liquid chromatography. Levels of O^6-methylguanine up to 1 adduct in 5 x 10^3 unmodified nucleotides were found, whereas levels of N^7-methylguanine adducts were more than 5 times higher (1 adduct in 10^3 unmodified nucleotides. Harris et al., (1985), Haugen et al., (1986), Manchester et al., (1988) and Weston et al., (1989a) have used synchronous fluorescence spectroscopy to obtain evidence of polycyclic aromatic hydrocarbon-DNA adducts in human tissues. Levels of polycyclic aromatic hydrocarbon-DNA adducts ranged between 1 in 10^7 to 1 in 10^6 depending on tissue type (peripheral blood lymphocytes or placenta) and exposure (occupational or non-occupational).

In order to obtain sufficient materials for chemically specific analyses of carcinogen-DNA adducts in humans, large quantities of DNA are often required. These DNA samples are then subjected to microchemical preparative techniques, since the overall sensitivity of any method is directly related to the total amount of DNA that can be introduced into a particular assay system. In pursuit of this goal, antibodies were elicited in rabbits against DNA that had been modified with benzo[a]pyrene-diol epoxide (Poirier et al., 1980; Santella et al., 1988). These antibodies have been shown to recognize a range of related polycyclic aromatic hydrocarbon-DNA adducts (Weston et al., 1987b), and have been immobilized on a Sepharose support matrix. They are being used to concentrate polycyclic aromatic hydrocarbon-DNA adducts prior to separation by high performance liquid chromatography and chemical analysis. In the experiments reported here a number of chemically specific methods have been used to identify and measure benzo[a]pyrene-diol epoxide-DNA adducts in human tissues.

MATERIALS AND METHODS

Chemicals

Racemic (±)-r-7,t-8-dihydroxy-t-9,10-epoxy-7,8,9,10-tetrahydro[1,3-^{3}H]benzo[a]pyrene was obtained from the National Cancer Institute Chemical Carcinogen Reference Standard Repository (Bethesda, MD 20892). Non-labeled authentic r-7,t-8,t-9,c-10-tetrahydrobenzo[a]pyrene (benzo[a]pyrene-7,10/8,9-tetrahydrotetrol; for nomenclature of tetrols and related compounds see Yang et al., 1978) and r-7,t-8,t-9-trihydroxy-7,8,9,10-tetrahydrobenzo[a]pyrene (benzo[a]pyrene-7/8,9-tetrahydrotriol) were also obtained from this source. Antibody isolation columns (IgM/IgG Quik-Step) were obtained from Isolab (Akron, OH 44321), and cyanogen bromide-activated Sepharose 4B was from Pharmacia (Piscataway, NJ 08854). Calf thymus DNA was obtained from Sigma (Sigma Chemical Co., St. Louis, MO 63178) and was repurified before use by phenol extraction and ethanol precipitation. Redistilled phenol was purchased from Bethesda Research Laboratories (Gaithersberg, MD 20877). Tri-Sil/bovine serum albumin in silylation grade pyridine was obtained from Pierce (Rockford, IL 61105). Isoamyl alcohol (analytical grade) was procured from Mallinckrodt (Paris, KY 40361). Tetrahydrofuran was obtained from Aldrich (Milwaukee, WI 53233). Water and methanol (both high performance liquid chromatography grade) were obtained from Baker (Phillipsburg, NJ 08865). Trimethylchlorasilane and hexamethyldisalazane were obtained from Aldrich, and pyridine (analytical grade) was obtained from FSA Laboratory Supplies (Loughbrough, UK).

BPDE-Modified DNA

Preparation of benzo[a]pyrene-diol epoxide-DNA was performed by using calf thymus DNA and tritium labeled diol epoxide as described previously by Tierney et al., (1977) and Pulkrabek et al., (1979). Briefly, benzo[a]pyrene-diol epoxide was dissolved in tetrahydrofuran (1 mg/ml), and the solution was made up to 5 ml with ethanol. The diol epoxide solution was mixed with 10 ml of a DNA solution (1 mg/ml in Tris 10mM buffer at pH 7.4). The mixture was incubated at room temperature overnight and was extracted the next day with an equal volume of water-saturated diethyl ether (eight times) and water-saturated isoamyl alcohol (four times) to remove unreacted polycyclic aromatic hydrocarbon residues. The DNA was precipitated by the addition of sodium chloride (100 mM) and ethanol (2.5 vol). The precipitated DNA was then washed in 70% ethanol and redissolved in water. The adduct level was determined to be 1.3% (36 pmol of hydrocarbon per μg of DNA) by UV absorption spectroscopy (ϵ_{347} = 29 x 10^3) and liquid scintillation counting.

Human Lymphocyte DNA

Lymphocytes were isolated by gradient centrifugation from 50 ml aliquots of heparinized whole human peripheral blood samples from coke-oven workers as previously described (Harris et al., 1985). DNA was extracted from the peripheral blood lymphocytes as follows: cells were treated with lysis buffer (0.6% SDS; 20 mM EDTA; Tris-HCl 10 mM pH 7.5 and RNase A 100 μg/ml Sigma) for 60 min, Proteinase K was added and the mixture was incubated for a further 2 hr. The lysate was extracted with phenol, phenol:chloroform (1:1) and chloroform and DNA was precipitated with ethanol. DNA recoveries were determined by measurement of the absorbance of the solutions at 260 nm, the samples were purified to an absorbance ratio (260nm/280 nm) of >1.7.

Human Placental DNA

Placentas from term, uncomplicated pregnancies were collected at delivery at University Hospital, Denver. Maternal histories and blood samples were obtained on the first postpartum day. Smoking histories included use of tobacco and marijuana. Active smoking was defined as daily use of cigarettes. Women who smoked less often or who quit smoking during pregnancy were excluded from the study. Placental nuclei were prepared by using the technique described by Resendez-Perez et al., (1984). For each placenta studied, fractions containing syncitial nucleii (NFIV, Resendez-Perez et al., 1984) were prepared from ≈40 g of freshly obtained placental villous tissue. Nuclear fractions were treated with RNase A (100 μg/ml) in buffer containing sodium dodecyl sulfate (SDS 0.6%), EDTA (10 mM), and Tris·HCl (10 mM; pH 7.5) at 37°C for 60 min. Proteinase K (Sigma) was added (100 μg/ml), and the mixture was incubated for an additional 20 min. The digest was extracted with equal volumes of phenol, phenol/chloroform (1:1), and chloroform; DNA was precipitated by the addition of 2.5 volumes of ethanol in the presence of NaCl (100 mM).

Immunoaffinity Chromatography

Immunoaffinity columns were prepared as a batch from rabbit polyclonal anti-benzo[a]pyrene-diol epoxide-DNA antibodies as described by Tierney et al., (1986). One column was used for calibration with radiolabeled benzo[a]pyrene-diol epoxide-DNA and the others were reserved for use with human placental DNA exclusively to avoid potential contamination with standard materials. DNA samples were digested with DNase I under the conditions described by Tierney et al., (1986). Up to

2 mg of digested DNA was applied to a single column at one time. Each placental DNA sample was added in 2 ml (1 void volume) and the columns washed with phosphate-buffered saline (KH_2PO_4, 1.7mM; Na_2HPO_4, 5mM; NaCl, 150mM; pH 7.4). The retained oligonucleotides were then eluted with 10 void volumes of NaOH (50 mM). It was necessary to repeat this cycle five times for each DNA sample (2 mg) loaded in order to recover all of the DNA that was applied. Columns were washed extensively with phosphate-buffered saline between applications of DNA to achieve neutral pH. Column eluates were collected in 2 ml fractions, and DNA contents were determined spectrophotometrically (A_{260}), and approximately 3% of the DNA applied was eluted with NaOH. DNA fragments bound by the antibodies (i.e., eluted with NaOH) were pooled, adjusted to pH 1.5 with HCl, hydrolyzed (90°C for 3 hr), and subjected to organic solvent extraction prior to chemical analyses as described below.

Hydrolysis to Tetrahydrotetrols

Previous experience with synchronous fluorescence spectroscopy in biological samples suggests the presence in human DNA of complex mixtures of fluorophores (Harris et al., 1985; Weston et al., 1987b). To resolve benzo[a]pyrene-derived signals from these mixtures, putative diol epoxide-DNA adducts were acid hydrolyzed to the corresponding tetrahydrotetrols, extracted with isoamyl alcohol, dried in vacuo, re-dissolved in water, and subjected to high performance liquid chromato-graphy as previously described (Weston et al., 1989a). Briefly, DNA from individual placentas was acidified by addition of HCl to a final concentration of 100 mM or in the case of immunoaffinity concentrated fractions to pH 1.5 and heated at 90°C for 3 hr. Each sample was then extracted three times with equal volumes of isoamyl alcohol. The organic phases were then washed with an equal volume of water and evaporated to dryness under reduced pressure, and the residues were dissolved in 600 μl of water. Under these conditions, recovery of radioactivity from a tritium labeled standard was found to be >99% (Weston et al., 1989a).

High Performance Liquid Chromatography

Reverse-phase high performance liquid chromatography was conducted at room temperature with Vydac C18 columns (25 cm x 4.6 mm). Samples were eluted with linear methanol/water gradients (30-60% over 10 min, followed by 60-100% over 5 min) at a flow rate of 1 ml/min. Eluates were collected in 0.5 ml fractions. Labeled benzo[a]pyrene-tetrahydrotetrol that was extracted from hydrolyzed tritium labeled benzo[a]pyrene-diol epoxide modified DNA eluted in a major peak at 14.5-15.0 min with a final recovery of 60% of the radioactivity.

Second Derivative Synchronous Fluorescence Spectroscopy

Synchronous fluorescence spectroscopy is described in detail elsewhere (Vo-Dinh, 1982; Vahakangas et al., 1985) and has previously been used as an assay for benzo[a]pyrene-diol epoxide-DNA adducts in cells and tissues from humans exposed to polycyclic aromatic hydrocarbons. More detailed analysis of the specific fluorescence spectral characteristics of polycyclic aromatic hydrocarbon residues that were isolated from human DNA was obtained upon generation of second deriva-tive synchronous fluorescence spectra (Weston et al., 1989b). The Savitsky-Golay algorithm (Savitzky and Golay, 1964) was used to convert spectral data acquired by driving the excitation emission monochromators of a fluorescence spectrophotometer (Perkin Elmer Corp., Rockville, MD 20850) simultaneously with a fixed-wavelength difference of 34 nm.

Gas Chromatography/Mass Spectroscopy

Placental DNA extracts that had been subjected to fluorescence analysis either with or without immunoaffinity chromatography were analyzed by gas chromatography/mass spectroscopy under the following conditions: samples were converted to trimethylsilyl derivatives by treatment with timethylchlorosilane/hexamethyldisilazane/pyridine, 1:3:9 (v/v, 60°C for 30 min) and analyzed by selected ion monitoring for the presence of the molecular ion m/z 608$^+$ and a base peak m/z 404$^+$. Split-less injection was used to introduce materials onto the column (OV-1, 25 m x 0.25 mm), which was eluted with a temperature gradient of 70°C - 290°C (30°C/min). Ions were detected by using a Vacuum Generators (VG) analytical 70-SEQ GC/MS instrument in the electron-ionization mode. Alternately, samples were evaporated under nitrogen, and a known volume of methanol was added. An aliquot of benzo[a]pyrene-7/8,9-triol (final concentration of 100 pg/μl) was added as an internal standard, and the samples were silylated in a total volume of 100 μl of Tri-sil/bovine serum albumin (2.5 milliequivalents per ml) for 2 hr in a sand bath at 100°C. The treated samples were evaporated under nitrogen and redis-solved in 20 μl of bistrifluoracetamide/toluene, 1:10 (v/v). Portions of these samples (2 μl) were isothermally chromatographed on a 30 m DB-1 capillary column (J & W Scientific, Folsom, CA) at 280°C by using helium as carrier. The column effluent was directed into the source of a VG MM-16 low-resolution mass spectrometer. Ions were formed by using a 20 eV (1 eV = 1.602 x 10^{-19}J) electron ionizer and characteristic germinal-diol fragment ions were detected with a VG 2000 system in the selected ion monitoring mode.

RESULTS

The spectra shown in Fig. 1 were generated by synchronous fluorescence spectroscopy. These spectra were determined by driving the excitation and emission monochromators of the fluorimeter with a fixed

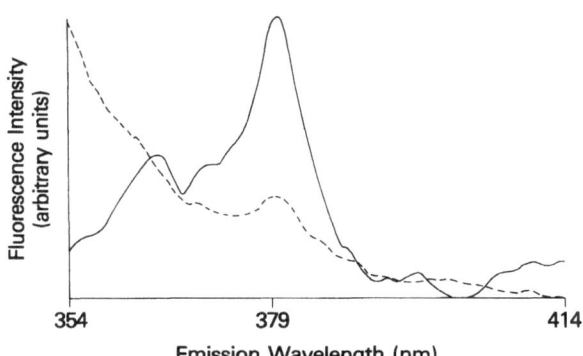

Figure 1. Synchronous fluorescence spectra of high perfomance liquid chromatography eluates of acid hydrolysates of DNA that had been modified with (±)-r-7,t-8-dihydroxy-t-9,10-epoxy-7,8,9,10-tetrahydro[1,3-^{3}H]benzo[a]pyrene. An original spectrum for 27 pg (90 fmol) of the tetrol (-----) and the same spectral data following subtraction of background light-scatter (———).

wavelength difference of 34 nm. These spectra were observed following high performance liquid chromatography of tritium-labeled benzo[a]pyrene-diol epoxide residues that were extracted, using an organic solvent (isoamyl alcohol), from mild acid hydrolysates of synthetically-modified calf-thymus DNA. High performance liquid chromatography and synchronous fluorescence spectroscopic analyses of the synthetically modified calf-thymus DNA were performed at the same time as identical analyses of non-radiolabeled human samples that were extracted from the peripheral blood lymphocytes of coke oven workers. The data shown in Fig. 1 indicate the presence of fluorescent materials that have the same chromatographic and spectral characteristics as benzo[a]pyrene-7,10/8,9-tetrahydrotetrol. The high performance liquid chromatography eluates were then analyzed by liquid scintillation counting. The data shown in Fig. 2 indicate that fluorescence emissions (synchronous spectral peak 379 nm, using a wavelength difference of 34 nm) and the presence of benzo[a]pyrene-residues as detected by the radiolabel were coincident. Since 150 fmol (45 pg) of tritium labeled benzo[a]pyrene-diol epoxide, bound to the calf thymus DNA, gave a yield of 90 fmol (27 pg) of benzo[a]pyrene-7,10/8,9-tetrahydrotetrol the efficiency of the extraction was determined, by liquid scintillation counting, to be 60%.

Samples of DNA that were extracted from the peripheral blood lymphocytes of 41 coke oven workers were hydrolysed with acid (0.1N HCl, 90°C, 3 hr) and then examined by synchronous fluorescence spectroscopy. Fluorescence signals were found in thirty-one of these samples (Harris et al., 1985), however, the majority of these fluorescence signals were broad and consistent with the presence of a mixture of fluorescent materials. Thirteen of the fluorescence positive samples were further analyzed by synchronous fluorescence spectroscopy following extraction with an organic solvent (isoamyl alcohol) and high performance liquid

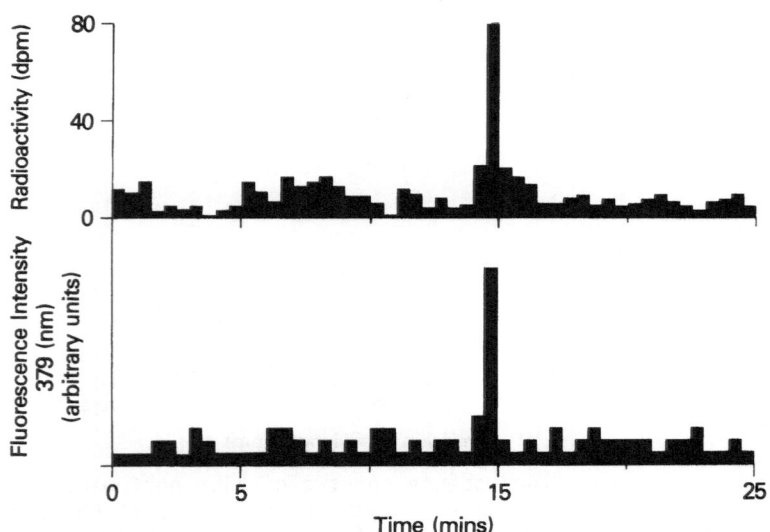

Figure 2. Liquid scintillation counting and synchronous fluorescence spectroscopy of high performance liquid chromatographs of radiolabeled benzo[a]pyrene-diol epoxide-DNA acid hydrolysates.

chromatography. The data show that specific synchronous fluorescence signals, indicating the presence of benzo[a]pyrene-diol epoxide residues were present in three samples (Fig. 3). These materials were confirmed by gas chromatography/mass spectroscopy in two cases. When benzo[a]pyrene-tetrahydrotetrol is treated with a mixture of trimethyl-chlorosilane, hexamethyldisilazane and pyridine in the ratio of 1:3:9 at 60°C for 30 minutes a molecular ion of 608^+ is formed. Following elution from the gas chromatograph, destruction of this ion in the mass spectrometer leads to the formation of a large fragment ion the base peak (m/z 404^+) and a geminal-diol (m/z 191^+). For two of the three DNA samples from coke-oven workers that contained fluorescent emissions that were specific for benzo[a]pyrene-diol epoxide adducts it was possible to detect the base-peak (m/z 404^+, Fig. 4a), but not the molecular ion (Fig. 4b). The inability to detect the molecular ion in these experiments is not entirely unexpected since this fraction constitutes only 2% of the materials that reach the detector in the mass spectrometer.

Quantitative comparison of the synchronous fluorescence spectra generated from radiolabeled samples and those produced from DNA samples obtained from coke-oven workers indicated that benzo[a]pyrene-diol epoxide-DNA adduct levels, in positive samples, ranged between 1 adduct in 5×10^7 - 5×10^6 unmodified nucleotides. These values correspond to as much as 1.5 fmol benzo[a]pyrene residues per microgram of DNA.

Samples of DNA (500 μg) from 28 human placentas were hydrolysed with acid (0.1N HCl, 90°C, 3 hr), extracted into isoamyl alcohol and analyzed by high performance liquid chromatography and synchronous fluorescence spectroscopy. Among these samples 10 were found to contain fluorescent materials that were indistinguishable from benzo[a]pyrene-7,10/8,9-tetrahydrotetrol. Smoking histories on all 28 mothers showed that 6 positive samples originated from current smokers, whereas 4 positive samples originated from non-smokers; the presence of benzo[a]pyrene-diol epoxide-DNA adducts in some of these samples was supported by the detection of putative chemical-DNA adducts by ^{32}P-nucleotide postlabeling (Table 1).

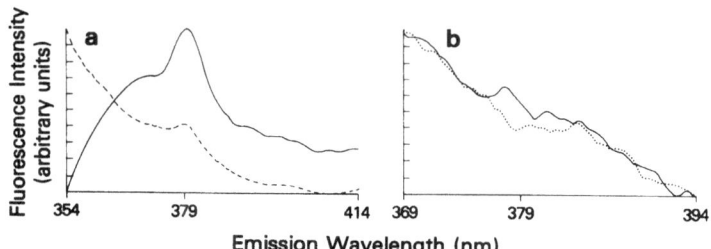

Figure 3. Synchronous fluorescence spectra of high performance liquid chromatography eluates of human DNA. a) An original positive spectrum (-----) and the same spectral data shown after subtraction of background light-scattering (———); b) two original spectra, one which is negative (.....) and one that has a small peak that could not be improved by subtraction of light-scatter (———).

Table 1. Detection of Polycyclic Aromatic Hydrocarbon-DNA
Adducts in Human Placenta by Synchronous Fluorescence Spectroscopy (SFS) and ^{32}P-Nucleotide Postlabeling (^{32}PNPL)

Sample Number	SFS	^{32}PNPL
Smokers		
1	+[a]	+
2	+	+
3	-	+
Non-Smokers		
4	-	-
5	+	+

[a] Symbols indicate whether a particular sample was considered
to be positive or negative; no attempt was made to
quantitate these adducts.

Further analysis of these placental DNA samples by high performance
liquid chromatography, second derivative synchronous fluorescence spectroscopy and gas chromatography/mass spectroscopy was undertaken in order
to corroborate these findings and seek evidence of other polycyclic
aromatic hydrocarbon-DNA adducts. Antibodies were elicited in rabbits
against DNA that had been modified at high level (28 pmol/μg) with
benzo[a]pyrene-diol epoxide. These antibodies were shown to recognize a
number of structurally related polycyclic aromatic hydrocarbon-DNA

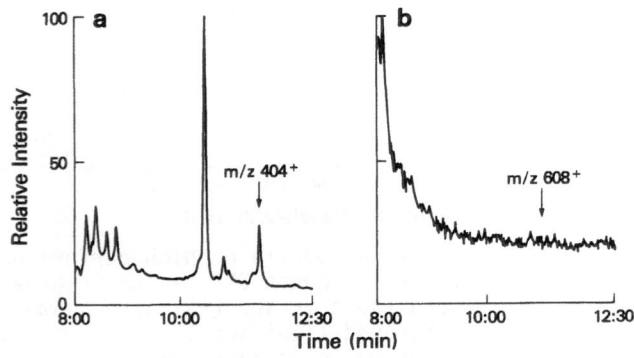

Figure 4. Gas chromatography traces of acid hydrolyzed human DNA
extracts produced using a VG analytical 70-SEQ instrument in
the single ion monitoring mode; a) m/z 404^{+} and b) 608^{+}

adducts (Santella et al., 1988), and were used in immunoaffinity chromatography experiments to concentrate adducts from large quantities of DNA, pooled from placental samples already known to be positive. Initially, DNase I partial hydrolysates of eight individual placental DNA samples (1 mg each) were applied to immunoaffinity chromatography columns. Materials that became specifically bound to the columns were eluted with sodium hydroxide (50 mM). Complete fluorescence excitation-emission matrices were generated in the synchronous spectral mode (Manchester et al., 1989); these spectra contained pyrene-like signatures as well as other highly complex information (data not shown). These observations are consistent with the data that define the broad specificity of the antiserum used to prepare the immunoaffinity chromatography columns, and suggest that the material concentrated by this procedure contains other as yet unidentified fluorescent adducts.

In order to concentrate larger amounts of DNA for further analyses, DNA (2-4 mg) was pooled from each of eight placental samples that were considered to be positive by synchronous fluorescence spectroscopy. This pool of DNA (30 mg) was divided, and half of it (15 mg) was digested with DNase I. The hydrolysate was applied to immunoaffinity chromatography columns and bound materials were eluted with sodium hydroxide (50 mM). Both the sample of adducts that had been concentrated by immunoaffinity chromatography and the remaining sample from the same placentas that had not were subjected to mild acid hydrolysis. The acid hydrolysates were then extracted into isoamyl alcohol, evaporated to dryness under reduced pressure and redissolved in water. These aqueous solutions of extracts of hydrolysed placental DNA were subjected to high performance liquid chromatography, typical chromatograms for each sample preparation are shown in Fig. 5. The high performance liquid chromatography eluates were monitored at wavelengths corresponding to absorbance peaks in the benzo[a]pyrene-7,10/8,9-tetrahydrotetrol ultraviolet spectrum (280 nm and 347 nm). These chromatograms suggest that the overall composition of each of the

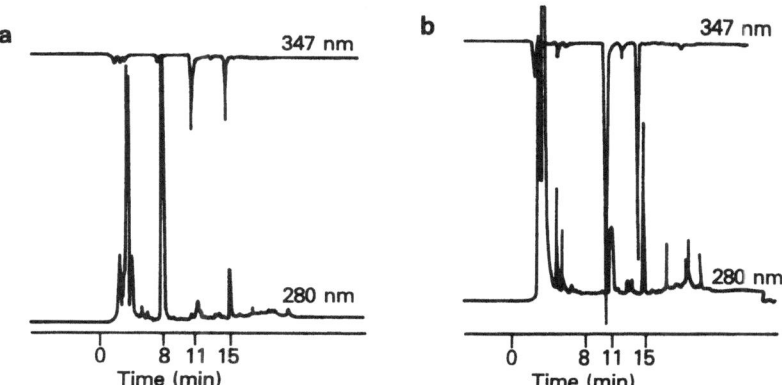

Figure 5. High performance liquid chromatograms monitored by ultraviolet light absorbance (280 nm and 347 nm) for extracts of acid hydrolysed human placental DNA (15 mg); a) without prior concentration by immunoaffinity chromatography and b) with prior concentration by immunoaffinity chromatography. Tracings for 280 nm and 347 nm are offset by 60 seconds.

mixtures of hydrolysis products is different. The retention time of
benzo[a]pyrene-7,10/8,9-tetrahydrotetrol was determined to be 14.5 -
15.0 minutes, and both Fig. 5a and 5b show the presence of ultraviolet
absorbing materials (280 nm and 347 nm) with this retention time. The
extracted mixture that was not concentrated by immunoaffinity chromatography also contained more polar components as evidenced by the peaks at
8 minutes and 11 minutes (Fig. 5a). It is also significant that the
component eluting at 8 minutes is absent from the mixture that was
extracted from the immunoaffinity chromatography concentrated DNA (Fig.
5b). This material may represent structurally unrelated adducts not
recognized by the anti-benzo[a]pyrene-diol epoxide-DNA antibodies.

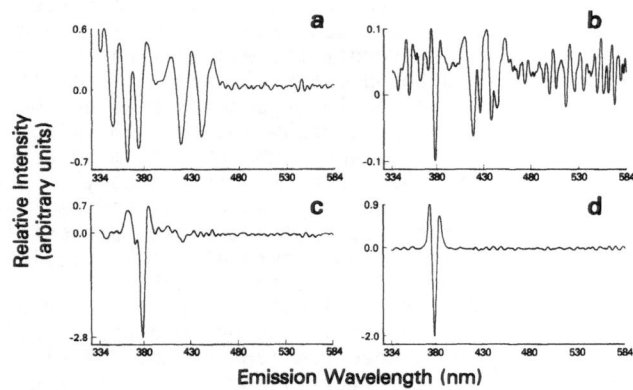

Figure 6. Second derivative synchronous fluorescence spectra (wavelength
difference 34 nm) generated for isoamyl alcohol extracts of
acid hydrolysed human placental DNA (15 mg): a) total
extractable materials, b) high performance liquid chromatography purified fractions of the total extractable materials
that had the same retention time as benzo[a]pyrene-7,10/8,9-
tetrahydrotetrol, c) total extractable material from adducts
that were concentrated by immunoaffinity chromatography using
antibodies directed against benzo[a]pyrene-diol epoxide-DNA
and d) material purified by immunoaffinity chromatography that
had the same retention time as benzo[a]pyrene-7,10/8,9-
tetrahydrotetrol when further purified by high performance
liquid chromatography.

    The preparation of these placental DNA extracts and the isolation
of benzo[a]pyrene-7,10/8,9-tetrahydrotetrol was also monitored by
synchronous fluorescence spectroscopy. These data were transformed
using the Savitsky-Golay algorithm (Savitzky and Golay, 1964) to the
second derivative because some studies have suggested the utility of
this approach for the resolution of components of complex mixtures.
Fig. 6a shows the second derivative synchronous fluorescence spectrum
(wavelength difference 34 nm) for the isoamyl alcohol extract of
hydrolysed human placental DNA. These data are indicative of the

presence in this sample of multiple fluorescent components. Comparison with the second derivative synchronous fluorescence spectrum that was generated for an authentic sample of benzo[a]pyrene-7,10/8,9-tetra-hydrotetrol (data not shown) indicated that this technique alone is not capable of allowing the resolution of components of this mixture, or to identify the presence of benzo[a]pyrene residues. A synchronous fluorescence signal at 374 nm was found in the complex spectrum (Fig. 6a), which is 5 nm from the signature signal (379 nm) for the benzo[a]pyrene-tetrahydrotetrol. It is possible that chemiluminescent interactions among multiple compounds in these potentially complex mixtures shift the benzo[a]pyrene-tetrahydrotetrol signal, but it is impossible without further experimentation to determine whether this in fact occurred. Even if it were possible to assign the origin of this or other fluorescent signals present in the spectrum to benzo[a]pyrene-7,10/8,9-tetrahydrotetrol, then the position of the signal in the spectrum and its relative magnitude may be variable depending on the composition of the mixture. Simplification of spectra can be achieved by further purification using high performance liquid chromatography. Fractions eluting from the chromatograph with the retention time expected for benzo[a]pyrene-7,10/8,9-tetrahydrotetrol were concentrated, dissolved in water and the resulting second-derivative synchronous fluorescence spectrum is shown in Fig. 6b. These data reveal the presence of a dominant peak at 379 nm, indicating the presence of the pyrene fluorophore. However, the spectrum remains complex indicating the continued presence of other unidentified materials.

Hydrolysates of DNA that had been concentrated by immunoaffinity chromatography were also analyzed by second-derivative synchronous fluorescence spectroscopy, and the results are shown in Fig. 6c. These data show a remarkable reduction in the level of spectral complexity that was achieved using anti-benzo[a]pyrene-diol epoxide-DNA antibodies to concentrate polycyclic aromatic hydrocarbon-DNA adducts. These apparently less prevalent chemiluminescence interactions are consistent with the decreased concentration in the immunochromatography purified fraction of more polar compounds detected by ultraviolet absorbance in the total extract (Fig. 5). However, the signature signal in this case is not perfect, and multiple minor peaks are present (340 nm, 370 nm, 385 nm and 425 nm). Since the antibodies used to prepare the immunoaffinity columns have been shown to possess broad specificity for related polycyclic aromatic hydrocarbon-diol epoxide-DNA adducts then this result is not unexpected. Fig. 6d shows the results of purifying hydrolysed immunoaffinity column eluates by high performance liquid chromatography. These data demonstrate a significant degree of purification since a single sharp signature signal is present, which was found to be indistinguishable from that generated from an authentic sample of benzo[a]pyrene-7,10/8,9-tetrahydrotetrol.

The same samples, for which second-derivative synchronous fluores-cence spectra are shown in Fig. 6b and 6d, were further analyzed by gas chromatography/mass spectroscopy. Selected ion monitoring was used to seek the molecular ion (m/z 608^+), the base peak (m/z 404^+) and a smaller fragment ion (m/z 191^+) of trimethylsilyl-derivatives in gas chromatography eluates of the placental samples. For each sample, clear signals for both the molecular ion and base peak were found with retention times that were identical to those for the trimethylsilyl-derivative of authentic benzo[a]pyrene-7,10/8,9-tetrahydrotetrol (data not shown). A smaller fragment ion of molecular weight 191^+, thought to be a geminal diol [$(CH_3)_3$-Si-O-CH$_2$-CH$_2$-O-Si-$(CH_3)_2$], was also sought. Benzo[a]pyrene-7/8,9-terahydrotriol was mixed with the samples prior to derivatization as an internal standard because its trimethylsilyl-derivative is easily resolved from that of the tetrol by gas chromatography and yields a small fragment ion of mass 191$^+$ (presumably a common geminal diol). The ratio of the tetrol to the triol was then used for quantitative analysis. Fig. 7 shows the results of these analyses, where Fig. 7a is an authentic chemical standard, Fig. 7b is an extract of human placenta shown to contain fragment ions (m/z 191$^+$) corresponding to the trimetylsilyl-derivative of benzo[a]pyrene-7,10/8,9-tetrahydrotetrol and Fig. 7c is a solvent control containing benzo[a]pyrene-7/8,9-tetrahydrotriol. The experimental points are plotted on the calibration curve as solid symbols (Fig. 7d). The results of quantitative analysis by gas chromatography/mass spectroscopy and those obtained by comparing zeroth order synchronous fluorescence spectra with a linear fluorescence calibration curve are given in Table 2. Data obtained using these two independent and chemically specific methods show levels of benzo[a]pyrene-adducts between 1 in 10^8 - 10^7 unmodified nucleotides to be present in the human syncitiotrophoblast DNA. The data show good agreement for the samples that were prepared by both immunoaffinity chromatography and high performance liquid chromatography, these samples were the most pure preparations by spectroscopic criteria. The samples that were purified by high performance liquid chromatography alone were in less good agreement. Substantial quenching is apparent in the high performance liquid chromatography purified fraction. Lack of quenching in the immunoaffinity concentrated sample suggests that quenching in the total extract results from interactions from contaminants and is not due to concentration dependent non-linear fluorescence.

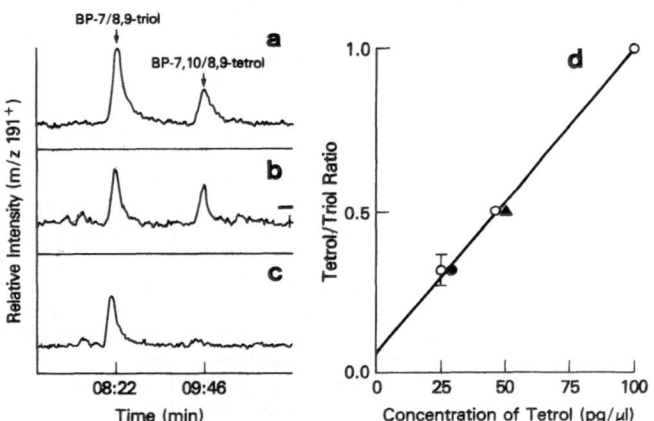

Figure 7. Gas chromatograph/mass spectroscopy analyses of the trimethylsilyl derivatives of extracts of acid hydrolysed human placental DNA samples. Eluates were monitored using a VG 2000 in the single ion mode (m/z 191$^+$), benzo[a]pyrene-7,10/8,9-terahydrotriol was added to each sample as an internal marker: a) a sample of authentic benzo[a]pyrene-7,10/8,9-tetrahydrotetrol, b) a placental DNA extract, c) solvent control and d) the calibration curve for authentic benzo[a]pyrene-7,10/8,9-tetrahydrotetrol, including experimental data points for high performance liquid chromatography purified placental extract (•) and immunoaffinity chromatography and high performance liquid chromatography purified extract (▲).

Table 2. Quantitative Analysis of Placental DNA Extracts by
Gas Chromatography/Mass Spectroscopy (GC/MS) and
Synchronous Fluorescence Spectroscopy (SFS)

Sample Preparation	SFS	GC/MS
HPLC	0.038[a]	0.140
IAC[b] and HPLC	0.253	0.206

[a] All values are expressed as fmol benzo[a]pyrene per microgram DNA
[b] Immunoaffinity chromatography

DISCUSSION

The data show that benzo[a]pyrene-DNA adducts are present in human tissues at levels of up to 1 adduct in 5×10^6 unmodified nucleotides. These data corroborate other methods that have reported the presence of aryl adducts in human tissues but which are less specific for these chemical-adducts (Perera et al., 1982; Poirier et al., 1985; Harris et al., 1985; Haugen et al., 1986; Everson et al., 1986; 1988; Phillips et al., 1988; Hemminki et al., 1988). The data also indirectly indicate that complex mixtures of hydrolyzable polycyclic aromatic hydrocarbon-DNA adducts are present in human DNA. The approach that has been taken here to the measurement of specific adducts has focused on isolation and purification of the chemical materials prior to their measurement. Low levels of carcinogen-DNA adducts in human DNA challenge the detection limits of conventional adduct assay systems, and complex mixtures of adducts that are present in human samples confound simple assay systems (Weston et al., 1987a). Fluorescence detection of lesions in human DNA following environmental exposure to chemical agents has previously been limited to the detection of high levels of methylation in cases of dimethylnitrosamine poisoning that were fatal (Herron and Shank, 1980). Methods that have previously been used to detect polycyclic aromatic hydrocarbon-DNA adducts in humans, which include ^{32}P-postlabeling and enzyme immunoassays, have either failed to detect benzo[a]pyrene-DNA adducts or lack chemical specificity for precise determination of adduct levels (Everson et al., 1986; 1988; Santella et al., 1988). Laser-based fluorescence spectroscopic methods provide powerful tools for the analysis of chemical carcinogens in the environment (Jeffrey et al., 1977; Jankowiak et al., 1988), however, these methods have not yet been used to measure carcinogen-DNA adducts in humans and they are still under development. Any method that is to be used for the precise measurement of specific chemical-DNA adducts in humans must technically address the problems of sensitivity and specificity. Synchronous fluorescence spectroscopy and mass spectroscopy, which are both inherently chemically specific techniques, have been used here to measure chromatographically purified benzo[a]pyrene-DNA adducts found in human tissues.

Analysis of human peripheral blood lymphocyte or placental DNA by simple acid hydrolysis and synchronous fluorescence spectroscopy generally showed non-specific spectra that were not easily interpreted. Separation of materials prior to synchronous fluorescence spectroscopic analysis provided for the elucidation of specific chemical identification that was corroborated by gas chromatography/mass spectroscopy. In the experiments reported here only the benzo[a]pyrene-7,10/8,9-tetrahydrotetrol was observed, which suggests that the major form of benzo[a]pyrene-diol epoxide metabolite that forms covalent adducts with DNA in human peripheral blood and placenta is the r-7,t-8-dihydroxy-t-9,10-epoxy-7,8,9,10-tetrahydrobenzo[a]pyrene (BPDE I) (Cooper et al., 1983). These data correspond to those generated in other biological systems that have been studied under experimental conditions and indicate involvement of cytochrome P450IA1 in humans (Conney, 1982). In rat-liver microsomal systems (Thakker et al., 1977) and in mouse skin (Phillips et al., 1978) the major stereochemical route of metabolic activation of benzo[a]pyrene leads to formation of r-7,t-8-dihydroxy-t-9,10-epoxy-7,8,9,10-tetrahydrobenzo[a]pyrene, this has also been shown to be true for a variety of human tissues treated with benzo[a]pyrene (Autrup et al., 1982; Autrup and Harris, 1983; Weston et al., 1983).

The qualitative mass and fluorescence spectroscopic analyses that are described in this report clearly demonstrate the presence of benzo[a]pyrene residues as chemical-DNA adducts in human DNA samples, and these data are consistent with enzyme immunoassay data (Perera et al., 1982; Harris et al., 1985; Santella et al., 1988) and other attempts to measure carcinogen-DNA adducts in humans (Phillips et al., 1988). However, quantitative analyses (Table 2) are not so clear. There is good correspondence between both fluorescence spectroscopy and gas chromatography on the most purified samples but a poorer correlation between more complex samples. Fluorescence spectroscopy detected only 27% of the material that was detected by mass spectroscopy in high performance liquid chromatography eluates of hydrolysed DNA. It is clear from the spectrum shown (Fig. 6b) that this preparation is a mixture, therefore loss of fluorescence signal specific for benzo[a]pyrene residues may be in part due to fluorophore interaction and fluorescence quenching. The increase in values that are observed when detection techniques are combined with immunoaffinity chromatography may be related to an increase in the efficiency of acid hydrolysis. In samples isolated by immunoaffinity chromatography a larger proportion of materials present will be adducted nucleotides.

The goals of our current studies are the further development, standardization and application of techniques for human cancer risk assessment. These studies fall into three broad categories: Methods for the identification and measurement of carcinogen-macromolecular adducts in humans (Hsu et al., 1980; Poirier et al., 1980; Manchester et al., 1988; Vahakangas et al., 1988; Weston et al., 1989a; 1989b), measurement of other forms of internal human exposure to carcinogens (Harris, 1987b) and determination of the contribution of genetic polymorphisms of xenobiotic metabolism to DNA damage (Ayesh et al., 1984; Law et al., 1989). The application of these complementary techniques within the framework of well designed cancer case-control studies should add to the understanding and prevention of human chemical carcinogenesis.

ACKNOWLEDGMENTS

We are indebted to P.V. Fennessey of the Department of Chemistry, University of Colorado, Denver, CO 80218 and P.B. Farmer of the Toxicology Laboratories, M.R.C. Unit, Carsharlton, Surrey SM5, U.K. for providing gas chromatography/mass spectroscopy analyses. We also acknowledge the skillful technical assistance of N.B. Parker. Our thanks to R.A. Julia for skillful editorial assistance.

REFERENCES

Anonymous, 1972, Particulate polycyclic organic matter: biological effects of atmospheric pollutants, Proc.Natl.Acad.Sci.USA.,

Autrup, H., Grafstrom, R. C., Brugh, M., Lechner, J. F., Haugen, A., Trump, B. F., and Harris, C. C., 1982, Comparison of benzo(a)pyrene metabolism in bronchus, esophagus, colon, and duodenum from the same individual, Cancer Res., 42:934.

Autrup, H., and Harris, C. C., 1983, Metabolism of chemical carcinogens by cultured human tissues, in: "Human Carcinogenesis," C. C. Harris, and H. Autrup, eds., Academic Press, New York.

Ayesh, R., Idle, J. R., Ritchie, J. C., Crothers, M. J., and Hetzel, M. R., 1984, Metabolic oxidation phenotypes as markers for susceptibility to lung cancer, Nature, 312:169.

Conney, A. H., 1982, Induction of microsomal enzymes by foreign chemicals and carcinogenesis by polycyclic aromatic hydrocarbons: G. H. A Clowes Memorial Lecture, Cancer Res., 42:4875.

Cooper, C. S., Grover, P. L., and Sims, P., 1983, The metabolism and activation of benzo[a]pyrene, in: "Progress in Drug Metabolism," J. W. Bridges, and L. Chasseaud, eds., Wiley and Sons, Ltd., England.

Doll, R., and Peto, R., 1981, "The Causes of Cancer," Oxford Press, New York.

Everson, R. B., Randerath, E., Santella, R. M., Cefalo, R. C., Avitts, T. A., and Randerath, K., 1986, Detection of smoking-related covalent DNA adducts in human placenta, Science, 231:54.

Everson, R. B., Randerath, E., Santella, R. M., Avitts, T. A., Weinstein, I. B., and Randerath, K., 1988, Quantitative associations between DNA damage in human placenta and maternal smoking and birth weight, JNCI, 80:567.

Floyd, R. A., Watson, J. J., Wong, P. K., Altmiller, D. H., and Rickard, R. C., 1986a, Hydroxyl free radical adduct of deoxyguanosine: sensitive detection and mechanisms of formation, Free Radical Res. Commun., 1:163.

Floyd, R. A., Watson, J. J., Harris, J., West, M., and Wong, P. K., 1986b, Formation of 8-hydroxydeoxyguanosine, hydroxyl free radical adduct of DNA in granulocytes exposed to the tumor promoter, tetradecanoylphorbolacetate, Biochem.Biophys.Res.Commun., 137:841.

Foiles, P. G., Miglietta, L. M., Quart, A. M., Quart, E., Kabat, G. C., and Hecht, S. S., 1989, Evaluation of 32P-postlabeling analysis of DNA from exfoliated oral mucosa cells as a means of monitoring exposure of the oral cavity to genotoxic agents, Carcinogenesis, 10:1429.

Gupta, R. C., Reddy, M. V., and Randerath, K., 1982, 32P-postlabeling analysis of non-radioactive aromatic carcinogen--DNA adducts, Carcinogenesis, 3:1081.

Harris, C. C., Yolken, R. H., and Hsu, I. C., 1982, Enzyme immunoassays: Applications in cancer research, in: "Methods in Cancer Research," H. Busch, and L. C. Yeoman, eds., Academic Press, New York.

Harris, C. C., Vahakangas, K., Newman, M. J., Trivers, G. E.,
    Shamsuddin, A. K. M., Sinopoli, N. T., Mann, D. L., and Wright, W.
    E., 1985, Detection of benzo[a]pyrene diol epoxide-DNA adducts in
    peripheral blood lymphocytes and antibodies to the adducts in serum
    from coke oven workers, Proc.Natl.Acad.Sci.USA, 82:6672.

Harris, C. C., Weston, A., Willey, J. C., Trivers, G. E., and Mann, D.
    L., 1987a, Biochemical and molecular epidemiology of human cancer:
    indicators of carcinogen exposure, DNA damage, and genetic
    predisposition, Environ.Health Perspect., 75:109.

Harris, C. C., 1987b, Biochemical and molecular effects of N-nitroso
    compounds in human cultured cells: an overview, in: "9th
    International Meeting on N-Nitroso Compounds," H. Bartsch, ed.,
    IARC, Lyon.

Haugen, A., Becher, G., Benestad, C., Vahakangas, K., Trivers, G. E.,
    Newman, M. J., and Harris, C. C., 1986, Determination of polycyclic
    aromatic hydrocarbons in the urine, benzo(a)pyrene diol epoxide-DNA
    adducts in lymphocyte DNA, and antibodies to the adducts in sera
    from coke oven workers exposed to measured amounts of polycyclic
    aromatic hydrocarbons in the work atmosphere, Cancer Res., 46:4178.

Hemminki, K., Perera, F. P., Phillips, D. H., Randerath, K., Reddy, M.
    V., and Santella, R. M., 1988, Aromatic DNA adducts in white blood
    cells of foundry workers, in: "Methods for Detecting DNA Damaging
    Agents in Humans: Applications in Cancer Epidemiology and
    Prevention," H. Bartsch, K. Hemminki, and I. K. O'Neill, eds.,
    IARC, Lyon.

Herron, D. C., and Shank, R. C., 1980, Methylated purines in human liver
    DNA after probable dimethylnitrosamine poisoning, Cancer Res.,
    40:3116.

Hsu, I. C., Poirier, M. C., Yuspa, S. H., Yolken, R. H., and Harris, C.
    C., 1980, Ultrasensitive enzymatic radioimmunoassay (USERIA)
    detects femtomoles of acetylaminofluorene-DNA adducts,
    Carcinogenesis, 1:455.

Jankowiak, R., Cooper, R. S., Zamzow, D., Small, G. J., Doskocil, G.,
    and Jeffrey, A. M., 1988, Fluorescence
    line-narrowing-nonphotochemical hole burning spectrometry:
    femtomole detection and high selectivity for intact DNA-PAH
    adducts, Chem.Res.Toxicol., 1:60.

Jeffrey, A. M., Weinstein, I. B., Jennette, K. W., Grzeskowiak, K.,
    Nakanishi, K., Harvey, R. G., Autrup, H., and Harris, C. C., 1977,
    Structures of benzo(a)pyrene--nucleic acid adducts formed in human
    and bovine bronchial explants, Nature, 269:348.

Law, M. R., Hetzel, M. R., and Idle, J. R., 1989, Debrisoquine
    metabolism and genetic predisposition to lung cancer, Br.J.Cancer,
    59:686.

Manchester, D. K., Weston, A., Choi, J. S., Trivers, G. E., Fennessey,
    P., Quintana, E., Farmer, P. B., Mann, D. L., and Harris, C. C.,
    1988, Detection of benzo[a]pyrene diol epoxide-DNA adducts in human
    placenta, Proc.Natl.Acad.Sci.USA., 85:9243.

Manchester, D. K., Wilson, V. L., Weston, A., Choi, J. S., Hsu, I. C., Parker, N. B., Mann, D. L., and Harris, C. C., 1989, Polycyclic aromatic hydrocarbon-DNA adducts detected in human placenta, Carcinogenesis. In press.

Perera, F., Mayer, J., Jaretzki, A., Hearne, S., Brenner, D., Young, T. L., Fischman, H. K., Grimes, M., Grantham, S., and Tang, M. X., 1989, Comparison of DNA adducts and sister chromatid exchange in lung cancer cases and controls, Cancer Res., 49:4446.

Perera, F. P., Poirier, M. C., Yuspa, S. H., Nakayama, J., Jaretzki, A., Curnen, M. M., Knowles, D. M., and Weinstein, I. B., 1982, A pilot project in molecular cancer epidemiology: determination of benzo[a]pyrene--DNA adducts in animal and human tissues by immunoassays, Carcinogenesis, 3:1405.

Phillips, D. H., Grover, P. L., and Sims, P., 1978, The covalent binding of polycyclic hydrocarbons to DNA in the skin of mice of different strains, Int.J.Cancer, 22:487.

Phillips, D. H., Hewer, A., Martin, C. N., Garner, R. C., and King, M. M., 1988, Correlation of DNA adduct levels in human lung with cigarette smoking, Nature, 336:790.

Poirier, M. C., Santella, R. M., Weinstein, I. B., Grunberger, D., and Yuspa, S. H., 1980, Quantitation of benzo(a)pyrene-deoxyguanosine adducts by radioimmunoassay, Cancer Res., 40:412.

Poirier, M. C., Reed, E., Zwelling, L. A., Ozols, R. F., Litterst, C. L., and Yuspa, S. H., 1985, Polyclonal antibodies to quantitate cis-diamminedichloroplatinum(II)--DNA adducts in cancer patients and animal models, Environ.Health Perspect., 62:89.

Pulkrabek, P., Leffler, S., Grunberger, D., and Weinstein, I. B., 1979, Modification of deoxyribonucleic acid by a diol epoxide of benzo[a]pyrene. Relation to deoxyribonucleic acid structure and conformation and effects on transfectional activity, Biochemistry, 18:5128.

Randerath, E., Avitts, T. A., Reddy, M. V., Miller, R. H., Everson, R. B., and Randerath, K., 1986, Comparative 32P-analysis of cigarette smoke-induced DNA damage in human tissues and mouse skin, Cancer Res., 46:5869.

Randerath, K., Reddy, M. V., and Gupta, R. C., 1981, 32P-labeling test for DNA damage, Proc.Natl.Acad.Sci.USA., 78:6126.

Randerath, K., Randerath, E., Danna, T. F., van Golen, L., and Putman, K. L., 1989, A new sensitive 32P-postlabeling assay based on the specific enzymatic conversion of bulky DNA lesions to radiolabeled dinucleotides and nucleoside 5'-monophosphates, Carcinogenesis, 10:1231.

Resendez-Perez, D., Barrera-Saldana, H. A., Morales-Vallerta, M. R., Ramirez-Bon, E., Leal-Garza, C. H., Feria-Velazco, A., and Sanchez-Anzaldo, F. J., 1984, Low-speed purification of human placental nuclei, Placenta, 5:523.

Santella, R. M., Weston, A., Perera, F. P., Trivers, G. E., Harris, C. C., Young, T. L., Nguyen, D., Lee, B. M., and Poirier, M. C., 1988, Interlaboratory comparison of antisera and immunoassays for benzo[a]pyrene-diol-epoxide-I modified DNA, Carcinogenesis, 9:1265.

Savitzky, A., and Golay, M. J. E., 1964, Smoothing and differentiation of data by simplified least squares procedures, Anal.Chem., 36:1627.

Shugart, L., Holland, J. M., and Rahn, R. O., 1983, Dosimetry of PAH skin carcinogenesis: covalent binding of benzo[a]pyrene to mouse epidermal DNA, Carcinogenesis, 4:195.

Thakker, D. R., Yagi, H., Akagi, H., Koreeda, M., Lu, A. H., Levin, W., Wood, A. W., Conney, A. H., and Jerina, D. M., 1977, Metabolism of benzo[a]pyrene. VI. Stereoselective metabolism of benzo[a]pyrene and benzo[a]pyrene 7,8-dihydrodiol to diol epoxides, Chem.Biol.Interact., 16:281.

Tierney, B., Hewer, A. J., Walsh, C., Grover, P. L., and Sims, P., 1977, The metabolic activation of 7-methylbenz(a)anthracene in mouse skin, Chem.Biol.Interact., 18:179.

Tierney, B., Benson, A., and Garner, R. C., 1986, Immunoaffinity chromatography of carcinogen-DNA adducts with polyclonal antibodies directed against benzo[a]pyrene diol epoxide-DNA, JNCI, 77:261.

Vahakangas, K., Haugen, A., and Harris, C. C., 1985, An applied synchronous fluorescence spectrophotometric assay to study benzo[a]pyrene-diolepoxide-DNA adducts, Carcinogenesis, 6:1109.

Vahakangas, K., Pelkonen, O., and Harris, C. C., 1988, Synchronous fluorescence spectrophotometry of benzo[a]pyrene diol epoxide-DNA adducts: a tool for detection of in-vitro and in-vivo DNA damage by exposure to benzo[a]pyrene, in: "Methods for Detecting DNA Damaging Agents in Humans: Applications in Cancer Epidemiology and Prevention," H. Bartsch, K. Hemminki, and I. K. O'Neill, eds., IARC, Lyon.

Vo-Dinh, T., 1982, Synchronous luminescence spectroscopy: methodology and applicability, Appl.Spectroscopy, 36:576.

Vo-Dinh, T., 1985, Development of a dosimeter for personal exposure to vapours of polyaromatic pollutants, Environ.Sci.Technol., 19:997.

Weston, A., Grover, P. L., and Sims, P., 1983, Metabolic activation of benzo[a]pyrene in human skin maintained in short-term organ culture, Chem.Biol.Interact., 45:359.

Weston, A., Newman, M. J., Vahakangas, K., Rowe, M. L., Trivers, G. E., Mann, D. L., and Harris, C. C., 1987a, Measurement of carcinogen-macromolecular adducts and serum antibodies recognizing DNA adducts in biological specimens from people exposed to chemical carcinogens, in: "Short-Term Bioassays in the Analysis of Complex Environmental Mixtures V," S. S. Sandhu, D. M. DeMarini, M. J. Mass, M. M. Moore, and J. L. Mumford, eds., Plenum Press, New York.

Weston, A., Trivers, G. E., Vahakangas, K., Newman, M. J., Rowe, M. L., Mann, D. L., and Harris, C. C., 1987b, Detection of carcinogen-DNA adducts in human cells and antibodies to these adducts in human sera, in: "Progress in Experimental Tumor Research," F. Homburger, ed., S. Karger, Basel.

Weston, A., Rowe, M. L., Manchester, D. K., Farmer, P. B., Mann, D. L., and Harris, C. C., 1989a, Fluorescence and mass spectral evidence for the formation of benzo[a]pyrene anti-diol-epoxide-DNA and -hemoglobin adducts in humans, Carcinogenesis, 10:251.

Weston, A., Manchester, D. K., Poirier, M. C., Choi, J. S., Trivers, G. E., Mann, D. L., and Harris, C. C., 1989b, Derivative fluorescence spectral analysis of polycyclic aromatic hydrocarbon-DNA adducts in human placenta, Chem.Res.Toxicol., 2:104.

World Health Organization, 1973, "IARC Monographs on the Evaluation of Carcinogenic Risk of the Chemical to Man: Certain Polycyclic Aromatic Hydrocarbons and Heterocyclic Compounds. Vol. 3," IARC, Lyon.

World Health Organization, 1983, "IARC Monographs on the Evaluation of the Carcinogenic Risk of Chemicals to Humans: Polynuclear Aromatic Compounds, Part 1, Chemical, Environmental and Experimental Data. Vol. 32," IARC, Lyon.

Yang, S. K., Deutsch, J., and Gelboin, H. V., 1978, Benzo[a]pyrene metabolism: activation and detoxification, in: "Polycyclic Hydrocarbons and Cancer," H. V. Gelboin, and S. K. Yang, eds., Acad. Press, New York.

SOLAR RADIATION INDUCED SKIN CANCER AND DNA PHOTOPRODUCTS IN HUMANS

Paul T. Strickland, Benjamin C. Vitasa, Magnus Bruze,
Edward A. Emmett, Sheila West, and Hugh R. Taylor

The Johns Hopkins Medical Institutions
615 N. Wolfe Street
Baltimore, Maryland 21205

INTRODUCTION

Solar radiation is a ubiquitous environmental carcinogen and the major
cause of skin cancer in caucasians (Scotto et al., 1981; Urbach, 1984).
Experimental studies indicate that the ultraviolet-B (UV-B, 290-320 nm)
portion of the solar spectrum is primarily responsible for the carcinogenic
properties of sunlight (Forbes et al., 1989). This waveband encompasses the
short-wavelength end of the solar spectrum that reaches the earth's surface.

A recent study of non-melanoma skin cancer in Maryland watermen
examined personal UV-B exposure-prevalence and age-prevalence relationships
(Strickland, et al., 1989). Prevalence of squamous cell carcinoma (SCC),
was strongly correlated with average annual UV-B exposure, while prevalence
of basal cell carcinoma (BCC) or actinic keratosis (AK) was poorly
correlated. In addition, two small groups of apparently hypersusceptible
individuals were identified in the population. Preliminary studies of solar
UV damage in DNA (Bruze et al., 1989) have examined cyclobuta-dithymidine
(T<>T) photoproduct induction and persistence in skin of (non-watermen)
volunteers exposed to simulated solar UV radiation.

SKIN CANCER IN MARYLAND WATERMEN

We have completed a cross-sectional prevalence study of skin cancer
among 843 licensed watermen aged 30 years and older who live and work on
the lower Eastern Shore of Maryland (Somerset and lower Dorchester
counties). The study was designed to examine the relationship between solar
UV exposure and a number of skin (Vitasa et al., 1987) and eye conditions
(Taylor et al., 1988). Watermen were contacted through the Maryland
Department of Natural Resources, which is the state licensing authority.

Watermen are primarily involved in traditional fishing tasks that are
regulated by state laws which have undergone few changes this century.
Therefore, an accurate estimate of cumulative lifetime UV-B exposure could
be constructed for each individual (Rosenthal et al., 1988). The exposure
estimate was based on data from three sources: i) field measurements of
daily ambient UV-B radiation in the geographical region collected by
stationary monitors, ii) field measurements of individual UV-B exposure
under working conditions using polysulphone personal dosimeters, and iii)
personal history of occupation and outdoor activities (Rosenthal et al.,

DNA Damage and Repair in Human Tissues
Edited by B. M. Sutherland and A. D. Woodhead
Plenum Press, New York, 1990

1988; Berger and Urbach, 1982). Annual ambient UV-B radiation measurements from Robertson-Berger meters at various locations in the United States are correlated with latitude, altitude and sky cover (Scotto et al., 1976). This information was used to estimate the annual UV-B radiation for two towns in the study area in collaboration with Hugh Pitcher of the U.S. Environmental Protection Agency. The average annual ambient UV-B radiation for Cambridge, MD (38.6°N,76.1°W) was 1.13×10^6 J/m^2 and for Crisfield, MD (38.0°N,75.9°W) was 1.15×10^6 J/m^2 in the R-B meter response range. These values are equivalent to approximately 3260 MED/year (assuming 350 J/m^2 per MED). For comparison, direct measurements in two locations with similar latitudes, Philadelphia, PA (40.0°N) and Oakland, CA (37.7°N), yielded annual ambient UV-B values of 2441 and 3426 MED/year, respectively (Berger and Urbach, 1982). The average annual UV-B exposure to facial skin was calculated for each individual as the mean of all yearly exposures from age 15 to the year of interview. Personal average annual exposures to facial skin ranged from approximately 1 to 8% of ambient UV-B radiation, equivalent to 33 to 260 MED per year. See Taylor et al. (1988) for details of identification, recruitment, and demographics of the study population. Each waterman (n=808) was examined for skin neoplasms, and a history of previous skin neoplasms was obtained. Clinical diagnoses of SCC and BCC were confirmed by histopathologic examination of biopsy material when available; diagnoses of previously removed lesions were verified from original pathology reports in all cases (Vitasa et al., 1988).

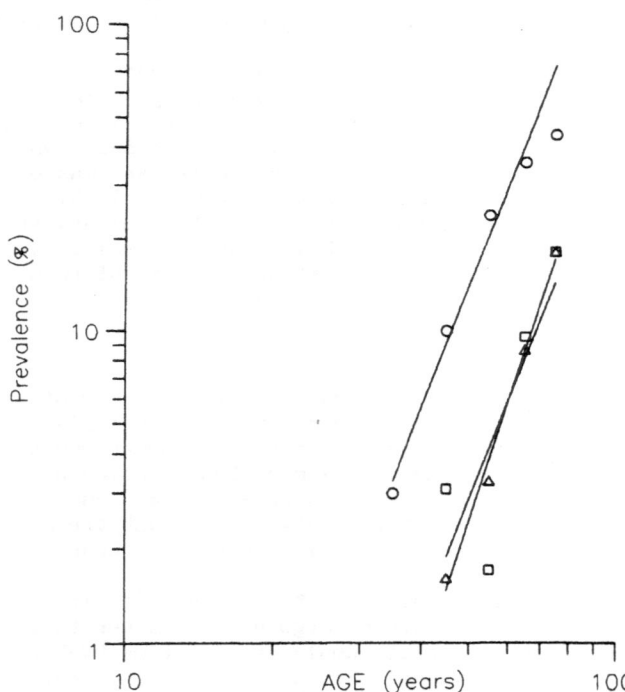

Fig. 1. Age dependence of skin neoplasm prevalence. Age-specific prevalence of skin neoplasms was deterimined for each decade of life from age 30 (30-39, 40-49, etc.). Simple power functions of the form y=mx^b were fitted by regression analysis to describe the relationship between age and prevalence of AK (0), SCC (Δ), or BCC (□).

Among the Caucasian watermen population (n = 808), 35 individuals had a total of 47 SCCs, 33 individuals had 60 BCCs and 202 individuals had 344 AKs. Cumulative UV-B exposure was positively correlated with age (r=0.7, p<.001) and more than 80% of the watermen had received at least 3300 minimal erythema doses (MED's) of cumulative UV-B radiation on exposed facial skin.

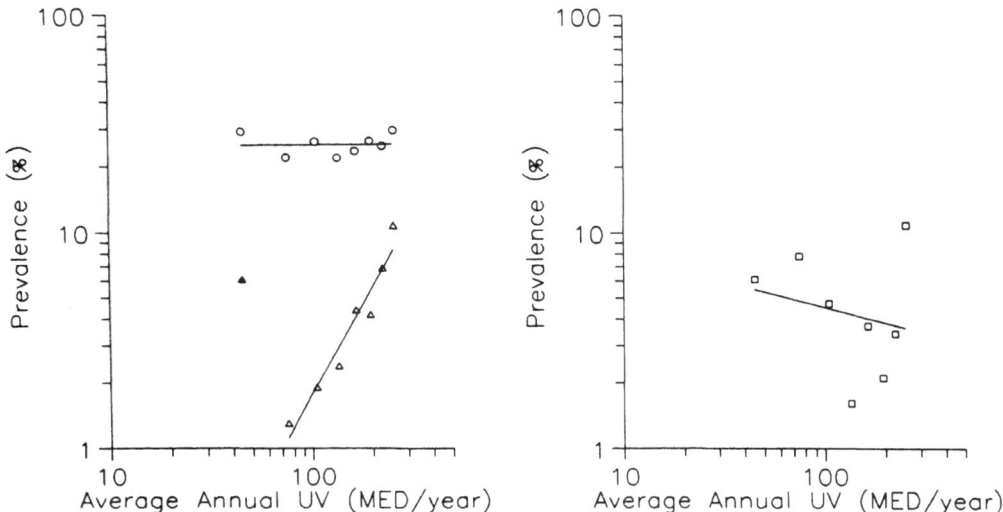

Fig. 2   Relationship of skin neoplasm prevalence to individual average annual UV-B exposure. The personal annual exposure to UV-B of each subject was determined by combining field measurements of UV-B under working conditions and published ambient UV-B data from stationary monitors with personal exposure histories obtained in interviews (Rosenthal et al., 1988). Prevalence of skin neoplasms was determined for 30 MED intervals of average annual exposure (<60, 61-90, 91-120, 121-150, etc.). Simple power functions were fitted by regression analysis to describe the relationship between average annual UV-B exposure and prevalence of AK (O), SCC (△), or BCC (□). The lowest exposure point for SCC (▲) was not included in the regression analysis and may represent hypersusceptible individuals (see text).

Previous studies (Fears and Scotto, 1983; Slaper et al., 1986) have demonstrated that simple power functions can be used to describe the relation between skin cancer incidence and terrestrial UV-B radiation. We have used this approach to relate prevalences of skin lesions to age (A) and average annual exposure (E) by a power function of the form:

$$\text{Prevalence} \backsim E^a \ A^b$$

Since A and E are independent of each other, their associations with prevalence were analyzed separately (Figs. 1 and 2). The values for the exponent b of age were 4.9 (SCC), 4.0 (BCC) and 4.1 (AK) as shown in Fig. 1. Prevalences of SCC and AK were also associated with cumulative lifetime exposure; this association is confounded by age since cumulative UV-B exposure is strongly age-dependent. When the average annual UV-B exposure was used as an age-independent measure of exposure, prevalence of SCC, but not BCC or AK, was clearly associated with UV-B exposure (Fig. 2). The values for the exponent a of average annual exposure were 1.7 (SCC), -0.2 (BCC) and 0.005 (AK). The lowest exposure point for SCC (4 cases) was excluded for the estimation of a. A similar association is observed when logarithmic or exponential functions are used to model the data (not shown).

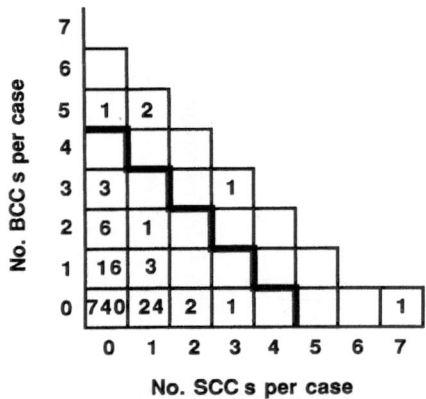

Fig. 3. Distribution of SCC and BCC among individuals. Number of study individuals with indicated numbers of SCC and BCC is tabulated in each cell. Cells above bold stepped line have 5 or more total SCC's and BCC's. In order to determine if the lesions were randomly distributed among the population, the expected distribution of lesions was calculated assuming a Poison distribution. Normal deviations of observed numbers of lesions (O) from expected numbers of lesions (E) were estimated by $(O-E)^2/E = Z^2$. Cases with 3 or more lesions per case would not be expected (p <.001) if the lesions were randomly distributed.

Interestingly, four cases of SCC occurred in the group of 64 individuals with very low average annual exposures ($\leq$60 MED/year) indicated in Fig. 2. The records of these four cases were reviewed in detail. None of the phenotypic characteristics (such as inability to tan, freckling, eye or hair color) which are believed to be related to individual skin cancer risk (Urbach, 1984) were consistently found in these cases. However, all 4 individuals had multiple AK (between 5 and 11 each) and, in addition, one individual had 5 BCC and 1 SCC. In the total Caucasian study population (n=808), 25% of participants had at least one AK, but only 4.3% had 5 or more. Thus, multiple AK in all four of these cases would not have been expected by chance (p<0.001). This finding suggests that the four cases may represent a hypersusceptible subgroup that is sensitive to lower doses of solar UV-B.

Multiple SCC and BCC were not uncommon and occurred in 19 of 68 total SCC and BCC cases (Fig. 3). Multiple BCC occurred more frequently (14 of 33 BCC cases) than multiple SCC (5 of 35 SCC cases) (X^2 = 5.36, p < 0.005). Both cancer types had more multiple lesion cases than would be expected by chance, assuming a Poisson distribution. Five individuals had 5 or more SCC and/or BCC (Fig. 3). The average annual and cumulative lifetime UV-B exposures of these five individuals (132 $\pm$ 64 MED/year; 6352 $\pm$ 3313 MED lifetime) were not statistically different from those of similarly aged individuals in the population (141 $\pm$ 59 MED/year; 6642 $\pm$ 2784 MED lifetime). These findings further support the concept of hypersusceptibility to skin cancer (in this case, multiple cancers) in subgroups of the study population, and are consistent with the frequent appearance of multiple lesion skin cancer cases in the general population (Teppo et al., 1985).

This study indicates that average annual UV-B exposure strongly influences the prevalence of SCC, but not AK or BCC, in a well-defined cohort with substantial solar exposure. While the study confirms a strong solar UV-B dependence of SCC, it does not refute the etiologic role of solar UV-B in BCC and AK. Evidence for such a role is quite convincing (Scotto et al., 1981; Urbach et al., 1981; Urbach, 1984), including anatomical distribution of BCC, protective effect of pigmentation, moderate latitude-dependence of BCC incidence, and high prevalence of BCC in DNA repair-deficient individuals. In addition, AK is weakly associated with cumulative UV-B exposure after adjustment for age and phenotypic characteristics (Vitasa et al., 1989). The absence of a detectable solar UV-B dose-dependence of BCC (and AK) in the present study suggests a dose saturation effect for these lesions at the relatively high doses of solar UV-B experienced by the study population. The prevalences of BCC and AK observed in the study population are considerably higher than those reported in the general population. Prevalence of AK in the general male population with "low to moderate sunlight exposure" is 5.6-9.6% (Engle et al., 1988), whereas the watermen population exhibited 25% (202/808) prevalence of AK. Similarly, prevalence of BCC in the general male population is 0.1-0.8% (Engle et al., 1988) compared to 4.1% (33/808) in the watermen. Thus, a saturation of the dose-prevalence relationship might not be observed in the U.S. population due to moderate exposure levels. Interestingly, in a recent study of skin cancer and actinic keratosis in Australia (Giles et al, 1988; Marks et al., 1988), BCC and SCC prevalence was not affected by latitude, whereas AK prevalence increased with decreasing latitude.

A saturation effect is further supported by the unusually high ratio of SCC:BCC of approximately 1:1 found in the study population (Strickland et al., 1989) compared to a ratio of 1:4 in the general population of the United States (Scotto et al., 1981). A similar increase in SCC:BCC ratio is observed in populations residing at lower latitudes which experience higher levels of ambient solar UV-B (Scotto et al., 1981; Fears and Scotto, 1983; Urbach, 1969). In this situation the increased ratio is due to a more rapid increase in numbers of SCC cases than BCC cases.

The biological reason for the saturation of BCC and AK prevalence at high doses is unclear. Also, the underlying mechanism of the apparently hypersusceptible subgroups has not been determined. In order to examine these findings in terms of mechanism, we have initiated studies directed at assessing UV-induced DNA damage and repair in human populations.

CYCLOBUTA-DITHYMIDINE INDUCTION IN HUMAN SKIN BY SOLAR-SIMULATING
UV RADIATION.

The interaction of UVB (290-320 nm) or UVA (320-400 nm) radiation with
epidermal DNA in human skin in situ has been demonstrated in previous
studies by the detection of cyclobuta-dipyrimidine photoproducts (Sutherland
et al., 1980; D'Ambrosio et al., 1981a; Freeman et al., 1987). In human
skin, repair of these lesions occurs either in the absence or presence
(D'Ambrosio et al., 1981b) of visible light. Solar radiation contains both
UVA and UVB radiation in a ratio of approximately 15:1 to 50:1 (UVA:UVB)
depending on a number of factors including atmospheric conditions, latitude,
altitude, time of day, time of year, etc. We have recently examined
cyclobuta-dithymidine (T<>T) photoproduct induction and repair in human skin
exposed in situ to environmental levels of sunlight (Bruze et al., 1989).
In order to accomplish this, we used a solar-simulating UV apparatus which
approximates both the spectrum and intensity of the UV portion of summer
midday sunlight at 39°N latitude (Strickland and Creasey, 1989).

Informed consent was obtained from 19 healthy volunteers between the
ages of 23 and 49. A brief interview was conducted with each volunteer to
ascertain sunburning and tanning characteristics. The solar-simulated light
source consisted of one UVB (Westinghouse, FS40) bulb and 2 UVA (Sylvania,
FR40T12 PUVA) bulbs filtered through 0.38 mm of cellulose triacetate

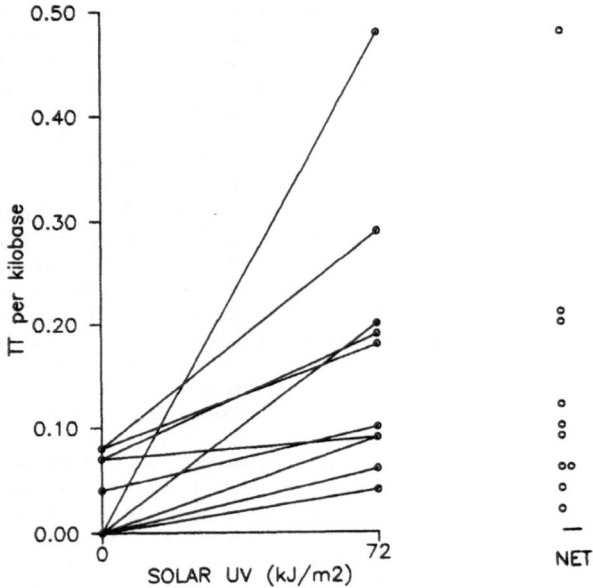

Fig. 4. T<>T photoproducts in skin of 10 individuals before and after
        exposure to 72 KJ/m² solar UV. DNA was extracted from epidermis of
        4 mm punch biopsies and T<>T content determined by ELISA as
        described in Materials and Methods. NET yields of T<>T are the
        difference between exposed (72 KJ/m²) yield and unexposed (0 J/m²)
        yield for each individual. Average variation between repeat assays
        was less than 25% of mean.

(Kodacel TA401) as previously described (Strickland and Creasey, 1989). The spectral output of this source closely approximates the spectrum and intensity of summer mid-day sunlight at 39°N latitude. The total UV fluence (290-400 nm) at the exposure site (10 cm from source) was 20 J/m^2/sec as measured by an Optronics 742 spectroradiometer (Optronics Lab, Orlando, FL). Untanned gluteal skin was exposed to solar UV in a pattern of five squares using a template. Four small squares (1.5 x 1.5 cm) received graded exposures of 15, 30, 45, or 60 minutes (18, 36, 54, 72 KJ/m^2) of solar UV for determination of minimal erythema dose (MED), and a fifth square (2.0 x 2.0 cm) received a single 60 minute exposure (72 KJ/m^2) for determination of T<>T photoproducts. The single exposure (72 KJ/m^2) is approximately equivalent to 60 minutes of midday summer sunlight at 39°N latitude.

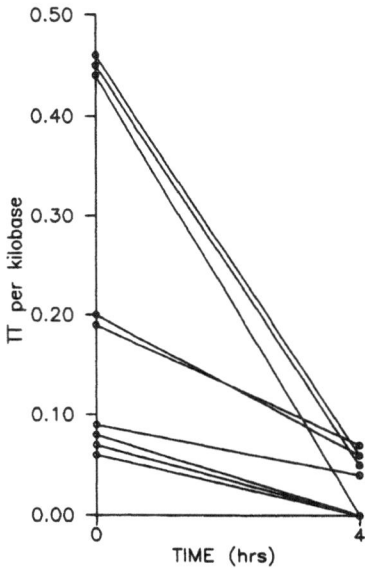

Fig. 5. T<>T photoproducts in skin of 9 individuals immediately or 4 hrs after exposure to 72 KJm/m^2 solar UV. Exposed skin was shielded from visible light during the 4 hr post-exposure period. Skin biopsy and ELISA procedures as in figure 4. Yields of T<>T immediately after exposure and not adjusted for background (unexposed) yields of T<>T as in figure 4.

Individual MEDs were determined 24 hrs. after exposure, as the minimum dose producing uniform erythema with clearly defined template margins. In ten individuals, skin biopsies were collected from exposed (72KJ/m^2) and unexposed skin immediately (<5 minutes) after irradiation for assessment of T<>T induction. In the remaining nine individuals, biopsies were collected from exposed (72 KJ/m^2) skin both immediately (<5 minutes) and 4 hours after irradiation for assessment of T<>T repair. During the 4 hour post-irradiation period, skin was covered by clothing, thereby preventing exposure to visible light. Punch biopsies (4 mm diameter) were taken after intradermal injection of 1% xylocaine with epinephrine, and immediately frozen at -135°C.

Table 1. Mean Yields of T<>T Photoproducts in
Individuals Exhibiting Different MEDs

T<>T per Kilobase[a]

MED[b] (KJ/m^2)	Unadjusted (n = 19)	Net (n = 10)	4 hr. residual (n = 9)	% Repair[d] (n = 9)
36	0.13 ± 0.06 (2)[c]	0.06 (1)	0.07 (1)	63 (1)
54	0.23 ± 0.16 (7)	0.16 ± 0.17 (5)	0.04 ± 0.03 (2)	84 ± 14 (2)
72	0.19 ± 0.14 (10)	0.13 ± 0.04 (4)	0.03 ± 0.02 (6)	82 ± 12 (6)

[a] All photoproduct measurements used DNA from skin irradiated with 72KJ/m^2 solar UV. Mean ± standard deviation (or range if n=2).

[b] Minimal erythema dose (solar UV)

[c] ( ) = number of individuals.

[d] % repair in 9 individuals tested.

The epidermis was removed from thawed skin biopsies and DNA was extracted as previously described (Bruze et al., 1989, Maniatis et al., 1982). Antibodies specific for T<>T photoproducts were used to assess photoproduct levels by enzyme-linked immunosorbent assay as previously described (Bruze et al., 1989; Strickland and Creasey, 1989).

Solar UV radiation (72 KJ/m^2) induced detectable amounts of T<>T in all individuals tested (Figures 4 and 5). In the first group (Figure 4), unexposed as well as exposed skin was assayed, and in 5 of 10 individuals some inhibition was detected by ELISA analysis of DNA from unexposed sites. This background level was subtracted from the unadjusted levels of T<>T (in exposed skin) to determine the net level of T<>T photoproduct induced in each case (Figure 4). Most of the samples (7 of 10) contained T<>T levels clustered between 0.02 and 0.12 T<>T per Kb. Three samples contained higher levels (0.20, 0.21, and 0.48 T<>T per Kb).

Repair of T<>T was examined in a second group of individuals (Figure 5). Unadjusted levels of T<>T ranged from 0.06 to 0.46 T<>T per Kb immediately after irradiation, and declined to between undetectable (≤0.01 T<>T per Kb) and 0.07 T<>T per Kb. Background levels of T<>T were unavailable from these individuals since the protocol was limited to two biopsies per person. Percentage loss of T<>T photoproducts at 4 hours ranged from 56 to 98% (80.2 ± 14.0%; mean ± SD). This rate of T<>T loss is equivalent to a half-time of about 100 min. and is comparable to previous measurements in human skin irradiated with UVB (Sutherland et al., 1980) or broad band UV (D'Ambrosio et al., 1981). These studies indicate that loss of cyclobuta-dipyrimidines occurs more rapidly in human skin cells in vivo than in cultured human keratinocytes or fibroblasts (Regan et al., 1978; Mellon et al., 1986; Keyse et al., 1987) which exhibit much slower repair kinetics. Thus repair rates measured in cultured cells may not accurately reflect absolute repair rates in vivo. Similar differences have recently been reported for repair rates of pyrimidine dimers in rat skin cells (Mullaart et al., 1988).

The amounts of T<>T photoproducts measured in skin samples irradiated with 72 KJ/m^2 of solar UV were compared with erythemal skin response characteristics of the individuals tested (Table I). MEDs varied from 36 KJ/m^2 (30 minute exposure) to 72KJ/m^2 (60 minute exposure) of solar UV. Most individuals exhibited solar MEDs of 54KJ/m^2 or 72 KJ/m^2. The mean unadjusted yield of T<>T photoproducts (induced by 72KJ/m^2 solar UV) in 7 individuals with MEDs of 54KJ/m^2 was not significantly different from the mean yield in 10 individuals with MEDs of 72KJ/m^2 (modified t-test). In two individuals with MEDs of 36KJ/m^2, the mean unadjusted yield of T<>T photoproducts was not different from either of the other two groups with higher MEDs (Table I). Thus, no consistent relationship between MED and unadjusted T<>T photoproduct yield was observed. However, the small range of MEDs observed and the large increments of dose administered prohibits a definitive statement regarding the association between photoproduct yield and skin sensitivity.

Freeman et al. (1986) have demonstrated an inverse relationship between UVB-induced erythema and yield of cyclobuta-dipyrimidines in skin. This effect was most clearly demonstrated in individuals who were very sensitive (skin type I) or very resistant (skin type V) to UVB radiation. All of the individuals in our study were assessed as intermediate skin types II or III, and therefore would not be expected to display a wide range of responses. The other major difference between the two studies was the duration and intensity of irradiation. Freeman et al. used a high intensity UVB lamp with exposures of short duration (0.3-3.9 min), whereas our exposures lasted 60 min. This difference may influence both MED and T<>T yield. Although we did not observe an association between individual MED and net T<>T yield, our value for T<>T photoproducts formed per MED by solar UV of 0.06 $\pm$ 0.04 T<>T per Kb per MED (in the 7 clustered samples) is similar to that found by Freeman et al. using UVB radiation. This suggests that the ratio of cyclobuta-dipyrimidines to MED does not differ substantially in UVB- and solar UV-irradiated skin. However, it should be noted that, under conditions of induced pigmentation, a constant ratio of cyclobuta-dipyrimidine content to MED is not observed (Gange et al., 1985).

FUTURE STUDIES

We are planning to assess DNA repair efficiency in cells of watermen with skin cancer for comparison with cells from watermen without skin cancer but matched for age, skin type, phenotypic characteristics, and solar UV exposure. In addition, DNA repair efficiency will be compared in SCC and BCC bearers to examine the relative importance of DNA repair in susceptibility to these neoplasms. These studies will use several methods for assessing repair efficiency, including UV (or solar) radiation cytotoxicity assays, photoproduct immunoassays to measure repair kinetics in keratinocytes and fibroblasts, and plasmid reactivation assays in lymphocytes or fibroblasts to measure efficiency of restoration of gene function.

ACKNOWLEDGEMENTS

The authors wish to acknowledge the assistance of Sharon Stainback for manuscript preparation and the volunteers who participated in these studies. Research supported in part by DHHS grants EYO4547, ESO3841, AR38884 and the World Health Organization. Figures 1-3 reprinted with permission from the

National Cancer Institute; figures 4 and 5 and Table I reprinted with permission from Elsevier Press.

REFERENCES

Berger, D.S., and Urbach, F.A. 1982. A climatology of sunburning ultraviolet radiation. Photochem Photobiol 35:187-192.

Bruze, M, Emmett, EA, Creasey, J., Strickland, P.T. 1989. Cyclobuta-dithymidine induction by solar-simulating UV radiation in human skin. II. Individual Responses. J Invest Dermatol 93:341-344.

D'Ambrosio, S.M., Slazinski, L., Whetstone, J.W., Lowney, E. 1981a. Excision repair of UV-induced pyrimidine dimers in human skin in vivo. J. Invest. Dermatol. 77:311-313.

D'Ambrosio, S.M., Whetstone, J.W., Slazinski, L., Lowney, E. 1981b. Photorepair of pyrimidine dimers in human skin in vivo. Photochem. Photobiol. 36:461-464.

Engle A., Johnson, M.L., Haynes, S.E. 1988. Health effects of sunlight exposure in the United States. Arch Dermatol 124:72-79.

Fears, T.R., Scotto, J. 1983. Estimating increases in skin cancer morbidity due to increase in ultraviolet radiation exposure. Cancer Investigation 1:119-126.

Forbes, P.D., Davies, R.E., Urbach, F. 1978. Experimental ultraviolet photocarcinogenesis: Wavelength interactions and time-dose relationships. NCI Monograph 50:31-38.

Freeman, SE, Gange, RW, Matzinger, EA, and Sutherland, BM. 1986. Higher pyrimidine dimer yields in skin of normal humans with higher UVB sensitivity. J. Invest. Dermatol. 86:34-36.

Freeman, S.E., Gange, R.W., Sutherland, J.C., Matzinger, E.A., Sutherland, B.M. 1987. Production of pyrimidine dimers in DNA of human exposed in situ to UVA radiation. J. Invest. Dermatol. 88:430-433.

Gange RW, Blackett SD, Matzinger, EA, Sutherland, BM, Kochevar, IE. 1985. Comparative protective efficiency of UVA and UVB-induced tans against erythema and formation of endonuclease-sensitive sites in DNA by UVB in human skin. J. Invest. Dermatol. 85:362-364.

Giles GG, Marks R, Foley P. 1988. Incidence of non-melanocytic skin cancer treated in Australia. Brit Med J. 296:13-17.

Keyse, SM, Tyrrell, RM. 1987. Rapidly occurring DNA excision repair events determine the biological expression of uv-induced damage in human cells. Carcinogenesis 8:1251-1256.

Maniatis, T., Fritsch, E.F., Sambrook, J. 1982. Molecular Cloning: A Laboratory Manual. Cold Spring Harbor Laboratories, New York, pp. 458-468.

Marks, R., Rennie, G., Selwood, T. 1988. The relationship of basal cell carcinomas and squamous cell carcinomas to solar keratoses. Arch Dermatol 124:1039-1042.

Mellon, I, Bohr, VA, Smith, CA, Hanawalt, PC. 1986. Preferential DNA repair of an active gene in human cells. Proc. Natl. Acad. Sci. 83:8878-8882.

Mullaart, E., Lohman, PHM, Vijg, J. 1988. Differences in pyrimidine dimer removal between rat skin cells in vitro and in vivo. J. Invest. Dermatol. 90:346-349.

Regan, JD, Carrier WL, Smith, DP, Waters, R, Lee, WH. 1978. Pyrimidine dimer excision in human cells and skin cancer. Natl. Cancer Inst. Monogr. 50:141-143.

Rosenthal, F.S., Phoon, C., Bakalian, A.E., Taylor, H.R. 1988. The ocular dose of ultraviolet radiation to outdoor workers. Invest. Ophthalmol Vis Sci 29:649-656.

Scotto, J., Fears, T.R., Fraumeni, J.F. 1981. Incidence of nonmelanoma skin cancer in the United States. NIH Publication No. 82-2433, p.1-113.

Scotto, T., Fears, T., Gori, G. 1976. Measurements of ultraviolet radiation in the United States and comparisons with skin cancer data. NIH Publi. No. 76-1029, pp. 1-120.

Slaper, H., Schothorst, A.A., van der Leun, J.C. 1986. Risk evaluation of UVB therapy for psoriasis: Comparison of calculated risk for UVB therapy and observed risk in PUVA treated patients. Photodermatology 3:271-283.

Strickland, P.T., and Boyle, J.M. 1981. Characterization of two monoclonal antibodies specific for dimerised and non-dimerised adjacent thymidines in single stranded DNA. Photochem. Photobiol. 34:595-601.

Strickland, P.T. and Creasey, J.S. 1988. Immunoassay of dithymidine cyclobutane dimers in nanogram quantities of DNA. In: Detection Methods for DNA-Damaging Agents in Man. H. Bartsch, K. Hemminki, and I.K. O'Neill, eds., IARC Pub. No. 89, Lyon, France. pp. 341-344.

Strickland, P.T., Creasey, J.S. 1989. Induction and repair of cyclobuta-dithymidine photoproducts in hamster skin by solar-simulated UV radiation. J. Photochem. Photobiol. B: Biology 3:17-24.

Strickland, PT, Vitasa, BC, West SK, Rosenthal FS, Emmett EA, Taylor HR. Quantitative carcinogenesis in man: Ultraviolet dose-dependence of skin cancer in Maryland watermen. J. Natl. Cancer Inst. (in press).

Sutherland, B.M., Harber, L.C., Kochevar, I. 1980. Pyrimidine dimer formation and repair in human skin. Cancer Res. 40:3181-3185.

Taylor, H.R., West, S.K., Rosenthal, F.S., Munoz, B., Newland, H.S. Abbey, H.S., Emmett, E.A. 1988. The epidemiology of cataract: The effect of ultraviolet radiation. N Eng J Med 319:1429-1436

Teppo, L., Pukkala, E., Saxen, E. 1985. Multiple cancer-an epidemiological exercise in Finland. JNCI 75:207-217.

Urbach, F. Geographic pathology of skin cancer. 1969. In: Biologic Effects of Ultraviolet Radiation (F. Urbach, ed) Pergamon Press, Oxford; pp.635-650.

Urbach, F. 1984. Ultraviolet radiation and skin cancer. In: Topics in Photomedicine (K.C. Smith, Ed) New York: Plenum Press pp. 39-142.

Urbach, F., Witcop, C.J., Laerum, O.D. 1981. Skin cancer in man: Geographical and racial variations. In: Biology of Skin Cancer (eds: O.D. Laerum, O.H. Iverson) Geneva: UICC Press, pp. 58-86.

Vitaliano, P.P. 1978. The use of logistic regression for modelling risk factors with application to nonmelanoma skin cancer. Am J Epidemiol

108:402-414.

Vitasa, B.C., Emmett, E.A., Ng, S.K., Taylor, H.R., Rosenthal, F.S. 1987. Prevalence of skin diseases and solar UVB exposure in watermen. Photochem Photobiol 45:40S.

DEFECTIVE DNA REPAIR IN HUMANS: CLINICAL AND MOLECULAR STUDIES OF XERODERMA PIGMENTOSUM

Kenneth H. Kraemer[1], Saraswathy Seetharam[1], Michael M. Seidman[2], Anders Bredberg[1], Douglas Brash[3], Haywood L. Waters[1], Miroslava Protić-Sabljić[1], Gary Peck[4], John DiGiovanna[4], Alan Moshell[5], Robert E. Tarone[6], Gary Jones[7], Ram Parshad[8], and Katherine Sanford[7]

[1]Laboratory of Molecular Carcinogenesis, [3]Laboratory of Human Carcinogenesis, [4]Dermatology Branch, [6]Biometry Branch, and [7]Laboratory of Cellular and Molecular Biology, National Cancer Institute, Bethesda, MD; [5]National Institute of Arthritis, Musculoskeletal and Skin Diseases, Bethesda, MD; [8]Howard University, Washington, D.C.; and [2]Otsuka Pharmaceutical Co., Rockville, MD 20850

INTRODUCTION

Xeroderma pigmentosum (XP), is a rare autosomal recessive disorder with increased sun sensitivity, multiple pigmentary abnormalities and a more than 1000-fold increased frequency of cancer of the sun exposed portions of the skin and eyes. Cultured cells from XP patients are hypersensitive to the cytotoxic and mutagenic effects of UV radiation and have defective DNA repair (reviewed in Robbins et al, 1974; Kraemer and Slor, 1985; Kraemer, 1987; Cleaver and Kraemer, 1989).

The DNA repair defect was studied using plasmid vectors. XP cells were unable to repair both dimer and non-dimer photoproducts. In addition, both dimer and non-dimer photoproducts were mutagenic in XP cells. The major mutagenic changes involved cytosines, indicating that the major UV photoproducts (TT dimers) were not the major mutagenic lesions. The spectrum of mutations found in UV treated plasmids replicated in XP cells was reduced in comparison to that with normal cells. These mutagenic abnormalities may be related to the cancer susceptibility in XP.

A literature survey of more than 800 XP patients revealed a mean age of onset of skin cancer of less than 10 years, a 50 year reduction in comparison to the general population (Kraemer, Lee and Scotto, 1984, 1987). Thus XP patients are good candidates for studies of the prevention of skin cancer.

Carriers of the XP gene (XP heterozygotes) are clinically normal. The usual assays for DNA repair defects are also

DNA Damage and Repair in Human Tissues
Edited by B. M. Sutherland and A. D. Woodhead
Plenum Press, New York, 1990

normal with cells from XP heterozygotes. A new assay was
developed that has detected XP heterozygotes in affected
families.

This paper will cover three topics: 1. DNA repair studies
in XP cells with shuttle vector plasmids, 2. prevention of
skin cancer with oral 13-cis retinoic acid in XP patients and
3. detection of XP heterozygotes.

DNA REPAIR IN XP MEASURED WITH SHUTTLE VECTORS

Studies of host cell reactivation employed plasmid
shuttle vectors to measure DNA repair or mutations. In the
typical experiment the purified plasmid DNA is treated with UV
in vitro and transfected into the XP or control (repair
proficient) cells. Within the cell, the plasmid DNA is
repaired by the cell's DNA repair enzymes. RNA transcription
and DNA replication also utilize cellular functions. The
plasmid then is harvested and its status assessed by measuring
a product produced by the repaired plasmid or by transforming
indicator bacteria.

A non-replicating plasmid containing the chloramphenicol
acetyltransferase gene (cat) was used to measure DNA repair as
indicated by the extent of cat expression in the XP and repair
proficient cells (Protić-Sabljić and Kraemer, 1985, 1986a,
1986b). Mutagenesis was measured with a plasmid carrying a
mutagenesis marker gene, the bacterial supF transfer RNA, and
SV40 sequences to permit replication in mammalian cells, which
was developed by Seidman et al, (1985). After passing
through the mammalian cells, plasmid survival is assessed by
converting transfected bacteria to ampicillin resistance. The
functioning of the marker gene is measured by its ability to
suppress a mutation in the gene for β-galactosidase in the
bacteria (Kraemer and Seidman, 1989). On agar plates
containing an indicator dye colonies expressing β-
galactosidase are blue while those with an inactive (mutated)
marker gene are white or light blue. The plasmid can be
purified from the colonies containing mutants and the DNA
sequence of the marker gene determined.

DNA Repair Measured by cat Plasmid Inactivation

Using a non-replicating plasmid, pSV2catSVgpt, coding for
the bacterial cat gene we measured the ability of XP cells to
restore activity to UV damaged plasmid (Protić-Sabljić and
Kraemer, 1985). The plasmid was exposed in vitro to radiation
from a germicidal lamp (primarily 254 nm UV) to create
photoproducts and then transfected into XP cells from
complementation groups A and D. Two days later cell extracts
were prepared and assayed for cat activity by thin layer
chromatography. The cat expression as a function of UV dose
was about 12-fold less in the XP cells than in normal cells
(D_0 56 J.m^{-2} vs 680 J.m^{-2}).

The frequency of cyclobutane dimers formed was estimated
by measuring the ability of the enzyme T4 endonuclease V to
nick UV treated supercoiled plasmid thereby converting it to a
relaxed circular form. After treating plasmids with a series
of increasing doses of UV, nicking with T4 endonuclease V,
separating the supercoiled DNA from relaxed circular DNA on a

neutral agarose gel, and scanning the photographic negative, the proportion of supercoiled (form I) molecules remaining was determined as a function of UV dose. The D_0 represents the dose that produces one lethal hit per plasmid (or in this case one T4 endonuclease V sensitive site i.e. one cyclobutane dimer). For the 7268 base pair plasmid pSV2catSVgpt the D_0 was 7 $J.m^{-2}$.

The results of <u>cat</u> inactivation and dimer induction indicate that one cyclobutane pyrimidine dimer inhibits expression in xeroderma pigmentosum (XP) group A cells.

Treatment of the plasmid with UV followed by enzymatic photoreactivation creates a damaged plasmid containing primarily non-dimer photoproducts (Protić-Sabljić and Kraemer, 1986a). This plasmid may serve as an indicator of the ability of the XP group A cells to repair non-dimer damage. If the XP group A cells could repair non-dimer damage then the D_0 of the UV inactivation slope of CAT activity should increase to the value of the repair proficient cells. If non-dimer photoproducts are not repaired by the XP cells then they also should be persistent blocks to transcription and the D_0 would not increase to the normal level. The reduced expression of a UV damaged transfecting plasmid in XP complementation group A cells is only partially reversed by photoreactivation. After photoreactivation, the D_0 increased to 168 $J.m^{-2}$, a value intermediate between that with the normal lines and that found with the plasmid treated with UV without photoreactivation, indicating that 25% to 37% of the lethal hits per <u>cat</u> gene remained after photoreactivation. This residual inhibition corresponds to the fraction of non-dimer photoproducts induced by UV. This result implies that XP12BE(SV40) cells do not repair most of the non-dimer photoproducts in DNA.

<u>DNA Mutagenesis Measured with Shuttle Vector Plasmid</u>

UV treated plasmid pZ189 was passed through XP group A or D cells and then used to transform bacteria (Bredberg et al, 1986, Seetharam et al, 1987; Seidman et al, 1987). The relative number of bacterial colonies recovered as a function of UV dose to the plasmid was much less with the XP-A and the XP-D cells than with normal cells. This hypersensitivity is similar to the relative sensitivity of XP and normal cells to killing by UV. This result is consistent with the earlier observations that UV photoproducts are not repaired as efficiently by XP as by normal cells and that UV photoproducts are lethal lesions.

This plasmid can also be used to measure the mutation frequency after UV treatment. There was a linear increase in mutation frequency with increasing UV exposure to the plasmid with the XP group D cells. This increase is greater than with the normal cells.

Table 1 shows the base sequence analysis of the mutants recovered after passage of UV treated pZ189 in XP and normal cells. With the normal cells, plasmids with single, tandem and up to 6 multiple base substitutions in the marker gene were found. In marked contrast, there were significantly fewer plasmids recovered with multiple base substitutions with the XP-A and XP-D cells.

TABLE 1. MUTATIONS in UV-TREATED and PHOTOREACTIVATED SHUTTLE
VECTOR pZ189 REPLICATED in XP CELLS[1]

| | XERODERMA PIGMENTOSUM | | | NORMAL |
| | XP-A | XP-A +PR | XP-D | GMO637 |
	Number of plasmids with base changes:			
Independent plasmids				
sequenced	61	42	69	90
Point Mutations				
Single base				
substitutions	47	38	59	48
Tandem base				
substitutions	12	3	4	16
Multiple base				
substitutions	1	1	6	25
Types of single or tandem base substitutions (number of changes):				
Transitions	67	29	59	61
G:C to A:T	66	29	57	59
A:T to G:C	1	0	2	2
Transversions	4	16	8	20
G:C to T:A	0	2	5	8
G:C to C:G	1	8	1	5
A:T to T:A	3	5	0	6
A:T to C:G	0	1	2	1

[1]Modified from Bredberg et al, 1986; Brash et al, 1987;
Seetharam et al, 1987; and Kraemer et al, 1988a.

Base sequence analysis of several hundred individual
mutant plasmids recovered from the XP and normal lines
revealed that more than half of the mutant plasmids had G:C to
A:T base substitution transition mutations (Table 1). Since
these mutations involve cytosine rather than thymine, this
implies that the major UV photoproduct, the 5'TT dimer, was
not the principal mutagenic lesion. This observation is
consistent with observations in prokaryotes more than 20 years
ago that the G:C to A:T transition was the major UV-induced
mutation (Drake, 1963; Howard and Tessman, 1964). More
recently this bias has been explained by the tendency of many
polymerases to insert an A opposite a non-instructional lesion
(the "A rule") (Boiteux and Laval, 1982; Strauss et al, 1982;
Schaaper et al, 1983) (Figure 1). In the case of a 5'TT dimer
this would result in insertion of the appropriate base. This
bias toward insertion of an A would be of evolutionary
advantage to organisms developing at a time of high UV
exposure before a significant protective layer of ozone was
established.

Despite their hypermutability, a restricted spectrum of mutations was recovered from the XP-A and XP-D lines. There were fewer plasmids with multiple base substitution mutations and with transversion mutations than with the normal cells. (Table 1).

When in Doubt Put in an "A"

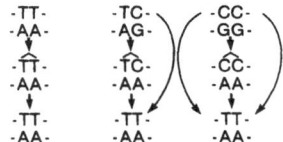

Figure 1. The "A" rule. Many polymerases tend to insert an adenine opposite a non-instructional lesion in DNA. Thus A:T base pairs would mutate much less frequently than G:C base pairs after ultraviolet damage.

The distribution of mutations was non-random with the normal and with the XP cells. Hotspots for mutations were present in the mutagenic target. There was a G:C to A:T hotspot at base pair 156 with all 3 cell lines. There were unique hotspots present with the XP-A and XP-D cells. With the XP-D cells a hotspot was present at base pair 159 and a weaker hotspot at base pair 168. With the XP-A cells, hotspots were present at base pairs 168 and 169.

Photoreactivation

Treatment of the plasmid with E. coli photoreactivating enzyme and visible light following UV exposure removes the cyclobutane dimers while leaving the non-dimer photoproducts in the plasmid.

Transfection of XP group A cells with the photo-reactivated plasmid resulted in greater plasmid survival (Brash et al, 1987) indicating that cyclobutane dimers are lethal lesions in the plasmid. The fact that the survival curve did not rise completely to normal levels demonstrates that 20-23% of the lethal hits remained after photoreact-ivation. This finding indicates that non-dimer photoproducts were also lethal lesions in repair deficient XP cells.

Photoreactivation reduced the mutation frequency by about 90% implying that about 90% of the mutations are due to photoreactivatable lesions (i.e. cyclobutane dimers). Since about 10% of the mutations remained, non-dimer photoproducts were also mutagenic.

Pyrimidine dimers were selectively removed from pZ189 by use of E. coli photolyase and the mutational spectrum was again determined. Removal of more than 99% of the cyclobutane dimers by in vitro photoreactivation before transfection reduced the mutation frequency while preserving the mutation distribution, indicating that: 1) cytosine-containing cyclobutane dimers were the major mutagenic lesions at these sites; and, 2) cytosine-containing non-cyclobutane dimer photoproducts were also mutagenic lesions. With the XP cells, about 90% of the mutations were the result of pyrimidine dimers. Analysis of the transition mutation hotspots with the XP cells showed their distribution to be unchanged after photoreactivation implying that at 5'TC and 5'CC sequences both cyclobutane dimers and non-dimer photoproducts were mutagenic.

Photoreactivation of the plasmid altered the types of base substitution mutations observed with the XP group A cells. There was an increase in transversions and a decrease in transitions so that the resulting proportion was similar to that with the normal cells (Table 1). Although the overall ratio of 6-4 photoproducts to dimers was 15%, at 5'TC and 5'CC sequences the ratio was 70% and 30%, respectively. New transversion hotspots were present at base pairs 120 and 155. These results suggest that in the XP cells cyclobutane dimers play a major role in transition mutations while non-dimer photoproducts were major contributors to transversion mutations.

CHEMOPREVENTION OF SKIN CANCER IN XP

A collaborative 3-year clinical trial of skin cancer prevention was conducted utilizing oral 13-cis retinoic acid (isotretinoin, Accutane) in patients with XP to determine if human skin cancer could be prevented with a pharmacologic agent (Kraemer et al, 1988b). We studied patients with xeroderma pigmentosum who had multiple cutaneous basal cell or squamous cell carcinomas. All pre-existing tumors were surgically removed and high dose (2 mg/kg/day) oral 13-cis retinoic acid was given for 2 years. The drug was then stopped for an additional 1-year of observation. Before, during, and after treatment all suspicious lesions were biopsied and skin cancers were surgically removed.

Five xeroderma pigmentosum patients had a total of 121 tumors (mean 24, range 8-43) in the 2-years prior to treatment. During 2 years of treatment with 13-cis retinoic acid there were 25 tumors (mean 5, range 3-9), with an average 63% reduction in skin cancers (p=0.019). After stopping the drug, the tumor frequency increased a mean of 8.5-fold (range 2- to 19-fold) compared to the tumor frequency during treatment (p=0.007) (Table 2). Although all patients experienced mucocutaneous toxicity, and some developed triglyceride, liver function, or skeletal abnormalities, high dose oral 13-cis retinoic acid was effective in the chemoprevention of skin cancers. This is one of the first studies to demonstrate effective chemoprevention of cancer in humans.

TABLE 2. NUMBER of SKIN CANCERS in XERODERMA PIGMENTOSUM
         PATIENTS BEFORE, DURING and AFTER THERAPY with ORAL 13-
         CIS RETINOIC ACID (2 mg/kg/day)[*]

		NUMBER OF TUMORS [RATE/YEAR]		
PATIENT	AGE/SEX	BEFORE TREATMENT (2 YR)	DURING TREATMENT (2 YR)	AFTER TREATMENT (12-14 MO)
1.	19 YR/F	43 [21.5]	3 [1.5]	18 [18.0]
2.	12 YR/F	37 [18.5]	4 [2.0]	29 [38.7]
3.	17 YR/M	23 [11.5]	6 [3.0]	20 [20.0]
4.	39 YR/M	10 [5.0]	3 [1.5]	4 [3.4]
5.	10 YR/M	8 [4.0]	9 [4.5]	10 [10.0]

[*]Modified from Kraemer, et al, 1988b.

DETECTION OF XP HETEROZYGOTES

     Carriers of XP are generally clinically asymptomatic
despite having one defective gene for XP. Epidemiologic
studies hint that they may be at increased risk of skin
cancer. However, most of the assays for DNA repair result
in normal results for obligate XP heterozygotes (parents of
XP patients).

     The G_2 chromosome breakage assay has been developed by
K. Sanford and her co-workers at NIH and Howard University
(Parshad et al, 1983, 1985; Sanford et al, 1987, 1989).
This cytogenetic assay involves treatment of cells with X-
radiation followed at a short interval (less than 2 hr) by
preparation of metaphase chromosomes. The preparation is
then scored for chromosome breaks and gaps. The frequency
of chromosome breaks and gaps is initially elevated in all
cell types but rapidly falls to baseline with cells from
normal individuals. This assay has previously been shown to
detect carriers of ataxia-telangiectasia (Shiloh et al,
1986), and of dysplastic nevus syndrome (Sanford et al,
1987) by virtue of their persistent chromosome breaks and
gaps.

     XP homozygotes have an abnormally delayed fall in
chromosome breaks and gaps (Parshad et al, 1983, 1985).
This assay was applied to fresh blood of XP patients and
their parents in an attempt to detect carriers of XP
(Parshad et al, 1990). All samples were coded before
analysis. The frequency of chromosomal breaks and gaps
immediately after treatment with X-radiation (58 R) was
similar for all samples. The frequency of chromatid breaks
and gaps was measured at 1.3, 2.3, and 3.3 h after x-
radiation. Lymphocytes from XP heterozygotes had 2-fold
higher frequencies of breaks and gaps than normal ($p < 10^{-5}$)
when fixed 2.3 or 3.3 h after irradiation.

     This elevated frequency of chromatid breaks and gaps
after G_2 phase x-irradiation may provide the basis of a test
for identifying carriers of the XP gene within known XP
families.

REFERENCES

Boiteux, S., and Laval, J., 1982, Coding properties of poly(deoxycytidylic acid) templates containing uracil or apyrimidinic sites: In vitro modulation of mutagenesis by deoxyribonucleic acid repair enzymes, Biochemistry 21: 6746-6751.

Brash, D.E., Seetharam, S., Kraemer, K.H., Seidman, M.M. and Bredberg, A., 1987, Photoproduct frequency is not the major determinant of ultraviolet mutation hotspots or coldspots in human cells, Proc. Natl. Acad. Sci. USA 84: 3782-3786.

Bredberg, A., Kraemer, K.H., and Seidman, M.M., 1986, Restricted mutational spectrum in an UV-treated shuttle vector propagated in xeroderma pigmentosum cells, Proc. Natl. Acad. Sci. USA 83: 8273-8277.

Cleaver, J., and Kraemer, K.H., 1989, Xeroderma pigmentosum. In Scriver, C.R., Beaudet, A.L., Sly, W.S., and Valle, D. (Eds.) The Metabolic Basis of Inherited Disease, Sixth Edition. New York, McGraw Hill, pp. 2949-2971

Drake, J.W., 1963, Properties of ultraviolet-induced rII mutants of bacteriophage T4, J Mol Biol 6: 268-283.

Howard B.D., and Tessman, I., 1964, Identification of the altered bases in mutated single-stranded DNA III Mutagenesis by ultraviolet light. J Mol Biol 9: 372-375.

Kraemer, K.H., Lee, M.M., and Scotto, J., 1984, DNA repair protects against cutaneous and internal neoplasia: Evidence from xeroderma pigmentosum. Carcinogenesis 5: 511-514.

Kraemer, K.H., and Slor, H., 1985, Xeroderma pigmentosum. Clinics in Dermatol. 3: 33-69.

Kraemer, K.H., Lee, M.M., and Scotto, J., 1987, Xeroderma pigmentosum: Cutaneous, ocular and neurologic abnormalities in 830 published cases, Arch. Dermatol. 123: 241-250.

Kraemer, K.H., 1987, Heritable diseases with increased sensitivity to cellular injury. In Fitzpatrick, T.B., Eisen, A.Z., Wolff, K., Freedberg, I.M., and Austen, K.F. (Eds.): Dermatology in General Medicine. New York, McGraw Hill, pp 1791-1811.

Kraemer, K.H., Seetharam, S., Protić-Sabljić, M., Brash, D.E., Bredberg, A., and Seidman, M.M., 1988a, Defective DNA repair and mutagenesis by dimer and non-dimer photoproducts in xeroderma pigmentosum measured with plasmid vectors. In Friedberg, E. and Hanawalt, P. eds. Mechanisms and Consequences of DNA Damage Processing, UCLA Symposia on Molecular and Cellular Biology, New Series, Vol 83. Alan R. Liss, Inc, New York, N.Y., pp 325-335.

Kraemer, K.H., DiGiovanna, J.J., Moshell, A.N., Tarone, R.E., and Peck, G.L., 1988b, Prevention of skin cancer with oral 13-cis retinoic acid in xeroderma pigmentosum, N. Engl. J. Med. 318: 1633-1637.

Kraemer, K.H., and Seidman, M.M., 1989, Use of supF, an Escherichia coli tyrosine suppressor tRNA gene, as a mutagenic target in shuttle vector plasmids, Mutat. Res. 220: 61-72.

Parshad, R., Sanford, K.K., and Jones, G.M., 1983, Chromatid damage after G_2 phase x-irradiation of cells from cancer-prone individuals implicates deficiency in DNA repair, Proc Natl. Acad. Sci. USA 80: 5612-5616.

Parshad, R., Sanford, K.K., and Jones, G.M., 1985, Chromosomal radiosensitivity during the G_2 cell cycle period of skin fibroblasts from individuals with familial cancer. Proc Natl. Acad. Sci. USA 82: 5400-5403.

Parshad, R., Sanford, K.K., Kraemer, K.H., Jones, G.M., and Tarone, R.E., 1990, Carrier detection in xeroderma pigmentosum, J. Clin. Invest. 85: 135-138.

Protić-Sabljić, M., and Kraemer, K.H., 1985, One pyrimidine dimer inactivates expression of a transfected gene in xeroderma pigmentosum cells. Proc. Natl. Acad. Sci. USA 82: 6622-6626.

Protić-Sabljić, M. and Kraemer, K. H., 1986a, Reduced repair of non-dimer photoproducts in a gene transfected into xeroderma pigmentosum cells. Photochem. Photobiol. 43: 509-513.

Protić-Sabljić, M. and Kraemer, K.H., 1986b, Host cell reactivation by human cells of DNA expression vectors damaged by ultraviolet radiation or by acid-heat damage. Carcinogenesis 10: 1765-1770.

Robbins, J.H., Kraemer, K.H., Lutzner, M.A., Festoff, B.W., and Coon, H.G., 1974, Xeroderma pigmentosum - An inherited disease with sun sensitivity, multiple cutaneous neoplasms and abnormal DNA repair, Ann. Intern. Med. 80: 221-248.

Sanford, K.K., Parshad, R., Greene, M.H., Tarone, R.E., Tucker, M.A., and Jones, G.M., 1987, Hypersensitivity to G_2 chromatid radiation damage in familial dysplastic nevus syndrome. Lancet ii: 1111-1116.

Sanford, K.K., Parshad, R., Gantt, R., Tarone, R.E., Jones, G.M., and Price, F., 1989, Factors affecting and significance of G_2 chromatin radiosensitivity in predisposition to cancer. Int. J. Radiat. Biol. 55: 963-981.

Schaaper, R.M., Kunkel, T.A., and Loeb L., 1983, Infidelity of DNA synthesis associated with bypass of apurinic sites, Proc Natl Acad Sci USA 80: 487-491.

Seetharam, S., Protić-Sabljić, M., Seidman, M.M. and Kraemer, K.H., 1987, Abnormal ultraviolet mutagenic spectrum in DNA replicated in cultured fibroblasts from a patient with the skin cancer-prone disease, xeroderma pigmentosum, J. Clin. Invest. 80: 1613-1617.

Seidman, M.M., Dixon, K., Razzaque, A., Zagursky, R., and Berman, M.L., 1985, A shuttle vector plasmid for studying carcinogen-induced point mutations in mammalian cells, Gene 38: 233-237.

Seidman, M.M., Bredberg, A., Seetharam, S. and Kraemer, K.H., 1987, Multiple point mutations in a shuttle vector propagated in human cells: Evidence for an error-prone polymerase activity. Proc. Natl. Acad. Sci..USA. 84: 4944-4948.

Shiloh, Y., Parshad, R., Sanford, K.K., and Jones, G.M., 1986, Carrier detection in ataxia-telangiectasia. Lancet i: 689-690.

Strauss, B.S., Rabkin, S., Sagher, S., and Moore, P., 1982, The role of DNA polymerase in base substitution mutagenesis on non-instructional templates. Biochimie 64: 829-838.

5-MOP INDUCED PROTECTION AGAINST EPIDERMAL DNA

DAMAGE BY ULTRAVIOLET RADIATION IN HUMAN SKIN

Antony R Young[1], Christopher S Potten[2], Caroline
A Chadwick[2], Gillian M Murphy[1], and A Jeffrey
Cohen[3]

[1]Photobiology Unit, Institute of Dermatology,
United Medical and Dental Schools of Guy's and St
Thomas's Hospitals, University of London, UK.

[2]Epithelial Biology Department, Paterson
Institute for Cancer Research, Christie Hospital
and Holt Radium Institute, Manchester, UK.

[3]Toxicology Advisory Services, Sutton, Surrey,
UK.

INTRODUCTION

It is now well recognized by the dermatological community
that solar exposure results in an increased risk of skin
cancer, especially in individuals of skin types I and II who
sunburn easily and have a limited ability to tan (MacKie et
al., 1987). In the last few years this information has been
widely publicized in the press and other media. Despite this,
a suntan is still a prized social asset and epidemiological
data indicate a continued rise in the incidence of skin
cancers. It also seems reasonable to suppose that the
possible depletion of the stratospheric ozone layer, over
populated areas of the earth's surface, would result in a
further long-term increase of skin cancer (van der Leun,
1988).

Ultraviolet radiation (UVR) induced damage of the skin
results in tanning and, in some cases, stratum corneum
thickening which are generally believed to offer subsequent
photoprotection from such damage. This view has been
supported by studies which show that a tan induced by UVB
(280-315 nm) or UVA (315-400 nm) protects against erythema
and/or DNA damage (Gange et al., 1985). However, such studies
do not necessarily represent what happens when a tan is
induced by solar UVR. It has also been demonstrated that a tan
acquired with UVR plus 8-methoxypsoralen (8-MOP) or 5-
methoxypsoralen (5-MOP) results in photoprotection from damage
such as erythema and sunburn cell formation by subsequent UVR
exposure (Cripps, 1981; Gschnait et al., 1978; Sambuco et al.,
1987).

DNA Damage and Repair in Human Tissues
Edited by B. M. Sutherland and A. D. Woodhead
Plenum Press, New York, 1990

An important, and as yet unanswered, question is whether a tan acquired by solar exposure offers any protection from skin cancer from UVR. It is difficult, if not impossible, to answer this question directly, at least in humans. One approach would be to study protection against UVR-induced DNA damage, which is believed to be an important marker of malignancy.

We report on human studies which were designed to investigate the relative protective effects of different tans from DNA damage induced by solar simulated radiation (SSR). The damage was estimated from the levels of unscheduled DNA synthesis (UDS) in epidermal cells, assuming that levels of DNA repair reflect levels of DNA damage. The tans were acquired by repeated exposure of normal human skin to sub-erythemogenic doses of SSR in the presence or absence of 5-MOP preparations containing UVB sunscreens. 5-MOP is present in natural citrus oils, especially Citrus bergamia, that have been added to some commercial sunscreen preparations to enhance tanning.

The data presented here are an extension of previously published studies (Young et al., 1988; Potten et al., 1988) in which we showed, in individuals of skin type II, that a tan induced by 5-MOP containing sunscreens plus SSR offered superior protection against SSR induced DNA damage when compared with a tan induced by SSR alone. We have now compared the responses of individuals of skin types I and II (poor tanning ability) with those of types III, IV, and V (progessively good tanning ability) and studied the onset and duration of photoprotection in skin type II.

MATERIALS AND METHODS

Sunscreen Preparations

Sunscreens were supplied by Laboratoires Bergaderm SA (France) and contained final concentrations of 0, 15, 30, or 45 ppm 5-MOP in citrus oils and a combination of UVB sunscreens; 2-3% Parsol MCX (2-ethylhexyl 4'-methoxycinnamate) with 1-2% Eusolex 6300 (1,7,7-trimethyl-3-(4-methyl-benzylidene) bicyclo [2.2.1]-2-heptanone). The concentrations of 5-MOP and UVB sunscreens in the test preparations were confirmed by Laboratoires Bergaderm.

SSR Source

The SSR source was a 2.5 kW Kratos (Westwood, N.J.) solar simulator with an air mass 1 filter (sun at 90° elevation). UVA irradiance was monitored with an International Light IL442A radiometer calibrated at 366 nm and was 11.25 mW.cm^{-2}. UVB irradiance was not determined.

Experimental Procedure

The test sites were previously untanned buttock skin of normal healthy subjects aged between 20-30, all of whom gave informed consent. Prior to the tanning protocol, the 24 hour SSR minimal erythema dose (MED) (just perceptible erythema) was determined for each subject using a $\sqrt{2}$ based incremental series of exposure times. Skin type was also assessed, based on skin coloration and tanning history.

The tanning protocol was as follows. Test preparations were applied to the buttock skin and 30 minutes later, the sites were exposed to 0.70 MED (barely perceptible) of SSR. This procedure was repeated 5 days/week (Mon-Fri) for 2 consecutive weeks unless otherwise stated. The preparations were spread over 1 cm^2 sites, defined with an adhesive foil template, with a gloved finger so that there was no excess of preparation. It was estimated (by tests over larger areas) that the amount of preparations applied was of the order of 2 µl/cm^2. It can be assumed that any variation would be randomized over the two-week treatment. After a lapse of one week (day 19 after the beginning of the treatments), control and treatment sites were challenged with 2 MED SSR. No test preparations were applied immediately before this challenge.

The degree of erythema and tan on each site was noted on a daily basis, and on the day of challenge.

Tissue Handling

After treatment, biopsies were taken under local anesthesia using a 3 mm full thickness dermal punch. Excess tissue was removed with a scalpel blade and the remaining circular piece of epidermal tissue was sliced into approximately 1 mm thick strips. Within 10-15 minutes of SSR challenge, the biopsy samples were placed in 5-10 ml balanced salt solution containing 370 kBq (10 µCi)/ml of methyl ^{3}H-thymidine (^{3}HTdR) (sp act 185 GBq (5 Ci)/mM). The samples were left to incubate for 1 hour at 37°C with manual agitation every 5 minutes and were then placed in Carnoy's fixative for not less than 20 minutes before being placed in 70% ethanol for storage.

Sectioning and Autoradiography

A single 1 mm strip was then carefully embedded in paraffin and sectioned at right angles to the surface (5 µm). The sections were dewaxed, hydrated, and dipped in K5 liquid emulsion (Ilford Ltd) diluted 1:1 with water. After air drying at not more than 20°C, the slides were exposed for two weeks at 4°C after which they were developed and stained with hematoxylin and eosin.

Microscopy and Counting of UDS

The slides were analysed using a Zeiss planapo x40 oil immersion lens. Six randomly selected areas of epidermis were used on each section. The number of silver grains overlaying each nucleus was counted and recorded. If S phase cells had more than 50 grains over their nuclei the number was not counted. Counts were kept separate for the basal layer (which contained most of the S cells) and the suprabasal layers of which there were generally more than 3-4. Generally about 15 basal cells were observed per field and about 50 suprabasal cells which provided about a total of about 100 basal cells and about 300 suprabasal cells per section. Generally, only one section per biopsy was scored. The average grain count for each volunteer was obtained excluding the S phase nuclei which were defined as having more than 30 grains per nucleus.

Scoring of Melanin and Stratum Corneum Thickness

Additional slides were stained using the Masson-Fontana silver reaction for melanin which also resulted in swelling of the stratum corneum. In this swollen state the number of cell layers was counted at 10 points in the section. The level of pigmentation was assessed by three independent assessors using an arbitary scale ranging from 0 (no detectable melanin at all) through to 6 (very high levels of pigmentation). The melanin levels in the basal layer and the suprabasal layers were determined separately.

RESULTS

The type I and some type II volunteers showed low grade erythema with confluent borders on some of the SSR only and some of the 5-MOP sunscreen sites during the treatments. In the type II subjects, erythema was usually restricted to the first week of treatment. Erythema was not seen on the suncreen without 5-MOP sites. In general the intensity and duration of erythema for the 5-MOP (30 and 45 ppm) sunscreens was similar to that of SSR alone which was greater than 5-MOP at 15 ppm. Some of the type I subjects showed erythema on the challenge day. This was not seen with type II, III, IV, or V subjects. Transient erythema was very occasionally seen in some of the type III, IV, and V subjects during the treatment period.

Visual tanning was absent or barely perceptible on the challenge day in the type I subjects. In general, the type II subjects started to show evidence of tanning on the SSR alone and 5-MOP sunscreen sites at the begining of the second week. Type III, IV, and V subjects started to show evidence of tanning after 1 to 3 days. Detailed results of visual tan on challenge day are not given here as, in general, they correlated very well with histologically observed tans described later in this section. The tans obtained in skin types II, III, IV, and V with the 5-MOP (30 ppm) sunscreen were similar to those obtained with SSR alone. Skin type IIs tanned minimally with the sunscreen only preparations, but skin types III, IV, and V showed some tanning with this treatment.

The UDS data presented in Table 1 are from counts in the basal layer. In general, the counts from the suprabasal layers showed the same trends.

Non-irradiated sites

Analysis of data from completely untreated sites of 30 skin type II volunteers showed a background UDS value (grains/basal cell nucleus) of 0.45 ± 0.16 (SD). In general, individual values ranged between 0.2 and 1.0.

Non-pretreated; 2 MED irradiated sites

2 MED was the standard challenge dose. Analysis of data from 20 skin type II volunteers showed a UDS value (grains/basal cell nucleus) of 5.6 ± 1.3 (SD).

The results are presented in seven annotated tables. With the exception of Table 6, each table has three columns. The first column shows the increase in pigmentation of each volunteer which is the treated value (melanin score) minus the non-treated control value. In general, the control value was in the region of 1.5 in skin type II volunteers. The second column shows the increase in cell layers of each volunteer which is the treated value (stratum corneum cell layers) minus the control value. In general, the control value was in the region of 15 layers in all skin types. The third column shows the UDS ratio which is the protection factor (PF) for each volunteer. The PF value is calculated by dividing the UDS value obtained by 2 MED challenge of the pretreated site by the UDS value obtained from the challenge of the non-pretreated site in each volunteer. As indicated above, the mean value of the latter for 20 volunteers was 5.6.

Table 1. Pretreament with SSR
Alone on Skin Type II

	Increase in pigmentation	Increase in cell layers	UDS ratio (PF)
	2.5	10.2	0.94
	3.3	3.7	1.07
	3.7	6.3	1.09
	1.8	8.6	0.75
	3.0	9.3	0.52
	2.0	5.8	1.62
	2.5	9.1	1.00
	0.3	9.0	1.03
	3.5	8.4	1.02
	4.0	20.0	0.62
	4.0	4.5	1.24
	4.5	18.5	0.62
	3.5	7.7	0.42
	3.3	10.9	0.62
	3.9	3.6	0.58
	3.5	5.3	0.89
Mean±SD	3.1±1.1(16)	8.8±4.7	0.88±0.31

The data in Table 1 show the results of 16 type II volunteers (4 experiments) in which subjects had 10 pretreatments of SSR alone prior to challenge with 2 MED SSR 7 days later. Despite evident increases in skin pigmentation and stratum corneum layers the PF value observed (0.88) is modest.

The data in Table 2 show the results of 23 volunteers (type II) from a total of 6 experiments in which the 10 pretreatments were UVB sunscreen without 5-MOP, followed by SSR exposure. It is evident that the increase in pigmentation and number of stratum corneum cell layers is much lower when compared to pretreatment with SSR alone. There is no evidence of protection from a 2 MED challenge dose; indeed, there is a suggestion that the level of DNA damage has increased as the PF is 1.11.

Table 2. Pre-treatment with UVB Sunscreen + SSR on Skin Type II				Table 3. Pre-treatment with 5-MOP + UVB Sunscreen + SSR on Skin Type II		
Incrs. in pig.	Incrs. in cell layers	UDS ratio (PF)		Incrs. in pig.	Incrs. in cell layers	UDS ratio (PF)
2.2	4.5	1.27		1.7	4.4	0.54
0.5	6.8	1.42		4.2	8.0	0.54
0.5	1.8	1.26		4.0	8.5	0.57
-2.0	3.1	-		2.0	7.7	0.66
0.5 *	1.8	1.03		4.7	8.3	0.20
1.0	5.4	0.79		4.9	11.4	0.28
2.7	- 0.5	0.78		4.7	-	0.56
0.0	6.7	1.30		4.0	-	0.41
1.2	-	1.28		3.4	5.3	0.40
0.5	5.4	1.57		3.1	9.9	0.41
1.0	1.5	1.54		3.5	4.6	0.23
-1.0	-0.4	0.95		1.0	3.3	0.93
2.0	1.5	1.15		2.2	4.5	0.71
1.3	3.8	0.91		3.0	5.8	0.33
1.2	2.0	0.92		2.5	2.6	0.73
0.0	3.2	1.23				
3.0	4.3	1.03		Means±SD (n=15)		
2.3	4.1	0.69				
2.9	6.1	0.87		3.3±1.2	6.5±2.7	0.50±0.20
2.2	2.5	1.14				
0.8	3.8	0.89				
2.2	1.6	0.99				
1.1	2.5	1.39				

Means±SD (n=23)

1.1±1.2	3.3±2.1	1.11±0.25

The data in Table 3 are from 15 skin type II volunteers (4 experiments) given pretreatments with a 5-MOP (30 ppm) containing sunscreen and SSR. It can be seen that the increase in pigmentation is similar to that observed in Table 1 (pretreatment with SSR alone). The increase in stratum corneum layers is less than seen with pretreatment with SSR alone but good protection is afforded with a PF value of 0.50 compared with that of 0.88 when pretreatment was with SSR alone.

Table 4 Effect of 5-MOP Concentration on Skin Type II

	Increase in Pigmentation	Increase in cell layers	UDS ratio (PF)
15ppm	3.7 ± 0.8 (4)	5.3 ± 3.9 (4)	0.57 ± 0.16 (4)
30ppm	3.3 ± 1.2 (15)	6.5 ± 2.7 (13)	0.50 ± 0.20 (15)
45ppm	3.6 ± 1.5 (8)	11.8 ± 4.3 (7)	0.36 ± 0.18 (8)

Table 5   Onset of 5MOP Protection on Skin Type II

No. daily pre-treat-ments	Increase in Pigmentation	Increase in cell layers	UDS ratio (PF)
3	1.0 ± 0.9 (3)	1.0 ± 0.9 (3)	1.03 ± 0.15 (3)
5	1.3 ± 0.7 (3)	1.5 ± 1.3 (3)	0.91 ± 0.02 (3)
8	2.4 ± 1.0 (3)	3.9 ± 1.1 (3)	0.64 ± 0.02 (3)
10a	2.6 ± 0.4 (3)	4.4 ± 1.6 (3)	0.59 ± 0.23 (3)
10b	3.3 ± 1.2 (15)	6.5 ± 2.7 (13)	0.50 ± 0.20 (15)

Table 6. Effect of Skin Type

Details of subjects		UDS Ratio (PF)		
MED (mins)	Skin Type	SSR only	S+SSR	5-MOP+S+SSR
14	I	1.43	1.07	0.70
14	I	1.00	0.80	0.33
14	I	0.89	1.23	0.93
14	I	1.12	0.98	0.39
14	I	1.07	1.39	0.27
mean±SD		1.10±0.20	1.03±0.29	0.52±0.28
14	II	0.81	0.88	0.61
14	II	1.27	1.03	0.73
14	II	1.34	1.38	0.60
14	II	1.14	0.80	0.33
mean±SD		1.14±0.23	1.02±0.26	0.56±0.17
20	III	0.41	1.15	0.40
20	III	0.62	0.91	0.41
20	III	0.58	0.92	0.23
20	III	0.90	1.03	0.48
mean±SD		0.63±0.20	1.00±0.11	0.38±0.11
*14(19)	IV	0.49	0.59	0.62
*28(37)	IV	0.73	1.18	0.39
*28(37)	IV	0.57	0.96	0.48
>40	IV	0.54	0.84	0.42
mean±SD		0.58±0.10	0.89±0.25	0.48±0.10
*40(53)	V	0.43	0.70	0.24

*In these subjects a higher irradiance (x 1.33) was used. Value in parenthesis indicates "equivalent MED".

The data in Table 4 show the effect of 5-MOP concentration on skin type II volunteers. Mean data are presented with the number of volunteers in parenthesis. The degree of pigmentation is independent of 5-MOP concentration, but there is a 5-MOP dose trend for increase in cell layers and PF.

Table 5 shows the mean data for the time of onset of increase in pigmentation, increase in cell layers, and UDS ratio in skin type II subjects treated with 5-MOP (30 ppm). The last 2 lines show (a) data obtained in same subjects as the first 3 lines, and (b) pooled data obtained from other experiments with the standard protocol. The number of subjects in given in parenthesis.

Table 6 shows the influence of skin type on MED and UDS ratios with pretreatment with SSR alone, UVB sunscreen (S) plus SSR, and 5-MOP (30 ppm) containing sunscreen plus SSR. The results show that pretreatment with SSR only shows no protection in skin types I and II but gives protection with skin types III plus. The application of the UVB sunscreen blocked the protection shown with skin type III and reduced that shown with skin types IV and V. Types I and II showed protection after treatment with the 5-MOP containing sunscreen and improved protection, compared with SSR only, is seen with skin types III plus.

Table 7. Duration of Protection

Post treat. challenge time	Increase in Pigmentation	Increase in cell layer	UDS ratio (PF)
SSR tan			
1 week	3.1 ± 1.1 (16)	8.8 ± 4.7 (16)	0.88 ± 0.31 (16
13 weeks	2.4 ± 1.9 (4)	3.1 ± 1.5 (4)	0.95 ± 0.10 (4)
13*weeks	2.8 ± 1.7 (4)	4.4 ± 1.5 (4)	0.95 ± 0.19 (4)
5-MOP tan			
1 week	3.3 ± 1.2 (15)	6.5 ± 2.7 (13)	0.50 ± 0.20 (15)
13 weeks	3.0 ± 1.5 (4)	3.9 ± 2.0 (4)	0.83 ± 0.16 (4)
13*weeks	3.3 ± 1.6 (4)	6.1 ± 1.4 (4)	0.68 ± 0.08 (4)

*plus 1 week retan with SSR alone

Table 7 compares the protection of tans induced by SSR alone and with 5-MOP at 1 week and 13 weeks after the last tanning treatment. In this experiment, both types of tan were also re-exposed to 1 week of SSR alone 13 weeks after the last of the initial tanning exposures and then challenged with 2 MED SSR 1 week later. With the SSR only treatment, virtually no

protection was seen at any of the sites. As previously
indicated, the 5-MOP site showed good protection at 1 week.
At 13 weeks this was much reduced but was better than the
equivalent SSR only site. However, re-exposure, at week 13,
of the 5-MOP site to SSR offered evidence of improved
photoprotection when compared with the non-re-exposed site.

DISCUSSION

     UVB-induced pyrimidine dimers have been shown to persist
in human skin for at least 24 hours (D'Ambrosio et al., 1981).
Hönigsmann et al. (1987) have shown that UDS is still apparent
at this time after a 2 MED exposure. We have delivered the
challenge dose of 2 MED SSR 7 days after the last tanning
exposure in order to eliminate the occurence of UDS as a
consequence of the tanning protocol itself. No UDS was seen
at 7 days in sites that were pretreated but not challenged
(data not shown). Almost all of the basal cells would have
undergone a cell division in 7 days (Potten, 1987) under
normal steady-state conditions. The increase in the number of
layers of the stratum corneum indicates a shorter turnover
time.

     Our skin type II data (Table 3) show that pretreatment
with a 5-MOP containing UVB sunscreen preparation plus SSR
offers good protection from DNA damage (about a 50% reduction
in UDS) caused by a challenge dose of 2 MED SSR. Associated
with this photoprotection was an increase in the number of
layers of the stratum corneum and an increase in pigmentation.

     Pretreatment with a UVB sunscreen without 5-MOP plus SSR
did not offer any photoprotection (Table 2). This is not
surprising as this protocol resulted in minimal increases in
skin pigmentation and number of stratum corneum layers.
However, pretreatment with SSR alone (Table 1) offered minimal
photoprotection despite increases of skin pigmentation and
number of stratum corneum layers which, in general, were
comparable to those that were obtained with the 5-MOP
protocols.

     These data indicate qualitative differences between the
SSR alone and the 5-MOP plus SSR groups, despite the
morphological similarities in tanning and stratum corneum
thickening that were observed in skin type II. These
differences may be in melaninization itself or other unrelated
biochemical processes that may be important in
photoprotection. The photoprotection obtained with 5-MOP in
the 4 skin type I volunteers was the same as that observed in
the skin type II subjects. The increase in pigmentation seen
in this group (Type I) after 5-MOP pretreatment was minimal
(other unpublished studies have shown 5-MOP induced tanning in
skin type I under different conditions). Thus, the type I
data, along with the discrepancy between pigmentation (with
SSR alone and 5-MOP plus SSR) and photoprotection in skin type
II suggest that induced pigmentation per se may not be the
determining factor in photoprotection. In addition, there
appears to be a relationship between 5-MOP dose and
photoprotection but not with increase in pigmentation (Table
4). The skin type III, IV and V subjects also showed good
photoprotection with the 5-MOP pretreatments but unlike the

other skin types also showed photoprotection with SSR alone pretreatment.

Gange et al. (1985) reported that both a UVA- and a UVB-induced tan offered about a 45% reduction in UVB-induced (1 MED with well defined margins) DNA damage as measured by endonuclease sensitive sites. The authors did not define skin type but stated that the subjects were Caucasian with good ability to tan. We conclude that these subjects were probably skin type III (or more), and that these data are in good agreement with our skin type III plus subjects whose tan was obtained by SSR alone.

The time of onset of photoprotection (Table 5) appears to be about 5-8 days in skin type II and there is some evidence this it will last for up to 3 months (Table 7). However, re-exposure, at this time, of a site previously treated with 5-MOP plus SSR to SSR alone for one week results in enhanced photoprotection which was not observed in the sites previously treated with SSR alone.

Any discussion on the use of 5-MOP containing sunscreens must acknowledge that, in the presence of UVA, 5-MOP is a potent mutagen (Ashwood-Smith et al., 1980) and a carcinogen in albino mouse skin (Zajdela and Bisagni, 1981; Young et al., 1983). Based on these studies, the use of 5-MOP in sunscreens has been taken to present a potentially enhanced risk of cancer in human skin. However, photocarcinogenicity of 5-MOP is significantly inhibited if UVB sunscreens are also present (Young et al., 1987). Thus, the risk associated with the use of 5-MOP in sunscreen preparations containing UVB filters is considerably lower than was previously estimated on data obtained with 5-MOP without UVB filters.

If a tan is the desired objective of a holiday it may be achieved by several means. Sunbathing without any sunscreen protection carries the risk of a sunburn and substantial DNA damage, especially in skin types I and II. The use of low SPF UVB sunscreens will allow a longer period in the sun but may not, unless carefully used, prevent sunburn or DNA damage. The use of effective high SPF (eg > 15) UVB sunscreens will prevent sunburn and, in all probability, reduce DNA damage but the desired tan may not be achieved in a reasonable time. Any tan obtained by such sunscreens is likely to have been partly induced by solar UVA. Recent data have shown that UVA is a skin carcinogen in mice and it has been noted that the UVB-UVA action spectra for human tanning and mouse skin photo-carcinogenesis are similar (Roza et al, 1989). Thus, a UVA tan, whether obtained by sunlight or a sunbed, is likely to carry a risk similar to that of a UVB tan. Our data indicate that the judicious use of 5-MOP-containing sunscreens is a further option. This approach has the advantage of offering protection against DNA damage induced by sunlight which was not noted with the other options except in skin type III plus. Our data also indicate that after use of 5-MOP containing sunscreens, type II skin behaves more like type III plus in response to solar ultraviolet radiation.

It is likely that obtaining a tan by whatever means enhances the risk of a skin cancer. Current knowledge does not allow us to predict with assurance the safest way of

obtaining a tan. We believe that our data show that the use
of 5-MOP containing sunscreens offers potential benefits which
may outweight potential risks. Our data also indicate that the
use of susncreens with UVB filters alone is not necessarily
safer than the use of UVB sunscreens containing 5-MOP.
However, quantitative risk/benefit analysis cannot be
undertaken without a considerable amount of further research.

ACKNOWLEDGMENTS

This work was supported by a grant from Laboratoires
Bergaderm SA, France. We thank John Havlin, Pam Elliot and
Judith Kinley for excellent technical assistance.

REFERENCES

Ashwood-Smith, M.J., Poulton, G.A., Barker, M. and
      Mildenberger, M., 1980, 5-methoxypsoralen, an
      ingredient in several suntan preparations, has lethal,
      mutagenic and clastogenic properties, Nature, 285:407.
Cripps, D.J., 1981, Natural and artificial photoprotection, J.
      Invest. Derm., 76:154.
D'Ambrosio, S.M., Slazinski, L., Whetstone J.W., and Lowney,
      E. 1981, Excision repair of UV-induced pyrimidine
      dimers in human skin in vivo, J Invest. Derm., 77:311.
Gange, R.W., Blackett, A.D., Matzinger, E.A. Sutherland, B.M.,
      and Kochevar, I.E. 1985, Comparative protection
      efficiency of UVA-and UVB-induced tans against erythema
      and formation of endonuclease-sensitive sites in DNA by
      UVB in human skin, J. Invest. Derm., 85:352.
Gschnait, F., Brenner, W., and Wolf, K., 1978, Photoprotective
      effect of a psoralen-UVA-induced tan, Arch. Dermatol.
      Res., 263:181.
Hönigsmann, H., Brenner, W., Tanew, A., and Ortel, B., 1987,
      UV-induced unscheduled DNA synthesis in human skin:
      Dose response, correlation with erythema, time course,
      and split dose exposure in vivo, J. Photochem.
      Photobiol. (Section B.) 1:33.
MacKie, R.M., Elwood J.M., and Hawk, J.L.M., 1987, Links
      between exposure to ultraviolet radiation and skin
      cancer, A Report of the Royal College of Physicians,
      J.Royal Coll. Phys., 21(2):1.
Potten, C.S. 1987, Possible defects in the proliferative
      organization and control mechanisms in psoriasis, in:
      "Proceedings of 4th International Symposium on
      Psoriasis, 1986 at Stanford University, California",
      Elsevier, New York.
Potten, C.S., Chadwick, C.A., Young, A.R., Murphy, G.M., and
      Cohen, A.J., 1989, A 5-methoxypsoralen-induced tan
      protects against DNA damage from a subsequent exposure
      to solar simulated radiation in human skin, in
      "Psoralens; Photochemoprotection and Other Biological
      Activities", T.B Fitzpatrick, P. Forlot, MA Pathak,
      and F Urbach, eds., John Libbey Eurotext, Paris.
Roza, L., Baan, R.A., van der Leun, J.C., and Kligman, L.,
      1989, UVA hazards in skin associated with the use of
      tanning equipment, J. Photochem. Photobiol.
      (Section B.) 3:281.
Sambuco, C.P., Forbes, P.D.,Davies, D.E., and Urbach, F.,

1987, Protective value of skin tanning induced by ultraviolet radiation plus a sunscreen containing bergamot oil, J. Soc. Cosmet. Chem., 38:11.

van der Leun, J.C., 1988, Ozone depletion and skin cancer, J. Photochem. Photobiol. (Section B), 1:493.

Young, A.R., Magnus, I.A., Davies, A.C., and Smith, N.P., 1983, A comparison of the phototumorigenic potential of 8-MOP and 5-MOP in hairless albino mice exposed to solar simulated radiation, Br. J. Derm., 108:507.

Young, A.R., Potten, C.S., Chadwick, C.A., Murphy, G.M., and Cohen. A.J., 1988, Inhibition of UV radiation-induced DNA damage by a 5-methoxypsoralen tan in human skin, Pig. Cell. Res., 1:350.

Zajelda, R., and Bisagni, E., 1981, 5-Methoxypsoralen, the melanogenic additive in sun-tan preparations, is tumorigenic in mice exposed to 365 nm u.v. radiation, Carcinogenesis, 2:121.

VARIABILITY IN DNA REPAIR IN HUMAN SKIN

Steven E. Freeman

Lovelace Medical Foundation

Albuquerque, NM

INTRODUCTION

Solar UV-Induced DNA Damage and Skin Cancer

Ultraviolet radiation (UV) from sunlight is the major etiologic factor in the genesis of skin cancer. For squamous and basal cell carcinoma, the correlation of rates of incidence with latitude and, presumbably, solar exposure (Scotto, 1986), occurence on sun-exposed body regions (Scotto, 1986) and higher incidence in individuals who spend more time outdoors (Urbach et al., 1972) point to the sun as a major etiologic agent. For melanoma, there is a good correlation of rates of mortality with latitude (Mason and Mckay, 1974). However, the relationship between solar UV radiation exposure and cutaneous melanoma is not simple (Sober, 1987).

A number of observations support the hypothesis that DNA damage by UV is the initiating signal for the induction of cancer. Identification of the photoproducts involved in UV-carcinogenesis comes from experiments on in vitro transformation of Syrian hamster embryo cells (Doniger et al., 1981) and human and embryonic skin and muscle fibroblasts (Sutherland et al., 1980; Sutherland et al., 1981). These studies suggest a causal relationship between cell transformation and UV-induction of DNA damage and the action spectra for these events were similar.

UV-Induced Pyrimidine Dimers in Human Skin

One significant UV-induced lesion is the cyclobutyl pyrimidine dimer formed between adjacent pyrimidines on the same DNA strand (Beukers and Berends, 1960). Pyrimidine dimers alter the biologic function of DNA and are a major cause of tumorigenic events in cells (Setlow and Hart, 1975; Hart et al., 1977; Ley et al., 1988).

Until recently, techniques were not available to measure DNA damage in small amounts of non-radioactive DNA (e.g. biopsies of human skin). Recently, however, alkaline agarose gel electrophoresis has provided a useful means of quantitating DNA damage in human skin irradiated with UV in situ. Gel electrophoresis in alkaline agarose disperses single-stranded DNA according to its molecular length (McDonnel et al., 1977). Achey et al. (1979) used alkaline agarose gel electrophoresis to detect

DNA Damage and Repair in Human Tissues
Edited by B. M. Sutherland and A. D. Woodhead
Plenum Press, New York, 1990

117

single-strand breaks induced at pyrimidine dimers by <u>Micrococcus luteus</u> UV endonuclease, and Sutherland and Shih (1983) improved the technique to quantitate such breaks. Sutherland et al. (1984) developed a computer-controlled scanner to quantitate rapidly the fluorescence of DNA on photographs of gels; this development has led to generalized methods of quantitating single-strand breaks in DNA by alkaline agarose gel electrophoresis (Freeman et al., 1986a; Freeman and Thompson, 1988). Futhermore, the sensitivity of this technique has been enhanced by the ability to image fluorescent gels with a charge coupled device (CCD) video camera (Sutherland et al., 1987a; Freeman and Thompson, 1989) and by better separation of DNA using pulsed field gel electrophoresis (Sutherland et al., 1987b).

Repair of Pyrimidine Dimers in Human Skin DNA

The alkaline agarose gel electrophoresis technique has been determined to be useful in the detection of dimers (Sutherland et al., 1980), the quantitation of the initial number of dimers (Sutherland and Shih, 1983; Gange et al. 1985; Freeman et al. 1986a; Freeman et al. 1986b; Freeman et al. 1987) and in assessment of repair (Sutherland et al. 1980b; Freeman, 1988) of pyrimidine dimers in human skin DNA. However, there is significant inter-individual variability in repair of UV-induced pyrimidine dimers in human skin (Freeman, 1987). Variability in initial dimer yields may be the cause of variability in observed repair kinetics.

MATERIALS AND METHODS

Selection of Volunteers

Volunteers were chosen based on their sunburn and tanning response and were characterized as either very sensitive (burn easily and do not tan - skin type I) or relatively insensitive (burn minimally and tan easily - skin type IV) (Pathak, 1985). Eight volunteers from whom informed consent was obtained were employed for this study.

Irradiation of Human Skin

Untanned gluteal skin sites were exposed to UV radiation from a 2500 W Hanovia high pressure Hg/Xe lamp in conjunction with a quarter-meter, diffraction-grating monochromator (Kratos Analytical Instruments, Inc.). The monochromator was set to deliver narrow bandwidth radiation centered at either 280, 297, 302, 313, or 334 nm. Ultraviolet radiation exiting the monochromator was filtered with Schott glass filters (Schott Glass Technologies, Inc., Duryea, Penn.) to reduce any scattered light of shorter wavelengths.

Dose rates were determined with an Optronic Model 742 spectroradiometer (Optronic Laboratories Inc., Orlando, FL). The dose rates were 40, 30, 20, 140, 260, and 170 W/m^2.

Exposures for each subject were chosen on the basis of the subject's minimal erythema dose (MED) at each wavelength. Minimal erythema doses were determined by exposing nine 1 cm^2 sites to a graduated series of UV doses, increasing geometrically by 25%. The MED was identified as the lowest exposure that induced uniform pinkness filling an exposure site with well-defined margins at twenty-four hours after irradiation.

Separate untanned gluteal skin sites (1 cm^2) were then exposed to at least two different exposures of UV in multiples of the MED (1/2, 1, 2, or 4 MED). After intradermal injection of 0.1 ml of 1% lidocaine, superficial shave biopsies (4 mm diameter) were excised immediately after irradiation using a number 11 sterile surgical scalpel. Individual biopsies were immediately immersed in 1.0 ml cold 0.25% trypsin (Difco) in phosphate-buffered saline (0.15 M NaCl, 0.01 M sodium phosphate buffer, pH 7.3) and incubated on ice in the dark for 12-24 h.

DNA Preparation

The epidermis was separated from the underlying dermis by gentle scraping and homogenized in a glass/glass micro-tissue grinder. Epidermal cells were then resuspended in a Tris buffer (0.05 M Tris, pH 8.0, 0.01 M EDTA, 0.04 M NaCl) and the cells were lysed by the addition of 75 μl of a 10% (w/v) solution of sodium dodecyl sulfate. Cells were incubated for 5 min at 55°C, then 10 μl of RNAse (10mg/ml) (Calbiochem, La Jolla, CA) was added and incubation continued for 30 min at 37°C. Twenty-five μl of proteinase K (10 mg/ml) was added to the solution, and incubation continued for 30 min at 37°C. High molecular weight DNA was then isolated (Gange et al., 1985) and the concentration determined with a spectrofluorometer (Hoefer Scientific Instruments, San Francisco, CA).

Aliquots of DNA (40-60 ng) were treated with M. luteus UV endonuclease (Carrier and Setlow, 1970) at sufficient concentrations to cleave quantitatively at pyrimidine dimer sites, while companion samples were incubated without endonuclease. Each DNA sample was denatured by treatment with alkali, added to one well of a .4% alkaline agarose gel. Samples were electrophoresed in a buffer of 2 mM EDTA and 30 mM NaOH for 2 h at 40V in a BioRad minigel (BioRAd, Richmond, CA) apparatus. Molecular length standards (bacteriophage DNA from: T4, 164 kb; T7, 40 kb; and a HindIII digest of λ DNA, 23, 9.4, 6.6, 4.4, and 2.3 kb respectively) were included in each gel. The gel was neutralized (0.1 M Tris, pH 8.0, 30 min), stained with ethidium bromide (1 μg/ml) in distilled water for 10 min and destained in distilled water for 1 h.

Video densitometry

The fluorescence of DNA in the gel was recorded with a monochrome CCD video camera (Model CAM5000, Fairchild Weston-Schlumberger, Sunyvale, CA). Video output from the camera is in the form of a standard RS-170A signal for 525 lines at a frame rate of 30 Hz. The sense head of the camera contains a 488 x 380 element CCD. The die temperature of the CCD is reduced about 20°C below ambient by a Peltier-effect thermo-electric cooler in the sense head. Cooling reduces the random temporal noise content in the signal output of the sensor and also reduces dark current non-uniformity or pixel pattern noise content of the sensor signal. Dry ice (CO$_2$) is packed around the sense head which is mounted in a fabricated plexiglass housing to further reduce sensor temperature.

Light input into the camera is transmitted through a 1 mm Schott KG-2 optical glass filter (Schott Glass Technologies, Inc., Duryea, Penn.) to give the camera a spectral sensitivity curve that is maximal for the 590 nm fluorescent wavelength of ethidium bromide-stained DNA.

A Fujinon CF25B 25 mm TV lens (Fuji Photo Optical Co., Japan) and a Cosimicar 5 mm extension tube (Cosimicar Lens Division, Asahi Precision Co., Japan) are attached to the sense head in order to use optically the field-of-view (FOV) within focal length restrictions. It is desireable to fill the available FOV with the image in order to maximize spatial resolution.

Frame Grabber and Computer

The monochrome RS-170A video signal from the camera is processed with a DT2651 high resolution frame grabber (Data Translation, Inc., Marlboro, MA). The DT2651 is a 512 x 512 x 8-bit frame grabber that processes digital images in real time at a rate of 30 frames per second. The frame grabber is interfaced on the Q-bus of a Microvax II microcomputer (Digital Equipment Corporation). The video image is digitized by the frame grabber and the image displayed at a resolution of 512 x 480 pixels on an ECM1912 high resolution color monitor (Electrohome, Kitchener, Ontario, Canada). The displayed image can be stored on magnetic disk or tape for later analysis.

Analysis of Video Images to Determine Pyrimidine Dimers

DNA fluorescence of the video acquired image is determined by superimposing movable cursors over the gel image displayed on the high resolution monitor at the lateral boundaries of the DNA fluorescence for a given lane and then computed by averaging the pixel values across the lane. We have shown that the CCD camera responds linearly to the amount of fluorescent light reaching the sense head, thus image intensity in a region containing DNA is a direct reflection of the amount of DNA within the region. Average pixel values are digitized with the frame grabber (8 bits), normalized and stored for later analysis (Freeman and Thompson 1988; Freeman and Thompson 1989).

The number-average molecular lengths, in 10^3 bases, for the UV endonuclease-treated and untreated samples were determined from analysis of the DNA digitization profiles (Freeman et al. 1988). The frequency of UV-endonuclease sensitive sites (ESS) (i.e. pyrimidine dimers) was calculated from these data (Freeman et al., 1986; Sutherland et al., 1987b; Freeman and Thompson, 1988; Freeman and Thompson, 1989).

RESULTS AND DISCUSSION

DNA Repair and Tumorigenesis

If one accepts the evidence that DNA damage (i.e pyrimidine dimers) leads to specific mutagenic events that may be carcinogenic, it follows that the ability of an individual to repair UV-induced DNA damage may influence that person's susceptibility to skin cancer. Studies on DNA repair properties of fibroblasts from cancer-prone xeroderma pigmentosum (XP) patients, indicate that depressed levels of DNA repair may responsible for the extreme sensitivity of these people to UV-induced skin cancer (Cleaver, 1983). However, the specific lesion involved is not known because XP cells are deficient in the repair of a wide range of DNA defects (Cleaver et al., 1987; Mitchell et al. 1985).

Cells from people with XP have been found to be defective in DNA repair as demonstrated by an inability to perform unscheduled DNA synthesis (UDS) (Cleaver, 1968). Since UDS has been shown to represent the polymerization step in excision repair of UV-induced DNA damage, a defect in such repair can thus be linked with a high risk of cancer from an environmental agent, i.e. sunlight. Is it possible that even in a so-called 'normal' population there might be subtle deficiencies in DNA repair that lead to an increased probability of carcinogenesis? One way to address this question is to determine the relative abilities of different members of the population to repair UV-induced DNA damage.

DNA Repair Estimates in Human Skin In Situ

A significant amount of variability was detected in people when UV-induced DNA repair was measured in skin irradiated in situ (Freeman, 1988). The average half-life for removal of pyrimidine dimers was 11.0 ($\pm$4.3) hours. However, there was significant inter-individual variability as evidenced by a 38% coefficient of variation. D'Ambrosio et al. (1981) found the rate of repair of UV-induced pyrimidine dimers in human skin to be much faster, with approximately 50% of the dimers removed in 58 min. Still, when the rate of removal among individuals is compared, the variability is quite large. Bruze et al. (1989) recently reported on repair of UV- induced DNA damage in human skin in situ using an antibody to detect pyrimidine dimers. They determined that an average of 80 $\pm$14% of the pyrimidine dimers were removed in 4 h.

Could the initial dimer levels influence the relative rate of repair? The results presented in Table 1 show that the average number of dimers at an erythemogenic dose of UV was .05 per 10^3 bases. However, the range of values was .024 to .072 per 10^3 bases, i.e. a 3.5 fold difference. The initial number of dimers ranged from 5.4 to 9.5 per 10^8 daltons (.018 to .031 per 10^3 bases) in the experiments of D'Ambrosio et al., (1981) and .06 to .45 per 10^3 bases in the experiments of Bruze et al., (1989). Although the number of volunteers in these studies was not sufficient to determine whether initial dimer yields affected the kinetics of repair, these studies did show that there is a wide variation in initial yields, with attendant variability in repair kinetics.

Variability in Initial Dimer Yields With Different UV Sources

We have shown that pyrimidine dimer yields vary with skin type, when people are exposed to a broadband UVB (290-320 nm) source. People of skin type I (sun sensitive) have greater yields than people of skin type IV (sun insensitive) (Freeman et al., 1986b). In addition, we find that the dimer yield correlates with the minimal erythema dose (MED).

When UV exposures are given in increments of the MED, we find that dimer yields are more consistent from person to person. This was the case when we recently determined an action spectrum for the frequency of pyrimidine dimer formation induced in the DNA of human skin per unit dose of monochromatic UV incident on the skin surface (Freeman et al., 1989). The skin types of the volunteers used this study were II (very sensitive, tan minimally with difficulty) and III (sensitive, tan gradually).

Action Spectrum for People of Skin Type I or IV

Determination of an action spectrum for pyrimidine dimer formation in DNA of the skin of people of different skin types requires measurement of dose-response curves for damage production in different volunteers over a wide wavelength range. To ensure that all exposures were in a biologically relevant range and induce similar dimer yields, we determined each person's MED for a particular wavelength. Then, volunteers were irradiated with increments of the MED, epidermal biopsies taken, the DNA was extracted and treated with UV endonuclease, and the number of pyrimidine dimers was determined from analysis of agarose gels. The dimer induction efficiencies (slopes of the lines relating dimer yield to UV exposure) were determined. The dimer induction efficiencies DIMERS/GENOME per photon/cm^2 for 280, 289, 297, 302, 313, and 334 nm for volunteers of skin type I or IV are shown in Figure 1.

This action spectrum is similar to the one generated for skin types II and III (Freeman et al., 1989) in that it varies over three orders of magnitude with a maximum around 302 nm. However the dimer yields for skin type I are consistently greater than for type IV.

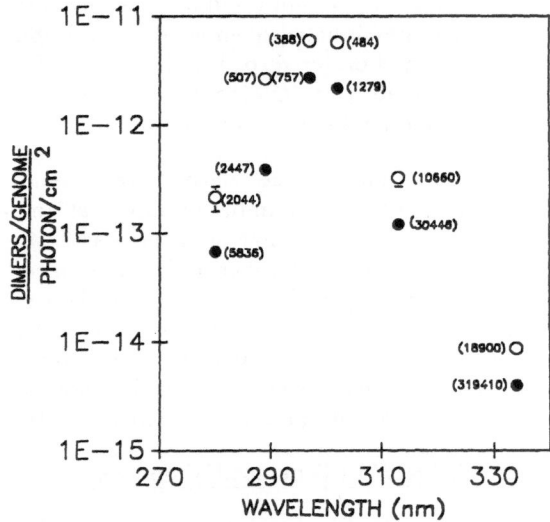

Fig. 1. Action spectrum for pyrimidine dimer formation in human skin for persons of skin type I (○) and skin type IV (●). Each point in the action spectrum represents the slope of the dose-response line for one volunteer at one wavelength, obtained from duplicate independent determinations. The error bars represent standard errors of the slopes. The numbers in parenthesis are the MEDs in J/m^2.

CONCLUSIONS

Due to the ease of dosimetry in a single layer of cells, initial dimer yields can be held fairly constant and thus, the extent of variability in DNA repair measurements using cells in vitro can be reduced. Since human skin has multiple cell layers, the dosimetry is much more complicated and thus adds to variability in intial dimer yields.

If we assume that enzymatic removal of pyrimidine dimers follows first order kinetics, then initial dimer yields should not affect the kinetics of removal (Roberts, 1977). However, this assumption holds true only if the concentration of pyrimidine dimers is much greater than the number of repair enzyme complexes. Since, we can only measure the number of pyridine dimers in this assay and we do not know the concentration of repair enzyme complexes, the proper manner for analysis of the kinetics of repair of pyrimidine dimers is to compare the kinetics of removal of dimers based on the same initial yield of dimers.

REFERENCES

Achey, P. M., Woodhead, A. D. and Setlow, R. B., 1979, Photoreactivation of pyrimidine dimers in DNA from thyroid cells of the teleost, Poecilia formosa, Photochem. Photobiol., 29:305.

Beukers, R. and Berends, W., 1960, Isolation and identification of the irradiation product of thymine, Biochim. Biophys. Acta.,41:550.

Bruze, M. Emmett, E. A., Creasey, J. and Strickland, P. T., 1989, Cyclobuta-Dithymidine induction by solar-simulating UV radiation in human skin: II. individual responses, J. Invest. Dermatol.,93:341.

Carrier, W. L. and Setlow, R. B., 1970, An endonuclease from Micrococcus luteus which has activity toward ultraviolet-irradiated deoxyribonucleic acid: Purification and properties, J. Bacteriology., 102:178.

Cleaver, J. E., 1968, Defective repair replication of DNA in xeroderma pigmentosum, Nature.,218:652.

Cleaver, J. E., 1983, Xeroderma pigmentosum, in "The Metabolic Basis of Inherited Disease, 5th edition," J. B. Stanbury, J. B. Wyngaarden, and D. S. Frederickson, ed., McGraw Hill, New York.

D'Ambrosio, S. M., Slazinski, L. M., Whetstone, J. W. and Lowney, E., 1981, Excision repair of uv-induced pyrimidine dimers in human skin in vivo, J. Invest. Dermatol.,77:311.

Doniger, J., Jacobson, E. D., Drell, K. and DiPaolo, J. A., 1981, Ultraviolet light action spectra for neoplastic transformation and lethality of Syrian hamster embryo cells correlate with the spectrum for pyrimidine dimer formation in cellular DNA, Proc. Natl. Acad. Aci. USA., 78:2378.

Freeman, S. E., 1988, Variations in excision repair of uvb-induced pyrimidine dimers in DNA of human skin in situ, J. Invest. Dermatol., 90:814.

Freeman, S. E., Blackett, A. D., Monteleone, D. C., Setlow, R. B., Sutherland, B. M. and Sutherland, J. C., 1986a, Quantitation of radiation-, chemical-, or enzyme-induced single strand breaks in nonradioactive DNA by alkaline gel electrophoresis: Application to pyrimidine dimers, Anal. Biochem. 158:119.

Freeman, S. E., Gange, R. W., Matzinger, E. A. and Sutherland, B. M., 1986b, Higher pyrimidine dimer yields in skin of normal humans with higher uvb sensitivity, J.Invest. Dermatol., 86:34.

Freeman, S. E., Gange, R. W., Matzinger, E. A., Sutherland, B. M. and Sutherland, J. C., 1987, Production of pyrimidine dimers in DNA of human skin exposed to uva radiation, J. Invest. Dermatol., 88:430.

Freeman, S. E., Hacham, H., Gange, R. W., Maytum, D. J., Sutherland, J. C. and Sutherland, B. M., 1989, Wavelength dependence of pyrimidine dimer formation in DNA of human skin irradiated in situ with ultraviolet light, Proc. Natl. Acad. Sci. USA., 86:5605.

Freeman, S. E. and Thompson, B. D., 1988, Evaluation of densitometry data using interactive computer graphics: Application to DNA agarose gels, Int. J. Biomedical Computing., 22:121.

Freeman, S. E., and Thompson, B. D., 1989, Comparative analysis of video and photographic densitometry: Quantitation of UV induced cyclobutyl pyrimidine dimers in DNA, Anal. Biochem., (In press).

Gange, R. W., Blackett, A. D., Matzinger, E. A., Sutherland, B. M. and Kochevar, I. E., 1985, Comparative efficiency of uva and uvb-induced tans against erythema and formation of endonuclease-sensitive sites in DNA by uvb in human skin, J. Invest. Dermatol., 85:362.

Hart, R. W., Setlow, R. B. and Woodhead, A. D., 1977, Evidence that pyrimidine dimers in DNA can give rise to tumors, Proc. Natl. Acad. Sci. USA., 75:5574.

Ley, R. D. Applegate, L. A., Fry, R. J. M. and Stuart T. D., 1988, UVA/Visible light suppression of ultraviolet radiation-induced skin and eye tumors of the marsupial Monodelphis domestica, Photochem. Photobiol.,47:45s.

Mason, T. J. and McKay, F. W., 1974, U.S. Cancer Mortality by County: 1950-1969 (U.S. Government Printing Office, Washington, DC) DHEW Pub. No. NIH 74-615.

McDonell, M., Simon, M. N. and Studier, F. W., 1977, Analysis of restriction fragments of T7 DNA and determinations of molecular weights by electrophoresis of neutral and alkaline gels, J. Mol. Biol., 110:119.

Mitchell, D. L., Haieh, C. A. and Clarkson, J. M., 1985, (6-4) Photoproducts are removed from the DNA of uv-irradiated mammalian cells more efficiently than cyclobutane pyrimidine dimers, Mutation Res., 143:109.

Pathak, M. A., 1985, Activation of the melanocyte system by ultraviolet radiation and cell transformation, in "The Medical and Biological Effects of Light, "R. Wurtman, M. Baum and J. Potts, Jr., ed., Ann. N. Y. Acad. of Sci.,Vol. 453, New York.

Roberts, D. V., 1977, "Enzyme Kinetics," Cambridge University Press,Cambridge.

Scotto, J., 1986, "Effects of Changes in Stratospheric Ozone and Global Climate", U.S. Environmental Protection Agency, Washington, D.C.

Setlow, R. B., Carrier, W. L. and Stewart, J., 1975, Endonuclease sensitive sites in uv-irradiated DNA, Biophs. J., 15:194a.

Sober, A. J., 1987, Solar exposure in the etiology of cutaneous melanoma. Photodermatol., 4:23.

Sutherland, B. M., Harber, L. C., Kochevar, I. E., 1980b,Pyrimidine dimer formation and repair in human skin, Cancer Res. 40:3181.

Sutherland, B. M. and Shih, A. G.1983, Quantitation of pyrimidine dimer content of non-radioactive deoxyribonucleic acid by electrophoresis in alkaline agarose gels, Biochemistry., 22:745.

Sutherland, J. C., Lin, B., Monteleone, D. C., Mugavero, J. H., Sutherland, B. M. and Trunk, J., 1987a, Electronic imaging for direct and rapid quantitation of fluorescence from electro phoretic gels: Application to ethidium bromide-stained DNA, Anal. Biochem., 163:446.

Sutherland, J. C., Monteleone, D. C., Mugavero, J. H. and Trunk, J. 1987b, Unidirectional pulsed-field electrophoresis of single- and double-stranded DNA in agarose gels: Analytical expressions relating mobility and molecular length and their application in the measurement of strand breaks, Anal. Biochem., 162:511.

Sutherland, J. C., Monteleone, D. C., Trunk, J. and Ciarrocchi, G., 1984, Two-dimensional, computer controlled film scanner: Quantitation of fluorescence from ethidium bromide-stained DNA gels, Anal. Biochem., 139:390.

Urbach, F., Rose, D. B. and Bonnem, M., 1972, "Environment and Cancer: A Collection of Papers," Williams and Wilkins, Baltimore.

EFFECTS OF CHEMICALS ON PHOTOBIOLOGIC REACTIONS OF SKIN

R. E. Davies, P. D. Forbes, and F. Urbach

The Center for Photobiology at Argus, Inc.[*]
905 Sheehy Drive
Horsham, PA 19044

INTRODUCTION

Human attitudes toward sunlight are equivocal. Almost everyone
experiences psychological, and possibly physical benefits from exposure
to the sun.   In contrast, most people recognize an imminent danger of
overexposure, with painful and, occasionally, serious consequences.

Sunlight is the most ubiquitous of environmental carcinogens. That
it is not also the most threatening is the result of two factors; its
carcinogenic efficacy is relatively low, and its biological consequences
are tolerable. Nevertheless, exposure to sunlight causes more human
cancer than any other single hazard, and the resulting economic and
emotional costs are substantial.

It has long been realized that some chemical agents can alter the
biological effects of sunlight exposure. Phototoxicity is sufficiently
well known that testing for this hazard is a routine part of toxicology.
Photoallergy, less well understood, is nevertheless recognized as a
possible and serious adverse effect. Much less understood, and the
subject of far less investigation, is the possibility of chemical contributions to long-term photobiological hazards. The most recognized,
and the most easily measurable of these hazards is photocarcinogenesis.
It is now known that several chemical agents can modify this process.
While the possible importance of such modification is difficult to
predict, exacerbation of an already significant health problem is a
serious concern.

It is possible to test the ability of chemicals to alter photocarcinogenesis, using available and documented animal test systems
(Epstein, 1977; Forbes et al., 1985; Urbach et al., 1988). Such testing
is difficult and expensive, however, and there are legitimate questions
about its proper place in the growing library of toxicologic procedures.
One such question, common to all model testing systems, concerns its
predictive relevance to human experience. A second question concerns
the possibility of substituting simpler models or in vitro procedures

---

[*]Formerly at The Skin and Cancer Hospital, Temple University,
Philadelphia, PA.

DNA Damage and Repair in Human Tissues
Edited by B M. Sutherland and A. D. Woodhead
Plenum Press, New York, 1990

for the prolonged and expensive animal tests. The most immediate concern for product developers involves the criteria which would make a particular product a likely candidate for this type of testing. Answers to these questions will come slowly, and will be influenced in unpredictable ways by such non-scientific factors as product liability law, regulatory decisions, and animal welfare legislation.

From the scientific viewpoint, the ability of chemicals to modify photocarcinogenesis is a challenging puzzle which our group has been examining for many years. A particular interest has been the development and standardization of quantitative animal models. One outgrowth of this type of investigation was the creation of "general-purpose" safety tests, which avoid the need for prior assumptions concerning the possible mechanisms of enhancement (Forbes et al., 1989).

An agent which enhances the photocarcinogenic process could do so by one of several types of mechanisms. If we limit the discussion to agents which exhibit no independent carcinogenicity, we can assume that the observed acceleration is not an artefact of separate processes generating separate but indistinguishable endpoints. What we are observing, then, is more "efficient" utilization of a carcinogenic stimulus for production of the same endpoint. One possible grouping of mechanisms would assume that the photocarcinogenic process begins with one (or more) low-probability interaction between a photon and a susceptible target (chromophore). Any process which could increase the probability of such an interaction would be acting "optically" in the sense that it would be facilitating an optical encounter. A topical sunscreen or other absorber would decrease the probability of an interaction, per unit of topical radiation delivery, by decreasing the number of photons capable of participating. Any agent which altered the transmissivity of skin superficial to the presumed chromophore (generally assumed to be in the lower epidermis), whether through its own optical properties or its effects on cutaneous structure, would similarly alter the effective delivery of photons and thus the probability of an interaction. Similarly, any agent which could alter the optical cross-section of the chromophore, e.g. by altering the number, size, or distribution of chromophoric organelles, could alter the probability of an effective encounter. Finally any agent which could facilitate or "sensitize" the interactive process (or induce a different but similarly carcinogenic process) would be acting as an optical amplifier of effective encounters.

Once the hypothetical interaction(s) has taken place, a sequence of events must occur before it is recognizable as a "carcinogenic" process. Any agent which can influence this sequence will also be seen as modifying the rate of photocarcinogenesis. The classic example is the "promoter" of chemical carcinogenesis, which is considered to facilitate the expression of occult but irreversible genetic damage. Any agent, however, which favored the selective survival or development of an altered cell, or of a clone of such cells, could enhance the rate of carcinogenesis as judged from the appearance of visible lesions.

For each of these mechanisms, there may be several molecular species which could produce alterations. The agent itself could affect incoming radiation, or some optically significant aspect of cutaneous structure. Direct photoproducts of the agent, or photoproducts of combinations of the agent with normal cutaneous constituents, similarly could influence radiation transmission. An agent could sensitize or participate in photobiological processes which themselves lead to carcinogenesis, as is thought to occur with psoralens. Finally the agent, its photoproducts, or the consequences of photosensitized injury could contribute to the successful evolution of a presumptive photoinduced tumor.

The testing system we employ would not differentiate between effects based on changes in the probability of carcinogenic events and those based on changes in subsequent evolution. Similarly it would respond to effects induced by the primary agent, its photoproducts, or the consequences of photosensitized biological damage. We consider this lack of specificity as a virtue; the safety testing protocol is designed to detect any adverse change in the effectiveness of an inevitable environmental hazard.

The present animal model for detecting enhancement of photocarcinogenesis is predicated on the acceleration of a clearly photocarcinogenic event, the production of squamous cell carcinomas and their precursors. For photoinduction of other major forms of skin cancer there are no satisfactory experimental models, so presently there is no way of determining how chemical agents may affect their progress.

Basal cell carcinomas in humans are clearly related to sun exposure. They can be induced experimentally in rats by chemical carcinogens or ionizing radiation, but are not consistently produced by UVR. With respect to one known chemical enhancer, the best experimental evidence relating to basal cell carcinomas comes from humans. In the prospective study of the effect of PUVA therapy on tumor incidence, the observed increase in tumor frequency was apparently confined to squamous cell carcinomas (Stern, 1989).

Although it is widely believed that solar UV radiation plays a part in the production of cutaneous malignant melanoma, experimental evidence for a causal association is weak. To the extent that melanotic tumors (not usually melanomas) have been produced experimentally, UV has been, at most, an adjunct to known chemical carcinogens such as DMBA. The poor correlation between anatomic distribution of melanomas and of UV exposure further weakens arguments for a causal association. However, it is fairly clear that those genetic groups of humans most likely to exhibit cutaneous photodamage are also most likely to develop melanoma, and the presence of pigmented nevi may be the best morphologic predictor of individual susceptibility. Possibly UV may be a modifier rather than an inducer of melanomagenesis, and the concept of "chemical modification of photocarcinogenesis" may not usefully apply to this type of tumor.

Measurement Endpoints

A carcinogen is an agent capable of eliciting cancer, an end-point diagnostic term referring to a malignant growth. The biological steps leading up to the diagnosis of cancer, which are generally poorly understood, are included in the term carcinogenesis.

Identification of a carcinogen is based on demonstrated cancer-producing activity in biological assays. These are usually referred to as carcinogen assays; it is the end result (cancer) rather than the process (carcinogenesis) which is measured. The diagnostic term cancer is usually reserved for situations in which histologic examination reveals abnormal, reproducing cells fitting predefined morphologic criteria. While the presence of cancer confirms the fact that carcinogenesis has occurred, terminology is less clear when "precancerous" changes are observed. Such changes are acceptable evidence of carcinogenesis only if it can be assumed that cancer would have been observed if histologic examination had been delayed. While it may be possible to follow the evolution of a potential cancer by a series of biopsies, this is not usually done in carcinogen assays, primarily because of the uncertain effect of the biopsy procedure on subsequent development of the growth. Thus, the usual assay procedure is designed to detect, rather than to measure, the process of carcinogenesis.

In experimental photocarcinogenesis, induced in mice by chronic but non-traumatic irradiation, the gross morphologic stages of the process are well established. Localized thickening of exposed skin is expressed as multiple small, discrete, usually symmetrical elevations. These progress to "wart-like" growths with increasingly abnormal surfaces, frequently in the presence of apparently normal surrounding skin. As the number and size of lesions increase, neighboring lesions merge into larger and more bizarre forms. The rate of progression of individual growths is quite variable, although merged masses usually continue to evolve relatively rapidly. Provided that the radiation stimulus is continuous and non-destructive, very few lesions disappear other than by merger or by local skin ulceration which may occur adjacent to necrotizing masses. Similar evolutionary patterns can be induced with a fairly wide range of radiation dose rates, with the difference being the time at which any stage is reached.

The histologic pattern at any specific stage of lesion evolution is quite consistent. Seen in isolation, the stages vary widely in their levels of "malignancy," and the resulting terminology may imply an expected degree of further evolution. This can lead to statements regarding the relative frequency of "non-malignant", "pre-malignant", "possibly malignant", and "malignant" tumors, and these statements may be interpreted as evidence for or against "carcinogenicity" of the treatment conditions. Experience suggests, however, that it is the time of observation, rather than any fundamental difference in the nature of the ongoing process, which determines the observed histologic pattern. There does not appear to be a qualitative discontinuity in the ability of various radiation doses to induce the sequence of morphologic changes which are implied by the term "carcinogenesis."

If some chemicals are introduced into a system in which photocarcinogenesis is known (from prior experience) to be occurring, they may alter the rate of the process. This effect is often indistinguishable from that produced by altering the radiation dose rate; similar numbers, sizes and types of lesions are produced, but at an earlier or later time. Particularly if the chemical is not known to produce cancer in the absence of radiation, these changes can be thought of as effects on the radiation dose rate, either increases or decreases. For some chemicals such an interpretation is obviously correct; cosmetic sunscreens can decrease the amount of radiation reaching the skin, and would thus be expected to reduce photocarcinogenesis. Other chemicals such as psoralens, which are known to "amplify" biological effects of radiation, may similarly increase the carcinogenic efficacy of a radiation load. In other cases the mechanism clearly does not involve changes in radiation dose rate nor efficacy; acceleration of the photocarcinogenic process by retinoic acid or croton oil probably indicates changes in later stages of tumor evolution. Nevertheless if only the rate of change is altered, rather than the observable nature of the change, it is possible to describe the alteration quantitatively, by equating it to the change of radiation dose rate which would have produced a similar alteration. It is this fact, and the consistently reproducible relationship between radiation dose rate and tumor evolution, which provides the basis for the "modi-fication of photocarcinogenesis" safety assay. Because of the assumption that such chemicals influence the rate, rather than the existence, of photocarcinogenesis, we avoid such terms as "photocarcinogenic chemical" (Forbes et al., 1985). In the assay we employ, the process of photo-carcinogenesis is ensured, while changes in its rate are measured by the time required to reach a predetermined morphologic state. Unless there are qualitative (rather than quantitative) changes in morphologic evolution, the measurement of time to equivalent response is a reasonable approach to the assessment of safety and of protective efficacy.

Response Quantitation

The type of skin cancer most readily induced by light is squamous cell carcinoma. These tumors are "dose-dependent" in the sense that the magnitude of the carcinogenic response is related to the magnitude of the radiative insult. This generalization refers to each of several indices of carcinogenic response; an increase in radiation dose will increase the number of affected individuals in the exposed population, the number of tumors present on each individual, and both the size and the histologic abnormality of those tumors. Moreover, the time required to reach any specified level of each of these criteria will decrease with increasing radiation exposure. While these various criteria are clearly inter-related, it is not certain that they all measure the same aspects of the carcinogenic process, nor that they all will be equally affected by modi-fications of that process. It could be useful to employ all of them in comprehensive tests of the carcinogenic process. For a variety of technical reasons, however, some of the measures are mutually exclusive, while others are difficult to evaluate. To quantify a photocarcinogenic stimulus the most useful response parameter is the frequency of affected individuals in an exposed population, where the term "affected" has some reproducible threshold definition. The most useful quantitative descrip-tion of that response, for repetitive stimulus conditions, is the time required to achieve a specified response frequency. Under appropriately controlled conditions of exposure, the rate of response is a remarkably consistent indicator of the magnitude of a stimulus. Within-group variability of the relative response, moreover, is acceptably small and virtually independent of magnitude of the stimulus. As a consequence, alterations in the magnitude or effectiveness of a photocarcinogenic stimulus can be measured with a sensitivity which is unusually high by biological standards.

Acute Responses as Predictors of Enhancement

Obvious similarities between the processes of phototoxicity and enhancement of photocarcinogenesis, together with the observation that some chemical carcinogens are phototoxic, led to investigation of acute phototoxicity as a predictive tool. An interesting contrast in the relationship between acute and chronic photoprocesses is provided by comparing several photoactive materials. A number of methoxylated furocoumarins (psoralens) can elicit acute photodamage when administered either orally or topically (Tables 1 and 2). Many aromatic compounds, such as anthracene, also are capable of inducing such "phototoxic" responses when administered topically. (There is little information concerning oral photosensitization by these frequently toxic compounds.) In contrast, several porphyrins (including hematoporphyrin) are highly phototoxic when delivered orally, but have no apparent effect topically. Members of the phthalocyanine family are photochemically active, and several have exhibited phototoxic effects in isolated systems (Zhou, 1989). One highly water-soluble phthalocyanine (zinc phthalocyanine sulfonate; ZPS) is locally phototoxic when delivered to sites which are washed slowly (subcutaneously in mice) or passively (vascular systems of invertebrate animals or plants), and produces transient phototoxic sensitization when administered intravenously, but is ineffective when delivered topically or orally to mice (unpublished data).

Neither anthracene nor hematoporphyrin appears to induce carcinogenic changes or to modify photocarcinogenesis when delivered chronically under potentially phototoxic conditions. In contrast, phototoxic psoralens, delivered orally or topically, can induce carcinogenic changes which represent either a different carcinogenic process (photochemical carcino-genesis) or a striking enhancement of photocarcinogenesis. ZPS, delivered

Table 1. Study Design: Treatment Groups (Identified by
          Arabic Numeral) in the 8-MOP Study

Level of 8-MOP	0	100mg/kg	250mg/kg	625mg/kg
No UV-A	1	2	3	4
2J* UV-A	5	6	7	8

*UV-A: 2 J/cm^2 each exposure; F74BL PUVA lamps,
        window glass filter.
        Mice were fasted overnight and then given the drug via "pulse
        feeding" of special pellets on Monday, Wednesday, and Friday
        each week for a year, followed by exposure to UV-A.

either topically (Table 3) or orally, did not induce carcinogenesis nor
modify photocarcinogenesis. We do not know whether it would do so when
delivered under photoxically effective conditions, or whether other, less
rapidly cleared, phthalocyanines could induce phototoxicity or modify
photocarcinogenesis.

Not all chemicals which enhance photocarcinogenesis exhibit
phototoxicity. Croton oil, and its active promotional constituent
tetradecanoyl phorbol acetate, is well known to "promote" photocarcinogenic changes, and can accelerate carcinogenesis induced by chronic UV
exposure. Similarly, retinoic acid, which is not phototoxic and which
is quite photosensitive, can also accelerate photocarcinogenesis (Davies
and Forbes, 1988).

Acceleration of photocarcinogenesis by non-phototoxic agents such
as croton oil and retinoic acid, and lack of acceleration by phototoxic
materials such as anthracene and (probably) hematoporphryin, indicate that
acute photoactivity is neither necessary nor sufficient to produce effects
on chronic photoprocesses. In addition to eliminating a possible method
for safety screening, this lack of correlation leaves us with no obvious
basis for deciding whether a chemical is a likely candidate for safety
testing. The following list suggests categories of materials for which
such testing should be considered:

1. Agents, no matter how delivered, which have as a known or intended
    consequence the alteration of skin or its appendages. Such agents
    could alter either optical or regenerative properties of skin, either
    of which could modify the probability or consequences of carcinogenic
    interactions. (The possible effects of nutrients known to modify skin
    health are largely unexplored.)

2. Agents intended for topical application, whether or not radiation
    exposure is expected. This category would include a variety of
    topical therapeutics and many cosmetic agents. The potential for
    hazard is likely to be greater if the expected use is prolonged,
    as with agents intended to be used for prophylaxis.

3. Agents intended to be exposed to radiation, including protectants
    (topical sunscreens), tan enhancers and skin lubricants. The photo-
    chemical properties of such materials are frequently poorly under-
    stood, and possible photoproducts should be considered as potential
    hazards.

Table 2. Results (8-MOP Study)

Endpoint Measure[1]

Group	Weeks to 0.2 Preval	Weeks to 0.5 Preval	Maximum Preval[2]	Longevity
1	nd[3]	nd	0.06	normal
2	nd	nd	0.07	normal
3	nd	nd	0.08	normal
4	nd	nd	0.15	normal
5	nd	nd	0.13	normal
6	nd	nd	0.14	normal
7	65	nd	0.39	reduced
8	23	30	1.00	reduced

[1]Animals were considered "affected" when they had one or more skin neoplasms ("tumors") measuring at least 1mm in diameter.

[2]Preval = prevalence (proportion affected).

[3]nd   = not determined (i.e., > 80 weeks).

Only group 8 showed cutaneous toxicity; skin inflammation was noted after 20 weeks of exposure, with no resolution until the end of treatment. Neither the drug nor the ultraviolet radiation alone produced a significant difference in time to tumor appearance nor in animal survival time. At the two higher levels of drug the combination treatment was carcinogenic, and animal survival time was reduced.

4. Biologically active agents not necessarily intended for application to skin, but for which the skin can reasonably be expected to be a secondary target (domestic, industrial, or agricultural chemicals).

Regulation of Enhancers of Photocarcinogenesis

If a material is phototoxic, that fact alone is sufficient to limit the conditions under which it can be employed, or the benefits which could justify its use. Similar, but even more restrictive considerations apply to the use of any material which is a demonstrated carcinogen. However, the concept of "acceleration of photocarcinogenesis" by materials which do not exhibit independent carcinogenicity presents a dilemma. It is possible that the level of hazard associated with such materials is proportional not only to exposure to the material itself, but also to the severity of the primary (photo)carcinogenic stimulus. If this is true, an appropriate regulatory stance will be difficult to define. The least intrusive response would be a requirement that producers of such material acknowledge a potential hazard, and define measures which would minimize its impact.

Accidental and deliberate exposure to carcinogenic radiation are hazards whose consequences are dimly perceived and long delayed. There is an impression, supported by some advertising claims, that measures which reduce the danger of acute sun damage will similarly reduce the danger of chronic damage. The existence of agents which are not phototoxic, but which, nevertheless, accelerate photocarcinogenesis, is one

Table 3. ZPS Study Design and Tumor Response

deterg[*]	Level of ZPS In Bath (grams/liter)		
	0	0.12	1.20
0	(no bath) 56.8 wks	---	56.2 wks
1g/l	60.3 wks	56.1 wks	60.0 wks

[*]deterg = detergent (a model granular laundry product).

UVR: 95 Roberston-Berger (R-B) counts each exposure;
      xenon 6500 Watt long-arc lamp with Schott WG345 filter.

Mice in five treatments were exposed daily (Mon-Fri) to a
xenon arc solar simulator. Before each exposure, four groups
were bathed for 2 min in a test solution (contents indicated
in Table). The fifth group, as shown, was not bathed before
exposure to UVR.

Median latent period (time to reach 0.5 prevalence for tumors
at least 1mm in planar diameter): time in weeks (wks). ZPS
did not enhance photocarcinogenesis.

line of evidence against this conclusion. Prudence suggests that at
least for the period during which such agents are employed, there should
be a concurrent reduction in exposure to carcinogenic radiation; whether
this is an adequate defensive response cannot be stated with certainty.

Special consideration must be given to cosmetic sunscreens. These
substances have, as their stated reason for use, the ability to attenuate
damaging UV radiation. For most such materials, specific testing demonstrates their ability to prevent acute radiation damage. In a few cases,
long-term protection has been demonstrated (Wulf et al., 1982; Forbes et
al., 1989). An extrapolation, not usually supported by documentation, is
that protection will be similarly afforded, by all such products, against
long-term damage including photocarcinogenesis. There are several reasons
to question the general applicability of such statements. Sunscreens,
unlike most other topical agents, are expected to be exposed to substantial levels of UV radiation, yet there is surprisingly little information
concerning the photochemistry of sunscreen chromophores. Furthermore,
indices of quantitative acute protection are employed to indicate tolerable levels of sunlight exposure much greater than those which would
normally be encountered. If less or no protection is afforded against
chronic damage, however, the implementation of such suggestions could be
disastrous. The situation would be analogous to the effect of an enhancer
of photocarcinogenesis, except that reduction of sunlight exposure would
not be a reasonable prophylactic step. An alternative approach might be
to add another chromophore with demonstrated chronic protective efficacy,
to provide a product with comparable acute and chronic protection. If
the sunscreen or its photoproducts also enhanced photocarcinogenesis,
of course, this type of solution would no longer be applicable.

As we have suggested, the enhancement of photocarcinogenesis is a quantitative rather than a qualitative hazard. Each of us experiences some exposure to carcinogenic UV radiation, and can thus be assumed to be experiencing the process of photocarcinogenesis. In the absence of other changes, an enhancer of photocarcinogenesis will exaggerate this process. It is appropriate to consider this exaggeration in the context of other quantitative variables. Much attention has been given to the possible carcinogenic contribution of a reduction in stratospheric ozone. While the probability of ecologic damage from such a reduction cannot be overstated, the magnitude of likely carcinogenic changes has been over-emphasized. Even the gloomiest scenarios suggest radiation increases of a few tens of percents, and relative carcinogenesis increases about twice as high. Some enhancers of photocarcinogenesis, in contrast, can amplify the carcinogenic efficacy of UV radiation by orders of magnitude. Conversely, relatively minor behavioral changes can reduce the carcino-genic hazard of environmental exposure by equally dramatic amounts. The fact that ozone changes would lead to inevitable and involuntary increases in the potential hazard level is an important consideration, but cannot justify overstatement of the problem.

If a chemical is known to enhance photocarcinogenesis, steps can be taken to mitigate that hazard. These steps include evaluating the usefulness or unavoidability of contact with the chemical, defining the hazard associated with use conditions, and modifying the concurrent or subsequent photocarcinogenic stimulus. None of these steps is possible, however, unless the possibility of hazard is recognized and its magnitude is measured.

REFERENCES

Davies, R. E., and Forbes, P. D., 1988, Retinoids and photocarcinogenesis, J. Toxicol. Cut. & Ocular Toxicol., 7:241.
Epstein, J. H., 1977, Chemicals and photocarcinogenesis, Australas. J. Derm., 18:57.
Forbes, P. D., Davies, R. E., and Sambuco, C. P., 1989, Drug products and photocarcinogenesis, in: "Photobiology," E. Riklis, ed., Plenum Publishing Corp., NY.
Forbes, P. D., Davies, R. E., Sambuco, C. P., and Urbach, F., 1989, Inhibition of ultraviolet radiation-induced skin tumors in hairless mice by topical application of the sunscreen 2-ethyl hexyl-p-methoxycinnamate, J. Toxicol. Cut & Ocular Toxicol., 8:209.
Forbes, P. D., Davies, R. E., Urbach, F., and Cole, C., 1985, Photo-carcinogenesis, J. Toxicol. Cut. & Ocular Toxicol., 4:219.
Stern, R., 1989, PUVA: Its status in the United States, in: "Psoralens: Past, Present, and Future of Photochemoprotection and Other Biological Activities," T. B. Fitzpatrick, P. Forlot, M. A. Pathak, and F. Urbach, eds., John Libbey Eurotext, Paris.
Urbach, F., Davies, R. E., and Forbes, P. D., 1988, Chemical modifiers of photocarcinogenesis, in: "The Target Organ and the Toxic Process," Arch. Toxicol., Suppl., 12:47.
Wulf, H. C., Toulsen, T., Brodthagen, H., and Hon-Jenson, K., 1982, Sunscreens for delay of ultraviolet induction of skin tumors, J. Amer. Acad. Dermatol., 7:194.
Zhou, C., 1989, Mechanisms of tumor necrosis induced by photodynamic therapy, J. Photochem. Photobiol., 3:299.

REPAIR OF 8-MOP PHOTOADDUCTS IN HUMAN LYMPHOCYTES

F. Gasparro, P. Bevilacqua, D. Goldminz, and R. Edelson

Photobiology Laboratory, Yale University
333 Cedar Street
New Haven, CT 06510

INTRODUCTION

Psoralen phototherapy in the form of psoralen plus long-wavelength
ultraviolet light (UVA, 320-400 nm) has been used in the treatment of a
variety of different skin disorders, including psoriasis (Parrish et al.,
1974), vitiligo (Parrish et al., 1976), and patch-plaque stage cutaneous
T-cell lymphoma (CTCL) (Gilchrest et al., 1976). More recently, photopheresis, a new form of psoralen photochemotherapy, has been developed
and successfully used to treat patients with the erythrodermic form of
CTCL (Edelson et al., 1987). In this treatment, a patient's lymphocytes
are extracorporeally irradiated with UVA in the presence of 8-methoxy-
psoralen (8-MOP), and then are reinfused.

Both psoralen plus UVA for the skin (PUVA) and photopheresis involve
the use of 8-MOP. The therapeutic efficacy of PUVA has been attributed
to the formation of psoralen-DNA photoadducts. For example, in psoriasis
the formation of photoadducts has been postulated to lead to decreased
DNA synthesis and inhibition of cell division, resulting in the clearing
of psoriatic skin lesions (Scott et al., 1976). The specific role and
relative importance of crosslink and monoadduct formation in psoralen
phototherapies have not been determined, however. In addition, the
persistence of DNA photoadducts may play a role in side effects, such
as phototoxicity and photocarcinogenicity (Gold et al., 1988). Although
these same photoadducts have been detected in the DNA of lymphocytes
treated extracorporeally, our working hypothesis is that other cellular
sites must also be affected since the response to reinfused cells appears
to be immune-mediated (Perez et al., 1989).

Furocoumarins are tricyclic aromatic compounds which occur
with either linear (psoralens) or angular (isopsoralens or angelicins)
arrangement of the three rings (Fig. 1). The absorption peak at 300 nm
is typical of these compounds (Fig. 2, upper portion). Depending on
the particular substitutions, other bands may be evident as shoulders
(Gasparro, 1988). In the dark, these molecules intercalate between DNA
base pairs with varying affinities, depending on the number and type of
substitutions and the DNA sequence (Gasparro, 1988). When exposed to
UVA, these dark-complexed molecules undergo 2+2 photocycloadditions with
pyrimidine bases (primarily thymine). Activation can occur at two carbon-
carbon double bonds, either in the 6-member pyrone ring or the 5-member

DNA Damage and Repair in Human Tissues
Edited by B. M. Sutherland and A. D. Woodhead
Plenum Press, New York, 1990

137

furan ring, leading to the formation of a 3,4-monoadduct (Fig. 3, upper right) or a 4',5'-monadduct (upper left). The latter photoproduct can absorb additional UVA radiation (Fig. 2, lower portion) which activates its pyrone double bond, and thus leads to the formation of a second cyclobutyl bond which results in the crosslinking of two DNA strands (lower structure in Fig. 3). The formation of these three photoadducts has been presumed to be the basis of psoralen plus UVA photochemotherapies.

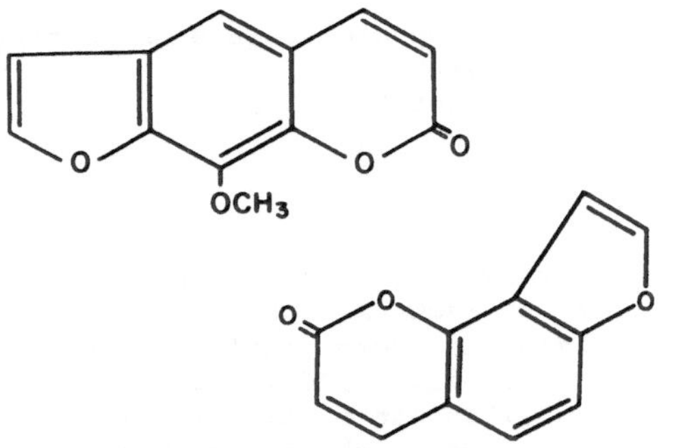

Fig. 1. Furocoumarins: 8-methoxypsoralen (left); angelicin (right).

The assay of UV-induced damage in the DNA of cells treated with psoralen and UVA using monoclonal antibodies raised against specific photoadducts offers the potential of developing highly sensitive methods to characterize the repair of these adducts. The primary advantage of using monoclonal antibodies arises from their specificity: the only potential drawback relates to the sensitivity of the assay method. Ultimately, this is related to the number of adducts formed during a therapeutic exposure. For example, thymine dimers form to the extent of 30 per megabase after a minimal erythema dose (Freeman et al., 1987). On the other hand, using [^{3}H]8-MOP we have shown that during the course of extracorporeal photochemotherapy for CTCL (photopheresis), psoralen photoadduct formation falls in the range of 0.1-10 adducts per megabase. This number of adducts can be detected using an enzyme linked immuno absorbent assay (ELISA) with monoclonal antibodies characterized by Santella et al. (1985). The question that remains to be answered is whether these adducts can be detected at the level at which cellular repair mechanisms are operative.

In this report we describe experiments designed to determine the doses of 8-MOP and UVA which abrogate the ability of a cell to either respond to mitogen stimulation or repair DNA damage. HPLC has been used to determine the distribution of 8-MOP photoadducts in DNA isolated from lymphocytes after treatment with 8-MOP and UVA (Gasparro et al., 1985). In addition, preliminary results using one of our monoclonal antibodies to determine specific adduct repair are described.

RESULTS AND DISCUSSION

8-MOP AND UVA Dose-Response Effects in Human Lymphocytes

Experiments were performed on human lymphocytes to assess the effects of 8-MOP and UVA on their functional activity. In addition, we wished to correlate this activity with the actual number of photoadducts formed in the DNA of the treated lymphocytes. Normal human lymphocytes were treated with different doses of 8-MOP plus UVA (Fig. 4). Tritiated thymidine (dThd) incorporation into newly formed DNA is a sensitive measure of cell proliferation. The data are plotted versus the product of the UVA dose and the concentration of 8-MOP to emphasize the reciprocal relationship that exists between the amount of 8-MOP and UVA used. The filled symbols are for data obtained by exposing the cells to a fixed dose of 8-MOP dose (100 ng/ml) and various UVA doses (0.1-5 J/cm^2). The open symbols were obtained in experiments in which the amount of 8-MOP

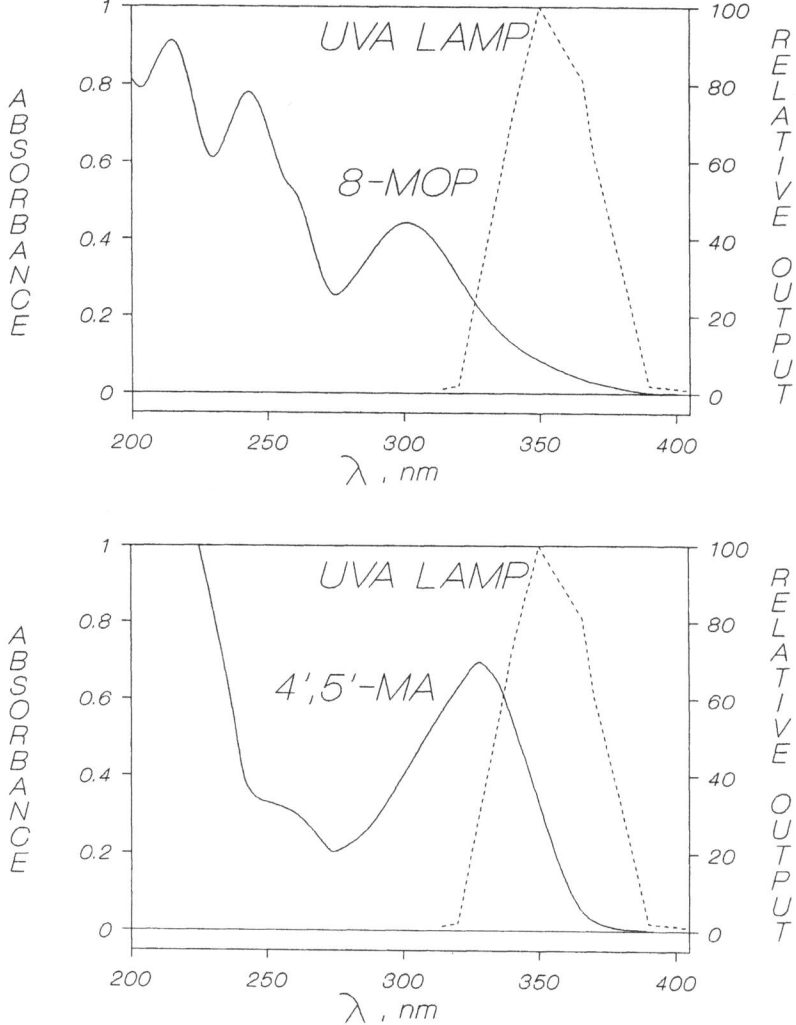

Fig. 2. UV spectra (8-MOP, upper; monoadduct, lower) compared to the UVA lamp output.

(0.1-1000 ng/ml) was varied, and the dose of UVA (either 1, 3 or 6 J/cm^2) held constant. Similar effects are obtained as long as the product of 8-MOP and UVA doses is the same. The complete reciprocity demonstrated in these data indicate that the likelihood of crosslink formation is very low.

The second-order regression analysis of the data from the Fig. 4 is also included in Fig. 5 for comparison to two other parameters: cell viability as measured by trypan blue exclusion (TBE), and DNA photo-adducts. The data depicted by the open squares represent the number of adducts formed per million base pairs as a function of the combined doses of 8-MOP and UVA. Increasing doses of 8-MOP and UVA led to an increased number of 8-MOP photoadducts. At the lower doses (1-50 combined dose units) the numbers of adducts formed increased monotonically. However, at greater doses of 8-MOP and UVA the actual number of adducts was less than that expected by extrapolation (data not shown). This effect may arise from a kind of 'inner filter' effect at the higher 8-MOP concentrations.

At 100 ng/ml 8-MOP and 1 J/cm^2 of UVA, 3.5 adducts per million bases were detected and the cells showed only 1% of control response to PHA stimulation, as measured by ^{3}H-dThd incorporation (Fig. 5, dThd). At a tenfold lower dose of 10 ng/ml of 8-MOP, the number of photoadducts is approximately tenfold lower (0.4) and the ability of lymphocytes to respond to PHA was 70% of control cells. Therefore, 1 J/cm^2 of UVA and 10 ng/ml of 8-MOP represent sublethal doses and these were the doses used in the repair experiments described below. Only at very high 8-MOP con-centrations do other cellular effects appear. For example, the ability of cells to exclude trypan blue (Fig. 5, TBE) is affected to an appreciable extent only at 8-MOP concentrations greater than 200 ng/ml.

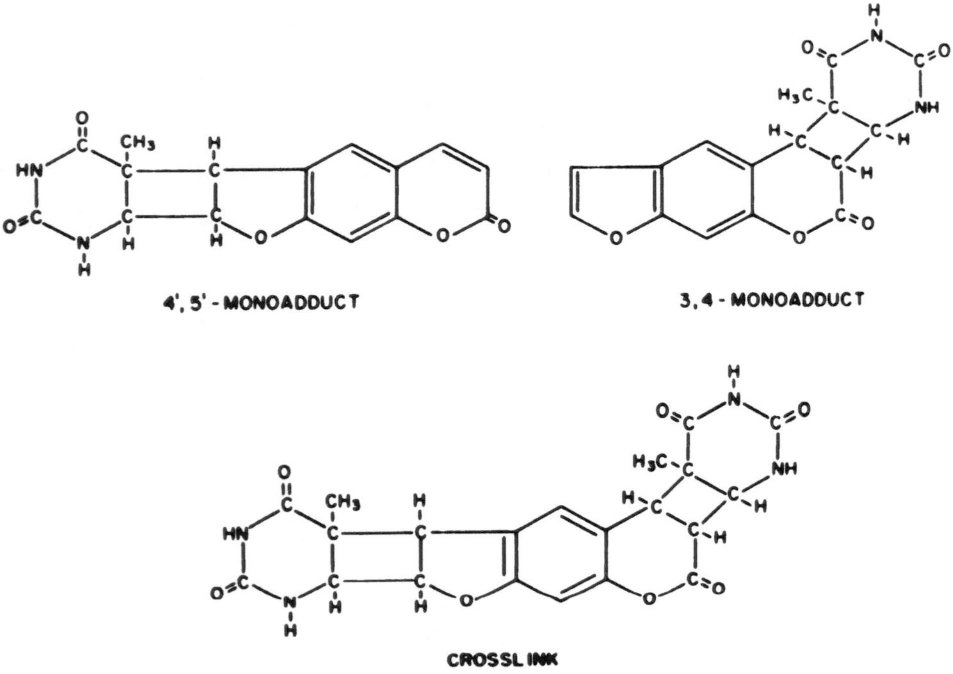

Fig. 3. Photoadduct structures.

140

Repair of 8-MOP Photoadducts in Lymphocytes

After treatment with 10 ng/ml 8-MOP and 1 J/cm^2 UVA (sublethal doses) normal human lymphocytes were incubated for up to 96 hours at 37°C in RPMI 1640 medium with 10% fetal bovine serum. To minimize any tendency for the lymphocytes to repair newly formed 8-MOP photoadducts, the cells were kept at 4°C during UVA treatment and during all subsequent manipulations until the cells were lysed or incubated. Treated cells showed a 22% reduction in photoadducts at 24 hours, and 27% at 48 hours (Fig. 6). By day four there was no evidence of further adduct removal. At 100 ng/ml and 1 J/cm^2, no removal of 8-MOP photoadducts was seen over a four-day incubation period. Therefore, lymphocytes are capable of photoadduct removal at sublethal doses of UVA and 8-MOP.

Photoadduct removal was associated with the recovery of cell proliferation as measured by [^{3}H]dThd incorporation after PHA stimulation (Fig. 7). Lymphocytes treated with either 3 or 10 ng/ml of 8-MOP and 1 J/cm^2 showed complete recovery of proliferative activity after three days, while cells treated with the greater dose of 20 ng/ml showed a slower rate and lower extent of recovery. At 100 ng/ml there was nor recovery. In contrast to normal lymphocytes, a malignant lymphocytic cell line did not demonstrate removal of adducts or recovery of cell proliferation when exposed to sublethal doses of 8-MOP and UVA (data not shown).

Previously, scintillation spectrometry and high performance liquid chromatography (HPLC) were used to analyze 8-MOP adduct formation in enzymatically hydrolyzed synthetic polynucleotides (Gasparro, 1988). These methods have now been used to detect psoralen photoadduct formation in human lymphocytes treated _in vitro_ with 8-MOP and UVA (10 ng/ml and 1 J/cm^2). DNA was isolated from cells immediately after treatment and after a repair period of 48 hours. The DNA was hydrolyzed enzymatically and analyzed by HPLC. HPLC fractions were collected and radioactivity was measured. Fig. 8 shows a plot of radioactivity versus fraction number. The peaks centered at fractions 38, 42, and 59 correspond to the crosslink (49%), the 3,4-monoadduct (10%) and 4',5'-monoadduct (41%), respectively.

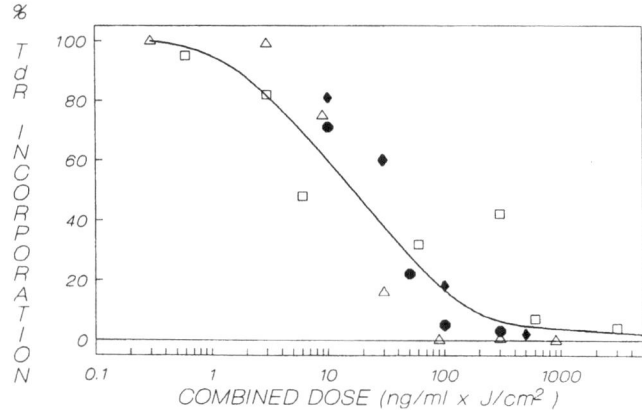

Fig. 4. Dose reciprocity of 8-MOP and UVA doses. (Symbols defined in text.)

We realized early in our studies that it would be invaluable to
be able to determine the in vivo levels of 8-MOP photoadduct formation in treated lymphocytes and keratinocytes (the target cells of
PUVA photochemotherapy). The method just described requires the use
of radioactive 8-MOP and is impractical for assay of samples obtained
from humans. Therefore, we initiated a program for the production of
monoclonal antibodies that would recognize 8-MOP photoadducts in DNA
isolated from human lymphocytes and keratinocytes.

Furocoumarin Photoadduct Monoclonal Antibodies

Balb C mice were immunized with DNA modified with 8-MOP or with
6,4,4'-trimethylangelicin (TMA) (Santella et al., 1985; Miolo et al.,
1989). Monoclonal antibodies were produced that specifically recognized
DNA modified with 8-MOP or TMA (Table 1). The sensitivities and specificities of the antibodies, reported as femtomoles of adduct in Table 1,
were obtained by competitve ELISA. In this type of ELISA assay, a known
amount of competitor is added to block the antibody binding to the DNA
attached to the assay plate. Thus, the lower the number of femtomoles,
the greater the sensitivity or specificty of the antibody or competitor.
In the early studies with 8-MOP, antigenic DNA was prepared using large
doses of light and an excess of 8-MOP. Under these conditions, greater
than 95% of the adducts formed were monoadducts. Competitive ELISA with
the most sensitive antibody obtained from immunization with 8-MOP modified
DNA, 8G1, demonstrated that one 8-MOP-DNA adduct in 10 million bases could
be reliably detected.

No cross reactivity with unmodified DNA or free 8-MOP was found.
The primary specificity of the 8G1 antibody was shown to be the 4',5'
thymine monoadduct. The apparent cross reactivity with 8-MOP crosslinks
in defined oligonucleotide sequences (oligo(AT)-XL and Kpn-XL in Table 1)
may be an artifact. The crosslinked oligonucleotides were isolated by
denaturing polyacrylamide gel electrophoresis, which requires the use of

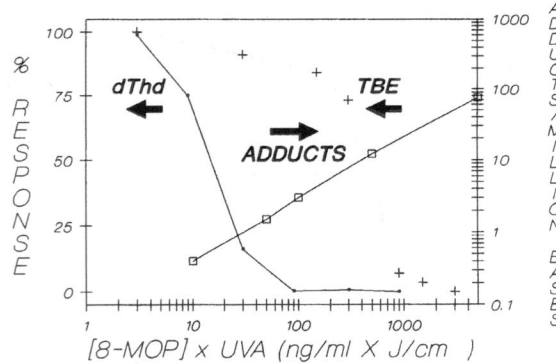

Fig. 5.   Effects of 8-MOP and UVA on lymphocytes: Tritiated thymidine
          incorporation (dThd), viability by trypan blue exlcusion (TBE)
          and photoadduct formation; arrows indicate the axis to be read.

8.3 M urea. Although the samples were purified, it is difficult to remove all of the urea. Remaining urea could affect antibody recognition and might be responsible for the greater amount of oligo(AT)-MA needed for 8G1 recognition.

Similarly, monoclonal antibody 7E3 was highly specific for TMA-DNA and demonstrated very little cross-reactivity with DNA modified with other angelicins. The data showed that the antibody preferentially recognized the 4',5' monoadduct and that one adduct in 10 million bases could be detected. To produce a monoclonal antibody with specificity for 8-MOP-DNA crosslinks, the self-complementary polynucleotide poly(dA-dT) and 8-MOP were irradiated. Poly(dA-dT) was chosen because every base pair is a potential crosslinking site. However, the resulting monoclonal antibodies were also shown to have specificity for the alternating A-T sequence itself and were not useful for the detection of 8-MOP crosslinks in other DNA sequences (Table 1). Work is underway to develop a crosslink antibody. Oligonucleotides containing a single 8-MOP-DNA crosslink will be prepared and used to immunize mice.

<u>Uses of Furocoumarin Photoadduct Monoclonal Antibodies</u>

The monoclonal antibody 8G1 has been used to detect the presence of 8-MOP photoadducts in biological samples. Indirect immunofluorescence was used to study human skin biopsies obtained from psoriasis patients undergoing PUVA therapy (Yang et al., 1989). Keratinocytes from three of five skin biopsies were positive for photoadducts using this method. The extent of DNA modification in these samples was estimated to be one adduct in one million bases. Epidemiologic studies have shown that patients undergoing long-term PUVA therapy have a dose-dependent increased risk of cutaneous squamous cell carcinoma (Stern et al., 1984). Cumulative psoralen-induced DNA damage to basal keratinocytes (Fig. 9) may account for this increased risk, although this has not been proved.

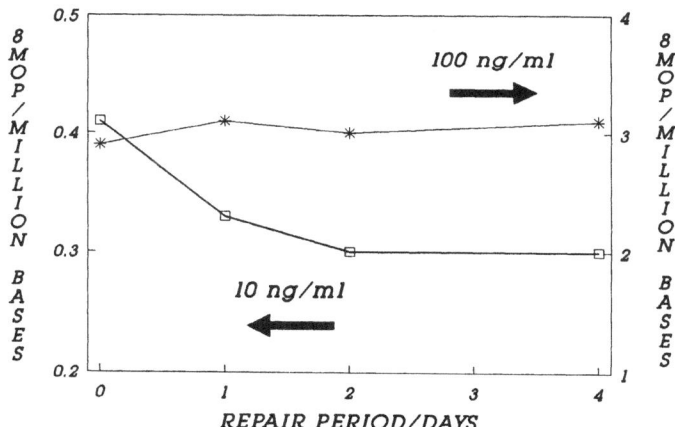

Fig. 6. Repair of photoadducts. (Arrows indicate axis to be read.)

Table 1.   8G1 - Recognition of Psoralen-Modified DNA and Oligonucleotides

Sample (specificity)	8G1 (4',5'MA)	10B12 (XL) femtomoles	7E3 (TMA)
8-MOP:DNA (calf thymus)[a]	17	430,000	--[e]
8-MOP:poly(dA.dT)[b]	13	6,500,000	--
8-MOP:poly(dA-dT)[c]	77	530	--
8-MOP:oligo(AT)-MA	1000	250,000	--
8-MOP:oligo(AT)-XL	1600	765	--
8-MOP:Kpn-MA	3600	360,000	--
8-MOP:Kpn-XL	7800	190,000	--
TMA-DNA[d]	--	--	112
TMA:Kpn-MA	--	--	9000

[a] original immunogen for 8G1: >95% 4',5'-monoadducts as shown by HPLC
[b] monoadducts only
[c] original immunogen for 10B12; crosslink enriched
[d] original immunogen for 7E3: >99% 4',5'-monoadducts as shown by HPLC
[e] dash indicates no test performed

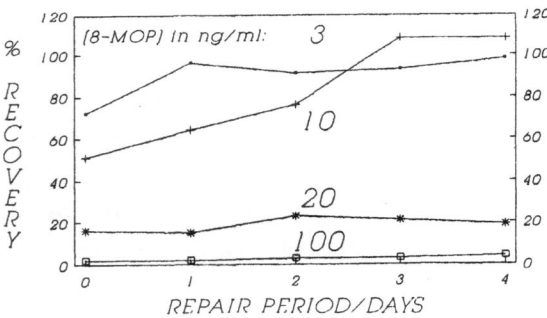

Fig. 7.   Recovery of lymphocyte PHA response after repair of adducts (1 J/cm^2).

Patients receiving PUVA can now be biologically monitored with the use of monoclonal antibodies to psoralen photoadducts. For example, a relationship between the number of specific adducts in basal keratinocytes and the increased risk of neoplasia may be found. If such a correlation is found, then modifications in the administration of PUVA with regards to type of psoralen, UVA wavelength, and UVA doses used could be made to make this therapy safer.

Monoclonal antibody 8G1 was also used to quantify the level of 8-MOP modification in the lymphocytes from patients treated with extracorporeal photopheresis. In one group of patients, adduct levels ranged from 0.55 to 0.75 adducts per million bases. More studies are being planned with the monoadduct monoclonal antibody and, when available, the crosslink monoclonal antibody.

These antibodies will afford us the unique opportunity of studying in vivo the formation and fate of these psoralen photoadducts, which could be important for several reasons. First, the level of adduct formation in the lymphocytes of treated patients may be important in determining clinical response. For example, a correlation between cis-platinum-DNA adducts in the leukocytes of ovarian cancer patients and their response to platinum-based chemotherapy has been found (Reed et al., 1987). Second, no studies have been performed to date to determine whether crosslinks or monoadducts are preferentially formed or repaired in treated lymphocytes. If the clinical response was found to correlate with the level of one adduct in particular, this information could be used to design safer and more efficacious psoralens for use in phototherapy. Third, there are no studies on the repair of photoadducts in human lymphocytes treated with photopheresis. The repair or lack of repair of these adducts may be ultimately responsible for the fate of a particular cell. Studies in other mammalian systems have shown that both monoadducts and crosslinks can be repaired. Existing methods for studying repair of 8-MOP photo-adducts measure the rates at which adducts are repaired, not the identity of the adduct being repaired. Also, kinetic studies cannot indicate whether a particular adduct may go unrepaired. Ongoing studies in our laboratory with psoralen monoclonal antibodies are aimed at answering some of these questions.

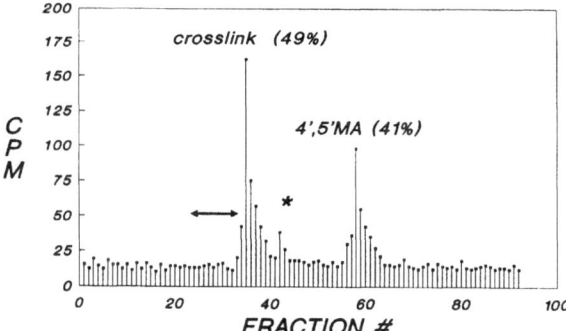

Fig. 8. HPLC separation of crosslink and monoadduct. The double-headed arrow indicates the region where unmodified bases elute; the asterisk shows the likely location of the 3,4-monoadduct.

Table 2. Distribution of 8-MOP Photoadducts in Lymphocyte DNA

Day	Total Adducts (a)	4',5'-MA (b)	XL (c)
		adducts per million base pairs	
0	0.40	0.13	0.27
2	0.32	0.17 (53%)	0.15 (47%)

[a] scintillation spectrometry
[b] 8G1 ELISA assay
[c] the extent of crosslink (XL) formation was obtained by taking the difference between (a) and (b)

     In preliminary studies, we have used 8G1 to determine which fraction
of the 8-MOP photoadducts measured by scintillometry are 4',5'-mono-
adducts. Table 2 summarizes these results. The HPLC chromatogram shown
in Fig. 8 was obtained by hydrolyzing 7 μg of the DNA sample collected
on day two (Gasparro et al., 1985). The adduct percentages based on CPM
areas corresponding to crosslink and 4',5'-monoadduct agree with the percentages obtained from the ELISA data shown in Table 2. These results,
indicating that 4',5'-monoadducts may escape repair, are consistent with
the results of experiments reported by Vos and Hanawalt (1987) who studied
the repair of psoralen photoadducts in the dihydrofolate reductase (DHFR)
gene of HeLa cells. They found that DNA damage in the sense strand was
repaired first. Ultimately, the adducts in the other DNA strand were

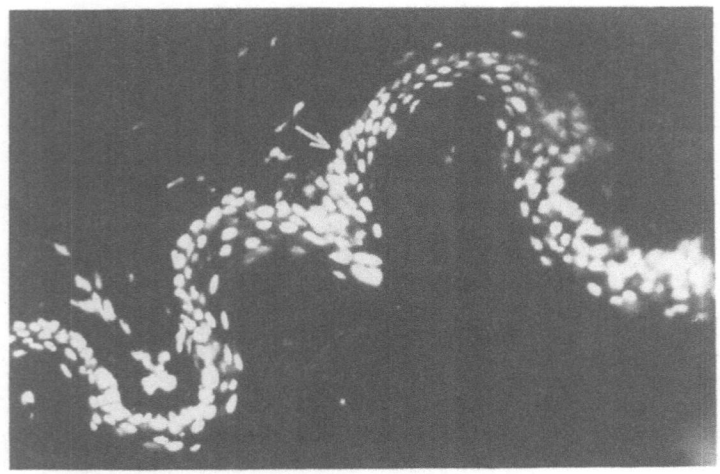

Fig. 9. Photomicrograph of human skin stained with 8G1. 30 μL 0.1%
         8-MOP was applied to a 2 cm square area of human skin. A 4-mm
         punch biopsy was obtained 30 min. later, and then while bathed
         in water, exposed to 2 J/cm^2 UVA.

146

repaired. In the DHFR gene, 80% of the crosslinks and only 45% of the monoadducts were eventually repaired. The repair of adducts in lymphocytes, which are normally in a resting state as compared to the active state of the DHFR gene, would be expected to differ.

The field of psoralen photobiology comprises diverse areas including psoralen photoadduct formation in DNA under both _in vitro_ and _in vivo_ conditions. The exact roles of the DNA photoadducts and the extent to which they are repaired remain to be determined. The unique ability of psoralen to intercalate between DNA bases and then photoreact would suggest that these photoadducts mediate significant events within a cell. Whether these DNA effects alone are responsible for the psoralen plus UVA effects in cells will only be determined by further experiments.

Given the 8-MOP concentrations typically achieved in patients and the low UVA doses that are actually delivered during photopheresis, lymphocytes are usually exposed to doses that fall in an intermediate region on the curve shown in Fig. 5, e.g. 100-200 (Edelson et al., 1987). Under these conditions, nuclear processes which control cell activity would be crippled. However, the cell membrane would remain intact, even though molecular modifications may begin to occur which are the precursors for the ultimate disintegration of the membrane. In photopheresis, for example, these cells would be reinfused in a patient and would circulate for a significant period during which time the immune system could respond to changes that might have been induced at the cell surface. These changes could include any one of the following: cell surface DNA modification (Bennett et al., 1985), protein photoadducts (Midden, 1988), and changes in cell membrane rigidity (Hornicek et al., 1985).

REFERENCES

Bennett, R. M., Gabor, R. T., and Merritt, M. M., 1985, DNA binding to human leukocytes: Evidence for a receptor mediated association, internalization and degradation of DNA, J. Clin. Invest., 76:2182.
Edelson, R. L., Berger, C., and Gasparro, F. P., 1987, Treatment of cutaneous T-cell lymphoma by extracorporeal photochemotherapy, New England J. Med., 316:297.
Freeman, S. E., Gange, R. W., Sutherland, J. C., and Sutherland, B. M., 1987, Pyrimidne dimer formation in human skin, Photochem. Photobiol., 46:207.
Gasparro, F., Bagel, J., and Edelson, R. L., 1985, HPLC analysis of 4',5'-monoadduct formation in calf thymus DNA and synthetic polynucleotides treated with UVA and 8-methoxypsoralen, Photochem. Photobiol., 42:95.
Gasparro, F. P., 1988, Psoralen-DNA interactions: Thermodynamics and photochemistry, in: "Psoralen-DNA Photobiology," F. P. Gasparro, ed., Vol. I, CRC Press, Boca Raton, FL.
Gilchrest, B. A., Parrish, J. A., Tanenbaum, L., et al., 1976, Oral methoxsalen photochemotherapy for mycosis fungoides, Cancer, 38:683.
Gold, R. L., Anderson, R. R., Natoli, S. M., and Gange, R. W., 1988, An action spectrum for photoinduction of prolonged cutaneous photosensitivity by topical 8-MOP, J. Invest. Dermatol., 90:818.
Hornicek, F. J., Malinin, G. I., Glew, W. B., Awret, U., Garcia, J. V., and Nigra, T. P., 1985, Photochemical crosslinking of eyrthrocyte ghost proteins in the presence of 8-methoxy and trimethylpsoralens, Photobiochem. Photobiophys., 9:263.
Miolo, G., Stefanidis, M., Santella, R. M., Dall'Acqua, F., and Gasparro, F. P., 1989, 6,4,4'-trimethylangelicin photoadduct formation in DNA: Production and characterization of a specific monoclonal antibody, J. Photochem. Photobiol., B:Biology, 3:101.

Midden, W. R., 1988, Chemical mechanisms of the bioeffects of furocou-marins: The role of reactions with proteins, lipids and other cellular constituents, in: "Psoralen-DNA Photobiology", F. P. Gasparro, ed, CRC Press, Boca Raton, FL.

Parrish, J. A., Fitzpatrick, T. B., and Tanenbaum, L., 1974, Photochemo-therapy of psoriasis with oral methoxsalen and longwave ultraviolet light, New England J. Med., 291:1207.

Parrish, J. A., Fitzpatrick, T. B., and Shea, C., 1976, Photochemotherapy of vitiligo using orally administered psoralens and high intensity longwave ultraviolet light system, Arch. Dermatol., 112:1531.

Perez, M., Edelson, R., Laroche, L., and Berger, C., 1989, Inhibition of antiskin allograft immunity by infusions with syngeneic photoinac-tivated effector lymphocytes, J. Invest. Dermatol., 92:669.

Reed, E., Ozols, R. F., and Tarone, R., 1987, Platinum-DNA adducts in leukocyte DNA correlate with disease response in ovarian cancer patients receiving platinum-based chemotherapy, Proc. Natl. Acad. Sci., 84:5024.

Santella, R. M., Dharmaraja, N., Gasparro, F. P., and Edelson, R. L., 1985, Monoclonal antibodies to DNA modified by 8-methoxypsoralen and ultraviolet A light, Nucl. Acids Res., 13:2533.

Scott, B. R., Pathak, M. A., and Mohn, G. R., 1976, Molecular and genetic basis of furocoumarin reactions, Mut. Res., 39:29.

Stern, R. S., Laird, N., Melski, J., Parrish, J. A., Fitzpatrick, T. B., and Bleich, H. L., 1984, Cutaneous squamous cell carcinoma in patients treated with PUVA, New England J. Med., 310:1156.

Vos, J. M. H. and Hanawalt, P. C., 1987, Processing of psoralen photo-adducts in an active human gene: Repair and replication of DNA containing monoadducts and interstrand cross-links, Cell, 50:789.

Yang, X. Y., Gasparro, F. P., DeLeo, V. A., and Santella, R. M., 1989, 8-methoxypsoralen-DNA photoadducts in patients treated with 8-methoxypsoralen and ultraviolet A light, J. Invest. Dermatol., 92:59.

DNA DAMAGE AND REPAIR IN HUMAN SKIN:

PATHWAYS AND QUESTIONS

Betsy M. Sutherland[a], Haim Hacham[a], Richard W. Gange[b],
Daniel Maytum[b] and John C. Sutherland[a]

[a]Biology Department, Brookhaven National Laboratory, Upton,
N.Y., and [b]Department of Dermatology, Harvard Medical
School, Boston MA.

INTRODUCTION

Skin, the principal barrier between human internal organs and the
external environment, is assaulted daily with physical and chemical
carcinogens, promoters, and modifiers of biological responses to such
agents. DNA is the principal target for most carcinogens, and DNA in skin
is particularly at risk. It is subject to damage not only from ingested
compounds and their metabolic products, but also from externally applied
or encountered chemicals, as well as from physical carcinogens such as
sunlight and cosmetic or medical sources of ultraviolet radiation. Three
major factors determine the balance between damage to DNA of skin and the
biological consequences of that damage: (1) the frequencies and types of
lesions, (2) the ability of the individual to repair a lesion, and (3) the
strategy that skin employs to deal with the different spectra of lesions
inflicted under varying environmental conditions. Thus, cellular
responses to DNA damage, including repair of DNA lesions, are critical
factors in determining the final level of damage and its consequences.

Human skin fibroblasts have allowed the collection of a vast
encyclopedia of information on repair in human cells in culture. Are
human cells in culture faithful representatives of human cells in the
body? The physical milieu is entirely different. For some organs, this
may not be a critical factor, but for skin, the presence of the overlying
keratinized layer changes both the quantity of sunlight reaching the
living cells of the epidermis and the spectrum of ultraviolet radiation
reaching those cells. For practical and economic reasons, human cells are
generally grown in culture using bovine serum, especially fetal bovine
serum. How the differences in composition of fetal bovine vs. adult human
serum affect repair is largely unknown. Are there inducible or otherwise
regulated repair enzymes, whose concentration or activities might be
changed in response to carcinogen exposure, nutrition, age, sex, or other
conditions?

Several lines of evidence indicate that--for whatever reasons--
repair in human skin fibroblasts in culture is quantitatively and
qualitatively different from that in human skin in situ. First, several
laboratories have shown that excision of pyrimidine dimers in skin in situ
is much more rapid than in most assays of excision in skin fibroblasts in

DNA Damage and Repair in Human Tissues
Edited by B. M. Sutherland and A. D. Woodhead
Plenum Press, New York, 1990

149

culture (Sutherland et al., 1980; D'Ambrosio et al., 1981a). Second, although photorepair is present in human fibroblasts only under special culture conditions, it seems to be a major repair pathway in intact skin (Sutherland et al., 1980; D'Ambrosio et al., 1981b; Eggset et al., 1983).

Although it may be possible to develop culture conditions which will allow repair responses in vitro comparable to those in situ, at present there are major differences between these situations. To have an accurate picture of the true levels of damage inflicted by carcinogens, the capacity of skin to remove, reverse or bypass such damage, and the residual levels of damage remaining after repair is complete, we must study these processes in skin itself.

Although many methods had been developed for measuring lesions in DNA and their repair, most of these methods required either radioactively labelled DNA or large quantities of non-radioactive DNA. Since it is not generally possible to obtain large quantities of human skin from volunteers nor to label their DNA with radioactive precursors, this posed a major problem impeding the quantitation of lesions in skin, and the study of repair in situ. The development of methods to quantitate lesion frequencies, to measure repair, and to evaluate strategies for lesion removal have provided powerful new methods for determining the carcinogenic potential of current and altered environmental conditions.

LESIONS IN DNA

Several new methods now allow quantitation of lesions in DNA of human organs. It is essential to consider the properties of the tissue of interest, the type of lesion to be measured, and its probable frequency (if such an estimate can reasonably be made) to allow selection of the most suitable method. For pyrimidine dimers produced by biologically realistic doses of ultraviolet radiation human skin (those to which people are routinely exposed in recreational, occupational, cosmetic or medical applications), analysis by alkaline agarose gel electrophoresis is quite useful.

Lesion Type and Detection Strategy

The frequency of DNA lesions may be quantitated by methods which count the increase in the number of DNA molecules due to induction of single- or double-strand breaks, for example, alkaline sucrose gradient centrifugation and alkaline agarose gel electrophoresis. The lesions measured by these methods may (1) be present immediately after the damaging treatment or (2) may serve as sites for induction of a break by an analytical reagent such as the pyrimidine dimer-specific UV endonucleases from T4 bacteriophage-infected Escherichia coli or from Micrococcus luteus (Carrier and Setlow, 1970).

Accurate quantitation of lesions of the first class demands that the extraction and other pre-analysis treatment of all DNAs be exactly reproducible, so that the number of molecules reflects only the breaks induced by the damaging agent. This is technically quite demanding, and poses a limitation on the measurement of these lesions at low frequencies.

Measurement of lesions of the second class is technically easier, as the number of lesions is determined by comparing the number of molecules in a sample of a given DNA with and without digestion by the lesion-specific agent. Since the quantitation of the lesions depends directly on the specificity of the cleaving agent and on its stoichiometric activity, its properties and optimum reaction conditions must be determined. An ideal cleaving agent must meet two criteria: first, it must be specific for the lesion of interest, with known substrate range under the conditions of the experiment, and second, in those conditions, cleavage must be stoichiometric.

Selection of a cleavage agent with appropriate specificity is a critical factor, determining the validity of the resulting assays. Naturally occurring enzymes with specificity for a single lesion type are rare, as most cells employ endonucleases of broad specificity able to deal with a spectrum of DNA lesions. For example, even the pyrimidine dimer-specific UV endonucleases recognize all classes of pyrimidine dimers: thymine-thymine, cytosine-cytosine, thymine-cytosine, cytosine-thymine, uracil-uracil, etc.

For accurate quantitation of lesions, the cleaving agent must induce a strand break quantitatively at each lesion. This requirement has two aspects: first, the enzyme must be able to recognize as substrate its specific lesion in a broad range of DNA sequences and tertiary structure; second, if the enzyme is capable of stoichiometric cleavage, it must be present at sufficient concentrations for each.sample (which may have different concentrations of inhibitors, for example, traces of DNA extraction agents) to achieve complete cleavage. It is essential that stoichiometric cleavage be attained before quantitation is attemped.

What about useful enzymes or other cleaving agents which do not cleave completely at all substrate lesions because of the context of sequence or tertiary structure in DNA surrounding the lesion? Although the use of such agents may be fraught with problems, in some cases their use makes possible at least the semi-quantitative measurement of otherwise unrecognizable lesions. In this case, it is essential to determine the specificity of the enzyme, to allow assessment of the fraction of the total lesions.

Production of DNA Lesions in Human Skin by Broad-spectrum Sources

Sunlight produces lesions in skin which can lead to short term damages (e.g. erythema) and long-term effects (e.g. skin cancers). What frequency of lesions corresponds to biological levels of damage? When we began this work in the late 1970s (Sutherland et al., 1980), the methods available for detection of pyrimidine dimers in human skin were not adequate for quantitation of lesions in human skin: they required either radioactive labeling of the DNA, or the use of large DNA quantities unavailable from small biopsies, or were not sufficiently sensitive for measuring the dimer levels produced by UV exposures encountered in everyday recreational, cosmetic or medical use. However, we soon found that the gel electrophoresis method allowed detection of dimer levels produced by even sub-erythemal doses of UV radiation.

Table 1 shows the frequency of pyrimidine dimers in DNA in skin of healthy human volunteers produced by a broad spectrum UVB source, and by contrast, representative data for dimer production by a UVA source. These data illustrate three important points: first, in humans whose minimal erythema doses (MEDs) vary over a large range, there seems to be a correlation between the MED and the yield of dimers induced by a given photon flux; second, for data obtained using one light source, the frequency of dimers per MED for different individuals varies rather little; third, the frequency of dimers per photon (or per MED) from a long wavelength UVA source is several orders of magnitude lower than from a UVB source.

Table 1. Pyrimidine Dimer Yields in Human Skin Irradiated In Situ
with Ultraviolet Radiation from Broad-spectrum UVB or UVA
Sources

UV Source	Volunteer	MED[a] (J/m^2)	Dimers/photon $(Dimers/Mb/J/m^2)$	Dimers/Mb/MED
FS-40[b]	A	240	11.5	32
	B	480	10.3	49
	C	600	6.9	50
	D	1460	2.6	40
UVASUN[c]	E	800,000	9.3×10^{-6}	8

[a]Minimal erythema dose; that quantity of radiation which produces
perceptible skin reddening with well-defined borders at 24 hr. after
exposure.
[b]Data taken from Freeman et al., 1986.
[c]Data from Freeman et al., 1987.

Wavelength Dependence of Pyrimidine Dimer Production in DNA in Human Skin: Biological Consequences

The data for production of pyrimidine dimers shown in Table 1
indicate the net yields of damages which are present shortly after
irradiation with broad-spectrum UV radiation. These data make clear that
radiation absorbed with high efficiency by DNA is much more effective in
dimer production than radiation of longer wavelengths. However,
calculation of the effectiveness of radiation of specific wavelengths--
and, therefore of the effect of changes in the spectrum of radiation
impinging upon human skin--requires knowledge of the efficiencies of
narrow wavebands of radiation in producing damage in skin in situ.

Determination of the relative efficiencies of different wavelengths
requires the measurement of the lesion yields at several UV doses in each
individual, thus permitting the calculation of the efficiency, defined as
the frequency of lesions (dimers/megabase) per photon/m^2 produced by the
wavelength of irradiation. Thus, data from many volunteers are necessary,
not only due to the large number of skin samples required, but also for
evaluation of the range of photoproduct yields in different individuals.

Figure 1 shows the wavelength dependence of production of pyrimidine
dimers in human skin irradiated in situ (Freeman et al., 1989). This
"action spectrum" is a plot of biological effect--in this case pyrimidine
dimer frequency/photon/cm^2--as a function of wavelength. These data
clearly show that the production of DNA damage is most efficient in the
300 nm range, decreases sharply at longer wavelengths, but is still
detectable at 365 nm. The decrease for wavelengths greater than 300 nm
results from absorption of incident light by protein and other components
of the strateum corneum. These data represent net yields of pyrimidine
dimers which are present after irradiation; excision occurring during

irradiation, and concomitant photorepair, which is driven by longer UV wavelengths, both will decrease the measured dimer yields.

From these data on DNA damage by narow waveband radiation, and assuming that the dimer yield in this dose range is linear with dose, we can calculate the total dimer yield induced by broad band sources of known wavelength composition. The product of the intensity of the source at each wavelength times the efficiency of that wavelength in producing damage, summed over all the wavelengths present in the broad spectrum source, gives the total damage of that type produced by that source. We can use this aproach to estimate the effect on pyrimidine dimer yield in human skin of alterations in the solar spectrum, for example through depletion of stratospheric ozone--with corresponding increases in shorter

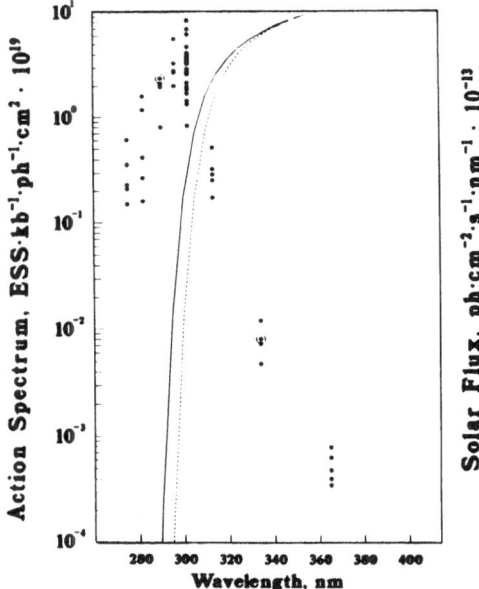

Fig. 1. Action spectrum for pyrimidine dimer formation in human skin
(o) and solar spectra at the surface of the earth for
stratospheric ozone levels of 0.32 cm ($\cdots$)and 0.16 cm (---)
(Shettle et al., 1975). Each point in the action spectrum
represents the slope of the dose-response line (dimer yields
at three exposures) for one volunteer at one wavelength,
obtained from triplicate independent determinations. A total
of 30 points occurs at 302 nm, although some points overlie
other values. There are five points at each wavelength;
points at 290 and 334 nm are circled to indicate that
identical dimer yields were recorded for two volunteers. (ph,
photon)

wavelength UV at the earth's surface. Figure 1 shows the shift in
spectral irradiance and wavelength distribution (Shettle et al., 1975) for
a 50% decrease in the ozone layer [similar to that observed in the
Antarctic ozone hole (Farman et al., 1985)]. Under such conditions, the
pyrimidine dimer yields in human skin would increase by more than 2-fold
(Freeman et al., 1989).

Furthermore, from knowledge of the correlation of skin cancer
incidence rates (Scotto, 1986) and sunlight exposure (generally, its UVB,
290-320 nm, component is measured because of its presumed importance in
cancer induction.), the dimer data can be used to estimate the increase in
incidence of human skin cancers (Freeman et al., 1989). For example, a
50% level of depletion of ozone, corresponding to greater than 2-fold
increase in dimers, would increase by 7- to 8- fold the incidence of nonmelanoma skin cancer in males of light pigmentation living in Seattle. The
new rate would be approximately that of a similar population living in
Albuquerque, New Mexico.

Hopefully, this is an extreme case of ozone depletion, and of
spectral shift. What would be the effect of smaller decreases in the
ozone column on dimer yield and skin cancer incidence? Use of the dimer
yield data in Figure 1, the data of Scotto (1986) and the spectral
calculations of Shettle et al. (1975) indicates that a 12.5% decrease in
ozone (to an effective ozone thickness of 0.28 cm would lead to a 17%
increase in DNA damage (as measured by pyrimidine dimers); the incidence
of skin cancer in male Caucasians living in Seattle would increase by some
23%. Similarly, a 25% decrease in the ozone column would be expected to
produce about 60% more DNA damage and results in over 2-fold increases in
human skin cancer rates.

REPAIR OF DNA

Knowledge of the damage inflicted on DNA in human skin by sunlight or
other carcinogens is only the beginning of the analysis of the biological
consequences of such damage. Through evolution in a world rife with DNA
damaging agents, cells in both procaryotic and eucaryotic organisms have
developed a variety of mechanisms to allow them to cope with alterations
in their genetic material.

Principally because of ease of manipulation, these repair pathways
have been elucidated principally in bacteria and in eucaryotic cells in
culture. Some simple eucaryotes (Saccharomyces cerevisae, Paramecium
aurelia, Tetrahymena pyriformis) are useful for simultaneous studies at
the organismal and molecular level.

However, for human cells in culture, early studies showed that repair
depends on culture conditions and, hence, might be significantly different
from that in the same type of cells in the intact organism. First,
independent investigators reported strikingly different rates of removal
of pyrimidine dimers in "normal human fibroblasts" in culture, with the
extremes ranging from about 1 hour (Amacher et al., 1977) to greater than
24 hours (Ahmed and Setlow, 1977) for removal of half the lesions.

Second, photorepair activity in cells in culture seemed to depend on the
medium in which the cells were grown (Sutherland and Oliver, 1976;
Mortelmans et al., 1977; Harm, 1980) or other regulatory factors, such as
stimulation of transcription (Henderson, 1978; Sutherland and Castellani,
1982).   Such findings suggested that repair in human cells in culture
might differ quantitatively or even qualitatively from that actually
carried out by those cells in the body, and stressed the importance of
determining the actual rates of repair in skin in situ.

Excision Repair

One of the first demonstrations of repair synthesis in human skin in situ was carried out by Epstein and his colleagues (Epstein et al., 1970), who injected ^{3}H thymidine into UV-irradiated skin of a normal volunteer and of a patient with xeroderma pigmentosum. They found that the normal individual incorporated the ^{3}H thymidine into non S-phase cells, thus carrying out unscheduled DNA synthesis (presumably repair synthesis) while the xeroderma patient did not. Although they did not carry out a detailed kinetic study, they found significant UDS by 1 hour.

In an early study of repair in human skin in situ, Kochevar, Harber and I (Sutherland et al., 1980) found very rapid exicision of pyrimidine dimers in human skin, with half the dimers removed in about one-half hour (Sutherland et al., 1980). D'Ambrosio and his colleagues (1981a) also found rapid excision in the skin of 11 healthy human volunteers, with a half-time of removal of about one hour. Recently, Bruze et al. (1989) (using only a zero time and a four-hour biopsy) found that about 70% were removed by that time, also suggesting rapid excision. In contrast, Freeman (1988) reported considerably slower excision rates, with an average half-time of about 12 hours.

What could be the source of the difference between the rapid repair rates found by Sutherland et al. (1980), D'Ambrosio et al. (1981a) and Bruze et al. (1989) and the much slower ones found by Freeman (1988)? One intriguing but unlikely possibility is that individuals in Albuquerque simply repair more slowly than those in New York, Columbus and Baltimore! We suggest that more plausible sources of these differences may be the age, skin type or history of sunlight exposure of the volunteers, or experimental differences between DNA extraction, dimer detection or analysis procedures. One experimental factor, the basic approach used for dimer quantation, does not seem likely to be a source of the difference: although several methods were used to measure the photoproducts-- D'Ambrosio et al., alkaline sucrose gradient sedimentation; Bruze et al., immunoassays-- both Freeman and Sutherland et al. analyzed dimer levels using alkaline agarose gel electrophoresis. The solution of this apparent discrepancy may well lead to interesting and important information on excision repair in skin in situ.

Photorepair

Most organisms can repair pyrimidine dimers in their DNA by photoreactivation, a one-enzyme repair pathway that uses long-wavelength UV or visible light as its energy source. The photoreactivating enzyme or photolyase binds to pyrimidine dimers in DNA, absorbs photoreactivating light, and reverses the dimer to two parental monomers. This process has three major advantages for the cell. First, since the energy source is light, no expenditure of cellular energy is required. Second, since most organisms are exposed to the damaging short UV wavelength radiation simultaneously with longer wavelength (more intense) UV and visible light, the energy source for repair is present immediately. Third, the process is error-free, unlike repair procedures in which new DNA synthesis is required.

Photorepair (PR) and the existence of photoreactivation in mammalian cells have been disputed for several years. Although Sutherland (1974) and Harm (1976) measured human leukocyte photoreactivating enzyme (PRE) in direct biochemical measurements or in competition experiments, respectively, and Henderson (1978) showed photoreactivation of UV-irradiated virus in human lymphocytes, contradictory data were obtained using human cells in culture. Although Sutherland et al. (1976) and Harm (1980) quantitated photolyase activity in several species of cultured mammalian cells, Cleaver (1976) did not detect any PRE activity. These contradictory results were apparently resolved by the finding that the level of photoreactivating enzyme activity in human cells in culture depended on the culture medium in which the cells were grown (Sutherland and Oliver, 1976; Mortelmans et al., 1977; Harm, 1980), suggesting that PRE levels are regulated in human cells, just as they are in E. coli (Nishioka and Harm, 1972), yeast (Boling and Setlow, 1967) and plant tissues (Saito and Werbin, 1969). The determination of photoreactivating enzyme levels in a tissue, then, is best carried out on the tissue itself, and measurement of the repair activity demands the measurement in the tissue in situ.

The most extensive recent study of photoreactivating enzyme in human tissues was carried out by Ogut et al. (1989), who examined the activity and characteristics of this enzyme in several different organs. They found the highest activity in the skin and brain, intermediate levels in the kidney and lung, and lowest in the intestine and liver. They also found evidence for the existence of at least two photoreactivating activities, both of which are heat- and protease-sensitive, act catalytically, and use light of wavelength greater than 320 nm in dimer photolysis.

In an early test for photorepair in human skin, we exposed untanned gluteal skin of healthy human volunteers to broad spectrum UVB radiation, then to visible light from an incandescent lamp (Sutherland et al., 1980). Dimers disappeared more rapidly in irradiated skin areas exposed to visible light than in those kept in darkness. These experiments indicated the presence of photorepair in skin in situ. D'Ambrosio and his colleagues carried out a more extensive study of the kinetics of photorepair (D'Ambrosio et al., 1981b); they exposed skin of healthy volunteers to UVB radiation, then to radiation greater than 455 nm. They found that about half of the dimers were removed in skin exposed to photoreactivating light in under 3 minutes (D'Ambrosio et al., 1981b). Removal of half the lesions by excision required about 1 hour (D'Ambrosio et al., 1981a, 1981b). Eggset et al. (1983) also observed photorepair in human skin by detecting binding of fluorescent antibodies to DNA damages in sections of skin; the antibodies used in the reactions were apparently specific for non-dimer lesions, but the disappearance of antibody binding upon post-UV illumination is clear.

Studies on the photoreactivability of UV-induced biological damage, such as erythema and other damages to skin have yielded variable results. In several such studies, investigators inflicted damage with radiation from a UVB source, then used radiation from a UVA source (320-400 nm) for photoreactivating light. (This choice was generally based on analogy with action spectra for yeast and E. coli cells, in which the wavelength of maximum effectiveness for photoreactivation was about 360 nm, with no activity at wavelengths greater than about 500 nm.) Such studies, by and large, gave either slight or no photorepair, or even increased damage from the "photoreactivating" light treatment. Our results on dimer yields in human skin irradiated in situ with radiation from UVA sources (Freeman et al., 1987) provide some insight into this problem: UVA induces detectable yields of dimers in the DNA of cells in normal human skin. Even though the cross section for dimer induction by radiation in the range 320-400 nm is lower than for photons of higher energy (280-320 nm), over the course of the illumination needed for photorepair, significant dimer frequencies are induced.

This finding would seem to pose a dilemma: how can photorepair be evaluated when the radiation required to drive the reaction also induces significant levels of dimers? One solution to this problem is provided by the wavelength dependence of the photoreactivating enzyme in mammalian cells. Action spectra for photoreactivation in human leukocytes (Sutherland and Sutherland, 1975), human fibroblasts in culture (Sutherland and Sutherland, 1975; Sutherland et al., 1976), and for marsupial cells in culture (Chiang and Rupert, 1979) indicate that the PR enzymes from these cells are able to use light of longer wavelength than are the photoreactivating enzymes from E. coli and yeast. The photoreactivation action spectrum in human cells extends to about 600 nm, and for Potorous tridactylus (marsupial) cells to at least 546 nm, indicating that long wavelength UV and visible radiation can be used as photoreactivating illumination in mammalian cells and tissues, including skin. Since radiation at 365 nm induces significant levels of pyrimidine dimers (Freeman et al., 1987) but photons in the wavelength range 385 to 405 nm do not (Hacham et al., 1989; Freeman et al., 1989), photoreactivating light sources for mammalian cells should include only radiation in the range 400-600 nm.

Examination of the current work on photoreactivation in human skin in situ indicates that several investigators used radiation greater than 400 nm as photoreactivating light sources: we (Sutherland, Kochevar, and Harber, 1980) used an incandescent light bulb, and D'Ambrosio and his colleagues (1981b) employed a broad spectrum light source filtered to remove radiation shorter than 455 nm. Our current results (Hacham et al., unpublished) indicate the apparent **necessity** for use of such a light source; we observed not only an apparent lack of photorepair in skin of volunteers exposed to 302 nm radiation and then to a high intensity, broad spectrum source containing UVB and UVA radiation, but even a net **increase** in the dimer content. With use of appropriate filters to remove dimer-inducing, shorter wavelength radiation, the rapid photorepair found by Sutherland et al. (1980) and by D'Ambrosio et al. (1981b) is easily observed. These results indicate that an in vivo action spectrum for pyrimidine dimer removal by photorepair is now imperative for understanding the role of this pathway in repair in skin exposed to sunlight.

STRATEGIES IN DNA REPAIR: PROSPECTS FOR THE FUTURE

At present our knowledge of repair in human skin in situ is fragmentary, with two pathways for removal of pyrimidine dimers found by several investigators (although even the basic properties of these pathways are not yet known). Fundamental questions yet to be answered include the number of other paths in human tissues for removal of dimers, other light-induced lesions and lesions induced by other agents, their possible interactions and degree of interrelationships with other pathways. In short, the basic strategies of repair in human skin in situ remain to be determined.

Priorities in Repair at the Molecular Level

Elegant methods for demonstrating the rapid repair of actively transcribed genes in human and rodent cells in culture have been developed by Hanawalt, Smith, Bohr and Okomoto (Bohr et al., 1985, 1986). In their cultured human skin fibroblasts, the time for removal of about half the pyrimidine dimers from genomic DNA was about 24 hours. Since the excision rate in human skin in situ is much faster, i.e., the removal of half the dimers in the overall genome in one hour or less, does skin still give preference to genes actively being transcribed?

Are there other priorities in repair which are employed by skin, but not accessible in studies on a single cell type in culture? New methods to distinguish among cell types, their repair pathways and the rates of repair are required for a full understanding of these priorities.

Human Repair Capacity

Many studies carried out by a large numbers of investigators have documented the repair deficiencies and their biological consequences in sun-sensitivity diseases such as xeroderma pigmentosum. Are other (non-xeroderma) individuals who are extraordinarily susceptible to damage by sunlight such as erythema and induction of skin cancer also deficient in repair of sunlight-induced lesions? Although the repair characteristics of cultured skin fibroblasts of these individuals may not be distinguishable from "normal" people when assayed in the laboratory, the striking quantitative and qualitative differences found so far between skin in situ and cells in culture indicates that possible differences in skin might not be observable in cells in culture.

Repair of Lesions Induced by Sunlight and by Chemicals

A final important area yet to be explored is the effect of lesions induced by chemicals on repair of sunlight-induced lesions. Could chemical adducts, for example, present blocks to the scanning of DNA sequences by repair enzymes which specifically or principally recognize UV-induced lesions? Would the presence of bulky, chemically-induced lesions successfully compete for repair enzymes at the expense of repair of UV-induced lesions?

What chemicals might be the culprits in such scenarios? Both ingested materials such as psoralens and externally applied cosmetics and environmental chemicals (e.g. tar deposits in highway or roofing workers) might pose such hazards. The elucidation of the true nature of the repair pathways present in human tissues in situ, the strategies cells use for deploying these paths to restore integrity to their genetic material, the effects of multiple lesions on repair, and the distribution of variability in repair among the human population will provide essential information for evaluating the effects of physical and chemical carcinogens in the environment.

ACKNOWLEDGMENTS

This research was supported by grants from the National Institutes of Health (CA 23096 to BMS, AR 35296 to RWG and GM 40936 to JCS), by a grant from the Wellman Foundation to RWG, and by the Office of Health and Energy Research of the Department of Energy.

REFERENCES

Ahmed, F. A. and Setlow, R. B., 1977, DNA repair in V-79 cells treated with combinations of ultraviolet radiation and N-acetoxyacetyl-aminofluorene, Cancer Res. 37:3414.

Amacher, D. C., Elliott, J. A., and Lieberman, M. W., 1977, Differences in removal of acetylaminofluorene and pyrimidine dimers from the DNA of cultured mammalian cells, Proc. Nat. Acad. Sci. 74:1533.

Bohr, V. A., Smith, C. A., Okumoto, D., and Hanawalt, P. C., 1985, DNA repair in an active gene: removal of pyrimidine dimers from the DHFR gene of CHO cells is much more efficient than in the genome overall, Cell 40:359.

Bohr, V. A., Okumoto, D. S., and Hanawalt, P. C., 1986, Survival of UV-irradiated mammalian cells correlates with efficient DNA repair in an essential gene, Proc. Natl. Sci. U.S.A., 83:3830.

Boling, M., and Setlow, J. K., 1967, Photoreactivating enzyme in log phase and stationary phase yeast cells, Biochim. Biophys. Acta 145:502.

Bruls, W. A. G., Slaper, H., van der Leun, J. and Berrens, L., 1984, Transmission of human epidermis and strateum corneum as a function of thickness in the ultraviolet and visible wavelengths, Photochem. Photobiol. 40:485.

Bruze, M., Emmett, E. A., Creasey, J. and Strickland, P. T., 1989, Cyclobuta-dithymidine induction by solar-stimulating UV radiation in human skin:II. Individual responses, J. Invest. Dermatol., in press.

Carrier, W. L. and Setlow, R. B., 1970. Endonuclease from Micrococcus luteus which has activity toward ultraviolet-irradiated deoxyribonucleic acid: purification and properties, J.Bacteriol. 102:178.

Chiang, T. and Rupert, C. S., 1979, Action spectrum for photoreactivation of ultraviolet irradiated marsupial cells in tissue culture, Photochem. Photobiol. 30:525.

Cleaver, J.E., 1976, Photoreactivation: a radiation repair mechanism absent from mammalian cells, Biochim. Biophys. Acta, 442:358.

D'Ambrosio, S. M., Slazinski, L., Whetstone, J. W. and Lowney, E., 1981a, Excision repair of UV-induced pyrimidine dimers in human skin in vivo. J.Invest. Dermatol. 77:311.

D'Ambrosio, S. M., Whetstone, J. W., Slazinski, L. and Lowney, E., 1981b, Photorepair of pyrimidine dimers in human skin in vivo, Photochem. Photobiol. 34:461.

Eggset, G., Volken, G, and Krokan, H., 1983, U.V.-induced damage and its repair in human skin in vivo studied by sensitive immunohistochemical methods, Carcinogenesis, 4:745.

Epstein, J. H., Fukuyama, K., Reed, W. B. and Epstein, W. L., 1970, Defect in DNA synthesis in skin of patients ·ith xeroderma pigmentosum demonstrated in vivo, Science 168:1477.

Farman, J. C., Gardiner, B. G. and Shanklin, J. D., 1985, Large losses of total ozone in Antarctica reveal seasonal ClO_x/NO_x interaction, Nature, 315:207.

Freeman, S. E., 1988, Variations in excision repair of UVB-induced pyrimidine dimers in DNA of human skin in situ, J. Inv. Derm. 90: 814.

Freeman, S. E., 1989, Wavelength dependence of pyrimidine dimer formation in DNA of human skin irradiated in situ with ultraviolet light, Proc. Natl. Acad. Sci. USA 86:5605.

Freeman, S. E., Gange, R. W., Matzinger, E. A. and Sutherland, B. M., 1986, Higher pyrimidine dimer yields in skin of normal humans with higher UVB sensitivity, J.Invest. Dermatol. 86:34.

Freeman, S. E., Gange, R. W., Sutherland, J. C., Matzinger, E. A., and Sutherland, B. M., 1987, Production of pyrimidine dimers in DNA of human skin exposed in situ to UVA radiation, J. Invest.Dermatol. 88:430.

Hacham, H., Freeman, S. E., Gange, R. W., Maytum, D. J., Sutherland, J. C. and Sutherland, B. M., 1989, Relationship between the minimal erythema dose and pyrimdine dimer formation in DNA of human skin irradiated in situ with ultraviolet radiation (275-405 nm),Photochem. Photobiol. 49S:70S.

Harm, H., 1976, Damage and repair in mammalian cells after ultraviolet and/or visible light treatment, in "Symposium on Biological Effects and Measurement of Light Sources, Proceedings," D. G. Hazzard, ed., HEW Publication (FDA) 77-8002, Rockville, Md.

Harm, H., 1980, Damage and repair in mammalian cells after exposure to non-ionizing radiations III. Ultraviolet and visible light irradiation of cells of placental mammals, including humans, and determination of photorepairable damage in vitro, Mutat. Res. 69:167.

Henderson, E. E., 1978, Host cell reactivation of Epstein-Barr virus in normal and repair defective leukocytes, <u>Cancer Res.</u> 38:3256.

Mortelmans, K., Cleaver, J. E., Friedberg, E. C., Paterson, M. C., Smith, B. P. and Thomas, G. H., 1977, Photoreactivation of thymine dimers in UV-irradiated human cells: unique dependence on culture conditions, <u>Mutat. Res.</u> 44:443.

Nishioka, H., and Harm, W., 1972, Analysis of photoenzymatic repair of UV lesions in DNA by single light flashes. Excess production of photoreactivating enzyme in E. coli BS-1-160 under different growth conditions and its suppression by adenine, <u>Mutat. Res.</u>, 16:121.

Ogut, S. E., D'Ambrosio, S. M., Samuel, M., and Sutherland, B. M., 1989, DNA photoreactivating enzyme from human tissues, <u>J. Photochem. Photobiol.</u>, in press.

Scotto, J., 1986, Nonmelanoma skin cancer--UVB effects in "Effects of Changes in Stratospheric Ozone and Global Climate," J. G. Titus, ed., United States Environmental Protection Agency, Washington, D. C., Vol. 2.

Saito, N. and Werbin, H., 1969, Evidence for a DNA-photoreactivating enzyme in higher plants, <u>Photochem. Photobiol.</u> 9:389.

Shettle, E. P., Nack, M. L., and Green, A. E. S., 1975, Multiple scattering and the influence of clouds, haze and smog on the middle UV reaching the ground, in "Impacts of Climatic Change on the Biosphere, Part 1," (National Technical Information Service, Springfield, Va. Department of Transportation DOT TST-76-55) Part 1.

Sutherland, B. M., 1974, Photoreactivating enzyme from human leukocytes, <u>Nature</u> 248:109.

Sutherland, B. M. and Castellani, A., 1982, Photoreactivating enzyme induction in human lymphocytes, <u>Photochem. Photobiol.</u> 35:275.

Sutherland, B. M. and Oliver, R., 1976, Culture conditions affect photoreactivating enzyme levels in human fibroblasts, <u>Biochim. Biophys. Acta</u> 442:358.

Sutherland, B. M., Oliver, R., Fuselier, C. O., and Sutherland, J. C., 1976, Photoreactivation of pyrimidine dimers in the DNA of normal and xeroderma pigmentosum cells, <u>Biochem.</u> 15:402.

Sutherland, B. M., Kochevar, I. and Harber, L., 1980, Pyrimidine dimer formation and repair in human skin, <u>Cancer Res.</u>, 40:3181.

Sutherland, J. C. and Sutherland, B. M., 1975, Human photoreactivating enzyme: action spectrum and safelight conditions, <u>Biophys. J.</u>, 15:435.

UNSCHEDULED DNA SYNTHESIS IN HUMAN SKIN

Herbert Hönigsmann

Division of Photobiology
Department of Dermatology I
University of Vienna, Vienna, Austria

INTRODUCTION

Present evidence suggests that the induction by UV radiation of cyclobutyl pyrimidine dimers (Setlow, 1966) in the DNA of human epidermis plays a major role in the initiation of UV carcinogenesis (Epstein, 1970; Robbins et al., 1974; Hart et al., 1977; Black and Chan, 1977). The repair of these DNA lesions has been widely studied in the recent past (Sutherland et al., 1980) but relatively little information is available on DNA repair in situ in human skin. Repair activity as a function of unscheduled DNA synthesis (UDS) can be measured by autoradiography (Epstein, 1970; Epstein et al., 1969). UDS is considered to be a measure for repair replication during the excision repair process of pyrimidine dimers. A more quantitative approach is the measurement of dimer loss by use of pyrimidine dimer-specific endonuclease assays (Setlow et al., 1975; Sutherland et al., 1980; Sutherland and Shih, 1983; D'Ambrosio et al., 1981a). However, these assays cannot give information on the distribution and localization of damage in epidermal cells in situ. For studies on skin carcinogenesis it may be important to know where DNA damage is located. UDS provides indirect information on the sites of DNA damage in skin and, within certain UV irradiation dose ranges, permits estimating the magnitude of the formation of dimers and other repairable lesions.

The present communication summarizes the results of several studies performed in our institution in order to obtain information on DNA damage and repair in human epidermis addressing various issues: We measured UDS to determine the magnitude of possible photoprotection against UVB-induced damage by orally administered carotenoids, by UVA-induced immediate pigment darkening (IPD), and by psoralen plus UVA-(PUVA) induced pigmentation. We further investigated the effects of equally erythemogenic doses of narrow-band UVA and UVB on the induction of UDS. Finally, we studied the dose response to UVB irradiation of UDS, its correlation with skin erythema, the time course over a period of 24 h, and the effect of dual exposures separated by 24 h.

DNA Damage and Repair in Human Tissues
Edited by B. M. Sutherland and A. D. Woodhead
Plenum Press, New York, 1990

MATERIAL AND METHODS

Subjects

Experiments were performed on healthy Caucasian volunteers (skin types II and III) with ages ranging from 20 to 72 years. Skin typing according to the subjects' ability to sunburn and acquire pigmentation revealed approximately 20 % type II and 80 % type III subjects. This distribution reflects the distribution of skin types in a central European population. The usually non-sun-exposed buttock skin was selected for phototesting and for biopsies. Informed consent was obtained.

Radiation sources

Experiments with UVA were performed with a high-intensity UVA source (Sellas Sunlight 2001, Sellas Medizinische Geräte GMBH, Gevelsberg-Vogelsang, FRG) equipped with a metal halogenide lamp and a 5-mm window glass filter. For narrow band UVA exposures a 6000 W Xe arc source (Optical Radiation Corp. V-4500) optically matched with a Jobin-Yvon HL 300 holographic grating monochromator at a half-band width of 30 nm between 335 and 365 nm was used.

Experiments with UVB were performed with an unfiltered water-cooled high-pressure XBF 6000 W xenon lamp (Osram GMBH, Munich, FRG) or with a high-pressure mercury lamp (Osram Ultra-Vitalux, Osram GMBH, Munich, FRG). At the irradiation doses used in these studies, the UVA fraction delivered by the lamps was considered biologically irrelevant, since earlier studies have shown that UDS does not occur at UVA doses which are far below the minimal erythema dose (MED). It has also been shown that suberythemogenic doses of UVA do not influence the incidence and the amount of UVB-induced UDS (Hönigsmann et al., 1981). However, traces of UVC may have contributed to some UDS in these experiments. For narrow-band UVB exposures the 6000 W Xe arc source with the Jobin-Yvon monochromator (as above) at a half-band width of 30 nm between 275 and 305 nm was used.

Detailed descriptions of the irradiation systems, fluence rates, filter equipment, and radiometric measurements have been published (Gschnait et al., 1978; Hönigsmann et al., 1981; 1987a; Wolf et al., 1988).

Experimental procedures

Before the experiments, the individual MED was determined in each volunteer by exposure of six or seven 6 cm²-circular test areas to increasing doses of UV. Dose increments corresponded to multiples of the square root of 2. The MED was defined as uniform pink erythema with well-defined borders and was read by two independent investigators 24 hours after exposure. With the radiation sources employed the MED values ranged from 14 to 56 mJ/cm² for UVB and from 40 to 112 J/cm² for UVA. Since there was no clear-cut correlation between clinical skin type and MED, the skin type was not considered relevant for the subsequent studies.

Throughout all experiments we used the individual MED as the baseline for UV dosimetry for each subject. Although the visual assessment of erythema may bear some risks of error, within a heterogenous study population of different skin types and, thus, different UV responsivenesses, the MED represents the only parameter that reasonably defines biologically equivalent doses.

Autoradiography

Shave biopsies of exposed skin and non-exposed control areas were secured under local anesthesia either immediately or, depending on the experimental protocol, up to 24 h after irradiation. The specimens were incubated immediately after biopsy with ^{3}H-thymidine (specific activity 5 Ci/mM; final concentration 20 μCi/ml in Medium 199) in vitro for 1 h at 37°.

Thereafter, 5 μ sections were dipped into Kodak Nuclear Track emulsion (NTB2) and stored in light tight boxes for 20 days at 4°C. The slides were developed using Kodak D 19 developer, fixed with Fixon Ultra Rapid (Daniel) and finally stained with hematoxylin-eosin. The coating and developing procedures were performed in complete darkness, no safety light was used.

Determination of unscheduled DNA synthesis

After the specimens had been processed they were examined with a light microscope. Epidermal cells of all viable layers usually exhibited sparse label, and, as observed previously (Hönigsmann et al., 1981), there was no obvious difference between the labels in the upper and the lower epidermal layers within a given specimen. In each section the number of sparsely labelled (3 - 25 silver grains per nucleus) cells (SLC) per 1000 basal and suprabasal epidermal cells (SLC index), and the number of grains per SLC (counted in 100 adjacent sparsely labelled basal and suprabasal epidermal cells per section) was determined. Three grains per nucleus were chosen as threshold count for defining sparse label since previous studies have shown that, with the specific activity employed, the average background count of control specimens remains below three. Densely labelled (S-phase) cells were not taken into consideration.

ASSESSMENT OF PHOTOPROTECTION

Carotenoids

Recently Mathew-Roth and Krinsky (1985) reported that dietary supplementation with carotenoids in relatively low doses could significantly decrease the number of UVB- induced skin tumors in hairless mice. How carotenoids exert this protective effect against photocarcinogenesis awaits clarification, but it is speculated that quenching of reactive oxygen species may be a decisive event (Mathews- Roth, 1986). It was thus interesting to evaluate whether the reported prevention of tumors by dietary carotenoids is possibly based on a reduction of UVB-induced DNA damage. Test subjects received an oral carotenoid preparation (Phenoro^R, Roche, Basle; 150 mg/day) for four weeks. After this time serum values usually reach levels known to suppress photosensitivity in protoporphyria. The UVB-MED was determined in all subjects before carotenoid treatment. They were irradiated with 1/2 MED (precarotenoid value) before and after four weeks of carotenoid intake. A dose of 1/2 MED was chosen, as previous studies have shown that UDS is not

TABLE 1.[*]   UDS Before and During Carotenoid
               Administration

day	Carotenoid serum level (µg/dl)	SLC index (x ± s)	Grains/SLC (x ± s)
0	130 ± 41	397 ± 94	6 ± 1.2
30	745 ± 243	441 ± 82	8 ± 2.0

There were no significant differences in SLC indices
and grains/SLC determined on day 0 and on day 30

[*]adapted from Wolf et al., 1988

saturated at this irradiation dose and, thus, differences may
not be obscured by plateau formation (Hönigsmann et al., 1987a)
(see also below).

Irradiation with 1/2 MED of UVB (precarotenoid value) induced measurable amounts of UDS in the epidermis before and after carotenoid medication. Quantitative assessment revealed no
statistically significant difference in the mean UDS activity
(Table 1).

Highly reactive forms of oxygen are suspected to contribute to DNA damage and, thus, to carcinogenesis (Mathews-Roth,
1986; Spikes, 1982). If this damage is repaired by excision
repair, a reduction of damage by carotenoids should be expressed by a reduction of UDS activity. Since this is not the
case, it appears unlikely that the antitumor activity of carotenoids operates by reducing the number of DNA lesions that are
repairable via the excision repair but may be based on other
mechanisms.

Immediate Pigment Darkening

The physiological function of immediate pigment darkening
(IPD) is unknown. It may have acted as a protection during
evolution but recent studies have demonstrated that IPD does
not protect against UVB-induced erythema (Black et al., 1985).

We tried to determine whether IPD provides substantial
protection against UV damage of DNA by measuring UDS in IPD-
positive and non-IPD skin exposed to UVB.

After determination of the UVB- and the UVA-MED, the IPD
reaction was induced by suberythemogenic doses of UVA. Immediately afterwards parts of the IPD area and an adjacent control
site were exposed to 1/2 MED and 1/4 MED of UVB. These doses
are known to induce measurable UDS and were considered low
enough not to obscure a possible weak protective effect of IPD
by massive UVB damage (Hönigsmann et al., 1987a).

After UVB irradiation, UDS was found to be not significantly different in IPD-positive skin as compared with non-IPD
skin. IPD skin alone did not exhibit UDS. This result indicates

that IPD neither prevents nor reduces the formation of DNA
lesions that can be detected by measuring UDS. Moreover, this
study showed that post-irradiation with UVB of UVA-exposed skin
does not give rise to photoadditive or photoaugmentative
effects with regard to UDS within the dose ranges used (Ortel
et al., 1986).

Psoralen-UVA-Induced Pigmentation

Pigmentation induced by the combined action of psoralens
plus UVA irradiation (PUVA) increases skin tolerance to subsequent exposures to sunlight. This effect appears to be of
particular importance in the preventive treatment of patients
with abnormal photosensitive reactions (for references see
Hönigsmann et al., 1987b). We investigated whether a PUVA-in-
duced tan can also protect against UVB damage on the macromolecular level.

After determination of the UVB-MED the test subjects were
given four PUVA treatments (8-methoxypsoralen, 0.6 mg/kg)
within a five-day period according to the European standard
procedure for treating psoriasis (Henseler et al., 1981). Ten
days after the last PUVA exposure, test areas were exposed to 1
pre-PUVA MED and UDS was measured in PUVA-treated pigmented
skin and in an adjacent non-PUVA- treated area. In PUVA-
pigmented skin a dramatic reduction of both SLC index (ˋ 60 %)
and grains/SLC (> 40 %)was observed as compared with non-
pigmented skin (Table 2).

TABLE 2.[*]   UDS With and Without
              PUVA-Induced Pigmentation

	SLC index $(x \pm s)$		Grains/SLC $(x \pm s)$	
untanned skin	500 $\pm$ 62		4.0 $\pm$ 0.7	
tanned skin	201 $\pm$ 101	$p < 0.005$	2.7 $\pm$ 0.2	$p < 0.005$

[*] adapted from Gschnait et al., 1978

Since it has been shown that therapeutic PUVA doses do not
infere with UDS after UVB exposure (Hönigsmann et al., 1981);
the decrease of SLC and grains/SLC does not seem to reflect
inhibition of excision repair but rather suggests a definite
reduction of UVB-induced DNA damage.

COMPARISON OF UVA AND UVB EFFECTS

Since the early studies of Epstein et al. (1969) who were
the first to employ autoradiographic methods to measure epidermal DNA sythesis after UVB exposure it was generally
accepted that UVB irradiation leads to UDS in human skin.
However, uncertainty remained with regard to UVA effects
(Willis et al., 1973; Bishop, 1979). This was partly due to

the fact that in earlier studies, the UVA sources were either contaminated with UVB or the UVA doses were too small to yield meaningful results. We determined the magnitude of UVA-induced DNA damage, as reflected by UDS in comparison to UVB damage.

Template areas of skin were irradiated with equally erythemogenic doses of UVA and UVB. Under these conditions UVA proved to induce about 50 to 60 % of the amount of UDS induced by UVB. The difference in the SLC index and in the grains/SLC was highly significant.

Erythemogenic doses of UVA produce morphological changes in the epidermis which are qualitatively similar to UVB-induced alterations (Kaidbey and Kligman, 1979; Rosario et al., 1979). Andrews (1980) demonstrated lethal (or growth inhibiting) effects of UVA in xeroderma pigmentosum cells but not in normal cells. Particularly, this latter observation suggested that UVA induces DNA lesions which require a proficient excision repair.

After completion of our study (Hönigsmann et al., 1981), more recently, Freeman et al. (1987) presented evidence that UVA induces the formation of pyrimidine dimers in human skin.

DOSE RESPONSE AND KINETICS OF UDS

Experiments with human fibroblasts have shown that following exposures to UVC (254 nm), UDS reaches a plateau above a certain threshold dose (Ahmed and Setlow, 1979). According to current concepts, this reflects saturation of the excision repair mechanism for cyclobutyl pyrimidine dimers (Ahmed and Setlow, 1979). For studies on UV carcinogenesis it is important to know whether exposure to UVB leads to a saturation of the excision repair in human skin and at what doses this might occur. Earlier studies, although not specifically addressing this issue have already suggested that repair activity in skin reaches a plateau (Bohnert et al., 1972). An exhaustion of excision repair capacity may lead to an accumulation of DNA damage which subsequently may be repaired by other, error-prone mechanism such as post-replication repair (Lehman et al., 1975).

In a series of experiments we investigated whether a similar saturation of UDS does occur in human skin in vivo with broad spectrum UVB and whether this plateau correlates with the degree of erythema. In addition we studied the time course of UDS in non-illuminated skin over a period of 24 h, and the effect of dual UVB exposures separated by 24 h.

Dose Response

The test areas were exposed to fractions and multiples of the individual MED in order to establish a dose-response curve from 1/16 up to 6 MEDs. The test subjects received 1/16, 1/8, 1/4, 1/2, 1, 2, 3, 4, 5, and 6 MEDs. Sparse label in the epidermis was found in all biopsy specimens from 1/16 to 6 MEDs. The smallest UVB irradiation applied was 1.25 mJ/cm², inducing an SLC index of 318 and a mean grain number/SCL of 5.3 which was clearly distinguishable from the background label present in non-irradiated control skin. UDS increased gradually with increasing UVB doses. This increase was not linear and tended to be lower with higher doses (Fig. 1).

Statistical analysis revealed a significant increase in both the SLC indices and the number of grains from 1/16 MED up to 1 MED. No statistically significant difference was found in both parameters between 1 MED and 6 MEDs (Fig. 1). These erythemogenic doses induced a sparse label in approximately 75 % of epidermal cells in all viable layers.

The UDS dose response curve followed a similar course in all test subjects and formed a plateau at 1 MED. However, there was no overall correlation between the relative exposure dose (expressed in MED) and the absolute exposure dose (expressed in mJ/cm²).

These results show that saturation of the excision repair expressed by UDS can be induced in human skin with broad-band UVB, similar to the saturation described for human fibroblasts with UVC in vitro (Ahmed and Setlow, 1979).

The dose response curves of both the grains per SLC and the SLC indices exhibit a gradual increase of UDS from suberythemogenic doses to erythemogenic doses. This increase is not

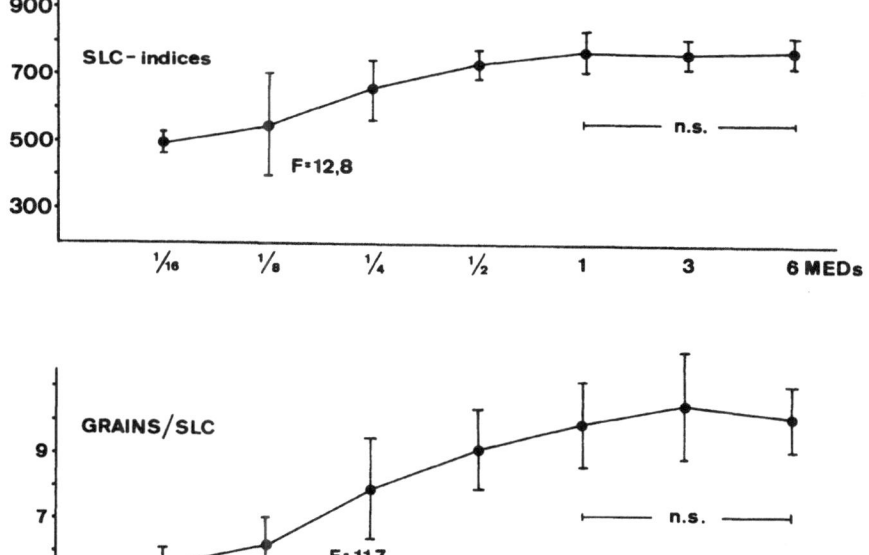

Fig. 1. Dose response of UDS to fractions and multiples of the MED. Mean values of 15 subjects. Vertical bars indicate standard deviations. a. sparse labelled cells per 1000 epidermal cells (SLC-index). b. number of grains per 100 sparse labelled cells. No significant difference is found between 1 MED and 6 MEDs.

linear and tends to become less marked with higher doses. At 1 MED a plateau is reached which remains unchanged up to 6 MEDs and this suggests exhaustion of the excision repair capacity.

One important finding is that even very low suberythemogenic doses of UVB induce considerable DNA damage. The lowest UVB irradiation used in this study which induced measurable UDS was 1.25 mJ/cm². From 1/16 to 1 MED UDS seems to be directly correlated with the relative UVB dose as expressed in fractions of the MED, and this is in keeping with the results of Freeman et al.(1986) who showed evidence that dimer formation correlates with erythemal response. A similar observation was also reported by Eggset et al. (1986) who employed an antibody technique to investigate DNA damage in human skin. No direct correlation was found with absolute doses as expressed in mJ/cm².

Time Course of the Response

In each individual two areas were exposed to 1/2 MED and 2 MEDs, respectively. Biopsies were secured immediately, and at 1, 3, 6, 12, and 24 h after exposure and processed for autoradiography. During the interval from exposure to biopsy the test areas were shielded in order to avoid possible repair of DNA lesions by photoreactivation.

As already reported above for the dose-response experiment, the SLC-indices of 1/2 MED were only slightly lower than that of 2 MEDs. This was again seen in this experiment. Starting at rather similar levels immediately after exposure, the curves of 1/2 MED and of 2 MEDs showed a gradual decline during the following hours. However, the 1/2 MED curve exhibited a steeper slope and reached the zero level between 12 and 24 h. In contrast, after 2 MEDs the mean grain and SLC values at 24 h were about 50 % of the initial value indicating that the repair activity is markedly prolonged after irradiation with 2 MEDs (Fig. 2a).

The grain counts per labelled cell revealed a similar time course. Both curves ran a parallel course until 6 h after exposure. Thereafter the 1/2 MED curve declined rapidly and reached zero between 12 and 24 h. There was a considerable number of grains still present 24 h after exposures to 2 MEDs, the values being again about 50 % of the initial levels (Fig. 2b).

The time course of UDS which revealed high UDS levels 24 h after exposure to 2 MEDs but no UDS after 1/2 MED represents another piece of evidence for the saturation phemomenon. This observation suggests that more repairable sites have been induced in the DNA with 2 MEDs than the repair mechanism is capable of eliminating within the 24 h period.

Dual Exposures

Test subjects were exposed to 2 MEDs. Twenty-four hours after the irradiation these test sites received a second exposure with either 1/8 or 1/4 MED. Biopsies were obtained immediately following the second exposure. For comparison, biopsies were taken also from areas exposed to single doses of 1/8, 1/4, and 2 MEDs immediately after irradiation, and of 2 MEDs 24 h after irradiation. In an additional experiment the

test sites were exposed 24 h after the first application of
1/8 and 1/4 MED to a second irradiation with the same doses.
Biopsies were taken in the same sequence as above.

Immediately after the first exposure, 2 MEDs induced more
UDS than 1/4 MED, which, in turn, induced slightly more UDS
than 1/8 MED. As already observed in the time-course study,
after 24 h UDS was still present in the 2 MEDs areas, whereas
UDS was absent from the 1/4 MED and the 1/8 MED sites. A second
exposure of the 2 MED area with 1/4 or 1/8 MED resulted in a

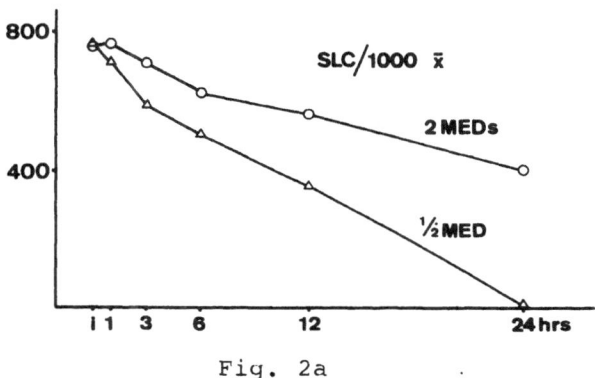

Fig. 2a

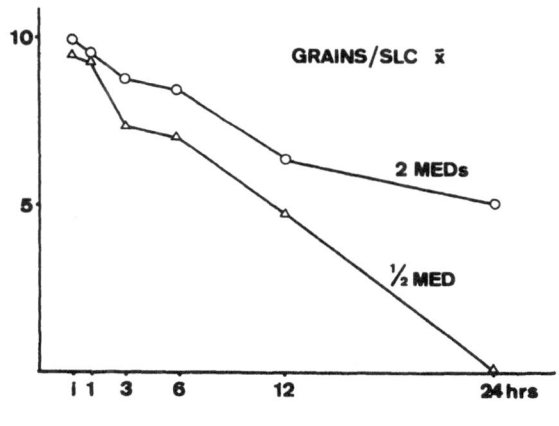

Fig. 2b

Fig. 2. Time course of UDS over 24 h after exposure (i) to 1/2 MED (Δ), and to 2 MEDs
(o). Mean values in 4 subjects. a. sparse
labelled cells per 1000 epidermal cells
(SLC). b. number of grains per 100 sparse
labelled cells.

minimal increase of UDS levels. These levels were even lower
than those after exposure with 1/4 or 1/8 MED alone in previously untreated test areas. However, a second hit of 1/4 MED
or of 1/8 MED 24 h after pre-irradiation of the test site with
1/4 MED or 1/8 MED produced UDS within the range found in untreated skin (Fig. 3).

Because of the persistence of UDS after 2 MEDs a second
exposure to fractions of the MED could be expected to add up
again to the previous UDS plateau. However, a new plateau de-
velops which is lower than that found in non-exposed skin.
Presently, there is no explanation why UDS cannot be increased
to previous levels by a second irradiation. It does not seem
very likely that the lower UDS levels reflect decreased dimer
formation, particularly since earlier experiments by Waters
(1980), with cultured human cells have indicated that split
doses of UV do not modify the incidence of pyrimidine dimers
but do reduce the amount of excision resynthesis. One could
speculate that large amounts of DNA damage may, in part, inhibit repair synthesis analogous to the observation of Tyrrell
and Webb (1973), who have shown that near-UV disrupts excision
repair of UVC-induced lesions in bacteria.

It is also unlikely that reduced dimer formation could be
the result of an inducible protective mechanism such as increased melanin pigmentation or stratum corneum thickening.
Twenty-four hours after one single UVB exposure, melanosome
formation and transfer of melanosomes into keratinocytes certainly has not reached a degree which could provide meaningful

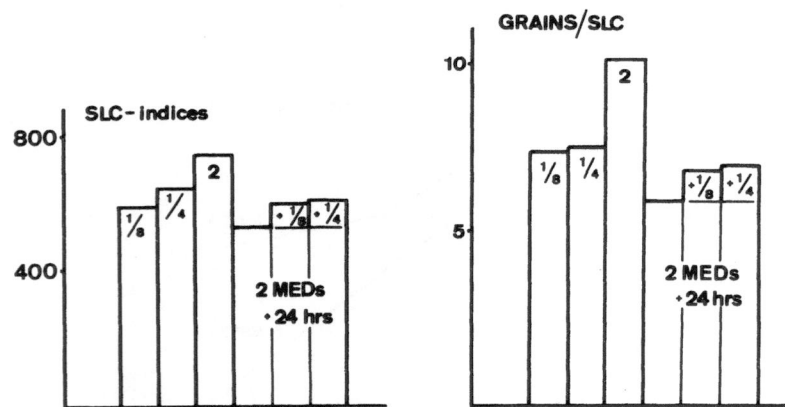

Fig. 3. Dual-dose study. Mean values in 4 subjects.
Note that there is only a minimal increase in UDS after the second exposure
of the 2 MEDs area to 1/8 MED and 1/4 MED
24 h after exposure to 2 MEDs. a. sparse
labelled cells per 1000 epidermal cells.
b. number of grains per 100 sparse labelled
cells.

UV protection. Trace amounts of UVA delivered to the skin during irradiation are too low to induce immediate pigment darkening. Moreover, immediate pigmentation does not protect against DNA damage. Radiation-induced stratum corneum thickening starts to develop much later. We cannot rule out, though, the possibility that biochemical events within the epidermal cells after UV exposure might reduce UV transmission and thus lead to a reduction of DNA damage. Direct measurement of dimers with quantitative methods such as determination of endonuclease-sensitive sites (Sutherland et al., 1980; Setlow et al., 1975; Sutherland and Shih, 1983; D'Ambrosio et al., 1981a; Freeman et al., 1986), and of repair by determination of cytosine arabinoside-induced single-strand breaks (Waters, 1979) will be required. Data from our laboratory obtained with human skin fibroblasts seem to confirm the in vivo observations on plateau formation and dimer persistence (Tanew et al., 1985).

CONCLUSIONS

The persistence of DNA lesions in the skin even after moderate sun exposure may be of significant importance for skin carcinogenesis. Repeated erythemogenic doses received within a certain period may induce cumulative damage which eventually will facilitate the formation of mutations. The clinical relevance of such cumulative damage as it may occur during sunbathing awaits clarification.

On considering our results from the time course and the dual-dose experiments the question arises how skin cells cope with an accumulation of DNA lesions without being either lethally damaged or producing overt mutations. There now exist data indicating that photoreactivation may occur in human skin (Sutherland and Sutherland, 1975; D'Ambrosio et al., 1981b; Sutherland et al., 1985). Our findings implicate that for maintaining skin integrity, mechanisms other than excision repair must protect human skin by error-free dimer removal from possibly mutagenic DNA lesions. Photoreactivation may be important in this respect.

ACKNOWLEDGEMENTS

Figures 1,2, and 4 were reproduced from Hönigsmann et al, 1987, with permission of Elsevier Sequoia, S.A., Lausanne, Switzerland.
The author gratefully acknowledges the contributions of W. Brenner, F. Gschnait, K.F. Jaenicke, B. Ortel, J.A. Parrish, W. Rauschmeier, A. Steiner, A. Tanew, C. Wolf, and K. Wolff to parts of the work presented in this chapter.

REFERENCES

Ahmed, F.E., and Setlow R.B., 1979, Saturation of DNA repair in mammalian cells, Photochem.Photobiol., 29:983.
D'Ambrosio, S.M., Slazinski, L., Whetstone, J.W., and Lowney, E., 1981a, Excision repair of UV-induced pyrimidine dimers in human skin in vivo, J.Invest. Dermatol., 77:311.
D'Ambrosio, S.M., Whetstone, J.W., Slazinski, and L., Lowney, E., 1981b, Photorepair of pyrimidine dimers in human skin in vivo, Photochem.Photobiol., 34:461.

Andrews, A.D., 1980, Sensitivity of xeroderma pigmentosum lymphoblasts to ultraviolet B (290-320 nm) and ultra-violet A (320-400 nm) light, J.Invest.Dermatol., 74:255.

Bishop, S.,1979, DNA repair synthesis in human skin exposed to ultraviolet radiation used in PUVA (psoralen and UV-A) therapy for psoriasis, Br.J.Dermatol., 101:399.

Black, H.S., and Chan, J.T., 1977, Experimental ultraviolet light carcinogenesis, J.Photochem.Photobiol., 26:183.

Black, G., Matzinger, E.A., and Gange, R.W., 1985, Lack of photoprotection against UVB-induced erythema by immediate pigmentation induced by 382 nm radiation, J.Invest. Dermatol., 85:448.

Bohnert, E., Asbach, W., and Jung, E.G., 1972, Replikation und Reparatur epidermaler DNA: Einflüsse von Lichtexposition und Alter, Arch.Dermatol.Forsch., 244:40.

Eggset, G., Krokan, H., and Volden, G., 1986, UV-induced DNA damage and its repair in tanned and untanned human skin in vivo, Photochem.Photobiophys., 10:181.

Epstein, J.H., 1970, Ultraviolet carcinogenesis, in: "Photo-physiology", vol 5, A.C. Giese, ed., Academic Press, New York.

Epstein, W.L., Fukuyama, K., and Epstein, J.H., 1969, Early effects of ultraviolet light on DNA synthesis in human skin in vivo, Arch.Dermatol., 100:84.

Freeman, S.E., Gange, R.W., Matzinger, E.A., and Sutherland, B.M., 1986, Higher pyrimidine dimer yields in skin of normal humans with higher UVB sensitivity, J.Invest. Dermatol., 86:34.

Freeman, S.E., Gange, R.W., Sutherland, J.C., Matzinger, E.A., and Sutherland B.M., 1987, Production of pyrimidine dimers in DNA of human skin exposed in situ to UVA radiation, J.Invest.Dermatol., 88:430.

Gschnait, F., Brenner, W., and Wolff, K., 1978, Photoprotective effect of a psoralen-UVA-induced tan, Arch.Dermatol.Res., 263:181.

Hart, R., Setlow, R.B., and Woodhead, A.D., 1977, Evidence that pyrimidine dimers in DNA can give rise to tumors, Proc. Natl.Acad.Sci., 74:5574.

Henseler, T., Hönigsmann, H., Wolff, K., and Christophers, E., 1981, The European PUVA study (EPS): oral 8-methoxy-psora-len photochemotherapy of psoriasis. A cooperative study among 18 European centres, Lancet, i:853.

Hönigsmann, H., Jaenicke, K.F., Brenner, W., Rauschmeier, W., and Parrish, J.A., 1981, Unscheduled DNA synthesis in normal human skin after single and combined doses of UV-A, UV-B and UV-A with methoxsalen (PUVA), Br.J. Dermatol., 105:491.

Hönigsmann, H., Brenner, W., Tanew, A., and Ortel, B., 1987a, UV-induced unscheduled DNA synthesis in human skin: dose response, correlation with erythema, time course and split dose exposure in vivo, J.Photochem.Photobiol., B: Biology, 1:33.

Hönigsmann, H., Wolff, K., Fitzpatrick, T.B., Pathak, M.A., and Parrish, J.A., 1987b, Oral photochemotherapy with psora-lens and UVA (PUVA): principles and practice, in: "Derma-tology in General Medicine", T.B. Fitzpatrick, A.Z. Eisen, K. Wolff, I.M. Freedberg, F.K. Austen, eds., McGraw-Hill Inc., New York.

Kaidbey, K.H., and Kligman, A.M., 1979, The acute effects of long-wave ultraviolet radiation on human skin, J.Invest. Dermatol., 72:253.

Lehmann, A.R., Kirk-Bell, S., Arlett, C.F., Paterson, M.C., Lohmann, P.H.M., de Weerd-Kastelein E.A., and Bootsma D., 1975, Xeroderma pigmentosum cells with normal levels of excision repair have a defect in DNA snythesis after UV irradiation, Proc.Natl.Acad.Sci., 72:219.

Mathews-Roth, M., and Krinsky, N., 1985, Carotenoid dose level and protection against UV-B induced skin tumors, Photochem.Photobiol., 42:35.

Mathews-Roth, M., 1986, Carotenoids quench evolution of excited species in epidermis exposed to UV-B (290-320 nm) light, Photochem.Photobiol., 43:91.

Ortel, B., Tanew, A., and Hönigsmann, H., 1986, Lack of protection against UVB-induced damage by immediate pigment darkening, J.Invest.Dermatol., 87:160.

Robbins, H.J., Kraemer, R.H., Lutzner, M.A., Festoff, B.W., and Coon, H.G., 1974, Xeroderma pigmentosum: in inherited disease with sun sensitivity, multiple cutaneous neoplasms, and abnormal DNA repair, Ann.Intern.Med., 80:221.

Rosario, R., Mark, G.J., Parrish, J.A., and Mihm, M.C., 1979, Histological changes produced in skin by equally erythemogenis doses of UV-A, UV-B, UV-C and UV-A with psoralens, Br.J.Dermatol., 101:299.

Setlow, R.B., 1966, Cyclobutane-type pyrimidine dimers in polynucleotides, Science, 153:379.

Setlow, R.B., Carrier, W.L., and Stewart, J., 1975, Endonuclease-sensitive sites in UV-irradiated DNA, Biophys.J., 194a.

Spikes, J.D., 1982, Photodynamic reactions in photomedicine, in: "The Science of Photomedicine", J.D. Regan, J.A. Parrish, eds., Plenum, New York/ London.

Sutherland, B.M., Harber, L.C., and Kochevar, I.E., 1980, Pyrimidine dimer formation and repair in human skin, Cancer Res., 40:3181.

Sutherland, B.M., and Shih, A.G., 1983, Quantitation of pyrimidine dimer content of nonradioactive deoxyribonucleic acid by electrophoresis in alkaline agarose gels., Biochemistry, 22:745.

Sutherland, B.M., Blackett, A.D., Feng, I .N., Freeman, S.E., Gange, and R.W., Sutherland, J.C., 1985, Photoreactivation and other ultraviolet/visible light effects on DNA in human skin, Ann.N.Y.Acad.Sci., 453:73.

Sutherland, J.C., and Sutherland, B.M., 1975, Human photoreactivating enzyme, Biophys.J., 15:435.

Tanew, A., Hönigsmann, H., Stampf, S., and Ortel, B., 1985, Kinetics of pyrimidine dimer formation and repair in human skin fibroblasts, Arch.Dermatol.Res., 277:428.

Tyrrell, R.M., and Webb, R.B., 1973, Reduced dimer excision following near ultraviolet (365 nm) radiation, Mutation Res., 19:361.

Waters, R., 1979, Repair of DNA in replicated and unreplicated portions of the human genome, J.Mol.Biol., 127:117.

Waters, R., 1980, The repair of human DNA following fractionated doses of ultraviolet irradiation, Carcinogenesis, 1:9.

Willis, I., Kligman, A.M., and Epstein, J.H., 1973, Effects of long ultraviolet rays on human skin: photoprotective of photoaugmentative, J.Invest.Dermatol., 59:416.

Wolf, C., Steiner, A., and Hönigsmann, H., 1988, Do oral carotenoids protect human skin against ultraviolet erythema, psoralen phototoxicity and ultraviolet-induced DNA damage, J.Invest.Dermatol., 90:55.

DNA REPAIR IN MAMMALIAN TISSUES AND CELLS

Hans E. Krokan[1], Lisbeth C. Olsen[2], Rein Aasland[2],
Gunnar Volden[3], Guri Eggset[4], Bjørnar Myrnes[4], Berit
Johansen[1], Åge Haugen[5], and Dag E. Helland[2]

UNIGEN Center for Molecular Biology, University of
Trondheim, Norway[1], Laboratory of Biotechnology,
University of Bergen, Norway[2], Department of
Dermatology, University of Trondheim, Norway[3],
Institute of Medical Biology, University of
Tromsø, Norway[4], Department of Toxicology, National
Institute of Occupational Health, Oslo, Norway[5]

INTRODUCTION

This article will mainly review the work of our
laboratories on the repair of DNA damage in human cells and
tissues and will include repair of damage caused by
ultraviolet light, uracil in DNA and alkylations due to N-
nitroso compounds. References to related work will be
restricted to those pertinent to the discussion and
interpretation of our own work.

The in depth study of the mechanism of DNA repair in
human cells has in general been limited by the lack of
suitable mutants and by the lack of detailed biochemical
information about the repair systems. Therefore, the molecular
genetics of mammalian DNA repair mechanisms is still virtually
unknown. However, a significant role of DNA repair systems in
the prevention of human disease was indicated more than 20
years ago when it was demonstrated that fibroblasts from
patients suffering from xeroderma pigmentosum (XP) were
defective in excision repair following exposure to ultraviolet
light (UV) (Cleaver, 1968). Since then defective DNA repair
has been demonstrated in a number of other human diseases,
although the evidence for a primary defect in the repair of
DNA damage is less well substantiated than in XP (Friedberg et
al. 1979).

In XP, there are at least 9 complementation groups, but
the biochemical defects in these groups have only been
partially resolved (Fischer et al., 1985, reviewed in
Friedberg, 1984). Patients suffering from Bloom's syndrome
(BS) show a strikingly low birth weight, stunted growth,
light-induced teleangiectasia on the facial skin and a highly
increased incidence of cancer. Fibroblasts from BS-patients
have high numbers of spontaneous chromosomal breaks and sister

DNA Damage and Repair in Human Tissues
Edited by B. M. Sutherland and A. D. Woodhead
Plenum Press, New York, 1990

chromatid exchanges (SCE) (Friedberg, 1984).

Uracil may appear in DNA as a result of incorporation of dUMP instead of dTMP during replication, or by deamination of cytosine residues in DNA. In both cases, uracil is removed by the DNA repair enzyme uracil-DNA glycosylase (UDG), (Wist et al., 1978; Lindahl, 1979). The presence of an immunologically abnormal form of UDG has been associated with BS (Seal et al., 1988). Furthermore, cells from individuals with BS were characterized by a temporal delay in the induction of UDG relative to the onset of the S-phase (Gupta and Sirover, 1984; Yamamoto and Fujiwara, 1986). The significance of these observations remains unclear. In normal cells, induction of UDG, as well as other DNA-glycosylases, an AP-endonuclease and a redoxyendonuclease, precede onset of the S-phase (Gupta and Sirover, 1980; Helland and Olsen, 1988). A physical association of UDG with the replication complex was indicated by the preferential association of UDG with replicating SV40 minichromosomes rather than with mature minichromosomes (Krokan, 1981), and by the possible association of UDG with the catalytic subunit of DNA polymerase alpha (Seal and Sirover, 1986).

Among the various DNA lesions caused by N-nitroso compounds, alkylation of the oxygen atom in guanine has attracted particular interest. This is because of the correlation between the presence of this lesion and the development of mutation and cancer in various tissues (Bartsch and Montesano, 1984; Bartsch et al., 1983). The mechanism for repair of O^6-alkylguanine in DNA is similar in Escherichia coli (Olson and Lindahl, 1980) and mammalian cells (Myrnes et al., 1982); the alkyl group is removed by an O^6-methylguanine-DNA methyltransferase (MT) that transfers the methyl or ethyl group from the O^6-position in guanine to a cysteine residue in the methyltransferase. The methylated MT appears to be a dead-end complex, thus each enzyme molecule is only used once and, therefore, consumed in the reaction. A significant number of established tumor cell lines lack MT activity (Yarosh, 1985), but, from our work, it seems likely that this is an in vitro phenomenon, since extracts of biopsies from human tumors infrequently are low in MT activity (Myrnes et al., 1984b).

The rare syndromes in which DNA repair is deficient are very instructive in demonstrating the biological significance of DNA repair processes. Furthermore, animal experiments have indicated a positive correlation between the persistence of O^6-ethylguanine in certain tissues and the development of tumors (Goth and Rajewsky, 1974). We have, therefore, studied various repair systems in a number of human and other mammalian tissues and cells to investigate whether large interindividual and interorgan variation exist. We have also studied biochemical properties of several mammalian DNA repair enzymes.

Our results clearly demonstrate that the capacity for repair of various DNA lesions varies widely not only between different organs, but also between different individuals and different species. Furthermore, our studies demonstrate that the molecular mechanisms of DNA repair are highly conserved through evolution, and at least in the case of uracil-DNA glycosylase, nucleotide sequences are highly conserved at the gene level.

RESULTS

Studies of UV-induced DNA Damage and Repair in Human Skin using Antibodies

Ultraviolet light (UV) is probably the most common mutagenic and carcinogenic agent with which living cells have to contend. The damaging effects of UV light on chromosomal DNA in skin cells are believed to be an important factor in skin carcinogenesis (Setlow, 1974). A number of lesions are induced by UV light. Major photoproducts include the classical cyclo-butane-type pyrimidine dimers and the more recently discovered pyrimidine-pyrimidine (6-4) lesion. Minor photoproducts include a number of monomeric base damages, such as 5,6 dihydroxy-5,6-dihydro-thymine (Friedberg, 1984). The quantitatively most important repair mechanism is excision repair. During excision repair, a short stretch of the DNA strand containing the damage is removed and replaced by new DNA synthesized using the undamaged complementary strand as template (Hanawalt et al., 1979). Reversal of the cyclo-butane type pyrimidine dimer by a light dependent photolyase has been demonstrated in mammalian cells, as well as in bacteria (Rupert 1975, Sutherland and Sutherland, 1975). Although the cyclo-butane type pyrimidine dimers have been assumed to be the most important premutagenic lesion, more recent studies suggest that, at least in E. coli, the (6-4) photoproduct may possibly be even more important (Franklin and Haseltine, 1986).

Immunoassays have been used for detection of a variety of DNA lesions (reviewed in Strickland and Boyle, 1984). Antibodies specific for UV-irradiated DNA can be used to detect DNA damage by radio immuno assay (RIA),(Lucas, 1972), or enzyme linked immuno sorbent assay (ELISA) (Leipold et al., 1983; Eggset et al., 1987). Antibodies can also be used for the in situ detection of DNA damage in cultured cells (Lucas, 1972; Cornelis et al., 1977; Mitchell et al., 1982; Wani et al., 1984) or in skin (Tan and Stoughton, 1969; Jarzabek-Chorelska et al., 1976; Eggset et al., 1983; Eggset et al., 1986; Olsen et al., 1989a). In many of these studies the specificity of the antibodies used was not determined.

We have applied affinity-purified polyclonal rabbit anti-UV-DNA antibodies and an improved immunohistochemical method to study repair of UV light induced DNA damage in human skin in vivo. Antibodies reacting with non-irradiated single stranded DNA was first removed on an ssDNA-Sepharose column and then the antibodies specific for irradiated DNA purified and concentrated on UV-irradiated ssDNA-Sepharose (Eggset et al., 1983). Initially, we assumed that the specificity of our affinity purified antibodies was directed towards cyclo-butane dimers. The rationale for this assumption was the preference of the antibodies for substrates with several adjacent pyrimidines, especially thymines. However, subsequent experiments suggested that photoproducts other than cyclobutane dimers were involved in antibody binding. Thus, DNA photosensitized with acetophenone and ultra violet light type A (UVA), (54 kJ/m^2, >360nm) to induce cyclobutane dimers did not bind the antibodies, as did smaller or similar amounts of UV-irradiated DNA (23 kJ/m^2, 254 nm). In addition, when crude extracts of E. coli photoreactivating enzyme were incubated with thin sections from irradiated skin during visible light illumination, no removal of antibody-binding sites was seen. Furthermore, induction of antibody-binding sites with increasing UV doses continued far beyond saturation doses for pyrimidine dimers. Finally, abrogation of the antibody-binding sites was demonstrated by non-enzymatic photolysis of (6-4) photoproducts. This result strongly indicated that (6-4) photoproducts were the major targets for the antibodies (Eggset et al., 1987).

Since the biological significance of (6-4) photoproducts was not realized until recently, the study of these photoproducts in biological systems is very limited. By our method (Eggset et al., 1983) we were able to study such damage in situ in human skin after irradiation with biologically relevant UV doses. Detectable amounts of mutagenic (6-4) photoproducts, thus, were detected already after irradiation with 0.5 minimal erythemal dose (MED) of UVB (225 J/m^2). To study the kinetics of repair in human skin, human volunteers were irradiated with 2 MED of UVB (maximum delivery at 310 nm), and antibody binding sites investigated in biopsies taken at different times post-irradiation (Eggset et al., 1983). The presence of DNA damage was demonstrated both by immunofluorescence (not shown) and by immunoperoxidase staining (Fig.1). To investigate the possible function of human photoreactivation enzyme in vivo, one area of the abdominal skin was exposed to visible light, whereas another area was kept in the dark. Removal of antibody-binding sites was well under way at 4-5 h post irradiation and essentially complete after 24 h. Visible light increased the rate of repair, indicating the involvement of a photoreactivating enzyme in human skin in vivo. However, dark repair appears to be dominating quantitatively. Repair was not restricted to proliferating cells in stratum basale; however, the damage in the deeper layers of epidermis seems to be more readily repaired than in the upper layers. In another study we found that the dose necessary to induce DNA damage was 4-6 times higher in tanned abdominal skin as compared to untanned abdominal skin from the same person (Eggset et al., 1986). Tanning and thickening of epidermis both contributed to reduced penetration of UV light in isolated human epidermis and probably explains the protective effect of tanning (Eggset et al., 1984).

Repair of DNA Damage Introduced by N-nitrosocompounds

The carcinogenicity of N-nitrosocompounds was first discovered in 1956 when it was shown that dimethylnitrosamine produced hepatic tumors in rats (Magee and Barnes, 1956). Since then the list of carcinogenic N-nitroso compounds has grown to become quite extensive (Magee and Barnes, 1967). Alkylation of nucleic acids by N-nitroso compounds was first described in 1962 (Magee and Farber, 1962) and later alkylations at several positions of DNA have been described (Hemminki, 1983). A striking organotropic effect of N-nitroso compounds has been described; furthermore, the sensitivity of

an animal is in general higher at the embryonal stage
(Druckrey et al., 1967; Kleihues et al., 1983). Alkylation at
the O^6-position in guanine was first proposed to be the major
site responsible for the mutagenic and carcinogenic effect of
N-nitrosocompounds by Loveless (1969). Subsequently, it was
shown that persistence of O^6-alkylation correlated well with
carcinogenesis (Goth and Rajewsky, 1974; Lawley, 1984). A
unique one-step repair process in which the methyl or ethyl
group is tranferred from the O^6-position in guanine to a
protein cysteine residue was first described in E.coli (Olson
and Lindahl, 1980). Subsequently, a very similar repair system

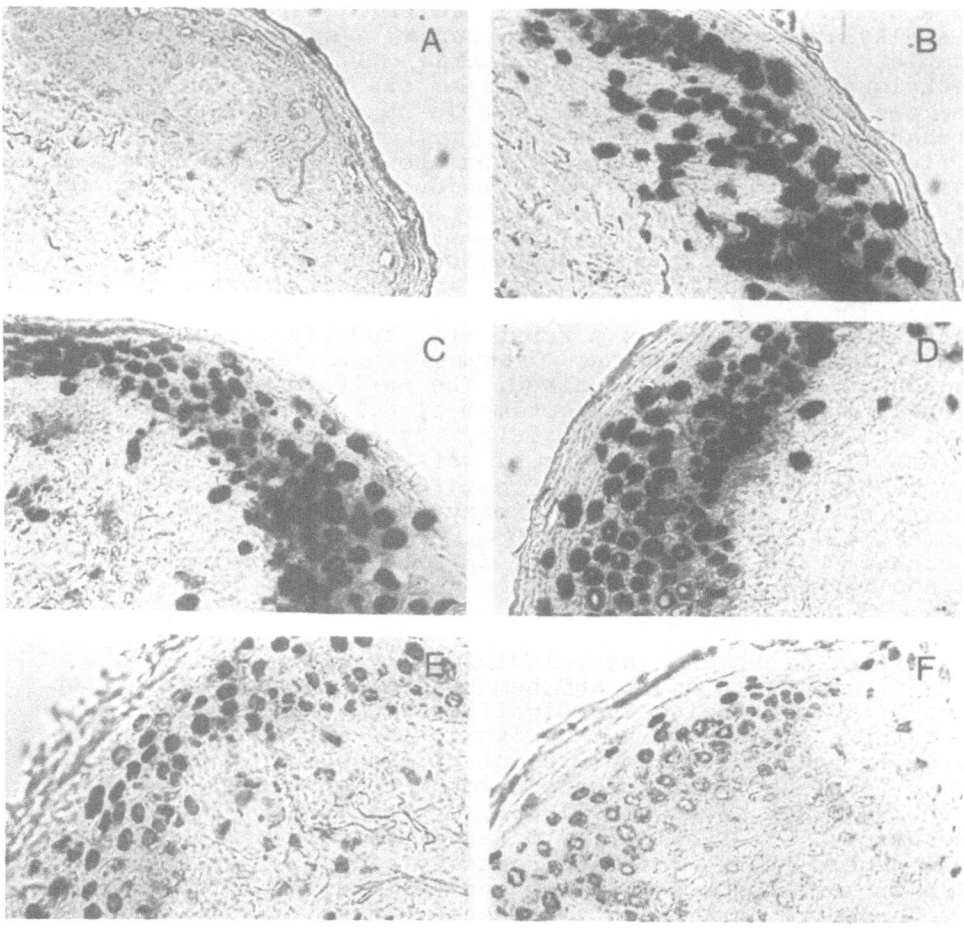

Fig. 1. Nuclear immunoperoxidase staining of <u>in vivo</u>
irradiated human skin after irradiation with 900
J/m^2 (2 MED) of UVB. A, unirradiated control; B,
immedi-ately after irradiation; C, 2 h post
irradiation, skin area kept in the dark; D, 2 h
post irradiation, skin exposed visible light; E, 4
h post irradiation, skin kept in the dark; F, 4 h
post irradiation, skin exposed to visible light
(from Eggset et al., 1983).

was found in human cells and tissues (Myrnes et al., 1982; Yarosh, 1985; Orren and Sancar, 1987).

We have studied the repair of alkylation lesions of DNA in human and other mammalian cells and tissues both with respect to the mechanism, the level of activity in different organs and cells, and the inter-individual and inter-organ capacity for repair. In most of these studies we also examined the activity of uracil-DNA glycosylase in the same extracts. The data accumulated allow certain predictions about the sensitivity of various organs to N-nitroso compounds.

The mechanism of alkylation repair. When extracts of HeLa S_3 cells, human liver, and rat liver were incubated with DNA alkylated with N-^{3}H-N-nitrosourea, a specific decrease or complete removal of O^6-methylguanine, N3-methyladenine, and N7-methylguanine was observed. Whereas the two latter alkylation lesions appeared to be removed by a DNA-glycosylase, the mechanism of repair of O^6-methylguanine residues was clearly different. Further investigations showed that the methyl group was transferred to a cysteine residue in an acceptor protein of apparent M_r 23,000, as shown by SDS-polyacrylamide gel electrophoresis (SDS-PAGE) (Myrnes et al., 1982). We later partially purified the MT some 2500-fold from HeLa S_3 cells to a specific activity of 2600 pmol/mg protein (Myrnes et al., 1986). The purified enzyme prefers double-stranded DNA rather than single-stranded as a substrate, and was specific for O^6-alkylations; thus, neither O^4-thymine residues nor phosphotriesters were repaired. The purified MT is inhibited by NaCl and KCl, has a pH optimum of 8.2, and does not require divalent cations for its activity. It is much more sensitive to heat inactivation and has slower kinetics than the corresponding enzyme from E. coli. HeLa S_3 cells, human fetal liver, spleen, lung, brain, kidney, colon, pancreas, and stomach all appear to repair O^6-alkylations by a similar mechanism, and only one enzyme species of approximately M_r 23,000 was found.

Inter-organ and inter-individual variation in MT and UDG activity in human adult and human fetal tissues. As a step towards understanding the significance of DNA repair enzymes in the protection against genotoxic and carcinogenic agents, we have examined the activity of MT and UDG in a number of human fetal and adult organs (Krokan et al., 1983; Myrnes et al., 1983; Myrnes at al., 1984a; Myrnes at al., 1984b). Presumably, the sensitivity of an organ to N-nitroso compounds will depend on the rate and capacity of repair relative to the rate of carcinogen activation and cellular proliferation. It was therefore surprising to us that MT activity was not higher in fetal tissues than in the corresponding adult tissues; in fact the activity in fetal liver was 7-fold lower than in adult. Extracts of 25 human placentae showed a 7-fold interindividual variation in activity (mean of 0.13 pmol/mg protein), which was a very significantly larger variation than in other fetal tissues. A number of control experiments precluded possible technical reasons for this variation (I. Lettrem, unpublished results). UDG was also lower in most fetal tissues. In extracts of adult tissues, liver had, on average, a 5 to 8-fold higher activity of MT (1.07 ± 0.62

pmol/mg protein) than the other organs (stomach, small intestine, and colon) and showed about an 8-fold inter-individual variation. A very significant inter-individual variation was observed in all tissues examined. The interindividual variation in MT and UDG activity was, in general, higher in adult tissues than in fetal. UDG also showed a very significant inter-organ and inter-individual variation. There was no correlation between MT and UDG activities, indicating that they are regulated differently.

The reports on the low or absence of MT activities in some 20% of human tumor cell lines from a number of different tumors (Yarosh, 1985) prompted us to examine the MT activity in fresh biopsies from human tumors (n=24) and the corresponding non-neoplastic tissues obtained during surgery (Myrnes et al., 1984b). On average, the MT activity was slightly higher in the extracts from tumors, but there were some exceptions; thus, 3 out of 7 stomach cancers had 1.8 to 3-fold lower activity than the corresponding non-neoplastic tissues, and one kidney tumor had a 7-fold lower activity of MT than the corresponding non-neoplastic tissue. Interestingly, the MT activity in a case of primary hepatocarcinoma was 5 to 7-fold lower in the tumor and in the corresponding non-neoplastic liver tissue than was previously found to be the case for the mean of 9 normal livers. In fact, the lowest activity of MT previously found in normal liver tissue was 2-fold higher than in non-neoplastic liver tissue from the individual carrying the hepatocarcinoma. These data indicate that a low level of MT activity is not a frequent event in human tumors. However, it is quite possible that some less common cancers, such as primary hepatocarcinoma, may more frequently be associated with a low repair capacity.

Such significant inter-individual and inter-organ variations in DNA repair capacity have later been verified and extended by several laboratories (Grafstrøm et al., 1984; Wiestler et al., 1984; Kyrtopoulos et al., 1984; Gerson et al., 1986; D'Ambrosio et al., 1987). However, D'Ambrosio et al. (1987), found higher levels of MT in human fetal liver than we did, but still less than found in adult liver. They also observed a greater inter-individual variation than we found. Values for other tissues were in excellent agreement with our results. In a study of age-and strain-dependence of hepatic MT activity in mice, significantly lower activity was found in young mice (3 or 8 weeks old) as compared to those of middle age (30-50 weeks) (Nakatsuru et al., 1989). Likachev (1985), reported lower levels of MT in the liver of 3-month old rats than in those aged 1 and 15 months.

The general conclusion that can be drawn from these studies is that the human fetus is likely to be more sensitive to certain alkylating agents than adult individuals. Fetal brain has the lowest activity, indicating that this organ may be highly sensitive to N-nitroso compounds, as previously found in animal experiments (Druckrey et al., 1965).

Cell specific differences in excision repair and MT and UDG activities. The measurements of DNA repair capacities in organs clearly does not give sufficient information on possible cell specific differences. To approach this question, we investigated DNA repair in various pulmonar cells of male

181

New Zealand white rabbits (Deilhaug et al., 1985). Clara cells (85% purity, 90% viability) and alveolar type II cells (95% purity, 85% viability) were isolated by centrifugal elutriation. Alveolar type II cells were further purified by Percoll gradient centrifugation. Alveolar macrophages were obtained by lavage. The extent of excision repair induced by direct acting alkylating agents (MMS, MNNG and ENU) was measured as unscheduled DNA synthesis (autoradiography) in cells in confluent primary cultures. Activities of MT and UDG in Clara cells and type II alveolar cells were measured in cell extracts after centrifugal elutriation. A dose dependent level of excision repair, and easily detectable MT activity was observed in alveolar type II cells. In contrast, Clara cells had 4 to 20-fold lower levels of excision repair, and non-detectable MT activity. The UDG activity was also lower in Clara cells. Alveolar macrophages had higher levels of MT and UDG activity than alveolar type II cells.

In a related study, Belinsky et al. (1988) examined alkylation of DNA and subsequent DNA repair in rat pulmonary cells after exposure to the tobacco-specific carcinogen 4-(N-methyl-N-nitrosamino)-1-(3-pyridyl)-1-butanone (NNK). Interestingly, the concentration of O^6-methylguanine in DNA was highest- and MT activity lowest in Clara cells. Furthermore, MT activity was essentially depleted in Clara cells after a 4 week exposure to NNK.

These observations are interesting, because Clara cells appear to be the primary site of cytochrome P-450 dependent monooxygenase reactions and have a capacity for proliferation (Serabjit-Singh et al., 1980; Jeffery and Reid, 1977). Furthermore, Clara cells have been shown to be progenitor cells of experimentally induced murine adenomas (Kauffman et al., 1979; Montes et al., 1966). Finally, evidence obtained from studies on human bronchiolo-alveolar carcinomas has strongly supported their origin from Clara cells (Kuhn, 1972; Greenberg et al., 1975; Jaques and Currie, 1977; Montes et al., 1977; Parsa and Kauffman, 1983). Assuming that DNA repair and xenobiotic metabolism follow similar patterns in rat, rabbit, and humans, one might speculate that low repair capacity and high metabolism of xenobiotics may be contributing factors to the development of bronchiolo-alveolar cancers in humans.

Cell specific differences in MT activity have also been observed in rat liver (Lewis and Swenberg, 1980).

Effect of various environmental agents on MT activity in mammalian cells. In E.coli the level of MT activity is highly inducible by some alkylating agents (reviewed in Lindahl et al., 1988). The picture is not as clear cut in mammalian cells. Thus, we found no increase in activity in HeLa cells after a single dose of MNNG (Myrnes et al., 1982). Furthermore, when normal human bronchial epithelial cells cultured in serum-free medium were exposed to non-toxic doses of MNNG at 6-8 h intervals for 4-5 days, MT activity did not increase. Neither did cell survival increase significantly following a range of challenge doses. These data suggest that human bronchial cells do not adapt to MNNG (Krokan et al., 1985a). Some evidence for an adaptive response to alkylating agents has, however, been obtained in other laboratories

(Waldstein et al., 1982; Laval and Laval,1984). Enhanced
activity of MT has also been observed after exposure to
various agents, such as the non-genotoxic drug phenobarbital
(O'Connor et al, 1988), or UV- or gamma-irradiation, and heat-
treatment as well as DNA damaging drugs (Lefebvre and Laval,
1986).

The picture that emerges from these findings and several
other observations is that some increase in MT activity can be
induced by a variety of agents in some cells, but not in
others. Furthermore, there appear to be species differences.
In mammalian cells the level of constitutive synthesis of MT
is in general significant, and the level of exposure
presumably fairly low. Therefore, a highly inducible system
like the one in E. coli may not be essential.

As already described, tobacco specific N-nitroso
compounds have been shown to deplete MT in pulmonary Clara
cells in rat (Belinsky et al., 1988). Other compounds, such as
lipid peroxidation aldehydes and the tobacco-smoke related
unsaturated aldehyde acrolein may contribute to the
inactivation of MT by reacting with an essential SH-group
(Krokan et al., 1985b). We found little effect of
formaldehyde, and no effect of acetaldehyde. In contrast
Espina et al. (1988), found a strong inhibitory effect with as
little as 10 nM acetaldehyde. We can not explain this
discrepancy, but if this strong effect of acetaldehyde is
correct, it is a very significant finding.

DNA glycosylases in human cells. Human cells have DNA
glycosylases that remove uracil (Wist et al., 1978) and
hypoxanthine (Jensen et al., 1982), which are deamination
products of cytosine and adenine, respectively, and alkylation
products such as 3-methyladenine (Myrnes et al., 1982; Male et
al., 1986) and 7-methylguanine (Myrnes et al., 1982).
Information from prokaryote organisms suggests that there are
several additional DNA glycosylases in human cells (Lindahl,
1979). Our work has concentrated mostly on uracil-DNA
glycosylase (UDG). SV40 minichromosomes is a good model for
studies on mammalian chromatin structure and replication. We
found that UDG is preferentially associated with replicating
minichromosomes rather than mature minichromosomes, indicating
that DNA repair is more active near the replication fork
(Krokan, 1981). Purification and biochemical characterization
of UDG have been complicated by an apparent tight association
of UDG with other proteins (Wittwer and Krokan, 1985).
However, we have recently succeeded in purification of human
UDG from HeLa cells (Myrnes and Wittwer, 1988) and human
placenta (Wittwer et al., 1989). In placenta, several
biochemically closely related forms of the enzyme were found,
but in HeLa cells only one form was apparent. A 131,000-fold
purification of UDG from placenta yielded a preparation
containing UDG of specific activity 8500 nmol uracil released
per mg protein per min at 30 °C. The apparent M_r was 29,000,
which was identical to the M_r found for UDG in HeLa cells. In
placenta, a tightly associated protein of M_r 26,500 could only
be separated from UDG by SDS-PAGE. UDG in placenta and HeLa
cells had an approximate molecular turnover number of 600 per
min, was stimulated 10-fold by 70 mM NaCl and had an apparent
K_m of 2 μM.

After separation on SDS-PAGE and blotting of UDG and the tightly associated protein onto Polybrene GF/C paper, a partial sequence of both proteins was obtained. This sequence allowed preparation of a mixed oligonucleotide probe on the basis of N-terminal amino acid residues 19-26 of the major form of UDG. The oligonucleotide probe was used to screen a lambda gt11 cDNA library from human placenta. Two of the positive clones, pUNG-15 and pUNG-40, were characterized by restriction enzyme mapping and DNA sequencing (Olsen et al, 1989). DNA sequencing revealed an open reading frame of 981 nucleotides (positions 38 - 1018). The first ATG-codon downstream from the in-frame stop codon at position 35 is

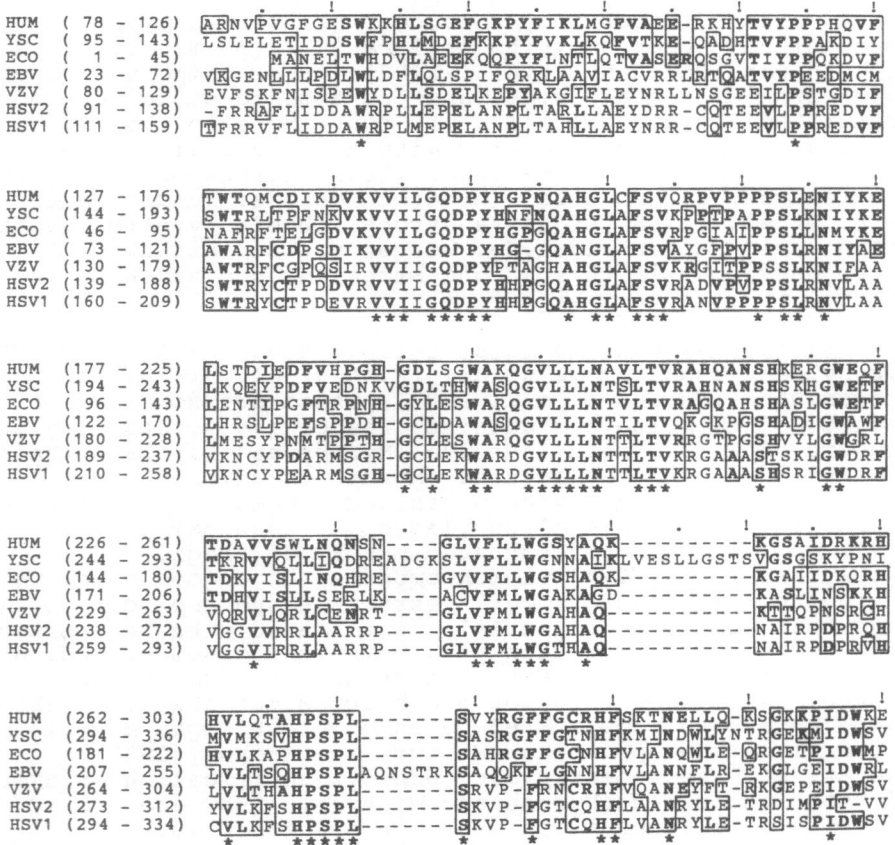

Fig. 2. Comparison of protein sequences of uracil-DNA glycosylases. Alignment of uracil-DNA glycosylase from humans (HUM), yeast (YSC, ung1-gene, Percival et al., 1989), E. coli (ECO, ung-gene, Varshney et al., 1988, Herpes Simplex Virus type 2 (HSV2, gene UL2, Worrad and Caradonna, 1988) and type 1 (HSV1, gene UL2, McGeoch et al., 1988), and the homologous sequences from Epstein-Barr Virus (EBV, gene BKRF3, Baer et al., 1984) and Varicella Zoster Virus (VZV, gene 59, Davison and Scott, 1986), (from Olsen et al., 1989).

found at position 107 and is a possible initiation codon. The
resulting reading frame encodes a translation product of 304
amino acids. The amino terminal amino acid sequence of the
purified protein (Wittwer et al., 1989) is found at residues
78-105 in the predicted protein sequence (fig. 2). This
suggests that the initial translation product is processed to
a mature protein which has an M_r 25,800. We can not explain the
discrepancy between the M_r values found by SDS-PAGE and the
predicted value from DNA sequencing. An amazing similarity to
recently cloned uracil-DNA glycosylases from E. coli, yeast,
Herpes Simplex virus type 1 and 2, Varicella Zoster virus and
Epstein-Barr virus was seen at the amino acid level (Fig. 2).
The similarity was 40.3%-55.7% identical amino acid residues.
Surprisingly, the proteins from human and bacterial origin
were most closely related, there was a 73.3% similarity when
conservative substitutions were included. The similarity
between different uracil-DNA glycosylase genes is confined to
several discrete boxes. We have now isolated several genomic
clones for UDG from an EMBL 3 human placenta library. By using
oligonucleotide probes specific for the 5' and the 3' ends of
UDG cDNA, we have found that at least two of our clones appear
to carry the whole gene on an 8 kb restriction fragment. These
clones are presently being further characterized.

Our findings strongly indicate that uracil-DNA
glycosylase from phylogenetically distant species are highly
conserved. It remains to be seen whether other DNA repair
enzymes are also conserved to a similar degree.

ACKNOWLEDGEMENT

This work was supported by the Norwegian Cancer Society
(Den Norske Kreftforening) and by the Norwegian Research
Council for Science and the Humanities (Norges
Allmenvitenskapelige Forskningsråd).

REFERENCES

Baer, R., Bankier, A.T., Biggin, M.D., Deininger, P.L.,
    Farrel. P.J., Gibson, T.J., Hatfull, G., Hudson,
    G.S., Satchwell, S.C., Seguin, C., Tuffnell, P.S., and
    Barrell, B.G., 1984, DNA sequence and expression of the
    B95-8 Epstein-Barr virus genome, Nature, 310:207.
Bartsch, H., and Montesano, R., 1974, Relevance of
    nitrosoamines in human cancer, Carcinogenesis 5:1381.
Bartsch, H., Terracini, B., Malaveille, C., Tomatis, L.,
    Waherndorf, J., Brun, G., and Dodet, B., 1983,
    Quantitative comparison of carcinogenicity,
    mutagenicity and electrophilicity of 10 direct-acting
    alkylating agents and of the initial O^6:7-alkylguanine
    ratio in DNA with carcinogenic potency in rodents,
    Mutat. Res., 110:181.
Belinsky, S.A., Dolan, M.E., White, C.M., Maronpot, R.R.,
    Pegg, A.E., and Anderson, M.W., 1988, Cell specific
    differences in O^6-methylguanine methyltransferase
    activity and removal of O^6-methylguanine in rat
    pulmonary cells, Carcinogenesis, 9:2053.
Cleaver, J.E.,1968, Defective repair replication in xeroderma
    pigmentosum, Nature, 218:652.

Cornelis, J.J., Rommelaere, J., Urbain, J., and Errera, M.,
1977, A sensitive method for measuring pyrimidine
dimers in situ, Photochem. Photobiol., 26:241.

D'Ambrosio, S.M., Samuel, M.J., Dutta-Choudhury, T.A., and
Wani, A.A., 1987, O^6-methylguanine-DNA methyltransferase
in human fetal tissues: Fetal and maternal factors,
Cancer Res., 47:51.

Davison, A.J., and Scott, J.E., 1986, The complete sequence of
Varicella-Zoster Virus, J. Gen. Virol., 67:1759.

Deilhaug, T., Myrnes, B., Aune, T., Krokan, H., and Haugen,
Aa., 1985, Differential capacities for DNA repair in
Clara cells, alveolar type II cells and macrophages of
rabbit lung, Carcinogenesis, 6:661

Druckrey. H., Ivankovic, S., and Preussmann, R., 1965,
Organotrope carcinogene Wirkungen bei 65 verschiedenen
N-Nitrosoverbindungen an BD-Ratten, Z. Krebsforsch.,
66:389.

Eggset, G., Volden, G., and Krokan, H., 1983, UV-induced DNA
damage and its repair in human skin in vivo studied by
sensitive immunohistochemical methods, Carcinogenesis,
4:745.

Eggset, G., Krokan, H. and Volden, G., 1986, UV-induced DNA
damage and its repair in tanned and untanned human skin
in vivo, Photobiochem. Photobiophys., 10:181.

Eggset, G., Volden, G., and Krokan, H., 1987, Characterization
of antibodies specific for UV-damaged DNA by ELISA,
Photochem. Photobiol., 45:485.

Espina, N., Lima, V., Lieber, C.S., and Garro, A.J., 1988, In
vitro and in vivo effect of acetaldehyde on O^6-
methylguanine transferase, Carcinogenesis, 9:751

Fischer, E.W., Keijzer, H.W., and Thielmann, H.W., 1985, A
ninth complementation group in xeroderma pigmentosum,
XPI, Mutat. Res., 145:217.

Franklin, W.A., and Haseltine, W.A., 1986, The role of the (6-
4) photoproduct in ultraviolet light-induced transition
mutations in E. coli, Mutat. Res., 165:1.

Friedberg, E.C., Ehman, U.K., and Williams, J.I.,
1979, Human diseases associated with defective DNA
repair, Adv. Rad. Biol., 8:85.

Friedberg, E.C., 1984, "DNA Repair", W.H. Freeman and Company,
New York.

Gerson, S.L., Trey, J.E., Miller, K., and Berger, N.A., 1986,
Comparison of O^6-alkylguanine-DNA alkyltransferase
activity based on cellular DNA content in human, rat
and mouse tissues, Carcinogenesis, 7:745.

Greenberg, S.D., Smith, M.N., and Spjut, J.H., 1975,
Bronchioalveolar carcinoma - cell of origin, Am. J.
Clin. Pathol., 63:153.

Gupta, P.K., ans Sirover, M.A., 1980, Sequential stimulation
of DNA repair and DNA replication in norman human
cells, Mutat. Res. 72:273.

Gupta, P.K., and Sirover, M.A., 1984, Altered temporal
expression of DNA repair in hypermutable Bloom's
syndrome cells. Proc. Natl Acad. Sci. USA, 81:757.

Hanawalt, P.C., Cooper, P.K., Ganesan, A.K., and Smith, C.A.,
1979, DNA repair in bacteria and mammalian cells, Ann.
Rev. Biochem., 48:783.

Helland, D.E., and Olsen, L.C., 1988, Cell cycle dependent
regulation of DNA repair enzymes. J. Cell. Biochem.
suppl. 12A:265.

Hemminki, K., 1983, Nucleic acid adducts of chemical
    carcinogens and mutagens, Arch. Toxicol., 52:249.
Jaques, J., and Currie, W., 1977, Bronchiolo-alveolar
    carcinoma: a Clara cell tumor?, Cancer, 40:2171.
Jarzabek-Chorelska, M., Zabreska, Z., Wolska, H., and Reza,
    G., 1976, Immunological phenomena induced by UV rays,
    Acta Dermatovener., 56:285.
Jeffery, P.K., and Reid, L.M., 1977, The respiratory mucous
    membrane, in: "Respiratory Defense Mechanisms", p. 193,
    J.D. Brain, D.F. Proctor, and L.M. Reid, eds, Marcel
    Dekker, New York.
Jensen, B.M., Guddal, P.H., and Krokan, H., 1982, Metabolism
    of dITP, incorporation into nuclear DNA and slow
    release of free hypoxanthine from DNA by a
    hypoxanthine-DNA-glycosylase, Nucl. Acids. Res.,
    10:3693.
Kauffman, S.L., Alexander, L., and Sass, L., 1979, Histologic
    and ultrastructural features of the Clara cell adenoma
    of the mouse lung, Lab. Invest., 40:708.
Kleihues, P., Hodgsen, R.M., Veit, C., Schweinsberg, F., and
    Wiestler, M., 1983, DNA modification and repair in
    vivo: towards a biochemical basis of organ specific
    carcinogenesis by methylating agents, in "Organ and
    Species Specificity in Chemical Carcinogenesis", R.
    Langenbach, S. Nesnow, and J.M. Rice, eds., Plenum
    Press, New York
Krokan, H.E., 1981, Preferential association of uracil-DNA
    glycosylase activity with replicating SV40
    minichromosomes, FEBS Lett., 133:89.
Krokan, H., Haugen, Å., Myrnes, B., and Guddal, P.H., 1983,
    Repair of premutagenic DNA lesions in human fetal
    tissues: evidence for low levels of O^6-methylguanine-DNA
    methyltransferase and uracil-DNA glycosylase activity
    in some tissues, Carcinogenesis, 4:1559.
Krokan, H., Lechner, J., Krokan, R.H., and Harris, C.C.,
    1985a, Normal human bronchial epithelial cells do not
    show an adaptive response after treatment with N-
    methyl-N'-nitro-N-nitrosoguanidine, Mutat. Res.,
    146:205.
Krokan, H., Grafstrøm, R.C., Sundqvist, K., Esterbauer, H.,
    and Harris, C.C.,1985b, Cytotoxicity, thiol depletion
    and inhibition of O^6-methylguanine-DNA methyl-
    transferase by various aldehydes in cultured human
    bronchial fibroblasts, Carcinogenesis, 6:1755.
Kuhn, C., 1972, Fine structure of bronchiolo-alveolar
    carcinoma, Cancer, 30:1107.
Kyrtopoulos, S.A., Vroutso, B., Golematis, B., Bonatsos, M.,
    and Lakiotis, G.,1984, O^6-methylguanine-DNA
    transmethylase activity in extracts of human gastric
    mucosa, Carcinogenesis, 5:943.
Laval, F., and Laval, J., 1984, Adaptive response in mammalian
    cells: Crossreactivity of different pretreatments on
    cytotoxicity as contrasted to mutagenicity, Proc. Natl.
    Acad. Sci. USA, 81:1062.
Lawley, P.D., 1984, Carcinogenesis by alkylating agents, in
    "Chemical carcinogens" 2nd edn., ACS Monograph, vol.
    182:325, Am. Chem. Soc., Washington DC.
Lefebvre, P., and Laval, F., Enhancement of O^6-methylguanine-
    DNA-methyltransferase activity induced by various
    treatments in mammalian cells, Cancer Res., 46:5701.
Leipold, B., Remy, W., and Adelmann-Grill, B., 1983,

Measurement of ultraviolet light-induced photolesions in mammalian DNA by microELISA, *J. Imm. Methods*, 60:69.

Lewis, J.G., and Swenberg, J.A., 1983, Differential repair of O^6-methylguanine in DNA of rat hepatocytes and nonparenchymal cells, *Nature*, 288:185.

Likachev, A.J., 1985, The effect of age on DNA repair in carcinogenesis due to alkylating agents, in: "Age related factors in Carcinogenesis", IARC Scientific. Publ. No. 58, p.239, A. Likachev, V. Anisimov, and R. Montesano, eds, International Agency for Research on Cancer, Lyon.

Lindahl, T.,1979, DNA glycosylases, endonucleases for apurinic/apyrimidinic sites, and base excision-repair, *Prog. Nucl. Acids Res. Mol Biol.*, 22:135.

Lindahl, T., Sedgwick, B., Sekiguchi, M., and Nakabeppu, Y., 1988, Regulation and expression of the adaptive response to alkylating agents, *Ann. Rev. Biochem.*, 57:133.

Loveless, A., 1969, Possible relevance of O^6-alkylation of DNA to the mutagenicity and carcinogenicity of nitrosamines and nitrosamides *Nature*, 223:206.

Lucas, C.J., 1972, Immunological demonstration of the disappearance of pyrimidine dimers from nuclei of cultured human cells, *Exptl. Cell Res.*, 74:480.

Magee, P.N., and Barnes, J.M., 1956, The production of malignant primary tumors in the rat by feeding dimethylnitrosamine, *Br. J. Cancer*, 10:114.

Magee, P.N., and Barnes, J.M., 1967, Carcinogenic nitroso compounds, *Avd. Cancer Res.*, 10:163.

Male, R., Helland, D.E., Lillehaug, J.R., and Kleppe, K., 1986, Properties of mammalian 3-methyladenine-DNA glycosylases, in: "Repair of DNA Lesions Introduced by N-nitroso Compounds",p. 230, B. Myrnes and H. Krokan, eds, Norweg. Univ. Press, Oslo.

McGeoch, D.J., Dalrymple, M.A., Davison, A.J., Dolan, A., Frame, M.C., McNab, D., Perry, L.J., Scott, J.E., and Taylor, P., 1988, The complete DNA sequence of the long unique region in the genome of Herpes Simplex Virus type 1, *J. Gen. Virol.*, 69:1539.

Montes, M., Adler, R.H., and Brennman, J.F., 1966, Bronchiolar apocrine tumor, *Am. Rev. Resp. Dis.*, 93:946.

Montes, M., Binette, J.P., Chaudhry, A.P., Adler, R.H., and Guarino, R., 1977, Clara cell adenocarcinoma. Light and electron microscope studies, *Am. J. Surg. Pathol.*, 1:245.

Myrnes, B., Giercksky,K.-E., and Krokan, H., 1982, Repair of O^6-methylguanine residues in DNA takes place by a similar mechanism in extracts from HeLa cells, human liver and rat liver, *J. Cell. Biochem.*, 20:381.

Myrnes, B, Giercksky, K.-E., and Krokan, H., 1983, Interindividual variation in the activity of O^6-methylguanine-DNA methyltransferase activity and uracil-DNA glycosylase activity in human organs, *Carcinogenesis*, 4:1565.

Myrnes, B., Eggset, G., Volden, G., and Krokan, H., 1984a, Enzymatic repair of premutagenic DNA lesions in human epidermis. Quantitation of O^6-methylguanine-DNA methyltransferase and uracil-DNA glycosylase activities,*Mutat. Res.* 131:183.

Myrnes, B., Norstrand, K., Giercksky, K.-E., Sjunneskog, C., and Krokan, H., 1984b, A simplified assay for O^6-

methylguanine-DNA methyltransferase activity and its application to human neoplastic and non-neoplastic tissues, <u>Carcinogenesis</u>, 5:1061.

Myrnes, B., Nilsen, I.W., Haugen, Aa., and Krokan, H., 1986, Molecular properties of O^6-methylguanine-DNA methyltransferase in human cells, <u>in</u>: "Repair of DNA Lesions Introduced by N-Nitroso Compounds" p. 112, B. Myrnes and H. Krokan, eds., Norweg. Univ. Press, Oslo.

Myrnes, B., and Wittwer, C.U., 1988, Purification of the human O^6-methylguanine-DNA methyltransferase and uracil-DNA glycosylase, the latter to apparent homogeneity, <u>Eur. J. Biochem.</u>, 173:383.

Nakatsuru, Y., Aoki, K., and Ishikawa, T., 1989, Age and strain dependence of O^6-methylguanine DNA methyltransferase activity in mice, <u>Mutat. Res.</u>, 219:51.

O'Connor, P.J., Fida, C.Y., Fan, C.Y., Bromley, M., and Saffhill, R.,1988, Phenobarbital: a non-genotoxic agent which induces the repair of O^6-methylguanine from hepatic DNA, <u>Carcinogenesis</u>, 9:2033.

Olsen, L.C., Aasland, R., Wittwer, C.U., Krokan, H.E., and Helland, D.E.,1989, Molecular cloning of human uracil-DNA glycosylase, a highly conserved DNA-repair enzyme. <u>EMBO J.</u>, 8, 3121-3125.

Olsen, W.M., Huitfeldt, H.S., and Eggset, G., 1989a, UVB-induced (6-4) photoproducts in hairless mouse epidermis studied by quantitative immunohistochemistry, <u>Carcinogenesis</u>, in press.

Olson, M., and Lindahl, T., 1980, Repair of alkylated DNA in Escherichia coli. Methyl group transfer from O6-methylguanine to a protein cysteine residue, <u>J. Biol. Chem.</u>, 255:10569.

Orren, D.K., and Sancar, A., 1987, New discoveries in the enzymology of DNA repair, <u>Cancer Rev.</u>, 7:5.

Parsa, I., and Kauffman, S.L., 1983, Malignant Clara cell line derived from ethylnitrosourea-induced murine lung adenomas, <u>Cancer Lett.</u>, 18:311.

Percival, K.J., Klein, M.B., and Burgers, M.J., 1989, Molecular cloning and primary structure of the uracil-DNA glycosylase gene from <u>Saccharomyces cerevisiae</u>, <u>J. Biol. Chem.</u>, 264:2593.

Rupert, C.S., 1975, Enzymatic photoreactivation: overview, in "Molecular Mechanisms for Repair of DNA", part A, P.C. Hanawalt and R.B. Setlow, eds., Plenum, New York, p. 73. Seal, G., Bretch, K., Karp, S.J., Cool, B.L., and Sirover, M.A., 1988, Immunological lesions in human uracil DNAglycosylase: Association with Bloom's syndrome. <u>Proc. Natl. Acad. Sci. USA</u>, 85:2339.

Seal, G., and Sirover, M.A., 1986, Physical association of the human base-excision repair enzyme uracil DNA glycosylasewith the 70,000-dalton catalytic subunit of DNApolymerase alpha. <u>Proc. Natl. Acad. Sci. USA</u>, 83:7608.

Serabjit-Singh, C.J., Wolf, C.R., Philpot, R.M., and Plopper, C.G., 1980, Cytochrome P-450: localization in rabbit lung, <u>Science</u>, 207:1469

Setlow, R.B., 1974, The wavelengths in sunlight effective in producing skin cancer: a theoretical analysis, <u>Proc. Natl. Acad. Sci. USA</u>, 71:3363.

Strickland, P.T. and Boyle, J.M., 1984, Immunoassays of carcinogen-modified DNA, <u>Prog. Nucl. Acid Res. Mol. Biol.</u>, 31:1.

Tan, E.M., and Stoughton, R.B., 1969, Ultraviolet light alteration of cellular deoxyribonucleic acid in vivo, Proc. Natl. Acad. Sci. USA, 62:708.

Sutherland, J.C., and Sutherland, B.M., 1975, Human photoreactivating enzyme: Action spectrum and safelight conditions, Biophys. J., 15:435.

Varshney, U., Hutcheon, T., and van de Sande, J.H., 1988, Sequence analysis, expression and conservation of Escherichia coli uracil DNA glycosylase and its gene ung, J. Biol. Chem., 263:7776.

Waldstein, E.A., Cao, E.-H., and Setlow, R.B., 1982, Adaptive increase of O^6-methylguanine-acceptor protein in HeLa cells following N-methyl-N'-nitro-N-nitrosoguanidine treatment, Nucl. Acids. Res., 15:4595.

Wani, A., Gibson-D'Ambrosio, R.E., and D'Ambrosio, S.M., 1984, Antibodies to UV irradiated DNA: the monitoring of DNA damage by ELISA and indirect immunofluorescence, Photochem. Photobiol., 40:465.

Wiestler, O., Kleihues, P., and Pegg, A.E., 1984, O^6-alkylguanine-DNA alkyltransferase activity in human brain and brain tumors, Carcinogenesis, 5:121

Wist, E., Unhjem, O., and Krokan, H.,1978, Accumulation of small fragments of DNA in isolated HeLa cell nuclei due to transient incorporation of dUMP, Biochim. Biophys. Acta, 520:253.

Wittwer, C.U., and Krokan, H., 1985, Uracil-DNA glycosylase in HeLa cells: Interconvertibility of an M_r 50,000 and an M_r 20,000 form of the enzyme, Biochim. Biophys. Acta, 83:308.

Wittwer, C.U., Bauw, G., and Krokan, H.E., 1989, Purification and Determination of the NH_2-Terminal Amino Acid Sequence of Uracil-DNA glycosylase from Human Placenta, Biochem., 28:780.

Worrad, D.M, and Caradonna, S., 1988, Identification of the coding sequence for Herpes Simplex Virus uracil-DNA glycosylase, J. Virol. 62:4774

Yamamoto, Y., and Fujiwara, Y., 1986, Abnormal regulation of uracil DNA glycosylase induction during cell cycle and cell passage in Bloom's syndrom fibroblasts, Carcinogenesis, 7:305.

Yarosh, D.B.,1985, The role of O^6-methylguanine-DNA methyltransferase in cell survival, mutagenesis and carcinogenesis, Mutat. Res., 145:1.

DAMAGE SPECIFIC MAMMALIAN ENDONUCLEASES

Bjørn-Ivar Haukanes, [1] Paul W. Doetsch [3],
Lisbeth C. Olsen,[1] Ikramul Huq, [1] Hans E.
Krokan [4] and Dag E. Helland [1,2]

[1]Laboratory of Biotechnology, University of
Bergen, Box 3152 Aarstad, N-5029 Bergen,
Norway
[2]Present address: Dana Farber Cancer
Institute, Harvard Medical School,
Department of Pathology, Division of Human
Retrovirology, Boston, USA
[3]Emory University Medical School, Atlanta,
Georgia, USA
[4]UNIGEN University of Trondheim, Trondheim,
Norway

INTRODUCTION

A broad spectrum of agents are known to react with DNA,
and the resulting changes in structure may have deleterious
biological consequences, if not removed. Modified bases in
DNA can be excised from DNA by different repair pathways.
The process of excision repair involves four major steps:
incision, excision, DNA synthesis, and ligation of the
repaired sequence. The enzymes responsible for the first
step in this scheme are damage-specific enzymes of which
several have been isolated and characterized both from
bacteria and eukaryotic cells. This group of enzymes is
known to recognize damage in double-stranded DNA induced by
a variety of agents, such as UV- and gamma-radiation, acid,
psoralen, and alkylating agents.
    To understand the complex reaction leading to repair of
DNA, the enzymes participating in this pathway must be
detected, isolated, and characterized. The damage-specific
enzymes can be classified as 1) Direct reversal of DNA
damage, 2) N-Glycosylases, and 3) Endonucleases (Friedberg,
1985). Here we will review what is known of the properties
of the mammalian damage-specific endonucleases, mainly
focusing on our own work, and discuss some of the techniques
used to characterize these enzymes and to deduce their
mechanisms of action. For a more complete and recent review

DNA Damage and Repair in Human Tissues
Edited by B. M. Sutherland and A. D. Woodhead
Plenum Press, New York, 1990

191

discussing all enzymes known to be important for DNA repair
see Wallace (1988) and Sancar and Sancar (1988).

At present, the mammalian damage specific endonucleases
can be grouped into three classes: apurinic/apyrimidinic
(AP) endonucleases, redoxyendonucleases, and a mammalian
analog to the E.coli uvrABC excision nuclease enzyme
complex. Of these, the redoxyendonucleases and AP-
endonucleases are the best characterized. The mechanisms of
action and base specificities of DNA cleavage mediated by
these two groups of enzymes have been deduced by DNA
sequencing techniques.

In addition to studying the mechanism of action of these
enzymes, we have also done experiments to study the activity
of these enzymes throughout the cell cycle, in order to
understand how the cell regulates its potential of repairing
damage in DNA in relation to DNA synthesis. We found that
enzyme activity is dependent upon the cell cycle.
The genes encoding these mammalian enzymes have not yet been
isolated, but work currently being carried out in our
laboratories as well as in others is directed towards this
goal.

RESULTS AND DISCUSSION

Apurinic/Apyrimidinic Endonucleases (AP-endonucleases)

An apurinic/apyrimidinic (AP) site in DNA can be formed
by spontaneous hydrolysis of the N-glycosidic bond, by
chemical or physical agents or by the action of a DNA
glycosylase (Friedberg, 1985). The deoxyribose residue in
such an abasic site exsists in an equilibrium between the
aldehyde form and the furanose form. Bypass of AP-sites
during DNA replication can lead to misincorporation (Randall
et al., 1987).

Enzymes recognizing AP-sites in DNA, called AP-
endonucleases, cleave the phosphodiester bond either 3' or
5' to the AP-site. At both the 3'-side and the 5'-side there
are two theoretical possibilities, making a total of four
theoretical classes of AP-endonucleases, as discussed by
Haukanes et al. (1988). Mammalian AP-endonucleases of which
the cleavage site has been determined, fall into class I or
class II (Fig. 1). Class II AP-endonucleases create a
deoxyribose-5'-phosphate at the 5'-termini and a 3'-hydroxyl
nucleotide terminus, which acts as a good primer for the DNA
polymerase. Class I AP-endonucleases produce a 3'-
deoxyribose and a 5'-phosphomonoester nucleotide termini and
are usually associated with a DNA glycosylase activity. It
has been suggested that class I AP-endonucleases act as
beta-elimination catalysts and not via enzymatic hydrolysis
(Bailly and Verly, 1987; Kim and Linn, 1988). Most class I

AP-endonucleases also have an associated glycosylase activity. Theoretically, class I and class II AP-endonucleases can work in concert, thus removing the baseless sugar-phosphate residue. Mammalian tissue usually contain both activities. However, the baseless sugar i.e. the deoxyribose-5'-phosphate at the 5'-terminus generated by the action of a class II AP-endonuclease, can also be removed by a DNA-deoxyribophosphodiesterase. This enzyme activity was recently detected, purified, and characterized from both bovine tissue and E.coli (Franklin and Lindahl, 1988).

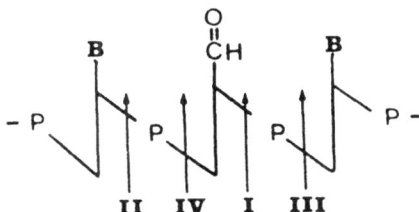

Fig. 1. Potentially sites for cleavage of phosphodiester bonds by AP-endonucleases at apurinic/apyrimidinic sites.

We developed a method by which the cleavage site produced by various DNA-repair endonucleases and other nucleases can be determined in one experiment. The method employ the Maxam-Gilbert DNA sequencing procedure, chemical modification with piperidine, the 3'-phosphatase activity of T_4-polynucleotide kinase, and enzymatic treatment with calf intestinal phosphatase (a 5'-phosphatase) in addition to separation on a DNA sequencing gel. The procedure allows the analysis of each single damaged site in the DNA-strand. Furthermore, the procedure distinguishes between all four theoretical classes of AP-endonucleases and can be used to study the nature of both DNA incision and excision (Haukanes et al., 1988). We have characterized two mammalian AP-endonucleases by this strategy. An AP-endonuclease from human placenta was found to act as a class I AP-endonuclease (Haukanes et al., 1989b), and an AP specific endonuclease present in mouse plasmacytoma cells was characterized as a class II AP-endonuclease (Haukanes et al., 1988; Haukanes et al., 1989a). Previous methods to distinguish between class I and class II were based on measuring the priming activity of DNA polymerase I from E.coli. However, these procedures will not give any
information about DNA excision nor the 3'-side of the AP-site. They will only measure the average values for all AP-

sites, and will most often give a rather high background due to non-specific nicking of the DNA, resulting in priming at other sites than those induced by the AP-endonuclease investigated.

A class II AP-endonuclease has been purified to homogeneity from calf thymus (Henner et al., 1987). This

	A				B			CLASS:
	1	**2**	**3**		**1**	**2**	**3**	
a	-----	-----	-----	a	-----	-XXX-	-XXX-	
b	-XXX-	-XXX-	-----	b	-XXX-	-----	-----	I
c	-----	-----	-XXX-	c	-----	-----	-----	
a	-----	-----	-----	a	-----	-XXX-	-----	
b	-XXX-	-XXX-	-XXX-	b	-XXX-	-----	-XXX-	II
c	-----	-----	-----	c	-----	-----	-----	
a	-----	-XXX-	-----	a	-----	-----	-----	
b	-XXX-	-----	-XXX-	b	-XXX-	-XXX-	-XXX-	III
c	-----	-----	-----	c	-----	-----	-----	
a	-----	-XXX-	-XXX-	a	-----	-----	-----	
b	-XXX-	-----	-----	b	-XXX-	-XXX-	-----	IV
c	-----	-----	-----	c	-----	-----	-XXX-	

Fig. 2. Strategy for classification of AP-endonucleases and other nucleases by separation of the cleavage products on a DNA-sequencing gel. The procedure allows detailed studies of the nature of phosphodiester bond breaks: (A) 5'-labeled DNA, analysis of the 5'-side of the cleavage site; (B) 3'-labeled DNA, analysis of the 3'-side of the cleavage site. (1) DNA containing eg. AP-sites cleaved by the enzyme to be examined; (2) as in (1) but in addition treated with 3'-phosphatase in (A) and 5'-phosphatase in (B); (3) treated as in (2) and then with piperidine in both (A) and (B) (Haukanes et al., 1988).

enzyme has no requirement for ring-opened or ring-closed deoxyribose moities. However, base fragments such as urea residues, or reduction of the C'-1 position of the abasic site abolish the activity (Sanderson et al., 1989). These experiments clearly distinguish this class II mammalian enzyme from the class I E.coli endonuclease III (Bailly and Verly, 1987; Kim and Linn, 1988) which cleaves DNA by an beta-elimination reaction, and the class II E.coli exonuclease III which cleaves DNA also at sites containing urea residues (Kow and Wallace, 1985).

Redoxyendonucleases

The redoxyendonucleases are a class of DNA damage-specific enzymes that are functionally highly conserved in prokaryotes and eukaryotes. Redoxyendonucleases are unusual DNA repair enzymes because that they possess both N-glycosylase and AP-endonuclease activities enabling them to mediate the first two steps in the base excision repair pathway (Doetsch et al., 1986). They are also unusual in that they appear to possess a broad substrate specificity directed against a variety of pyrimidine (and also probably purine) base damages that have lost aromaticity (Helland et al., 1986). This group of enzymes is named redoxyendonucleases due to the chemical mechanisms that produce substrates for them (reductions or oxidations). Such base damage products are produced by high doses of UV-light, ionizing radiation, and a variety of oxidizing agents.

In this respect the redoxyendonucleases behave like the other base excision repair N-glycosylases that do not possess AP-endonuclease activity. The biochemical implication of the Mg2+ independence of the redoxyendonucleases is difficult to deduce, but indicates that the interaction with DNA is different from that of the Mg2+ endonucleases, since Mg2+ interacts with the negatively charged phosphate groups on the DNA phosphodiester backbone. Do redoxyendonucleases act on intact chromatin? To carry out DNA repair in vivo, redoxyendonuclease must act on DNA organized into nucleosomal structures. We employed UV-irradiated SV40 minichromosomes as substrates for the mouse plasmacytoma redoxyendonuclease (Helland and Krokan, 1983). The UV-irradiated minichromosomes were cleaved by the enzyme and the rate appeared to be similar to that of the naked virus DNA. The UV-doses required to convert the SV40 minichromosomes to a substrate for redoxyendonuclease was also similar to that used for øX174 RFI DNA. We do not know at the present time whether the nicks introduced are in the linker region on the nucleosomes or whether they are randomly distributed through the DNA.

However, the uvrABC excision nuclease complex only produces nicks in irradiated SV40 DNA after the histones have been removed, indicating that the prokaryoric enzyme complex cannot use DNA organized in nucleosomal subunits as a substrate (E.Seeberg, personal communication). The implication of this observation would be that the defect in DNA repair following UV-light exposure in various xeroderma pigmentosum cell lines cannot be compensated for by introducing the E.coli genes encoding the UVRA, B, and C proteins.

Redoxyendonucleases have been found in a variety of mammalian sources including bovine, rodent, and human cells (Helland et al., 1982; Doetsch et al., 1986; Doetsch et al.,

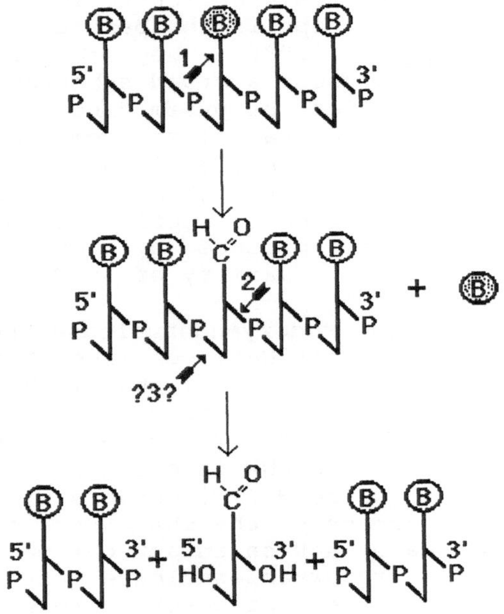

Fig. 3. Processing of oxidative base damage by redoxyendonuclease. An oxidative base damage product (shaded "B") is removed from the DNA strand by (1) an N-glycosylase activity to produce an apurinic/apyrimidinic (AP) site. The AP-site is incised at positions 3' (2) and 5' (3) to that site by a process that produces cleaved DNA fragments containing phosphoryl groups at both the 3'- and 5'-ends. Hence the initial step in the base excision repair of oxidative damage is carried out by a redoxyendonuclease-mediated two-step reaction.

1987). In addition, such an enzyme activity has been found in all systems studied so far including bacteria, yeast, and Drosophila (for a review, see Wallace, 1988). It is likely that most aerobic organisms will contain this activity, including plants. Our studies with the mammalian redoxyendonucleases have focused primarily on the bovine and human enzymes and we have obtained highly purified preparations from calf thymus and human lymphoblasts. We have used DNA sequencing techniques to characterize mammalian redoxyendonucleases. This approach can provide direct information at the level of individual nucleotides with regard to the base specificity of cleavage and mode of phosphodiester bond cleavage mediated by redoxyendonuclease. Different end-labelled, defined sequence DNA substrates containing various oxidative- (OsO_4, $KMnO_4$, H_2O_2, acid) and radiation- (UV and X-ray) induced DNA damages were incubated with redoxyendonuclease and the enzyme digestion products were analyzed on DNA sequencing gels (Doetsch _et al._, 1986; Helland _et al._, 1986; Doetsch _et al._, 1987). The results of such experiments together with HPLC analysis of radiolabelled base damage products released from various DNA substrates indicate that ring-saturated (e.g.thymine glycol) and ring-fragmented (e.g. urea) pyrimidines are substrates for the mammalian redoxyendonucleases and that the enzyme cleaves DNA by a combined N-glycosylase and AP-endonuclease activities (Fig. 3). The exact electrophoretic mobilities of redoxyendonuclease-generated DNA cleavage fragments relative to the corresponding Maxam-Gilbert base-specific DNA sequencing fragments indicates the nature (hydroxyl, phosphoryl, or modified sugar) of the 3'- and 5'-termini and provides insight into the mode of phosphodiester bond cleavage (Doetsch _et al._, 1986). Interestingly, under the conditions of _in vitro_ experiments, the mammalian redoxyendonucleases appear to produce both 3'- and 5'-phosphoryl groups on DNA following cleavage, perhaps via combined beta- and delta-elimination reactions at the AP-site (Doetsch _et al._, 1986). It should be pointed out again that DNA sequencing approaches are a potentially powerful method for characterizing DNA repair endonucleases, and should be very useful in general for the discovery and characterization of other DNA repair endonucleases acting on other classes of damage. Because of the relative ease with which damage-specific, end-labelled substrates can be generated, the endonucleolytic "signature" of putative DNA repair endonuclease present in samples ranging from crude extracts to various types of purified column fractions can be precisely monitored.

Redoxyendonuclease preparations of various degrees of purity have been obtained from bovine, human, and yeast cells (Doetsch _et al._, 1986; Helland _et al._, 1986; Doetsch _et al._, 1987, Helland _et al._, 1987a; Gossett _et al._, 1988)

and show a pattern of base specificity and mode of DNA cleavage very similar to that of E.coli endonuclease III. Hence, although we cannot ascribe the observed N-glycosylase/AP-endonuclease activities to one protein in the eukaryotic preparations, on the basis of their close similarity to endonuclease III, it is likely that the observed activities are being mediated by a single or closely associated protein. The bovine enzyme was recently purified to homogeneity (Huq and Helland, unpublished results) and experiments to ascertain whether or not the N-glycosylase and AP-endonuclease activities remain associated are in progress. The bovine and human redoxyendonucleases are relatively small in size (30 to 60 kDa) and are fully active in the absence of divalent cations such as Mg^{2+} (Helland et al., 1987a; Lee et al., 1987).
Recently we found that human skin epidermis has a high specific activity of redoxyendonuclease compared to other tissues studied, indicating that this activity might be important in repair of UV-damage (Helland, unpublished observation).

Mammalian Repair Enzyme Activity Resembling the E.coli uvrABC Excision Nuclease Complex

Using a novel assay system, Wood, Robins and Lindahl (1988) recently described an enzyme activity in human lymphoid cells that incises covalently closed circular DNA containing bulky adducts such as pyrimidine dimers or psoralene.

This activity resembles the uvrABC enzyme complex present in E.coli. They were able to demonstrate that the activity was absent in extracts from xeroderma pigmentosum cell lines, but could be reconstituted by mixing extracts from group A and C. The mechanism of action of this activity has not yet been described, but the defined assay system developed should allow purification and further characterization of this activity.

Cell Cycle Regulation of Mammalian Redoxyendonuclease and AP-endonuclease Activities

In bacteria several studies have shown that at least some of the repair pathways can be induced following exposure to specific damaging agents. In mammalian systems, however, there is conflicting data on the inducability of known damage-specific enzymes like methyltransferases (see Krokan, this volume).

The mammalian cells could either produce their repair enzymes constitutively to ensure repair throughout the cell cycle or they could induce or increase the repair capacity before or at the same time as the onset of replication. Just

before and during replication, the DNA should be more
accessible to repair since, at that stage, the DNA is not
condensed as much as it is throughout the rest of the cell
cycle. To test these two possibilities, mouse L-cells (L-
929) growing in non-synchronous suspension cultures were
separated according to size by elutriation centrifugation
(Helland et al., 1987b). Following incubation of isolated
G_1-cell populations, fractions of cells were harvested at
different times of incubation and the activity of AP-
endonuclease and redoxyendonuclease measured in extracts of
these cells. As indicated in Figure 4, there is a 3-6 fold
increase in the specific activity of these enzymes in late
G_1-phase. Since the doubling time of the cells used here is
approximately 20 hrs., some activity should persist
throughout the whole cell cycle giving the cell some

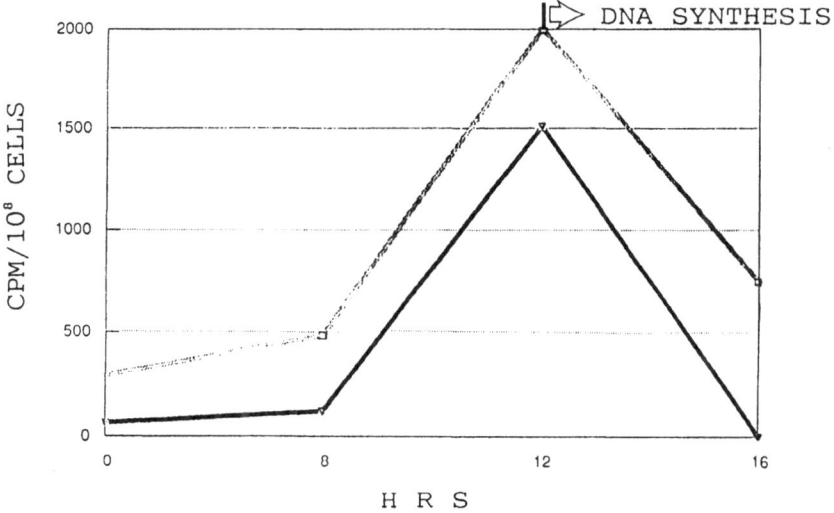

Fig. 4. Activity of damage-specific endonucleases throughout
cell cycle in synchronized mouse L-cells. Cells
growing in a non-sychronous suspension culture were
separated according to size by centrifugation
elutriation. G_1-cells (measured by flow cytometry)
were put back into culture and harvested at
different intervals. DNA synthesis was followed by
incorporation of ^{3}H-thymidine. Redoxyendonuclease and
AP-endonuclease activities were measured in cleared
lysates (100.000x g, 1 hr) by the nitro cellulose
filter assay using [3]H- X174 supercoiled DNA damaged
by UV light (▼: redoxy) or acid (□: AP-endonuclease)
(Helland et al., 1987b).

capacity to repair DNA also in other phases of its cycle. If the major repair enzymes are regulated in a cell cycle dependent manner, the control of these activities should be the same as the control of the other enzymes participating in replication.

CONCLUSION

In spite of the large amount of research done over the years on mammalian DNA repair enzymes, it is not known how important each of the enzymes discussed in this review are in the maintenance of an unmodified genome. The most important approach to address the role of these enzymes in DNA repair would be to isolate the genes for each of these activities. This should be possible by applying the same approach as we recently took to clone the human uracil-DNA glycosylase gene (Olsen et al., 1989).

REFERENCES

Bailly, V., and Verly, W.G., 1987, Escherichia coli endonuclease III is not an endonuclease but a beta -elimination catalyst, Biochem. J., 242: 565.

Doetsch, P.W., Helland, D.E., and Haseltine, W.A., 1986, Mechanism of action of a mammalian DNA repair endonuclease, Biochemistry, 25: 2212.

Doetsch, P.W., Henner, W.D., Cunningham, R.P., Toney, J.H., and Helland, D.E., 1987, A highly conserved endonuclease activity present in Escherichia coli, bovine, and human cells recognizes oxidative DNA damage at sites of pyrimidines, Mol. Cell. Biol., 7: 26.

Franklin, W.A., and Lindahl, T., 1988, DNA deoxyribophosphodiesterase, EMBO J., 7: 3617.

Friedberg, E.C., 1985, DNA repair, W.H. Freeman and Co., New York.

Gossett, J., Lee, K., Cunningham, R.P., and Doetsch, P.W., 1988, Yeast redoxyendonuclease, a DNA repair enzyme similar to Escherichia coli endonuclease III, Biochemistry, 27: 2629.

Haukanes, B.I., Helland, D.E., and Kleppe, K., 1988, Analysis of cleavage products of DNA repair enzymes and other nucleases. Characterization of an apurinic/apyrimidinic specific endonuclease from mouse plasmacytoma cells, Nucl. Acids Res., 16: 6871.

Haukenes, B.I., Helland, D.E., and Kleppe, K., 1989a, Action of a mammalian AP-endonuclease on DNAs of defined sequences, Nucl. Acids Res., 17: 1493.

Haukanes, B.I., Wittwer, C.U., and Helland, D.E., 1989b, Mechanism of incision by an apurinic/apyrimidinic endonuclease present in human placenta, <u>Nucl. Acids Res.</u>, 17: 5529.

Helland, D.E., Doetsch, P.W., and Haseltine, W.A., 1986, Substrate specificity of a mammalian DNA repair endonuclease that recognizes oxidative base damage, <u>Mol. Cell. Biol.</u>, 6: 1983.

Helland, D.E., and Krokan, H., 1983, UV-irradiated SV40 minichromosomes as substrates for DNA repair endonucleases. <u>Biochem. Biophys. Res. Commun.</u>, 113: 309.

Helland, D.E., Male, R., and Kleppe, K., 1987a, Separation of damage specific DNA endonuclease activities present in calf thymus, <u>FEBS Lett.</u>, 213: 215.

Helland, D.E., Male, R., Haukanes, B.I., Olsen, L.C., Haugan, I., and Kleppe, K., 1987b, Properties and mechanism of eukaryotic 3-methyladenine-DNA glycosylase, <u>J. Cell. Sci. Suppl.</u>, 6: 139.

Helland, D.E., Nes, I.F., and Kleppe, K., 1982, Mammalian DNA-repair endonuclease acts only on supercoiled DNA, <u>FEBS Lett.</u>, 142: 121.

Henner, W.D., Kiker, N.P., Jorgensen, T.J., and Munck, J.-N., 1987, Purification and amino-terminal amino acid sequence of an apurinic/apyrimidinic endonuclease from calf thymus, <u>Nucl. Acids Res.</u>, 15: 5529.

Kim, J., and Linn, S., 1988, The mechanism of action of <u>E.coli</u> endonuclease III and T$_4$ UV endonuclease (endo V) at AP-sites, <u>Nucl. Acids Res.</u>, 16: 1135.

Kow, Y.W., and Wallace, S.S., 1985, Exonuclease III recognizes urea residues in oxidized DNA, <u>Proc. Natl. Acad. Sci. USA</u>, 82: 8354.

Lee, K., McCray, W.H., and Doetsch, P.W., 1987, Thymine glycol-DNA glycocylase/AP-endonuclease of CEM-C1 Lymphoblasts: A Human analog <u>E.coli</u> Endo III, <u>Biochem. Biophys. Res. Comm.</u>, 149: 93.

Linn, S., 1982, Nucleases involved in DNA repair. In <u>"Nucleases"</u> (Ed.: S. Linn) pp 59-84. Cold Spring Harbor, New York.

Olsen, L.C., Aasland, R., Wittwer, C.U., Krokan, H.E., and Helland, D.E., 1989, Molecular cloning of human uracil-DNA glycosylase, a highly conserved DNA repair enzyme, <u>EMBO J.</u>, 8: 3121.

Randall, S.K., Eritja, R., Kaplan, B.E., Petruska, J., and Goodman, M.F., 1987, Nucleotide insertion kinetics opposite abasic lesions in DNA, <u>J.Biol.Chem.</u>, 262: 6864.

Sancar, A., and Sancar G.B., 1988, DNA repair enzymes. <u>Ann. Rev. Biochem.</u>, 57: 29.

Sanderson, B.J.S., Chang, C.-N., Grollman, A.P., and Henner,W.D., 1989, Mechanism of DNA cleavage and substrate recognition by a bovine apurinic endonuclease, <u>Biochemistry</u>, 28: 3894.

Wallace, S.S., 1988, AP-endonucleases and DNA glycosylases that recognize oxidized DNA damage, <u>Environment Mol. Mut.</u>, 12: 431.

Wood, R.D., Robins, P., and Lindahl, T., 1988,
    Complementation of the xeroderma pigmentosum DNA
    repair defect in cell-free extracts, _Cell_, 53: 97.

CHARACTERISTICS OF DNA EXCISION REPAIR IN NONDIVIDING XERODERMA

PIGMENTOSUM CELLS, COMPLEMENTATION GROUP C

G. J. Kantor

Department of Biological Sciences
Wright State University
Dayton, OH 45435

INTRODUCTION

Most of the cells in the human body are relatively quiescent, entering an active cell division cycle infrequently or in some cases not at all during the life span of an individual. In contrast, most studies of radiation effects and DNA repair mechanisms in human cells are done with cultured cell populations maintained in an active, proliferative state. In response to this contradiction, we have studied cultures of quiescent cells that exhibit the low levels of DNA replicative synthesis and cell division found in human skin. We find that radiation, in particular ultraviolet light (UV; 240 to 313 nm) and sunlight, produces changes in the quiescent cells that can be readily observed and quantified. DNA is the principal target for these changes and DNA excision repair can ameliorate them (Kantor, 1986). Studies employing cells that are deficient in DNA excision repair from patients with the genetic disease xeroderma pigmentosum (XP) have been useful in defining the molecular basis for these changes. Here we describe results obtained with XP cells from complementation group C (XP-C) that further extend our understanding of the cellular reaction to UV and of DNA excision repair processes and their significance in human cells.

The most readily observable change induced by UV is a lethal one evidenced by cell degeneration, cell detachment from the culture surface and eventual loss from the culture. That is, UV kills nondividing cells and the killing is evident without the need of a colony formation assay (Kantor et al., 1977). Nondividing cells from human strains with proficient DNA excision repair are more resistant to this UV-induced death than are those from strains with deficient repair mechanisms such as those from XP patients. The relative sensitivity of nondividing cells from specific XP strains is in general related to the amount of DNA repair activity detected in each strain (Kantor and Hull, 1984) and is also similar to that detected using proliferating cultures and a colony-formation survival assay (Kantor and Elking, 1988). XP-C cells are an exception to these generalizations. They exhibit very little DNA excision repair activity and are very sensitive to UV when colony forming ability is measured (Andrews et al., 1978) but are relatively resistant when they are in a nondividing state (Kantor and Hull, 1984; Kantor and Elking, 1988).

DNA Damage and Repair in Human Tissues
Edited by B. M. Sutherland and A. D. Woodhead
Plenum Press, New York, 1990

203

Table 1. Characteristics of DNA Excision Repair
in Nondividing XP-C Cells

---

1. Five to 10% of the dimers are excised in the first 24 h (1).

2. Very little additional repair occurs in subsequent periods
   (Fig. 1).

3. Saturation of repair occurs at the same DNA damage level as in
   normal cells (20 J/m^2) (1).

4. Repair occurs in localized regions (2, 3, 4).

5. Most of the repair is in relatively large domains (30 to 70 kb,
   minimum size) (4).

6. The repaired domains are the same specific ones in all cells
   (Fig. 2 and ref. 5).

7. The repaired domains represent 10 to 20% of the genome (Fig.
   4).

8. The repaired domains may represent transcriptionally active
   domains (5, 6).

9. None of the remaining DNA is repaired (Fig. 4 and ref. 7).

10. The domain-oriented repair is biologically significant (1).

Numbers in parentheses are references. (1) Kantor and Elking, 1988;
(2) Mansbridge and Hanawalt, 1983; (3) Karentz and Cleaver, 1986; (4)
Kantor and Player, 1986; (5) Kantor et al., 1990; (6) Mayne et al., 1988;
(7) Kantor and Hull, 1984.

With the dogma that UV sensitivity reflects DNA repair capabilities
in mind, we characterized the excision repair properties of XP-C cells in
search of reasons for the UV resistance of quiescent XP-C cells. The
purpose of this paper is to summarize the current knowledge of DNA
excision repair in these cells. We find that although the level of DNA
repair activity remains low in the quiescent cultures, specific chromatin
regions are exclusively and efficiently repaired. This unique feature of
XP-C repair could be responsible for the greater UV resistance of the
nondividing cells by promoting repair of genomic regions containing
information essential for cell survival. Our data suggest that these
same specific regions are rapidly repaired in normal cells (Kantor et
al., in press). The results are consistent with our model that the
lethal action of UV in all quiescent cell populations is caused by a
pyrimidine-dimer-affected transcription block (Kantor and Hull, 1979).

EXCISION REPAIR IN XP-C CELLS

The characteristics of excision repair in nondividing XP-C cells are
summarized in Table 1. The experimental results that support these
conclusions are discussed in the following paragraphs.

1) Only a small fraction of the pyrimidine dimers are excised in
UV-irradiated XP-C cells (Kantor and Elking, 1988). We estimate an
excision of 5 to 10% of the dimers in the initial 24 h following exposure
to 20 J/m^2 UV or less. This estimate is based on quantitative DNA repair
synthesis data and depends on the assumption that the repair patch size
in XP-C cells is the same as in normal and XP-A cells. Results of standard experiments to detect pyrimidine dimers as UV-endonuclease sensitive
sites (ESS) confirm that the excision repair activity is only a small
fraction of that found in normal human cells. The ESS data, however,
cannot be used to quantitate the remaining dimers after a repair period
because of the nonrandom nature of repair discussed in item 4 below.

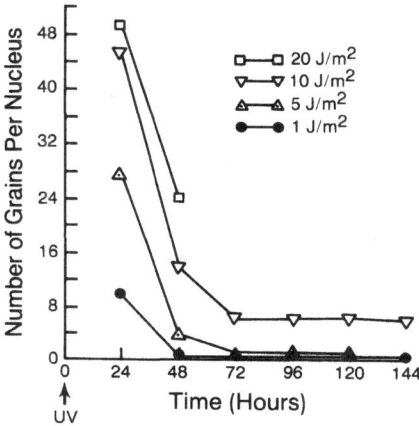

Fig. 1.   Time course for DNA repair in XP-C cells. Several cultures
          of nondividing XP4RO cells were UV-irradiated at time zero.
          Two cultures representing each UV dose were incubated with
          ^{3}H-thymidine (1 μCi/ml) and hydroxyurea (10 mM) for each 24
          h post-UV period. At the end of the period, cells were
          fixed and coated with photographic emulsion. Ten days
          later, the emulsion was developed and nuclei were scored
          for silver grains. Each datum point, plotted at the end of
          the appropriate 24 h period, is an average determined for
          at least 100 lightly-labeled nuclei. Background levels of
          2 grains per nucleus were subtracted. Symbol sizes
          approximate the standard error of the mean.

2) Very little additional repair occurs after the initial 24 h
post-UV period. This was determined by quantifying repair synthesis in
24 h periods by both autoradiographic and CsCl equilibrium sedimentation
procedures. Typical autoradiographic results are shown in Fig. 1.
Silver grains above lightly labeled nuclei from UV-irradiated cells were
counted to assess the amount of ^{3}H-dThd incorporated into DNA as a result
of repair synthesis activity. The results show that repair activity

declines rapidly after the first 24 h. Repair activity is detected in all cells, indicating that the limited repair detected in XP-C populations is a collective property of individual cells rather than an artifact created by cells with different repair activities.

3) Repair is saturated at the same DNA damage level as in normal cells. Even though repair activity is greatly reduced from normal values, the amount of repair in the first 24 h period increases with UV dose to about 20 J/m^2, as observed for normal cells (Kantor and Elking, 1988). Saturation of repair is at much lower UV doses (0-5 J/m^2) in XP-A strains, even in those strains that exhibit considerably more repair activity.

4) Repair occurs in localized regions. The original experimental protocol (Mansbridge and Hanawalt, 1983) used to detect nonrandom repair in XP-C has been employed with other XP strains to ascertain the uniqueness of this pattern (Karentz and Cleaver, 1986; Kantor and Player, 1986). Relatively large strands of DNA devoid of pyrimidine dimers but containing DNA repair patches are formed during a 24 h repair period in UV-irradiated nondividing XP-C cells. The large strands are detected by fractionating the extracted DNA digested with a UV-endonuclease specific for pyrimidine dimers in alkaline sucrose gradients, appearing as fragments larger than most of the DNA. A similar pattern of localized repair is not detected in normal, XP-A or XP-D strains (Kantor and Player, 1986; Karentz and Cleaver, 1986) nor in XP-C strains maintained in culture conditions that promote cell division (Cleaver, 1986).

5) Most of the repair is in relatively large domains. The sizes of the largest repaired DNA strands detected in our experiments as devoid of pyrimidine dimers range from 30 to 70 kb. These molecules contain 50% of the total repair synthesis. This size range represents a minimum of their actual size because the DNA has experienced some shear in the extraction and fractionation procedures. The number-average size of the remaining DNA (85%) after UV-endonuclease digestion is much smaller (about 6 kb; Kantor and Player, 1986; Kantor et al., in press). We assume that the repair synthesis activity is a direct measure of dimer excision activity and thus, that the large DNA molecules have experienced at least half of all the excision repair activity. Since the entire DNA population has experienced the same shear, some of the smaller DNA molecules that have some of the remaining repair synthesis associated with them must have been part of larger molecules. Thus, we estimate that a majority of the repair is in domains that are large and have this minimum size.

6) The repaired domains are specific ones. Samples of the large repaired DNA were isolated and probed for specific genes. We found more copies of some genes (β-actin, DHFR) but not all in the repaired DNA compared to the bulk unrepaired DNA. Results illustrating the enhanced representation of the β-actin gene in the repaired DNA are shown in Fig. 2. Data are obtained from blots on nitrocellulose membranes of repaired DNA and bulk unrepaired DNA hybridized to a probe unique to the transcriptionally active β-actin gene. The two DNA fractions, repaired and bulk unrepaired, are from XP-C cells uniformly labeled in DNA with [14]C. Both fractions have the same ^{14}C specific activity. After hybridization to a ^{32}P probe, sections of the membrane were cut out and assayed by liquid scintillation methods for ^{14}C and ^{32}P activity. The results show that a greater amount of β-actin is detected in the repaired DNA compared to bulk DNA. In a similar experiment done as a control with

UV-irradiated cells that experienced no repair period, and with DNAs from the fractionation procedure that represent the repaired and bulk DNAs in the previous experiment, we observed the same amount of the β-actin gene in each fraction (Kantor et al., in press). This indicates that initially dimers are distributed randomly throughout the β-actin repair domain. We interpret these results to mean that the greater amount of β-actin sequences in the large repaired DNA results from the preferential removal of dimers from the β-actin region. Evidently, the repaired DNA in XP-C cells is unique and represents the same specific regions in each cell. We have found one gene that is represented equally in both DNA fractions, an expected result for an unrepaired DNA region. This gene is transcriptionally inactive in the nondividing fibroblasts and is detected by a probe referred to as 754 (Kantor et al., in press).

7) The repaired domains represent 10-20% of the genome. Excision repair in nondividing XP-C cells is a limited but relatively efficient process directed at specific chromatin regions. The estimate of the fraction of the genome represented as repair domains is an upper limit derived both from experimental data and from computer modeling of those data. Experimentally, the small number of repaired DNA fragments are detected by size-fractionating on a single alkaline sucrose gradient two UV-endonuclease-digested DNA samples, one from UV-irradiated cells and

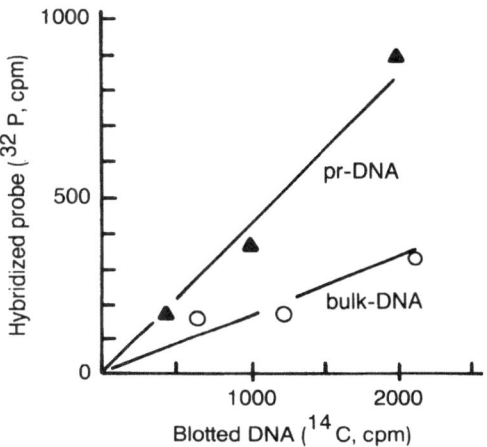

Fig. 2. Enhanced representation of the β-actin gene in the repaired XP-C DNA. UV-irradiated (20 J/m^2) XP10BE cells uniformly labeled in DNA with ^{14}C were incubated for 24 h. Preferentially repaired (pr) and unrepaired (bulk) DNA samples were then isolated using procedures that size-fractionated the extracted DNA after it was digested with a UV-endonuclease that nicks at sites of pyrimidine dimers. Samples of ^{14}C-labeled pr- and bulk-DNA were blotted onto nitrocellulose and hybridized to a ^{32}P-labeled probe specific for the β-actin gene. Blots were cut out and assayed for ^{32}P and ^{14}C activity. About 2000 ^{14}C cpm correspond to 1 μg of DNA.

one from UV-irradiated cells that have repaired their DNA for 24 h. Differences in the sedimentation patterns of the two DNAs, even if small, are indicative of the occurrence of repair. Experimentally, cells labeled in DNA with ^{14}C are UV-irradiated and incubated for 24 h while other cells labeled in DNA with ^{3}H are UV-irradiated only, experiencing no repair period. Cells from both cultures are combined and lysed and the DNA extracted. After digestion of the DNAs with UV-endonuclease, they are fractionated in an alkaline sucrose gradient. Typical results are presented in Fig. 3. The results are for the fractionated DNAs prior to endonuclease digestion (part A) to illustrate the co-sedimentation of the two co-extracted DNAs and after digestion (part B) to illustrate the divergence from co-sedimentation that is created by the small amount of DNA repair. The greater size of some of the DNA from the cells experiencing a repair period compared to those experiencing no repair indicates that fewer UV-endonuclease sensitive sites (ESS) are present in some DNA molecules. The sedimentation pattern is consistent with both the very limited and the localized repair activity found in these cells. The large fragments free of ESS seen near the bottom of the gradient are created by active excision repair in some domains and would not be observed as the only molecules repaired if repair occurred randomly. These large fragments represent about 5% more of the total DNA when compared to the resulting unrepaired DNA sample. This value is consistent with our estimate of repair of about 5% of the dimers in this period. An analysis of these sedimentation patterns by computer simulations provide approximations of the fraction of the genome that participates in domain repair.

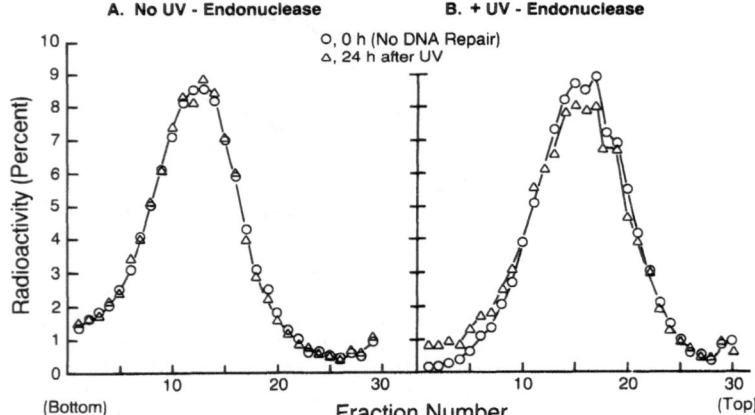

Fig. 3. Detection of the repaired DNA domains in XP-C cells. Nondividing XP4RO cultures containing cells uniformly labeled in DNA with either ^{3}H or ^{14}C were UV-irradiated (20 J/m^2). The ^{14}C cells were incubated for 24 h ($\triangle$) and then combined with unincubated ^{3}H cells (o). The DNAs were coextracted and (A) sedimented in an alkaline sucrose gradient (50,000 rpm, 70 min) or (B) digested with a UV-endonuclease and sedimented in a similar gradient (50,000 rpm, 140 min). Sedimentation is from right to left.

In brief, our computer program employs 10,000 DNA strands with a normal size distribution. The population has a number average molecular weight of 20 x 10^6 daltons (60 kb) and a range of (1 to 40) x 10^6 daltons. These parameters are observed experimentally (Fig. 3A). All strands are radioactively labeled with the same specific activity, so that simulations can be compared directly to the actual results. We assume dimers are distributed randomly, with 12 dimers per average strand (20 x 10^6 daltons) at 20 J/m^2 (Fig. 3B). These strands are cut at dimer sites resulting in a population with a number average molecular weight of about 1.5 x 10^6 daltons. For repair simulations, we select repair of any fraction of dimers, occurring either completely randomly or completely in selected domains. The size of the repaired DNA is then compared to the size of the unrepaired DNA in simulated alkaline sucrose gradients after both DNAs are nicked at dimer sites. Results are compared to the experimental results of Fig. 3. For domain repair, we assume a domain size of 20 x 10^6 daltons (60 kb), primarily because that is the number average size of our extracted DNA. This size coincides with our estimates of domain size and with estimates of sizes of transcriptional domains. We can select any fraction of the genome to be represented as repair domains. Once a strand is selected for repair, dimers are removed from it until the total number of dimers repaired equals the selected fraction. The selection that 10% of the genome is represented as repair domains and that 5% of the dimers are repaired implies that any strand has a probability of 10% of being selected for repair and that dimers are removed from the selected strands randomly until 5% of all the dimers are repaired.

Five simulations are shown in Fig. 4. These were chosen because they use repair parameters consistent with our data and illustrate the limits in this modeling exercise and the limits for defining the fraction of the genome represented as repair domains. Since our earlier repair synthesis data indicated that 5% of the total dimers were excised, we emphasize the simulations that use this value.

The conditions of the simulation in Fig. 4B, repair of 5% of all the dimers and limited to domains that represent 5% of the genome, imply that all of the domains are completely repaired, so that the repaired DNA fragments are large and located at the bottom of the gradient. We have never observed this sedimentation pattern in an actual experiment. The conditions of the Fig. 4C simulation, repair of 5% of all the dimers and limited to domains that represent 10% of the genome, create a sedimentation pattern that more closely approximates our actual results (Fig. 4A). The simulation of repair of 5% of all the dimers and limited to domains representing 20% of the genome (Fig. 4D) illustrates that as the repair activity remains low but distributed throughout a greater fraction of the genome, the sedimentation profiles approach that observed for repair of dimers at random locations (Fig. 4E). The simulation that best fits our experimental data, 10% of all dimers repaired with repair activity limited to domains that represent 20% of the genome, is shown in Fig. 4F. "Fit" is determined by visual comparison of the sedimentation profiles of simulations compared to actual results.

Based on repair synthesis data interpreted in terms of the fraction of dimers excised, on actual sedimentation data for repaired DNA and on simulations, we conclude that the repair activity is limited to 5 to 10% of dimers in domains that represent 10 to 20% of the genome.

8) The repaired domains may represent transcriptionally active domains. The genes with enhanced representation in the XP-C repaired DNA

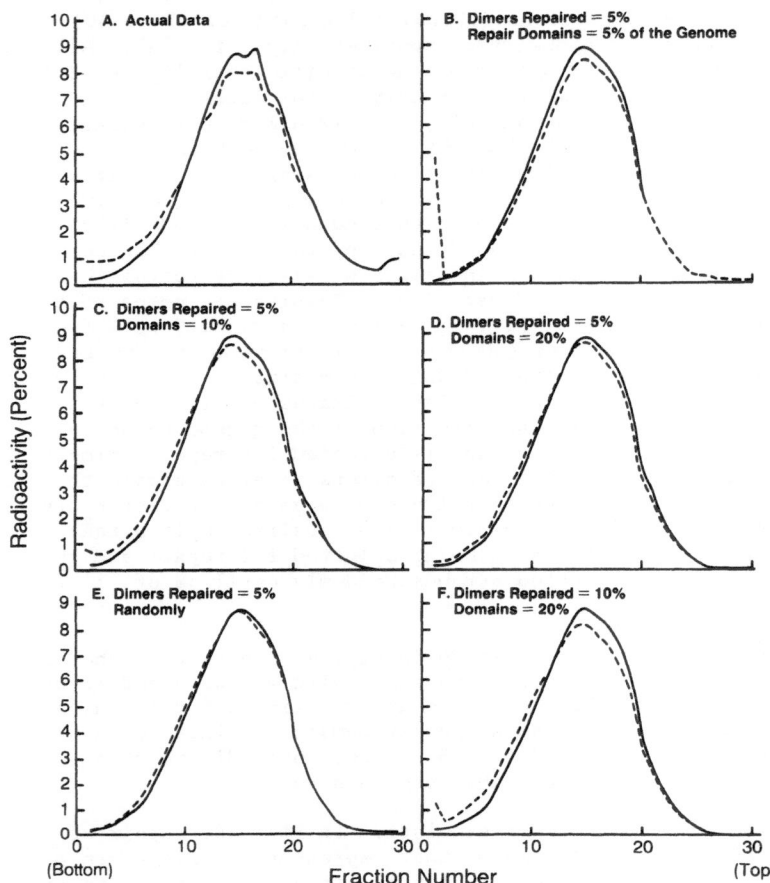

Fig. 4. Computer-generated simulations of domain-oriented repair in
XP-C cells. The simulations are for the experimental
protocol described in Fig. 3 and DNA fractionated in
alkaline sucrose gradients. The parameters used in the
computer program are described in the text. A. Curves are
those presented in Fig. 3B and represent experimental data.
B-F are simulations. B. Repair of 5% of the total dimers,
limited to domains representing 5% of the genome; C.
Repair of 5% of the total dimers, limited to domains
representing 10% of the genome; D. Repair of 5% of the
dimers, limited to domains representing 20% of the genome;
E. Repair of 5% of the dimers at random locations; F.
Repair of 10% of the dimers in domains representing 20% of
the genome. (——), sedimentation pattern for DNA extracted
from cells irradiated with 20 J/m^2 and digested with UV-
endonuclease; (----), DNA from irradiated cells (20 J/m^2)
incubated for 24 h, digested with UV-endonuclease.

210

(β-actin, DHFR) are transcriptionally active in the nondividing cells, while the 754 gene, which does not have an enhanced representation in the repaired DNA, is transcriptionally inactive (Mayne et al., 1988). Others (Mayne et al., 1988) have shown that a DNA restriction fragment containing the transcriptionally active adenosine deaminase gene is repaired rapidly in XP-C cells while a fragment containing the 754 gene is not repaired. Two other general lines of evidence, that the repaired DNA in XP-C cells is associated with the nuclear matrix (Mullenders et al., 1984) and has a greater sensitivity to endogenous nucleases than does the bulk DNA (Player and Kantor, 1987), provide support for this hypothesis. Matrix-bound DNA is thought to be transcriptionally active as is DNA hypersensitive to nucleases.

9) None of the remaining DNA is repaired. As mentioned earlier, most of the repair occurs in the first 24 h following exposure of cells to UV and very little occurs afterwards. Cells that survive the radiation insult do so with 90% or more of the original dimers. Repair of this large fraction of dimers never occurs. The same number of dimers can be detected even after a period of 50 days (Kantor and Hull, 1984). More specific gene-repair data confirm that specific genomic regions are probably not repaired. A DNA restriction fragment containing the 754 gene experiences no repair in nondividing XP-C cells in the immediate 24 h after UV exposure (Kantor, et al., in press). We conclude that nearly all of the repair activity is in a limited number of specific regions and little or none of the remaining DNA is repaired.

10) The domain-oriented repair in XP-C cells is biologically significant. Relative to normal cells, nondividing XP-C cells are more resistant to the lethal effects of UV than are proliferating XP-C cells (Kantor and Elking, 1988), even though the total amount of repair is the same in both conditions (Cleaver, 1986). The proliferating cells repair DNA in an apparent random fashion rather than in a few discreet regions. In addition, nondividing XP-C cells are more UV resistant than are nondividing XP-A cells that have more DNA excision repair activity (Kantor and Elking, 1988). The repair activity in the XP-A cells is distributed randomly throughout the genome rather than in localized regions. In these two cases, the distinguishing feature of DNA repair associated with the greater UV resistance of nondividing XP-C cells is the occurrence of domain-oriented rather than random genomic repair. The relative sensitivities of the XP-A strains are the same regardless of whether they are in a proliferative or nondividng state.

CONCLUSIONS

Quiescent cells in culture experiencing UV-induced DNA damage will degenerate and disappear from the culture if efficient repair of some of the damage does not occur. Efficient repair of the entire genome is not required for survival but evidently must occur in some specific genomic locations. For example, XP cells that execute no repair of DNA damage will degenerate and die, whereas normal and other XP cells that efficiently repair some of the damage can survive for very long periods (> 1 year) with a significant number of pyrimidine dimers remaining (Kantor and Hull, 1984).

The excision repair activity in quiescent XP-C cells is limited to a few chromatin regions representing less than 20% of the genome. Relatively large chromatin domains that are the site for most of the cellular repair activity are easily detected and consequently have been the object of initial studies. We recognize that smaller selectively repaired domains may exist and because of their small size, could represent a considerable fraction of the repaired domains. The repair in the large domains is slower than in normal cells but evidently complete and effective (Kantor et al., 1990). The level of repair increases with DNA damage, indicating that the reduced repair at low UV doses, compared to normal cells, is a result of limited substrate (i.e., DNA damage) in these repairable chromatin regions rather than a reduced level of repair enzymes. The transcriptional state of chromatin regions may be the determining factor for repair. A very limited amount of data lead to this suggestion. Whether or not all regions of a repaired domain or all repaired domains are transcriptionally active has not been determined. As an example, the transcriptionally active β-actin gene is 3.5 kb long (Ng et al., 1985), located in a significantly larger repaired DNA region (30-70 kb) that may or may not contain other transcriptionally active regions. The association between domain-oriented repair and a greater UV resistance probably indicates that the repair alleviates some DNA damage responsible for the lethal UV effects. Transcription is the major DNA-related activity in nondividing cells and its interruption is not tolerable. We suggest that selective repair alleviates lethal UV effects through the repair of transcription-inhibiting UV lesions in genes whose products are required for continued maintenance of the nondividing cells. The implication of this model is that repaired regions, which are evidently regions important to cell survival, contain transcriptionally active regions. The repair defect in XP-C is thus in a gene whose product promotes repair of bulk DNA, probably through some damage recognition process that isn't required in the repaired domains.

Some properties of excision repair in normal cells indicate that some of the characteristics of excision repair in XP-C cells may apply to normal cells as well. Repair domains are not detected in normal cells when the same technique used successfully with XP-C cells is employed. However, we propose that a similar domain repair mechanism for preferential repair of some genes exists in normal cells. The 3.5 kb β-actin gene resides in the middle portion of a 14 kb Eco Rl fragment (Ng et al., 1985). We have examined the repair of this fragment in both normal and XP-C cells. The fragment is repaired very rapidly in normal cells, with removal of about 80% of the ESS in 8 h. This is significantly faster than repair of the genome overall in normal cells, which is represented by a rate of about 60 to 80% in 24 h. In contrast, a 14 kb DNA restriction fragment containing the 754 gene is repaired efficiently but at a much slower rate (Kantor et al., in press). Based on the observations that all dimers can be repaired in normal cells and that DNA is repaired more rapidly in some regions than in others, we propose that the mechanisms leading to the efficient repair of domains in XP-C cells represent the remnants of a repair process in normal cells.

These studies with quiescent cells clearly suggest that repair of DNA damage in nonproliferating human cells in vivo is essential for the continuation of their functions. They also suggest that repair may follow a genome location pattern not predicted by studies using proliferating cells. The biological consequences of this repair may differ significantly from those predicted by such studies.

ACKNOWLEDGEMENTS

    The experiments described in Figs. 1 and 2 were done with assistance from C. F. Elking and L. S. Barsalou. The computer program for the

repair simulations was written by Daniel T. Voss, Mathematics and
Statistics Department, Wright State University. I gratefully acknowledge
many helpful discussions of this work with R.B. Setlow, P.C. Hanawalt and
C.A. Smith. This research has been supported by grants from the National
Science Foundation, the National Cancer Institute of NIH (grant no.
CA49411) and the Biological Sciences Department of Wright State
University.

REFERENCES

Andrews, A. D., Barrett, S. F., and Robbins, J. H., 1978, Xeroderma
   pigmentosum neurological abnormalities correlate with colony-forming
   ability after ultraviolet radiation, Proc. Natl. Acad. Sci. USA,
   75:1984.
Cleaver, J. E., 1986, DNA repair in human xeroderma pigmentosum group C
   cells involves a different distribution of damaged sites in confluent
   and growing cells, Nucleic Acids Res., 14:8155.
Kantor, G. J., 1986, Effects of UV, sunlight and x-ray radiation on
   quiescent human cells in culture, Photochem. Photobiol., 44:371.
Kantor, G. J., Barsalou, L. S., and Hanawalt, P. C., 1990, Selective
   repair of specific chromatin domains in UV-irradiated cells from
   xeroderma pigmentosum complementation group C, Mutat. Res., (in
   press).
Kantor, G. J., and Elking, C. F., 1988, Biological significance of
   domain-oriented DNA repair in xeroderma pigmentosum cells, Cancer
   Res., 48:844.
Kantor, G. J., and Hull, D. R., 1979, An effect of ultraviolet light on
   RNA and protein synthesis in nondividing human diploid fibroblasts,
   Biophys. J., 27:359.
Kantor, G. J., and Hull, D. R., 1984, The rate of removal of pyrimidine
   dimers in quiescent cultures of normal human and xeroderma
   pigmentosum cells, Mutat. Res., 132:21.
Kantor, G. J., and Player, A. N., 1986, A further definition of
   characteristics of DNA-excision repair in xeroderma pigmentosum
   complementation group A strains, Mutat. Res., 166:79.
Kantor, G. J., Warner, C., and Hull, D. R., 1977, The effect of
   ultraviolet light on arrested human diploid cell populations,
   Photochem. Photobiol., 25:483.
Karentz, D., and Cleaver, J. E., 1986, Excision repair in xeroderma
   pigmentosum group C but not group D is clustered in a small fraction
   of the total genome, Mutat. Res., 165:165.
Mansbridge, J. N., and Hanawalt, P. C., 1983, Domain-limited repair of
   DNA in ultraviolet irradiated fibroblasts from xeroderma pigmentosum
   complementation group C, in: "Cellular Responses to DNA Damage", pp.
   195-207, E.C. Friedberg and B.A. Bridges, eds., A.R. Liss, New York.
Mayne, L. V., Mullenders, L. H. F., and van Zeeland, A. A., 1988,
   Cockayne's syndrome: a UV sensitive disorder with a defect in the
   repair of transcribing DNA but normal overall excision repair, in:
   "Mechanisms and Consequences of DNA Damage Processing", pp. 349-353,
   E.C. Friedberg and P.C. Hanawalt, eds., A.R. Liss, New York.
Mullenders, L. H. F., van Kesteren, A. C., Bussmann, C. J. M., van
   Zeeland, A. A. and Natarajan, A. T., 1984, Preferential repair of
   nuclear matrix associated DNA in xeroderma pigmentosum
   complementation group C, Mutat. Res. 141:75.
Ng, S-Y., Gunning, P., Eddy, R., Ponte, P., Leavitt, J., Shows, T., and
   Kedes, L., 1985, Evolution of the functional human β-actin gene and
   its multi-pseudogene family:conservation of noncoding regions and
   chromosomal dispersion of pseudogenes, Mol. Cell. Biol., 5:2720.

Player, A. N., and Kantor, G. J., 1987, The endogenous nuclease sensitivity of repaired DNA in human fibroblasts, Mutat. Res. 184:169.

PROSPECTS FOR EPITHELIAL GENE THERAPY

Elizabeth S. Fenjves, Joseph I. Lee, Jonathan A.
Garlick, David A. Gordon, David L. Williams and Lorne
B. Taichman

School of Dental Medicine and School of Medicine, State
University of New York at Stony Brook, Stony Brook,
New York

INTRODUCTION

There is considerable excitement about the possibility of
somatic cell gene therapy, that is, the introduction and
expression of defined genes into cells for the purpose of
providing a needed gene product. Most current research on gene
therapy has been focused on the use of marrow stem cells as a
therapeutic vehicle (Belmont et al., 1986). Inherited
hematological disorders, such as severe combined immunodeficiency
caused by adenosine deaminase deficiency, are diseases that might
be amenable to this form of therapy (Kellems et al., 1985). A
possible approach would be through genetic transfer of a
recombinant adenosine deaminase gene into autologous marrow stem
cells, transplantation of the transformed cells into the patient,
and establishment of a population of stem cells that give rise to
immunologically competent lymphoid cells. Although many questions
need to be answered before we know the efficacy of such therapy,
the National Institute of Health has issued guidelines for its
use, and clinical trials have already begun (Culliton, 1989).

Another tissue being considered as a vehicle for gene
therapy is the epidermis. Epidermis is composed primarily of
a single cell type, the keratinocyte. Keratinocytes are easily
obtained by biopsy and can be maintained in culture in
semidefined media (Rheinwald and Green, 1975). Their culture
lifetime has been variably reported as between 50 to 150
doublings and addition of growth factors to the medium
considerably extends this number (Rheinwald, 1975). In serum-
containing medium, cultured keratinocytes form a partially
keratinized epithelium (Holbrook and Hennings, 1983) consisting
of replicating basal cells and differentiating suprabasal cells.

Keratinocytes can also be transfected (Lee and Taichman,
1989), or transduced (Morgan et al., 1988), and subsequently
transplanted as a graftable epidermis (Gallico et al. 1984).
Autologous grafts of keratinocytes cultured from burn victims
have been successfully used for long term wound coverage
indicating that the stem cell population survives in culture and
can reconstitute a useful epidermis.

DNA Damage and Repair in Human Tissues
Edited by B. M. Sutherland and A. D. Woodhead
Plenum Press, New York, 1990

Table 1.   Example of Substances Secreted by Cultured
Human Keratinocytes

Protein	First Author/ Page*	
Vitamin D	Holick, M.	14
	Bickle,D.	27
Steroids	Milewich, L.	66
Parathyroid Hormone-like peptide	Insogna, K.	146
Eicosanoids	Goldyne,M.	108
Apolipoprotein E	Fenjves,E.	160
Fibroblast Growth Factor	Halban, R.	180
Thymocyte Activating Factor	Sauder, D.	241
Transforming Growth Factor	Pittelkow, M.	211
Cytokines	Kupper, T.	262
	Tigelaar, R.	271
Interleukin 3	Yaar,M.	299
Lymphocyte Inhibitory Factor	Nickoloff, B.	312
Gamma Interferon	Mornen, V.	321
Thy-1 Protein	Chambers,D.	331
Collagenase	Lin, H.	333
Lymphokines	Thestrup-P, K.	348

* Compiled from articles in Annals of the New York Academy of Sciences, Vol. 548. Endocrine, Metabolic and Immunologic Functions of Keratinocytes, ed: L. Milstone and R. Edelson, 1988.

Although the function of epidermis is primarily protective, it is becoming evident that keratinocytes secrete a variety of cytokines and growth factors, as listed in Table 1. Since it is likely that cytokines elaborated by keratinocytes have local or even distant sites of action, it is possible that epidermal cells can be used to deliver defined proteins. As will be discussed, there is recent evidence that an epidermally secreted protein has a systemic fate.

What kinds of diseases may be amenable to treatment with epithelial gene therapy? In the context of this symposium, diseases such as xeroderma pigmentosum (XP) may be managed by this approach. It may be possible to introduce the normal gene for a missing or defective repair enzyme into cells cultured from a XP patient and then graft the patient's own epithelial cells at sites of high risk. In this case, epithelial gene therapy would be used for a disease confined to the epithelium. It may also be possible to utilize genetically transformed epithelia to treat diseases in distant sites. In such a case the epithelial cells would be engineered to produce a protein that is secreted and enters the systemic circulation. Systemic disorders such as hormone deficiencies or inborn errors of metabolism might be treated by such therapy. In large measure, the specific diseases that may be alleviated by epithelial gene therapy will depend on the capacity of epidermal cells to synthesize a foreign gene product, to secrete that product, and to continue to provide epidermal functions while doing so.

For the past several years we have been engaged in two projects related to epithelial gene therapy, the first addressing the question of synthesis, secretion, and fate of an epidermal protein, the second dealing with the expression of a foreign gene by keratinocytes.

SYSTEMIC FATE OF AN EPIDERMAL PROTEIN

To determine if an epidermally secreted protein is absorbed by the circulation we have been studying apolipoprotein E (apo E). Apo E is present on low density lipoproteins, high density lipoproteins and on chylomicrons. Unlike other apolipoproteins, apo E is produced in a variety of extrahepatic tissues in which it is thought to target lipoproteins for delivery to the liver or redistribute cholesterol among peripheral tissues (Mahley and Innerarity, 1983). Apo E is also synthesized by epidermal keratinocytes in culture and rapidly secreted into the media with the correct post-translational modifications (Gordon et al. 1989). When grafts of cultured epidermal keratinocytes are placed on excised sites on the backs of athymic mice, human apo E is detected in the sera of such mice as early as 4 days postgrafting and for as long as the graft is present (Fenjves et al. 1989). Furthermore, when split thickness skin is grafted onto athymic rats, apo E levels in the serum of the vein draining the graft are higher than levels in the venous serum from other sites on the animal. These results show that apo E produced by keratinocytes in epidermis has a systemic distribution and suggest that other proteins produced and secreted by keratinocytes might have a similar fate.

To determine if apo E encoded by a gene introduced into keratinocytes would also reach the systemic circulation, we

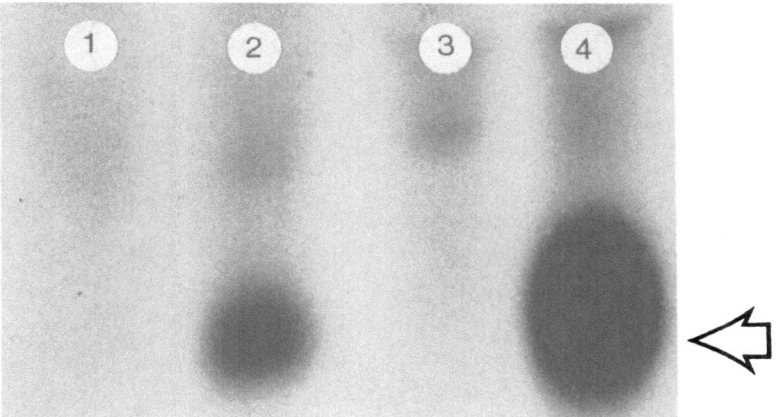

Fig. 1. Cultured SCC9 Cells Secrete Apo E after Introducion of the cDNA for ApoE. Aliquots of media from cells cultured for 4h in ^{35}S-methionine were immunoprecipitated with excess rabbit anti-human apoE as the primary antibody by the previously described procedure (Blue et al, 1983), and run on a 10% SDS-PAGE as described by Laemmli (1970). Lane 1: SCC9 parental (wild type), Lane 2: SCC 9-3 (a clone of SCC9 derived after transfecting with pLJ-ApoE DNA), Lane 3: negative control sample immunoprecipitated with pre-immune rabbit serum, Lane 4: positive control hepatoma cell line (HepG2). Arrow indicates position of apoE.

cloned the cDNA for human apo E into a retroviral vector pLJ (J. Morgan, Somatix, Cambridge Mass.) to form pLJ-Apo. PLJ-Apo was transfected into SCC9 cells (Rheinwald and Beckett, 1981); a line of keratinocytes derived from an oral squamous cell carcinoma. SCC9 cells contain mRNA for apo E (data not shown), but do not secrete detectable levels of the protein into the medium as shown both by immunoprecipitation (Fig. 1) and by an enzyme linked immunosorbent assay of the culture media (Table 2). In culture, SCC9 cells are phenotypically similar to keratinocytes but are blocked in their ability to undergo differentiation.

SCC9 cells transfected with the plasmid pLJApo were selected by their ability to grow in the presence of the aminoglycoside, G418, and then screened for apo E secretion. One clone, SCC9-3, was found to secrete 1.7 ng/h/million cells (Table 2). When one million SCC9-3 cells were injected intradermally into athymic mice, tumors were evident at the injection site within 10 days.

Upon gross inspection the tumors measured 1cm x 0.4cm. The tumor mass was composed of cysts lined by a well differentiated stratified squamous epithelium and surrounded by a connective tissue pseudocapsule. In most areas, the epithelial lining of the cyst had papillary projections extending into the lumen. In these sites, the epithelium was dysplastic and demonstrated basilar hyperplasia, pleiomorphism and keratin pearls (Fig. 2a).

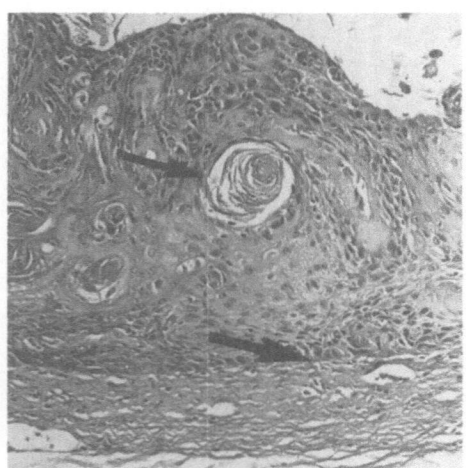
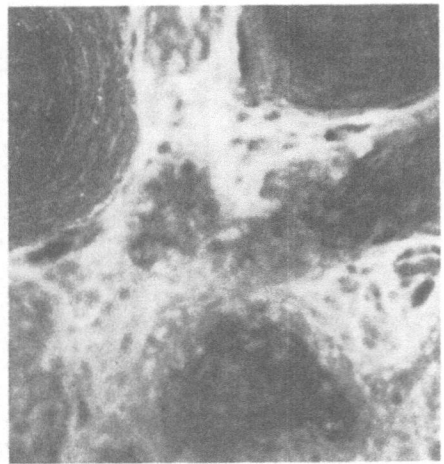

a   b

Fig. 2a) Photomicrograph of cyst lining showing epithelial dysplasia and keratin pearls (upper arrow). Note that basal cells are intact (lower arrow) and no epithelial cells are invading the subepithelial connective tissue (x40).
   b) Immunofluorescence microscopy of a cross section of the SCC9-3 tumor after incubation with rabbit anti-human apoE. Positive staining is seen in dysplastic spinous cells (x75).

| Cell Type | Culture | | Animals |
	Conc. media ng/ml	Rate ng/hr/10^6 cells	Conc. serum ng/ml
Keratinocytes	4.3	0.9	NA
SCC (parental)	0.07	ND	ND
SCC9-3	5.44	1.7	1.29
medium	0.044	ND	NA

Secretion of apoE in culture was measured by incubating cells in serum-free media for 12 h and carrying out ELISAs on aliquots of the media as previously described (Gordon et al., 1989). Data is normalized for cell number. Two to four weeks following intradermal injection of 10^6 cells levels of apoE were measured in the sera of tumor-bearing animals. NA (not applicable), ND (not detectable).

It is of interest to note that the basal cell layer was intact and no squamous cells were invading the subepithelial connective tissue. When examined with immunofluorescence using a polyclonal antibody to human apo E, cells derived from the SCC9-3 tumor were clearly shown to contain human apo E (Fig. 2b).

Sera from tumor-bearing mice were tested for the presence of human apo E using an ELISA assay. Apo E was detected in the sera of two mice bearing the SCC9-3 tumors but was undetectable in the sera of two mice bearing tumors derived from the nontransfected parental SCC9 cells (Table 2). These results show that apo E produced by a gene introduced into SCC cells can be synthesized and secreted by the cells and subsequently detected in the serum of tumor bearing mice.

EXPRESSION OF AN EXOGENOUS GENE IN KERATINOCYTES

A key element in achieving useful levels of production of a foreign protein is the choice of promoter. There is considerable interest in using keratinocyte-specific promoters in the hope that these will provide high level gene expression. However, while keratinocyte-specific promoters have been cloned, details of their regulatory elements remain unknown at the present time.

In the absence of keratinocyte-specific promoters, regulatory elements from viruses have been used. Morgan et al. (1987) noted expression of the human growth hormone gene in keratinocytes when the gene was regulated by the SV40 early promoter-enhancer complex (Lee and Taichman 1989). We have examined transient gene expression in keratinocytes with the use of the long terminal repeat (LTR) of Rous sarcoma virus. The LTR is known to be a strong promoter in a variety of eukaryotic cells. The reporter gene for chloramphenicol acetyltransferase (CAT) was linked to the LTR (Gorman et al., 1982) and the recombinant transfected into primary foreskin keratinocytes. Expression in these cells is considerably less than in established lines such as 3T3, probably due to the low number of competent cells (Lee and Taichman 1989). Expression is not

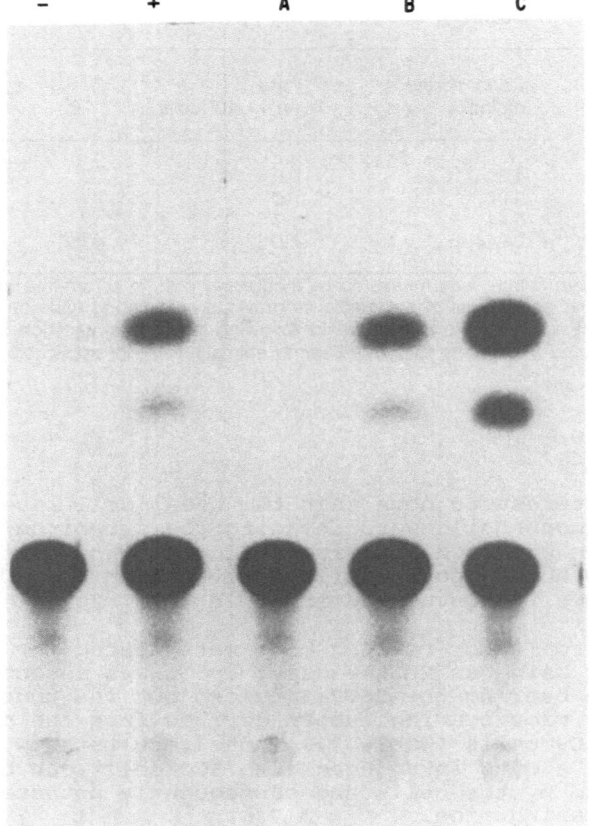

pRSVCAT

    –   +   A   B   C

Fig. 3. CAT activity per cell in differentiated and nondifferentiated keratinocytes following transfection with pRSVCAT. Cultured human keratinocytes were transfected in 10cm dishes with 15ug of pRSVCAT DNA. Two days later the cultures were disaggregated with trypsin and the single cell suspension was separated into 3 fractions on the basis of density on Ficoll 400: small nondifferentiated cells, larger more differentiated cells, and an intermediate fraction containing a mixture of the two cell types (Lee and Taichman, 1989). To determine the level of activity of CAT enzyme in differentiated and nondifferentiated cells, equal numbers of keratinocytes from each fraction were lysed in 100 ul of 0.25M Tris pH7.5 and 50 ul of the clarified supernatant assayed for CAT activity. Lane A: small cells, Lane B: intermediate cells, Lane C: large cells. The(-) and (+) lanes represent ^{14}C-chloramphenicol in the absence(-) and presence(+) of purified chloramphenicol acetyl transferase.

uniform in all cells of the culture. CAT expression on a per cell basis is 5 to 7 fold higher in the differentiated cell population (Fig. 3). The increased levels of CAT expression in the differentiated cells is associated with increased levels of steady state RNA (Fig. 4). This increase in expression might be useful for epithelial gene therapy since high levels of expression of a therapeutic gene might be less toxic to differentiating keratinocytes than to non differentiated replicating cells.

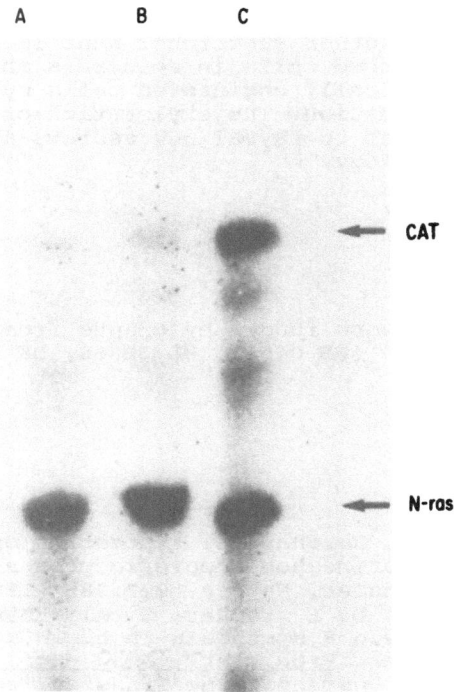

Fig. 4. Steady state levels of CAT mRNA in differentiated and nondifferentiated keratinocytes following transfection with pRSVCAT DNA. Keratinocytes were transfected with pRSVCAT and separated on gradients of Ficoll 400. Total cellular RNA was isolated from keratinocytes in each fraction. 100 ug of total RNA from each fraction was hybridized in solution to 200,000 cpm of ^{32}P-labelled RNA probes complementary to CAT mRNA and c-N-ras mRNA. After allowing hybridization to proceed for 24 h, the reaction mixture was treated with 75ug/ml of RNase A to digest all nonhybridized RNA. The hybridized RNA was electrophoresed on urea-polyacrylamide denaturing gels and visualized by autoradiography. RNA from small, intermediate and large keratinocytes are presented in lanes 1, 2 and 3 respectively. The upper band is the CAT mRNA. The c-N-ras mRNA (lower band) was used as an internal standard to assure that equal amounts of cellular RNA were assayed.

Additional experiments are underway to determine more precisely the mechanism of enhanced gene expression and to determine if a similar phenomenon is observed when the LTR is stably expressed in keratinocytes.

CONCLUSION

Epithelial gene therapy represents a new approach to medical therapeutics wherein the patient's own skin cells manufacture and deliver the needed product. Numerous questions in addition to those related to synthetic and secretory capacity, remain to be answered. For example, will an epidermis comprised of cells genetically engineered to produce a foreign protein continue to provide barrier and other functions? What is the behavior of genetically transformed cells in epidermis and are they stable or replaced? Are genetically engineered cells susceptible to neoplastic transformation. The exploration of epithelial gene therapy also promises to reveal new secrets about epidermal keratinocyte physiology.

ACKNOWLEDGEMENTS

These studies were funded by grants from the National Institutes of Health (DE 04511, HL 32868, DK 18171, DC 00203, HL 07891).

REFERENCES

Belmont, J., Tigges, J. Chang S. Expression of human adenosine deaminase in murine hematopoietic progenitor cells following retroviral transfer, Nature. 322:385 (1986).

Blue, M-L, Williams, D. L. Zucker, S. Ali Khan, S. and Blum, C. B. Apolipoprotein E synthesis in human kidney, adrenal gland, and liver. Proc. Natl. Acad. Sci. USA 80:283 (1983).

Culliton, B. News & Comment, Gene Transfer Test: so far so good. Science. 244: 913, 1325 and 1430 (1989).

Fenjves, E. S., Gordon, D. A., Pershing, L. K., Williams, D. L. and Taichman, L. B. Systemic distribution of apolipoprotein E secreted by grafts of epidermal keratinocytes: implication for epidermal function and gene therapy, Proc. Natl. Acad. Sci. USA (in press, 1989).

Gallico, G., O'Connor N., Compton, C., Kehinde, I. and Green, H. Permanent coverage of large burn wounds with autologous cultured human epithelium. N Engl. J. of Med. 311:448 (1984).

Gordon, D. A., Fenjves, E. S., Williams, D. L., and Taichman, L. B. Synthesis and secretion of apolipoprotein E by cultured human keratinocytes. J. Invest. Dermatol. 92:96 (1989).

Gorman, C., Moffat, L., Howard, B. Recombinant genomes which express chloramphenicol acetyltransferase in mammalian cells. Mol. Cell Biol. 2:1044 (1982).

Holbrook, K. and Hennings, H. Phenotypic expression of epidermal cells in vitro: a review, J. Invest. Dermatol. 81:11s (1983).

Kellems, R., Yeung, C. and Ignolia D., Adenosine deaminase deficiency and severe combined immunodeficiency, **Trends Genet.** 1:278 (1985).

Laemmli, U. K. Cleavage of structural proteins during the assembly of the head of bacteriophage T4, **Nature**, 227:680 (1970).

Lee, J.I., and Taichman, L. B., Transient expression of a transfected gene in cultured epidermal keratinocytes: implications for future studies, **J. Invest. Dermatol.** 92:267 (1989).

Mahley, R. W. and Innerarity, T. L. Apolipoproteins: Structure and function. **Biochim. Biophys. Acta.** 737:197, (1983).

Morgan, J., Barrandon, Y., Green, H. and Mulligan, R. Expression of an exogenous growth hormone gene by transplantable human epidermal cells, **Science.** 237:1476 (1987).

Rheinwald, J. G. Serial cultivation of normal human epidermal keratinocytes, **Methods Cell Biol.** 21A:229 (1975).

Rheinwald, J. G. and Beckett, M. Tumorigenic keratinocytes lines requiring anchorage and fibroblast support cultured from human squamous cell carcinomas. **Cancer Res.** 41:1657, (1981).

Rheinwald, J. G. and Green, H. Serial cultivation of strains of human epidermal keratinocytes: the formation of keratinizing colonies from single cells. **Cell.** 6:317 (1975).

THE SIGNIFICANCE OF DNA DAMAGE AND REPAIR MECHANISMS

IN HEALTH RISK ASSESSMENT*

Lorenz Rhomberg, Vicki L. Dellarco,
William H. Farland, and Roger S. Cortesi**

Office of Health and Environmental Assessment and
Office of Exploratory Research**
US Environmental Protection Agency, Washington, DC

INTRODUCTION

DNA is usually presumed to be the critical macromolecular target for carcinogenesis and mutagenesis. After an active chemical reacts with DNA to form the macromolecular adduct, DNA repair processes play an important role in removing this initial damage in an attempt to assure cellular proliferation and survival. There has been a rapid increase in our knowledge of DNA damage and repair mechanisms over the last several years, using the tools of molecular biology to study DNA repair at the level of the gene. Exciting findings include the discovery that particular genes may be preferentially repaired (Bohr and Wassermann, 1988). It is not our intent to discuss the advances made in the field of DNA damage and repair, but rather to provide a conceptual outline for considering how such information may be applicable or relevant to the assessment of health risks, particularly those posed by exposure to carcinogens and mutagens.

Estimations of human risk are generally based on animal studies, and thus require a species-to-species extrapolation. Such data are usually obtained at exposure levels much higher than those ordinarily encountered by humans; consequently, estimates of low-dose risk require a consideration of how the animal dose-response can be extrapolated to lower exposures. Information on mechanisms and rates of DNA repair and on similarities and differences among different cell types and species is important in the development of biologically based extrapolation models for quantitative risk assessment. Such information serves to guide or to provide insight into predicted shapes of dose-response curves at low exposures and how to extrapolate risk across species.

---

*The views expressed in this document are those of the authors and do not necessarily reflect the views and policies of the US Environmental Protection Agency.

DNA Damage and Repair in Human Tissues
Edited by B. M. Sutherland and A. D. Woodhead
Plenum Press, New York, 1990

Risk assessment in the past has focused on the correlation of grossly manifested disease (e.g., tumors) following some externally delivered exposure or dose. The exposure of toxicological concern is related empirically to the ensuing disease state. This relationship is then extrapolated from the observed circumstances (e.g., tumor induction in experimental animals given high, lifetime exposures) to the circumstances of concern (tumor incidence in humans exposed to low and perhaps intermittent levels), with the extrapolation method based largely on presumptions about how the "black box" linking exposure to disease should behave at different dose levels in different species.

Recently, attention has been concentrated on the use of our knowledge about the physiological processes that link exposure to disease in order to improve the scientific basis for extrapolating dose-response relationships (Fig. 1). By examining the underlying mechanisms--by opening the "black box" and examining the biological machinery--one can better understand how dose level and species differences might affect the magnitude and probability of disease following exposure.

In order to discuss this "mechanistic" basis for extrapolation of toxicological effects (and to highlight the role of DNA damage and repair), it is useful to develop a framework that recognizes its component parts. The following conceptual framework may be useful, since it identifies the individual aspects of xenobiotic-induced disease that tend to be investigated separately. Specifically, in the following discussion, this scheme will be described in terms of cancer risk assessment, but small and obvious modifications will allow it to apply to other toxic end points as well.

The mechanistic connection of exposure to tumor formation can be thought of as having three parts (Fig. 1), namely, pharmacokinetics, pharmacodynamics, and cell kinetics. *Pharmacokinetics* constitutes the processes of absorption of the agent into the organism, its distribution through the various tissues, its metabolism (biotransformation) into chemically modified forms (which may be more or less toxic than the parent compound), and its elimination from the body. The *input* to the pharmacokinetic component is the pattern of the individual's exposure to the agent of concern. The *output* is a pattern of exposure to the proximate toxin (which may be the parent compound or a metabolite) experienced by the site of toxic action (which may be an organ, tissue, subcellular organelle, or DNA). Essentially, the output of the pharmacokinetic process defines the "target dose" of the active chemical. Determination of target dose is an important factor in risk assessment because the toxic effects of a chemical are more precisely related to the delivered dose reaching the target cells than to the amount originally administered. Thus, methods to measure DNA or protein adducts (e.g., immunologic, fluorescent, and ^{32}P-postlabeling assays) are important tools in determining tissue dosimetry. Measurements of macromolecular adducts will help establish (1) the relationship of external exposure or administered dose to target tissue concentration; (2) how this relationship is modulated or influenced by route of administration, concentration, and pattern of exposure; and (3) how these relationships vary among species. Indirect methods of measuring the presence of DNA damage and repair (e.g., unscheduled DNA synthesis tests, alkaline elution assays for single strand breaks) may also be useful in establishing exposure-target dose relationships. However, these indirect approaches utilized end points that are one or

EXPOSURE TO ENVIRONMENTAL AGENTS

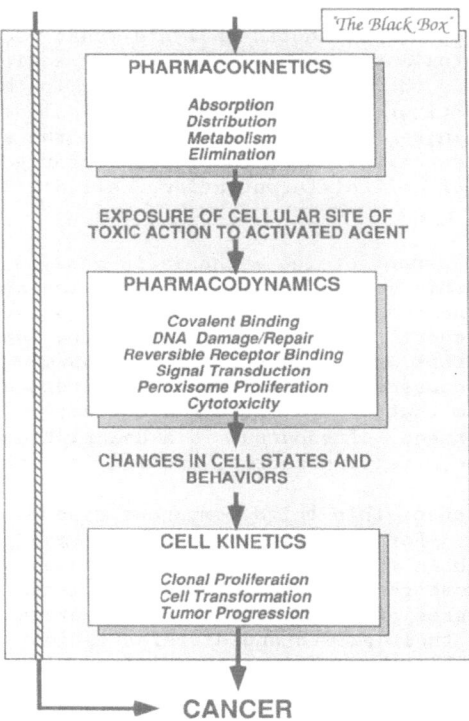

Fig. 1. A mechanistic conceptualization of the "processes"--namely, pharmacokinetics, pharmacodynamics, and cell kinetics--tieing carcinogen exposure to tumor formation.

several steps removed from initial target dose, and thus by their very nature add uncertainty in the determination of target dose. Nonetheless, methods to determine target dose, whether direct or indirect, are critical in establishing equivalency of dose across species.

The second component tieing exposure to response may be termed *pharmacodynamics*. As used in this context, pharmacodynamics consists of the processes whereby the proximate toxic agent acts on cells and cellular constituents to alter their states or behavior; that is, it treats the dynamics of the actual mechanisms of toxicity at the cellular level. Such processes include macromolecular covalent binding, reversible binding to receptors and the consequent tripping of signal transduction mechanisms, increased peroxisome proliferation, and cell death. The *input* to the pharmacodynamic component is the same as the *output* of the pharmacokinetic analysis, that is, the pattern of exposure to the proximate toxin at the site of action. The *output* of pharmacodynamics is the time-dependent changes in the affected cells. In the case of carcinogenesis, these outputs include rates of mutations or other changes in genetic material affecting the activation of proto-oncogenes or the deactivation of tumor suppressor genes, as well as effects on rates of cell differentiation, cell division, and cell survival.

The third component of the mechanistic analysis of the dose-response relationship can be termed *cell kinetics* and refers to the consequences of the changes in cell states and behaviors for the manifestation of overt disease. It takes as its *input* the descriptions of changed cells that are the result of the pharmacodynamic processes, and examines the consequences for the health state of the tissue and the whole organism that emerges from the collective effects of the cellular-level changes. Its *output* is a description of the risk of developing disease, its time-course, and its intensity.

The definition of this third component depends on the toxic end point of interest. For germ-line toxicity, it may concern the processes involved in fixing genetic damage and passing affected gametes on to future generations. For developmental toxicity, it may concern the processes of normal and abnormal ontogeny as mediated by effects on cells, their growth and differentiation. For carcinogenicity, this third component consists of modeling the probability of development of malignant cells as a consequence of rates of mutation, differentiation, and proliferation of target cells. The so-called "biologically based dose-response models" for carcinogenesis (e.g., Moolgavkar et al., 1988; Bogen, 1989) essentially separate two mechanisms of potential carcinogenic action by an agent: "initiation," that is, the induction of mutations and other genomic events that alter the action of loci mediating the regulation of cell division, and "promotion," increased clonal proliferation of initiated cells. Clearly, DNA damage and repair pathways play an important part in defining the parameters for initiation in biologically based modeling of cancer risk.

ROLE OF DNA DAMAGE AND REPAIR IN PHARMACODYNAMICS

Given this three-part scheme for examining underlying mechanisms of toxic effects, it is clear that knowledge of DNA damage and repair fits into the middle category, that of pharmacodynamics. It is the processes of DNA damage and repair that mediate the translation of target cell exposure to the consequent genetic lesions, and differences in this translation for different parts of the genome, for different target tissues, and for different species can profoundly affect the expected toxicity following exposure to an agent.

Recent research findings in DNA damage and repair have lead to an ever increasing appreciation of the degree of heterogeneity in types of processes and their rates across different biological situations. Clearly, the relationship of target cell exposure to incidences of genetic lesions is a complex one, the particulars of which must be taken into account in any successful application of mechanistic considerations to risk assessment. Unfortunately, this area is somewhat neglected in the current practice of risk assessment-- attention has been focused on species and dose-level differences in pharmacokinetics as a key to understanding high to low-dose and cross-species extrapolations. Cell kinetic models of carcinogenesis have not dealt with the complexities of predicting mutation rates at specific key loci (and projecting these rates across species and dose levels) from data on the exposure of tissues to carcinogens. The balance of this paper identifies and examines some of these complexities.

Dose-Level

Certain DNA repair pathways appear to be inducible by damage that reaches a sufficient level, and constitutive repair enzymes may become saturated at high levels of DNA damage. Such processes lead to nonlinear relationships between the amount of damage initially induced (which may be proportional to target tissue dose) and the risk of fixed lesions, which will in turn affect the low-dose shape of the dose-response curve. If low doses fail to induce repair enzymes, the consequent risk may be underestimated based on observations at higher doses. Conversely, if high doses saturate constitutive repair pathways, low doses may be safer than otherwise expected. A large number of DNA-damaging agents are found in the environment; it is possible that constitutive expression of inducible repair enzymes is the rule, affecting the expected shape of the dose-response relationship for any other further environmental exposures.

It has been argued that in some cases enzymatic repair may be able to remove all DNA lesions at low molecular doses, with the result that a "true threshold" exists for mutation. However, DNA repair processes are complex and heterogeneous over the genome. It is the balance among damage, repair, and mutation-fixing replication that determines mutation rates at particular loci. To the extent, however, that one can demonstrate effective error-free repair at very low measurable doses, the Agency would consider this fact in establishing a dose-response relationship for a given chemical, particularly highly DNA reactive agents. Additionally, it is possible that as the dose to the target decreases, the statistical probability of the induced effect becomes very rare. This may result in a dose-response trend that declines so steeply that a convex (sublinear) relationship is produced at low doses. Such a response might be described as a "practical threshold" (i.e., negligible risk), although not necessarily representing an absolute threshold at the molecular level.

Dose-Rate

The net genetic damage or risk that is achieved results from the balance of the rates of damage and repair in relation to the exposure concentration over time. The fixing of damage may depend on the timing relative to the cell cycle of target cells. To the degree that variations in "dose rate" (i.e., temporal pattern of administered total dose) can differentially affect these processes, there may be dose-rate effects on the damage realized by a given dose. Additionally, short-but-intense exposures may momentarily saturate repair processes (or fail to induce them), leading to damage out of proportion to the total dose.

Heterogeneity Over the Genome

Rates of DNA damage and repair differ for loci that are actively expressed versus ones that are quiescent, for different primary sequences, for transcribed and regulatory sequences, and even for the two complementary strands. Some agents cause very specific kinds of DNA damage, which may or may not be relevant to the specific mutations that may be involved in disease induction. The important practical consequence is that there is no generally measurable rate of DNA damage and repair that can be compared across targets distributed over the genome. If damage and repair are measured at other than the specific target of interest, the possible differences in susceptibility to damage between the surrogate target and the true target must be addressed.

Different Tissues and Cell Types

Since different parts of the genome are active in cells of different histological type, and since the expression of repair capacity and other defenses may differ, there is potential for differences across cell types in the relationship of target dose to induced genetic damage. This difference may affect site specificity of agents, and the extrapolation of expected effects across cell types. The targets of carcinogens may be the uncommon stem cells within a tissue, rather than the more common differentiated cells. Thus, measurement of damage and repair in the target tissue as a whole may be misleading.

Species Differences

In extrapolating across species it is conceivable that the molecular dose at the level of DNA is comparable but that the amount of resulting genetic damage may differ owing to differences in repair processes. Thus, interspecies variation in DNA repair may explain variations found in toxicological response among species. Species may also differ in their *relative* differences across tissues, dose levels, and inducibility/saturability of repair processes. In extrapolating from one species to another of different size (e.g., mice to humans), differences in the number of targets for damage must also be allowed for.

Inter-Individual Variation

Individuals may vary in their susceptibility to genetic damage, their defenses, and their capacities for repair. This is potentially a large determinant of inter-individual variation in susceptibility to toxic agents. There may be variation with age, sex, condition, and general health. Genetic differences in repair capacity are seen dramatically in repair-deficient syndromes that lead to high susceptibility to certain carcinogenic agents (e.g., xeroderma pigmentosum and skin cancer induced by ultraviolet light). In addition to such genetic variability, however, there may be quantitative

variability in repair processes that have important, although less
marked, influences.

SUMMARY

Clearly, the distinction of the three components in the underlying
mechanisms of toxicity--pharmacokinetics, pharmacodynamics, and cell
kinetics--is somewhat artificial. Together they form a continuous
process rather than a set of stages. But these components correspond
to the areas of studies that are often applied to the investigation of
toxic mechanisms. Moreover, the components identify *complexes* of
interacting processes, the consequences of which must be studied by
examining their actions in concert with one another--metabolic
activation must be examined as it competes with excretion, and rates of
DNA-adduct formation must be studied along with mechanisms and rates of
their repair.

By enumerating these components, it becomes evident that
clarification of the biological processes in only one realm, say
pharmacokinetics, leaves other parts of the "black box" unrevealed.
Components that are inadequately understood can be bridged either by
plausible assumptions or by empirical measurement, but at the cost of
some uncertainty in the risk extrapolations. For some processes, the
artificial division into components may be problematic. For example,
mutation rates clearly depend not only on the pharmacodynamic processes
of creation of DNA adducts and their removal via repair, but also on
the rates of cell division, allowing fixing of mutations, and on
survival of the affected cells.

The extrapolation of toxic effects across dose levels and across
species hinges on the changes in the proportionality of input to output
in each of the three components. Different degrees of metabolic
activation of a procarcinogen across species clearly affect the
comparative potency of an agent in experimental animals and human
beings. Likewise, differences among species, among tissues, among dose
levels, and among genetic loci in the balance struck between the
processes of DNA damage and repair will profoundly affect the degree to
which target-tissue doses are translated into genetic damage, which in
turn will affect the manifestation of disease. It is in this context
that comparative studies of DNA repair become important to risk
assessment. It is important to know the differences operating at the
cellular level in different species, in different tissues, and at
different levels or patterns of toxic insult. Such insights into DNA
repair will not in themselves dictate the proper extrapolation of risk
across species or dose levels, or even the proper understanding of
pharmacodynamics of DNA-affecting agents. These must be pursued by
investigating the interactions among a suite of simultaneous,
interdependent processes. Progress in the development of techniques
for detecting DNA damage and repair, and an enhanced understanding of
underlying mechanisms of such processes will increase the likelihood
that such information will influence health risk assessment, and thus
impact on regulatory decision making.

REFERENCES

Bogen, K.T., 1989, Cell proliferation kinetics and multistage cancer
    risk models, J. Natl. Cancer Inst., 81:267-277.

Bohr, V.A., Wassermann, K., 1988, DNA repair at the level of the gene, *Trends in Biochemical Sciences*, 13:429-433.

Moolgavkar, S.H., Dewanji, A., Venzon, D.J., 1988, A stochastic two-stage model for cancer risk assessment. I. The hazard function and the probability of tumor, *Risk Anal.*, 8:383-392.

MEASUREMENTS OF GENOMIC AND GENE-SPECIFIC DNA REPAIR OF ALKYLATION DAMAGE

IN CULTURED HUMAN T-LYMPHOCYTES

Jeanette N. Hartshorn, David A. Scicchitano,[†]
and Steven H. Robison

VRCC-Genetics Laboratory, 32 N. Prospect St, Burlington,
VT, 05401 and [†]American Health Foundation, Division of
Toxicology and Pathology, 1 Dana Rd, Valhalla, NY, 10595

INTRODUCTION

Due to the predominance of mutagens and carcinogens in the environment and the prevalence of cancers in the human population, there exists a need to understand the mechanism and efficiency of DNA repair in human cells. Most of the mechanisms which have been proposed for the repair of various types of damage in human cells has been based upon prokaryotic models (Friedberg, 1985); however, our knowledge of DNA repair processes in human cells is not as extensive as that of prokaryotic cells. Unlike bacterial systems, there have been no readily available repair deficient mutants in which to study DNA repair mechanisms until recently. In the past, lymphoblast and fibroblast cell lines have been established from individuals with disorders which have been attributed to a defect in or alteration of DNA repair and predispositions to cancer (such as xeroderma pigmentosum, ataxia telangiectasia, and Fanconi's anemia) in order to dissect the mechanisms of DNA repair. These cell lines have been instrumental in the characterization of the human DNA repair genes and have permitted the assignment of two human DNA repair genes to chromosome 19, ERCC I and ERCC II involved in excision repair (van Duin et al., 1986; Weber et al., 1988).

Autosomal recessive human disorders with purported etiologies in alterations of DNA repair capacity include xeroderma pigmentosum (XP), Cockayne's syndrome (CS), ataxia telangiectasia (AT), Fanconi's anemia (FA), and Bloom's syndrome (BS). Individuals with XP fail to repair UV-light induced damage to varying degrees and develop multiple skin cancers. To date, there have been nine complementation groups described in XP, as well as the XP variant characterized by an alteration in post-replication repair. It has been shown that individuals with XP have a higher incidence of other types of tumors as well (Kraemer et al., 1984; Kraemer et al., 1987), suggesting that the DNA repair deficit is a generalized phenomenon. XP-E cells have been found to lack two binding proteins which are responsible for the recognition of DNA damage induced by UV-irradiation (Chu and Chang, 1988). These binding proteins could be analogous to those found in the UVRabc complex of E. coli. Increased sensitivity to UV-light also is a characteristic in CS cells. Two XP patients have been found with features of CS as well (Lehman, 1982). This observation has led to the hypothesis that there may be overlapping DNA repair pathways affected in both XP and CS. A recent finding indicates

DNA Damage and Repair in Human Tissues
Edited by B. M. Sutherland and A. D. Woodhead
Plenum Press, New York, 1990

that CS cells are deficient in the repair of UV-lesions in actively transcribing genes (van Zeeland et al., 1988). These findings suggest the compexity of the excision repair process in human cells.

The arguments supporting a DNA repair defect in AT, FA, BS, and CS are controversial. In AT, there is an increased sensitivity to ionizing radiation as measured by cell survival (Cox and Masson, 1980). Also, these cells have "radioresistant DNA synthesis", a curious phenomenon which contributes, in part, to the radiosensitivity in AT. Cells from patients with FA have increased levels of spontaneous chromosomal breakage, and increased sensitivity to DNA crosslinking agents (Fujiwara, 1982) although there remains some controversy as to whether a true DNA repair defect for crosslinking agents exists in these cells (Kaye et al., 1980). The hallmark feature of BS cells is the occurrence of spontaneous chromosomal aberrations, the two most common being the symmetrical quadriradial and the sister chromatid exchange (Gianelli et al., 1982). It also has been reported that unscheduled DNA synthesis is defective following exposure of BS cells to UV-light (Gianelli et al., 1982) and that there are alterations in DNA repair associated with the cell cycle (Gupta and Sirover, 1984). Reports have suggested the existence of defects in both a DNA glycosylase (Seal et al., 1988; Vollberg et al., 1987) and a DNA ligase in these cells (Willis and Lindahl, 1987; Chan, 1987).

It is evident from the aforementioned diseases and the fact that levels of certain constitutive DNA repair proteins vary greatly among individuals (Waldstein et al., 1982) that considerable variation exists in the "normal" levels of DNA repair. We have evidence in our own laboratory (Bartlett and Robison, 1989) that different individuals have measurable, reproducible differences in O^6 methylguanine DNA-transferase levels. The relevance of this to disease is not fully appreciated, but we do know that cells which have lower levels of this protein are more sensitive to the effects of alkylating agents which induce the O^6-alkylguanine lesion.

There is also variation in the repair of UV-damage among normal individuals as measured by BrUrd photolysis or UDS (Setlow, 1983; Lambert et al., 1979; Madden et al., 1979). Weichselbaum et al. (1980), Arlett and Harcourt (1980) and Cox and Masson (1980) studied human cell strains for sensitivity to x-irradiation by cell survival. Their D_0 values ranged from 90 to 190 rads for normal cell strains. Also included were cells strains from a number of individuals with different diseases. Individuals with AT, FA and retinoblastoma were found to be more sensitive than normals. There is also evidence for differences in cell survival and strand break repair between normals after exposure to an alkylating agent (Scudiero et al., 1981; Munzer et al., 1988; Hartshorn and Robison, 1989).

Several recent advances have been made regarding the efficiency of DNA repair in mammalian cells. Using Southern blot and slot blotting techniques, it has been shown not only in Chinese hamster ovary (CHO) cells but also in human cells containing amplified copies of the dihydrofolate reductase (dhfr) gene that the repair of UV-dimers is more efficient in the constitutively expressed dhfr gene than in genomic DNA (Bohr et al., 1985, 1986) and that lesions on the actively transcribed strand of that gene are repaired more efficiently than those on the non-transcribed strand (Mellon et al., 1986, Mellon et al., 1987).

Human T-lymphocytes offer an ideal system in which to study DNA repair in response to various agents in normal and diseased states. These cells are easily obtained by non-invasive procedures. In addition, culture techniques have been established by which to maintain these cells for extended periods (Munzer et al., 1988; Hartshorn and Robison, 1989). Furthermore, T-cells have been utilized in investigations involving mutagenesis (Albertini, 1985), carcinogenesis and disease (Harris, G. et al., 1983; Lehman, 1982; Pedersen-Bjergaard and Olesen-Larsen, 1982; Setlow, 1978), and cytogenetics (Bender et al., 1988; Cimino et al.; 1986). However, before it is possible to detect and/or evaluate proficiencies and deficencies of DNA repair, one must dissect the potential variables present in the system under investigation. For these reasons, we have chosen to study DNA repair capacity in human T-lymphocytes cultured for extended periods of time, while also monitoring growth characteristics and evaluating the potential effects of modified culture conditions on DNA repair levels. Furthermore, because two major subpopulations of T-cells exist _in vitro_ (Hartshorn and Robison, 1989; Gullberg and Smith, 1986), we have been interested in determining whether the repair capacities of these two subtypes are comparable.

Previous studies in our lab have revealed the existence of a significant decline in genomic DNA repair in response to alkylating agent-induced damage during a 3 week culture period (Hartshorn and Robison, 1989). The current study describes an extension of previous experiments in which we were interested not only in measuring genomic repair during an additional 2-3 weeks of culture, but also in comparing genomic repair to gene-specific repair in the constitutively expressed _dhfr_ gene. The alkaline elution technique as described by Kohn et al (1981) was used to measure genomic repair in response to N-methyl-N'-nitro-N-nitrosoguanidine (MNNG) and methyl methanesulfonate (MMS) induced damage, while a Southern blot technique as described by Scicchitano and Hanawalt (1989) was used to measure gene-specific repair in response to MMS-induced damage. The primary adduct induced by MMS and MNNG is the addition of a methyl group at the N-7 position of guanine (which accounts for 66% and 81% of the total methylation respectively). Other adducts include 3-methyladenine (MMS 11%, MNNG 8%), and 1 & 7-methyladenine (MMS & MNNG 1-2%). The significant difference between the action of these two alkylating agents is the formation of phosphotriesters and O-6 methylguanine by MNNG (12% and 5%, respectively) while MMS induces only a small percentage of these lesions (0.8% and 0.25%, respectively) (Day et al, 1987). Base methylations and phosphotriesters produce alkali-labile sites (Hall et al., 1988; Lindahl, 1981; Teebor et al., 1981; Walker and Ewart, 1973) and therefore result in strand breaks which are detectable by alkaline elution. Studies of the repair of alkylation damage have revealed that there are two main mechanisms involved in the repair of these types of lesions. In a direct reversal mechanism, an alkyltransferase is responsible for the removal of alkyl groups from the O^6 position of guanine, a potentially mutagenic lesion (Friedberg, 1985). The remainder of the alkylation products are thought to be repaired by a base excision mechanism (Friedberg, 1985).

Research in our laboratory also has shown that during extended periods of _in vitro_ culture, there is a change in the ratio of the two major subpopulations of T-cells which occurs after approximately 18 days of culture. The two primary subtypes of mature peripheral T-lymphocytes in humans are the CD4+ and CD8+ subsets, bearing either the CD4 or the CD8 glycoprotein respectively (Reinherz and Schlossman, 1980). These glycoproteins are acquired as cortical thymocytes mature. T-cells bearing the CD4 marker comprise most of the helper/inducer cell population, while those bearing the CD8 marker comprise most of the suppressor/cytotoxic cells. In the peripheral blood, the ratio of CD4+/CD8+ T-cells is approximately 2:1 (Reinherz and Schlossman, 1980). In previous investigations undertaken in our laboratory, _in vitro_ ratios of CD4+/CD8+ T-cells were observed to range from 2:1 to 8:1 during the first 18 days of culture, after which the ratio changed to approximately 1:1 (Hartshorn and Robison, 1989). In the present study, we were interested in determining how the CD4+/CD8+ ratio was affected by extended in vitro culture beyond 3 weeks and whether or not any changes in the CD4+/CD8+ ratio correlated with changes in genomic DNA repair.

Using the alkaline elution technique, we have confirmed previous results indicating reduced levels of repair of MNNG and MMS-induced lesions in human T-lymphocytes which have been maintained in culture for 3 weeks. Repair levels measured for an additional 3 weeks stabilized or were somewhat increased from the levels determined between days 20-22. In addition, we have determined that the ratio of the two subtypes of T-cells, CD4+ and CD8+, changes over a 6 week culture period. In a preliminary investigation in which genomic repair levels were compared to repair in the transcriptionally active dhfr gene, we have found that the alkylation damage at the dhfr locus seemed to be repaired at a more rapid rate than in genomic DNA. These preliminary findings are interesting and merit further investigation.

METHODS

Cell Culture Lymphocytes were isolated from peripheral blood using ficol-hypaque density centrifugation (Munzer et al., 1988) and maintained in culture as described (Hartshorn and Robison, 1989). Mononuclear cell fractions were seeded at 10^6 cells/ml in RPMI/10% fetal bovine serum (FBS) and stimulated with 1μg/ml PHA for 2-3 days. Mass cultures of T-lymphocytes were routinely maintained in complete growth medium consisting of 20% HL1, 5% fetal bovine serum, 0.125μg/ml PHA, 20% lymphokine-activated T-cell growth factor (LAK-TCGF, at a final concentration of 300 units/ml), irradiated TK6 feeder cells (x-TK6, irradiated with 8000 rads of ionizing radiation delivered from a ^{137}Cesium source) and 55% RPMI. The LAK-TCGF was prepared in our laboratory as described previously (Hartshorn and Robison, 1989). Cells were seeded at 2×10^5/ml and subcultured every 3-4 days. For the comparison of growth characteristics, cells were seeded at either one of two densities: 10^5/ml or 2×10^5/ml and maintained using either one of two PHA concentrations: 0.125μg/ml or 0.25μg/ml.

Determination of lymphocyte cell surface markers In order to ascertain what proportion of T-cell subsets were present in each culture at various time points, lymphocytes were analyzed by fluorescence activated cell sorting (FACS) after reaction with surface marker specific monoclonal antibodies using the procedure described previously (Hartshorn and Robison, 1989). Two aliquots containing (0.5-1.0) x 10^6 cells of each lymphocyte culture at various days in culture were washed with saline G, pH 7.2 (phosphate buffered saline solution containing 6mM glucose). To one set of cell aliquots, 14μl of Simultest anti-CD4/anti-CD8 was added, and to the other set of aliquots, 14μl of anti-CD2 was added. Anti-CD4 and anti-CD2 were directly conjugated to fluorescein isothiocyanate (FITC), while anti-CD8 was directly conjugated to phycoerythrin (PE). Samples were incubated on ice in the dark for 30-45 minutes, after which they were washed twice with saline G containing 0.1% sodium azide. Samples were resuspended in 0.5ml saline G containing 1% paraformaldehyde and 2% heat-inactivated FBS, and stored at 4°C in the dark until FACS analysis. An Ortho Cytofluorograph 50 with a 2150 Data Acquisition Unit (Ortho Diagnostics, Westwood, MA) was used for the FACS analysis.

Alkaline Elution Cultured T-lymphocytes were labelled with 0.025μCi/ml of 2-[^{14}C]-thymidine for 2 days, followed by a 1 day chase period in fresh complete growth medium without radiolabel. Cell aliquots containing approximately 10^6 cells were washed with 5ml of serum free RPMI

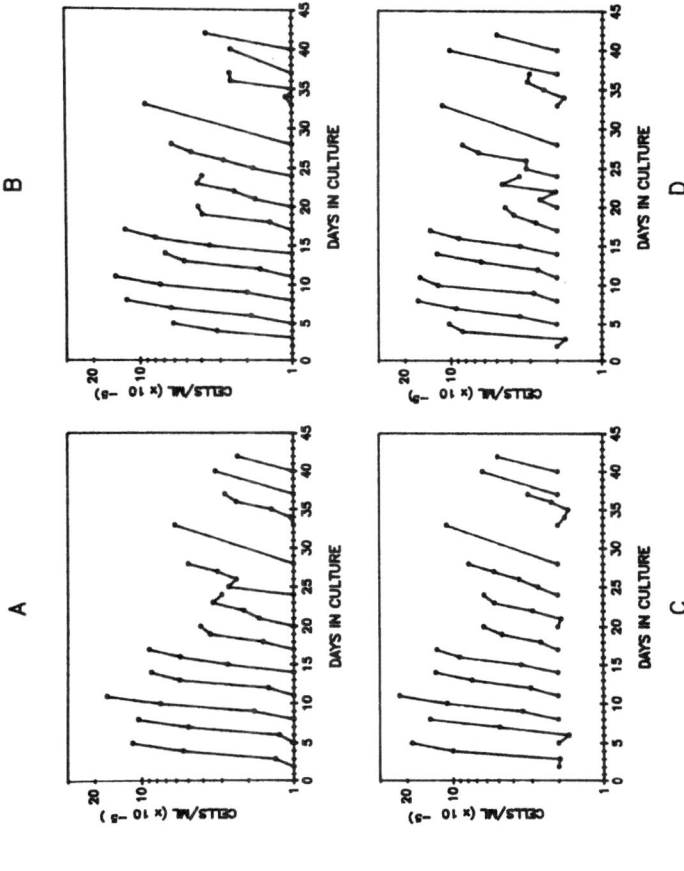

Figure 1A. In vitro growth characteristics of human T-cells. (A) Cells were cultured in IL-2 containing medium for up to 42 days as described in the methods section. Two seeding densities and two PHA concentrations were employed: Panel a) Cells were seeded at 10^5/ml every 3-4 days, with $0.125\mu g$/ml PHA; b) Cells were seeded at 10^5/ml with $0.25\mu g$/ml PHA; c) Cells were seeded at 2×10^5/ml with $0.125\mu g$/ml PHA; d) Cells were seeded at 2×10^5/ml with $0.25\mu g$/ml PHA;

(pH 7.2) before drug treatments, as well as after drug treatments and before repair periods. Cells were treated at a final concentration of either $4\mu M$ MNNG (Sigma Chemical Company, St. Louis, MO; CAS registry #70-25-7) or $400\mu M$ MMS (Aldrich Chemical Company, Milwaukee, WI; CAS registry #66-27-3) at 2×10^5 cells/ml in serum free RPMI for 1hr at $37^{\circ}C$. [In order to do a direct comparison between genomic and gene-specific DNA repair, cells were treated with 1.5mM MMS at 4×10^5 cells/ml in serum free RPMI for 30min at $37^{\circ}C$. Repair periods were 3, 6 and 24 hrs at $37^{\circ}C$.] After cell treatments or recovery periods, genomic DNA damage and its repair were determined using the alkaline elution technique as described (Munzer et al, 1988; Hartshorn and Robison, 1989). After 12 hours of elution, DNA contained on the filters and in the fractions was quantified by liquid scintillation counting using quench curves to convert counts per minute to disintegrations per minute. Strand break factors (SBF) were calculated as described previously (Munzer et al., 1988), as well as percent recovery (Hartshorn and Robison, 1989).

<u>Repair analysis by Southern blotting</u> This assay was an adaptation of that described by Scicchitano and Hanawalt (1989). T-lymphocytes were cultured in complete growth medium as described above with $0.02\mu Ci/ml$ of $2-[^{14}C]$-thymidine and $10^{-5}M$ cold thymidine for 2 days to radiolabel DNA, after which they were chased in medium without radiolabel for 1 day. Then, cells were treated at a concentration of 4×10^5 cells/ml in serum free RPMI at $37^{\circ}C$ for 30min with 1.5mM MMS, a concentration sufficient to induce 1 abasic site per 14kb of DNA. Repair periods consisted of 0, 3, 6, or 24hr after treatment, during which fresh medium containing $10\mu M$ Bromodeoxyuridine (BrdUrd) and $1\mu M$ Fluorodeoxyuridine (FdUrd) was present. Cells were then lysed for 14-16hrs in an SDS buffer containing $750\mu g/ml$ proteinase K in a $37^{\circ}C$ waterbath.

DNA was extracted by the addition of an equal volume of phenol, followed by 2hrs of continuous inversion. After centrifugation, the phenol layer was removed and a 50/50 (vol:vol) mixture of phenol/chloroform:isoamyl alcohol (CIAA, 24:1) was added, followed by 1hr of continuous inversion. Again, samples were centrifuged and the phenol layers were removed. Finally, an equal volume of CIAA was added, samples were inverted and centrifuged. The aqueous layers containing DNA were removed and DNA was precipitated with ice cold 100% ethanol. Precipitates were washed with cold 70% ethanol, and dissolved in 10mM Tris-1mM EDTA ($T_{10}E_1$), pH 8.0 for 24-48hrs. Samples then were digested with endonuclease Hind III at approximately 6 units/μg of DNA for 12-24hrs at $37^{\circ}C$.

After Hind III digestion, DNA was diluted to 4ml with $T_{10}E_1$ and sufficient cesium chloride was added to each sample to bring the density to 1.72gm/ml. The samples were centrifuged to equilibrium (36,000 rpm for 68hrs) in a Beckman L8-70M ultracentrifuge. Gradients were fractionated and fractions containing parental density DNA were pooled and dialyzed overnight in $T_{10}E_1$ followed by 1mM Tris-0.1mM EDTA ($T_1E_{0.1}$). DNA was quantified using a fluorometric assay employing Hoechst dye #33285. This assay is accurate to levels of $0.1\mu g$ DNA.

DNA samples were diluted to 10 μg per 30 μl of $T_{10}E_1$. A pair of aliquots from each sample was taken; to one, methoxyamine was added to a final concentration of 5mM, while to the other aliquot buffer was added. Samples were incubated at $50^{\circ}C$ for 6hrs to liberate N-methylpurines after which they were made alkaline with NaOH and incubated at $37^{\circ}C$ for 30min in order to induce strand breaks in samples not containing methoxyamine.

Alkaline loading dye was added to samples, after which they loaded onto 0.5% alkaline agarose gels and DNA was electrophoresed for 16-20hrs at

35V. Gels were washed first with an acid buffer (0.25N HCl), followed by
an alkaline buffer (0.4 M NaCl/0.5M NaOH), and finally a neutral buffer
(0.5M Tris-HCl/1.5M NaCl, pH 7.5). DNA was transferred to a nylon
membrane, after which it was washed with 0.1X Sodium chloride, sodium
phosphate EDTA-0.5% sodium dodecylsulfate (SSPE-SDS) at 65°C for 2hr.
Filters were prehybridized at 42°C with a solution containing 50%
formamide, 5X SSPE, 10X Denhardts solution, 0.4% SDS and 500μg/ml
denatured salmon sperm DNA for 2hr.

     Hybridizations were performed by combining 4ml of a solution
containing 50% formamide, 5X SSPE, 1X Denhardts solution, 1.2% SDS, and
200μg/ml denatured salmon sperm DNA with the labelled probe (see below).
The hybridization mixture was added to the nylon support membrane and
incubated at 42°C for 3 days. Following hybridization, membranes were
washed with 2X SSPE-0.2% SDS followed by 0.1X SSPE-0.1% SDS, each for 15
min at room temperature, and finally with 0.5X SSPE-0.2% SDS at 65°C for
25 min. Blots were overlaid onto Kodak XAR-5 X-ray film and exposure was
allowed for 3 days at -70°C.

Probe for gene specific DNA repair The human dhfr gene spans
approximately 29kb and contains 6 exons (Yang et al, 1984). Digestion of
genomic DNA with the restriction endonuclease HindIII produces a 23kb
fragment which contains the 5' flanking region, the first 3 exons and part
of intron 3. The plasmid used for this study was pBH31R1.8 which contains
a 1.8kb cDNA insert of the dhfr gene. This insert contains part of the 5'
transcribed region and spans the first 2 exons of the human dhfr gene.
Probe DNA (150ng per blot) was radiolabeled by nick translation using
α-[^{32}P]-dATP and used for hybridization.

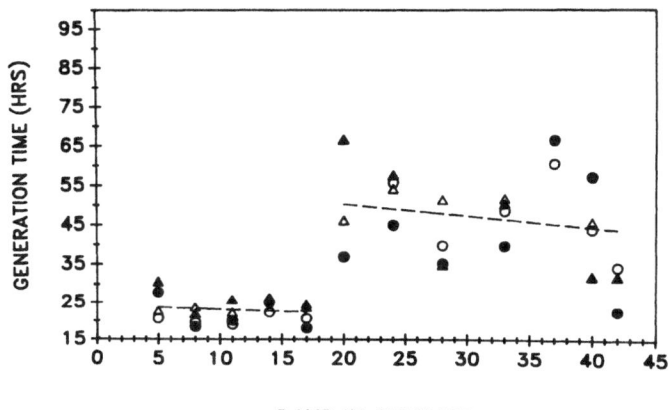

DAYS IN CULTURE

Fig. 1B.   In vitro growth characteristics of human T-cells. (B) Changes
          in the generation times of T-cells with sustained in vitro
          growth. The regression line represents the average generation
          time for all four cultures described in (A), since there were no
          significant differences between the groups (p<0.05): (O)
          seeding density: 10^5/ml, 0.125μg/ml PHA; (●) seeding density:
          10^5/ml, 0.25μg/ml PHA; ($\triangle$) seeding density: 2×10^5/ml, 0.125μg/ml
          PHA; (▲) seeding density: 2×10^5/ml, 0.25μg/ml PHA.

RESULTS

Growth Characteristics of Cultured T-cells Using culture conditions
as described in the methods section, mass cultures of T-lymphocytes

typically exhibited population doubling times ranging from 18-25hrs after PHA stimulation until approximately day 20. As the growth curves in figure 1A (panels A-D) show, it is at approximately day 20 when the doubling times of T-cells began to increase. Between days 20-35, the population doubling times of mass cultures ranged from about 35-65hrs, after which they decreased, appproaching initial values (Fig. 1B).

In a study undertaken to compare the growth characteristics of T-cells utilizing slightly different culture conditions, two seeding densities and two PHA concentrations were employed. As shown in figure 1A, neither the initial seeding density nor the PHA concentration employed had an effect on the final density to which the cells grew, the time at which the doubling time began to increase, the capacity of the mass cultures for extended <u>in vitro</u> growth, or the change in generation time. T-cells grew to approximately $1-2 \times 10^6$/ml after PHA stimulation until approximately day 20, at which time growth slowed until approximately day 37 when it began to approach initial rates.

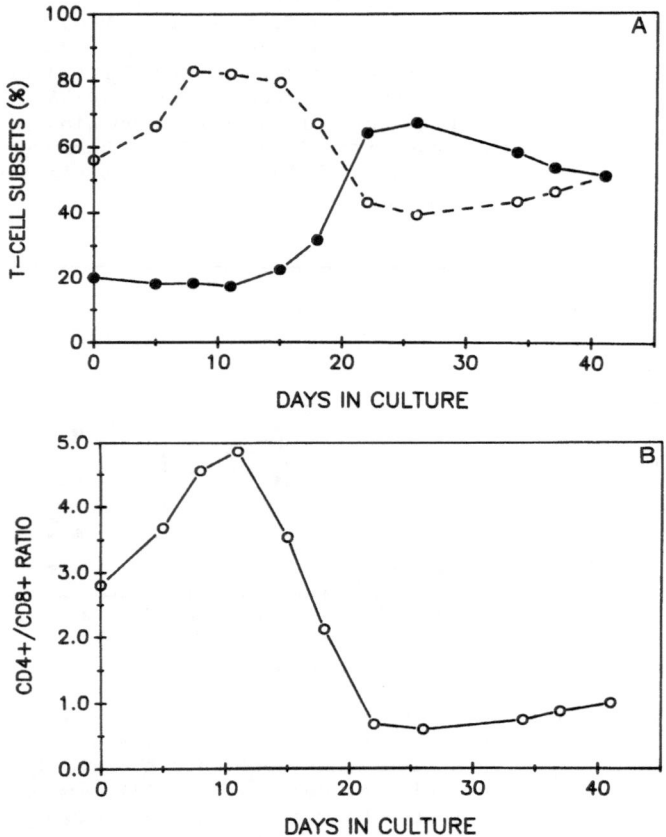

Fig. 2. Transition in the distribution of CD4+ and CD8+ T-cells in culture. Lymphocytes were cultured and prepared for FACS as described in the text: (A) percentage of (O) CD4+ T-cells and (O) CD8+ T-cells; (B) the ratio of CD4+/CD8+ T-cells.

<u>T-Cell Subsets during Extended Culture</u> As Fig. 2A shows, CD4+ T-cells predominate from the initial levels found in peripheral blood until approximately day 20, at which time there are approximately equal percentages of CD4+ and CD8+ cells. This transition in the CD4+/CD8+ ratio correlates with the abrupt increase in generation time shown in figure 1B. The CD4+/CD8+ ratio ranges from 3.7 on day 5 to approximately 5 on day 11, at which time it declines to and stabilizes at a value of approximately 1 from days 22 to 42 (figure 2B). The mean percentage of the sum of CD4+ and CD8+ cells is 100.25% ± 2.01 (standard error of the mean, SEM), while the mean percentage of CD2+ cells is 90.40% ± 2.57 (SEM). Statistical analysis using a paired t-test comparing the mean percentage of the sum of CD4+ and CD8+ cells to the mean percentage of CD2+ cells reveals that no significant difference exists between these two groups ($p < 0.01$).

<u>Measurement of Genomic DNA Repair during Extended Culture</u> Results of alkaline elutions performed on a control cell line (L87-083) during various times of <u>in vitro</u> growth confirmed previous findings of a significant decrease ($p < 0.05$) in the level of MNNG or MMS-induced repair occurring during the initial 3hrs after treatment as measured to day 22 of culture (Fig. 3). The relative decrease in the repair of MNNG-induced damage was found to be approximately 30%, while that of MMS-induced damage was approximately 40%. However, when repair during the initial 3hrs after treatment was measured in cells cultured beyond day 22, we found that, in the case of MMS-induced damage, repair increased to levels approaching initial levels, and in the case of MNNG-induced damage, repair stabilized at levels similar to those on day 22. Statistical analysis testing the quality of two regression lines revealed that the difference between the levels of repair of MNNG-induced lesions and MMS-induced lesions between days 5-44 was significant ($p < 0.05$). After a 24hr repair period, cells treated with MNNG exhibited a relative decrease in repair of approximately 20% between days 5-22 ($p < 0.05$) after which repair stabilized until the last determination on day 44. Furthermore, preliminary results on a second control cell line (L88-0324) support the results found on the first cell line (table 1). Genomic repair measured during the initial 3hrs after treatment with 4μM MNNG or 400μM MMS was reduced in cells cultured for 3 weeks as compared to cells cultured for 1 week.

Preliminary results on repair levels in cultured T-cells after treatment with the higher concentration of MMS used in the gene-specific repair assay (1.5mM) revealed that repair levels measured 3hr after treatment were lower than those measured after treatment with 400μM MMS (table 1, $p < 0.05$). After a 24hr repair period, however, repair levels in cells treated with 400μM MMS and 1.5mM MMS were not significantly different ($p < 0.05$). Repair in cells treated with the lower concentration of MMS was nearly complete by 24hr after treatment (x ± SEM = 91.6% ± 1.81) while the mean repair after treatment with 1.5mM MMS was 79.0% (SEM = 7.66).

<u>Gene-Specific DNA Repair</u> The dose of MMS used in conjunction with the 30min treatment time caused approximately 1 abasic site per 14kb in cultured T-cells. The average number of abasic sites per 14kb in untreated cells was found to be 0.07. Gene-specific repair was measured in different cell lines than was genomic repair, however all cell lines were from control individuals. Furthermore, repair was measured between days 10-15 of culture. Preliminary results demonstrate that repair at the <u>dhfr</u> locus ranges from 64% to nearly 100% complete by 6hr after treatment with 1.5mM MMS (x ± SEM = 82.9% ± 9.9). Although this mean repair value is higher than that of genomic DNA repair measured by alkaline elution using this same concentration of MMS (x ± SEM = 51.4% ± 15.9), the

TABLE 1. Genomic DNA Repair After Alkylating Agent Treatment

		PERCENT REPAIR AFTER						
		4μM MNNG		400μM MMS		1.5mM MMS		
CELL LINE	DAYS IN CULTURE	3HR	24HR	3HR	24HR	3HR	6HR	24HR
L87-083	7-11	62.1	93.1	82.2	96.0	4.0	35.5	83.1
	20-22	47.8	79.0	56.1	90.3	--	--	--
	35-36	43.2	73.4	69.6	92.4	6.8	40.0	68.2
L88-0324	10	58.4	88.0	74.4	97.6	38.2	67.3	100.0
	22	38.5	72.3	33.9	85.6	12.8	--	56.1
	36	51.7	84.0	60.3	89.4	42.6	--	87.7

difference is not statistically significant ($p<0.05$). As the number of determinations increases, the difference between the two groups may prove to be significant. The mean repair level at the dhfr locus after a 24hr repair period (90.1% ± 7.1) was not significantly greater than that at the 6hr repair period ($p<0.05$), ranging from 76% to 100%.

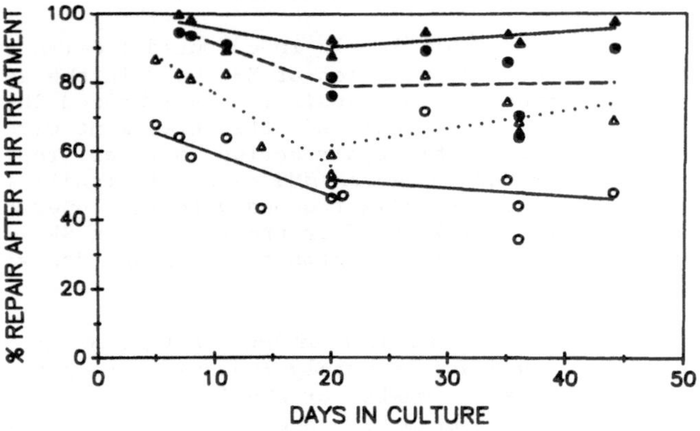

Fig. 3. Changes in genomic DNA repair of alkylating agent induced damage in T-cells during sustained culture. Cells were treated for 1hr at 37°C and then allowed the appropriated repair periods at 37°C: (O) 4μM MNNG/3hr repair; (O) 4μM MNNG/24hr repair; (Δ) 400μM MMS/3hr repair; (Δ) 400μM MMS/24hr repair. Regression lines have been drawn to include either day 5-22 data or day 22-44 data in order to demonstrate the biphasic nature of the data.

TABLE 2. DNA Repair at the DHFR Locus after Treatment with MMS

CELL LINE	ABASIC SITES/14 KB AFTER 1.5mM MMS			PERCENT REPAIR	
	0HR	6HR	24HR	6HR	24HR
L88-009	1.14	0.14	0.27	88.0	76.4
L88-012	0.94	0.01	0.00	97.0	100.0
L88-022	1.17	0.43	0.08	63.8	93.8
MEAN:	1.08			82.9	90.1

DISCUSSION

The purpose of this investigation was to extend a previous study in which we determined the existence of a reduction in the level of genomic DNA repair of alkylating agent-induced damage occurring over the course of 3 weeks of in vitro growth in human T-lymphocytes. In the present study, we sought to determine not only the levels of genomic DNA repair beyond 3 weeks of culture, but also to determine levels of DNA repair occurring in the active dhfr gene at an early time of in vitro growth (between days 10-15). Furthermore, we chose to quantify the subtypes of T-cells present in mass cultures at various times of in vitro growth beyond 3 weeks, since our previous study showed that a transition in the CD4+/CD8+ ratio occurred at approximately 3 weeks of culture. We also compared the growth characteristics of T-cells cultured under slightly modified conditions in order to determine whether these modifications may affect in vitro T-cell growth, which, in turn, may affect CD4+/CD8+ ratios and/or DNA repair levels. Because of the widespread use of lymphocytes in DNA repair studies, we have chosen to investigate the potential variables which may affect DNA repair capacity in cultured human T-cells.

In the present study of in vitro T-cell growth, we have shown that T-cells undergo a crisis at approximately 17-21 days of culture. Furthermore, analysis of the subtypes of T-cells present in mass lymphocyte cultures confirmed our previous finding that after approximately 15-20 days of culture, the ratio of CD4+ to CD8+ T-cells is approximately 1. The occurrence of this phenomenon was independent of the initial seeding density of T-cells as well as the PHA concentration used during culture. This crisis was characterized by an increase in the doubling times of the mass cultures which corresponded to the transition in the CD4+/CD8+ ratio. Until day 17, doubling times of mass cultures ranged from 18-25hrs, while the CD4+/CD8+ ratio ranged from 2.1 to nearly 5.0. However, after day 20 of culture, doubling times of mass cultures ranged from 35-65hrs and the CD4+/CD8+ ratio ranged from 0.6 to 1.0. Therefore, it appears that CD4+ T-cells are capable of optimal in vitro growth for approximately 2 weeks, while optimal growth of CD8+ T-cells is possible for a minimum of 6 weeks. Previously, Gullberg and Smith (1986) have shown that CD4+ cells cease to proliferate in vitro before CD8+ cells, whether cultured together or separately. Our study presented here also supports this hypothesis. The fact that neither the initial seeding density nor the PHA concentration used during culture had an effect on the occurrence of this crisis suggests that the transition in the CD4+/CD8+ ratio is not influenced by minor variations in cell culture conditions. Furthermore, the fact that cultures of T-cells seeded at either seeding density underwent a crisis at the same time of in vitro growth suggests that this crisis is independent of the number of doublings through which a T-cell divides and is more dependent on the number of days for which a culture is maintained. Cells seeded at a density of $2x10^5$/ml underwent approximately half the number of doublings as cells seeded at 10^5/ml because the final densities of both of these cultures were similar. All cultures exhibited a peak in the final density to which the cells grew between days 10-15, after which final densities were substantially lower until after day 30. The loss of high-affinity IL-2 receptors during sustained culture is the probable cause of this. Proliferation of T-cells is induced by the interaction of IL-2 with the high affinity IL-2 receptor (Smith and Cantrell, 1985). Investigators have found that during in vitro growth of T-cells, there is a significant loss of high affinity IL-2 receptors after the initial stimulation by lectin (such as PHA) or antigen (Cantrell and Smith, 1983; Depper et al., 1985; Gullberg and Smith, 1986). We have shown here that a higher concentration of PHA during sustained culture had no effect on the final density to which the cells grew and therefore probably had no effect on the level of high affinity IL-2 receptor expression. Therefore, we can also hypothesize that all cultures were losing the high affinity IL-2 receptors at equal rates.

Lymphocytes in mass cultures were analyzed not only for the CD4 and CD8 markers but also for the presence of the CD2 marker. The CD2 marker represents the T-cell lineage-specific receptor protein which binds with sheep red blood cells, resulting in the formation of T-cell rosettes. Statistical analysis revealed that the percentage of the CD2+ cells (90.40%) was not different from the sum of the percentages of the CD4+ and CD8+ cells (100.25%). Therefore, we have concluded that the mass lymphocyte cultures were a pure T-cell population comprised of only CD4+ and CD8+ T-cells.

In the study comparing the growth characteristics of mass cultures, we found that seeding density and PHA concentration had no effect on the doubling times and the final densities to which cells grew. Therefore, because the variations in culture conditions tested here showed no effects on the growth characteristics of T-cells, it is not likely that DNA repair capacity would be affected by subtle variations in culture conditions. Preliminary data comparing DNA repair levels in T-cells seeded at two densities (10^5/ml and $2x10^5$/ml) supports this hypothesis (data not shown).

Genomic DNA repair of MNNG or MMS-induced damage was measured over three intervals, 3hr, 6hr and 24hr, between days 5 and 44, using the alkaline elution technique. MMS and MNNG most predominantly cause methylations at the the N^7 position of guanine and the N^3 position of adenine (Day et al., 1987). MNNG also causes significantly more methylation at the O^6 position of guanine (5.4%) and phosphotriesters (12.1%) as compared to MMS (0.25% and 0.8% respectively for these two lesions) (Day et al., 1987). Base methylations (except O6-MeG) and phosphotriesters produce alkali-labile sites (Hall et al., 1988; Lindahl, 1981; Teebor et al., 1981; Walker et al., 1973), while neither the O6-MeG lesion nor the repair of this lesion produces an alkali-labile site. Results confirmed previous findings that a significant reduction in the repair measured during the initial 3hrs after treatment with either 4μM MNNG or 400μM MMS existed between days 5 and 22 of culture. Furthermore, the difference in the repair of MNNG and MMS-induced damage is likely to be due to the repair of phosphotriesters which are induced to a larger degree by MNNG than MMS. The repair of MMS-induced lesions was nearly complete after a 24hr incubation and was not effected by in vitro age when a 24hr repair period was allowed. However, the greater variance in 24hr repair levels after treatment with 1.5mM MMS as compared to 400μM MMS may suggest that in vitro age may have a significant effect on repair capacities after treatment with sufficient doses of MMS. On the other hand, the repair of MNNG-induced lesions after a 24hr repair period was still reduced at day 22 as compared to initial levels. At later times of in vitro growth, the repair of MNNG-induced lesions after a 24hr incubation approached initial levels. These results suggest that T-cells are not losing the capacity to repair alkylating agent-induced damage during their initial 2-3 weeks of culture but rather that the rate of repair of these lesions is slower.

Comparison of genomic repair levels and CD4/CD8 ratios suggest that reduced repair between initial levels and day 22 is attributable to the transition in the CD4/CD8 ratio. However, statistical analysis in a previous investigation has revealed that a negative correlation exists between the CD4/CD8 ratios and repair levels (Hartshorn and Robison, 1989). The observed decrease in repair (or slower rate) may be due to reduced protein and/or RNA synthesis in the CD4+ population which is undergoing both positive and negative selection pressures in vitro. If this were true, we would expect that when cultures undergoing this transition were treated with a higher concentration of alkylating agent (such as 1.5mM MMS), a more dramatic reduction in genomic DNA repair would be the result. Preliminary results indicate this to be true. Repair measured 24hr after treatment of day 22 cells with 1.5mM MMS was markedly reduced from that measured in cells treated with 400μM MMS. Furthermore, 24hr repair in day 10 and day 36 cells was not as effected by treatment with the higher concentration of MMS.

The recent finding of differential repair of UV-dimers in actively transcribed sequences (Bohr et al., 1986; Mellon et al., 1986) and on the actively transcribed strand (Mellon et al., 1987) indicates that the mechanism(s) for recognition and repair of DNA lesions must be reevaluated. A similar difference might exist for the repair of MMS or MNNG induced lesions in actively transcribed sequences. Until recently (Scicchitano and Hanawalt, 1989) there have been no techniques available to study the repair of alkylating agent-induced damage in specific DNA sequences. The repair of these lesions is particularly important since one of the intermediates in their repair is the apurinic (abasic) site. It has been estimated that a human cell undergoes 10^4 spontaneous depurinations and 10^2 depyrimidinations per day. Failure to recognize or repair these lesions would be catastrophic to the cell. Although there have been reports of the existence of a DNA insertase (Linn et al 1981), it is generally accepted that apurinic sites are repaired by a base excision mechanism. Results obtained after treatment of CHO cells with DMS indicate that although there were no differences in the overall repair of apurinic lesions in genomic DNA and the dhfr gene, there was a slight difference in the rate of repair between active sequences and non-transcribed regions (Scicchitano and Hanawalt, 1989).

Our studies of the repair of MMS-induced damage in the dhfr gene indicate that there may be a rate difference in the repair of damage in the transcriptionally active sequence as compared to bulk DNA in human T-lymphocytes. Alkaline elution studies after 3, 6 and 24hr of repair reveal that approximately 20%, 48% and 90%, respectively, of the damage is repaired in genomic DNA. When the repair of damage in the dhfr gene was examined, we found that after 6hr and 24hr of repair, approximately 80% and 90%, respectively, of the abasic sites were repaired. Repair measured at the dhfr locus during a 24hr period after treatment with MMS was not significantly greater than that measured after only 6hr, while genomic DNA repair after a 6hr period was significantly lower than that after 24hr. This suggests that the repair of alkylating-agent induced damage occurs more slowly in genomic DNA than in the constitutively expressed dhfr gene. This finding is in agreement with that of others, who have found that the repair of UV-light induced damage in CHO and human cells (Mellon et al., 1986) and the repair of alkylation damage in CHO cells (Scicchitano and Hanawalt, 1989) is more efficient at the dhfr locus than in bulk chromatin. This indicates that actively transcribed genes and/or housekeeping genes may have preferential repair of alkylated bases over bulk chromatin. It is generally accepted that alkylation damage does not block DNA replication or transcription (Friedberg, 1985). Therefore, unrepaired lesions may result in mutation. Because only 2-4% of the genome encodes for transcribed sequences (Friedberg, 1985), preferential repair of damaged bases would be an efficient system whereby mutational processes in transcriptionally active DNA would be minimized, resulting in enhanced cell survival and function.

In using the alkaline elution technique to measure genomic DNA repair, we have confirmed previous results indicating reduced levels of repair of MNNG and MMS-induced lesions in T-lymphocytes which have been maintained in culture for 3 weeks. In addition, we have determined that the ratio of the two subtypes of T-cells, CD4+ and CD8+, changes over a 6 week culture period. Initially, there are 2-5 times as many CD4+ cells as there are CD8+ cells. However, after 3 weeks of culture, the ratio of CD4+ to CD8+ cells is approximately 1:1 for the duration of the period under investigation. This transition is coordinated with the nadir of alkylating agent-induced repair. We have hypothesized that this decrease in repair observed between the initial levels and those at day 22 may be due to reduced protein synthesis in the CD4+ population which is being selected against in vitro. In a preliminary investigation in which genomic repair levels were compared to repair in the transcriptionally active dhfr gene, we have found that the alkylation damage at the dhfr locus seemed to be repaired at a more rapid rate than in genomic DNA. These preliminary findings are interesting and merit further investigation. Future experiments will focus, not only on the comparison of genomic DNA repair efficiency to that at the dhfr locus, but also on determining how gene-specific repair at the dhfr locus in cells cultured for extended periods of time compares to that of "younger" cultures. These studies confirm the complexity of DNA repair mechanisms in mammalian cells.

ACKNOWLEDGEMENTS

The authors would like to thank Philip Hanawalt for helpful discussions and for allowing one of us, SHR, to spend time in his laboratory, Vincent Falco, operator of the Fluorescence Activated Cell Sorter in the department of Microbiology at the University of Vermont for his expertise; Greg Magin in the Neurology Department, and Gary Badger in the Biostatistics Department for their statistical expertise. This research was supported by grants from the NIH-NIA (grant #RO1-AG-06163), the American Federation for Aging Research (AFAR), the Alzheimer's Disease and Related Disorders Association (ADRDA), and the ALS Association of America.

REFERENCES

Albertini, R. J., 1985, The use of human T-lymphocytes to monitor
          mutations in human populations, in: "New approaches in toxicity
          testing and their application in human risk assessments", A. P.
          Li, eds., Raven Press, New York, 51.
Arlett, C. F., and Harcourt, S. A., 1980, Survey of radiosensitivity in a
          variety of human cell strains, Cancer Res., 40:926.
Bartlett, J. D., and Robison, S. H., 1989, O^6-methylguanine-DNA
          methyltransferase activities from exponentially growing human

   T-lymphocytes: Similar activities in controls and Alzheimer's
   disease patients, Mutagenesis, (in press).
Bender, M. A., Viola, M. V., Fiore, J., Thompson, M. H., and Leonard, R.
   C., 1988, Normal G$_2$ chromosomal radiosensitivity and cell
   survival in the cancer family syndrome, Cancer Res., 48:2570.
Bohr, V., Smith, C. A., Ocumoto, D., and Hanawalt, P., 1985, DNA repair in
   an active gene: Removal of pyrimidine dimers from the DHFR gene
   of CHO cells is much more efficient than in the genome overall,
   Cell, 40:359.
Bohr, V. A., Okumoto, D. S., and Hanawalt, P. C., 1986, Survival of
   UV-irradiated mammalian cells correlates with efficient DNA
   repair in an essential gene, Proc. Nat. Acad. Sci. U.S.A.,
   83:3830.
Cantrell, D. A., and Smith, K. A., 1983, Transient expression of
   interleukin-2 receptors: Consequences for T cell growth, J.
   Expt. Med., 158:1895.
Cathcart, R., and Goldthwait, D. A., 1981, Enzymatic excision of
   3-methyladenine and 7-methylguanine by a rat liver nuclear
   fraction, Biochem., 20:273.
Chan, J. Y. H., Becker, F. F., German, J., and Ray, J. H., 1987, Altered
   DNA ligase I activity in Bloom's syndrome cells, Nature,
   325:357.
Chu, G., and Chang, E., 1988, Xeroderma pigmentosum group E cells lack a
   nuclear factor that binds to damaged DNA, Science, 242:564.
Cimino, M. C., Tice, R. R., and Liang, J. C., 1986, Aneuploidy in
   mammalian somatic cell in vivo, Mutation Res., 167:107.
Cox, R., and Masson, W. K., 1980, Radiosensitivity in cultured human
   fibroblasts, Int. J. Radiat. Biol., 38:575.
Day, R. S., Babich, M. A., Yarosh, D. B., and Scudiero, D. A., 1987, The
   role of O^6-methylguanine in human cell killing, sister chromatid
   exchange induction and mutagenesis: A review, J. Cell Sci.,
   suppl 6:333.
Depper, J. M., Leonard, W. J., Drogula, C. L., Kronke, M., Waldmann, T.
   A., and Green, W. C., 1985, Activators of protein kinase C and
   5-azacytidine induce IL-2 receptor expression on human T
   lymphocytes, J. Cell. Biochem., 27:267.
Friedberg, E. C. 1985. "DNA Repair". W. H. Freeman and Company, New York.
Fujiwara, Y., 1982, Defective repair of mitomycin C crosslinks in
   Fanconi's anaemia and loss in confluent normal human and
   xeroderma pigmentosum cells, Biochim. Biophys. Acta, 699:217.
Gallagher, P. E., and Brent, T. P., 1984, Further purification and
   characterization of human 3-methyladenine DNA glycosylase.
   Evidence for broad specificity, Biochim. Biophys. Acta, 782:394.
Gianelli, F., Botcherly, P. K., and Avery, J. A., 1982, The effect of
   aphidicolin on the rate of DNA replication and unscheduled DNA
   synthesis of Bloom syndrome and normal fibroblasts, Hum. Genet.,
   60:357-359.
Gullberg, M., and Smith, K. A., 1986, Regulation of T cell autocrine
   growth. T4+ cells become refractory to interleukin 2, J. Expt.
   Med., 163:270.
Gupta, P. K., and Sirover, M. A., 1984, Altered temporal expression of DNA
   repair in hypermutable Bloom's syndrome cells, Proc. Nat. Acad.
   Sci. U.S.A., 81:757-761.
Hall, J., Kataoka, H., Stephenson, C., and Karran, P., 1988, The
   contribution of O^6-methylguanine and methylphosphotriesters to
   the cytotoxity of alkylating agents in mammalian cells,
   Carcinogenesis, 9:1587.
Harris, A. L., Karran, P., and Lindahl, T., 1983, O^6-methylguanine-DNA
   transferase of huamn lymphoid cells: Structural and kinetic
   properties and absence in repair deficient cells, Cancer Res.,
   43:3247.

Harris, G., Lawley, P. D., Asbery, L. J., Chandler, P. M., and Jones, M. G., 1983, Autoimmune haemolytic disease in mice after exposure to a methylating carcinogen, Immunol., 49:439.

Hartshorn, J. N., and Robison, S. H., 1989, The relationship between DNA repair capacity after alkylation damage and in vitro aging in human T-lymphocytes, Mutation Res., (in press).

Kaye, J., Smith, C. A., and Hanawalt, P. C., 1980, DNA repair in human cells containing photoadducts of 8-methoxypsoralen or angelicin, Cancer Res., 40:696.

Kohn, K. W., Ewig, R. E., Erickson, L. C., and Zwelling, L. A., 1981, Chapter 29: Measurement of strand breaks and cross-links by alkaline elution, in, DNA Repair: A Laboratory Manual of Research Procedures, E. C. Friedberg, and P. C. Hanawalt eds., Vol. 1A, Marcel Dekker,Inc, New York, 379.

Kraemer, K. H., Lee, M. M., and Scotto, J., 1984, DNA repair protects against cutaneous and internal neoplasia: Evidence from xeroderma pigmentosum, Carcinogenesis, 5:511.

Kraemer, K. H., Myung, M. L., and Scotto, M. S. J., 1987, Xeroderma pigmentosum, Arch. Dermatol., 123:241.

Lambert, B., Ringborg, U., and Skoog, L., 1979, Age-related decrease of ultraviolet light-induced DNA repair synthesis in human peripheral leukocytes, Cancer Res., 39:2792.

Lehman, A. R., 1982, Xeroderma pigmentosum, Cockayne syndrome and ataxia-telangiectasia: Disorders relating DNA repair to carcinogenesis, Cancer Surv., 1:93.

Lindahl, T., 1981, Chapter 17: Measurement of sites of base loss, in, DNA Repair: A Laboratory Manual of Research Procedures, E. C. Friedberg, and P. C. Hanawalt eds., Vol. 1A, Marcel Dekker,Inc, New York, 213.

Linn, S., Demple, B., Masbaugh, D. W., Warner, H. P., and Deutsch, W. A., 1981, Enzymatic studies of base excision repair in cultured human fibroblasts and in Escherichia coli, in: "Chromosome Damage and Repair", E. Seeburg, and K. Kleppe eds., Plenum, New York, 97.

Madden, J. J., Falek, A., Shafer, D. A., and Glick, J. H., 1979, Effects of opiates and demographic factors on DNA repair synthesis in human leukocytes, Proc. Nat. Acad. Sci. U.S.A., 76:5769.

Mellon, I., Bohr, V., Smith, C. A., and Hanawalt, P., 1986, Preferential DNA repair of an active gene in human cells, Proc. Nat. Acad. Sci. U.S.A., 83:8878.

Mellon, I., Spivak, G., and Hanawalt, P., 1987, Selective removal of Transcription-blocking DNA damage from the transcribed strand of the mammalian DHFR gene, Cell, 51:241.

Munzer, J. S., Jones, S. K., O'Neill, J. P., Hartshorn, J. N., and Robison, S. H., 1988, Detection of DNA damage and repair by alkaline elution using human lymphocytes, Mutation Res., 194:101.

Pedersen-Bjergaard, J., and Olesen-Larsen, S., 1982, Incidence of acute nonlymphocytic leukemia, preleukemia and acute myeloproliferative syndrome up to 10 years after treatment of Hodgkins disease, New Eng J Med., 307:965.

Reinherz, E. L., and Schlossman, S. F., 1980, The differentiation and function of human T-lymphocytes, Cell., 19:821.

Scicchitano, D. A., and Hanawalt, P. C., 1989, Repair of N-methylpurines in specific DNA sequences in Chinese hamster ovary cells: Absence of strand specificity in the dihydrofolate reductase gene, Proc. Nat. Acad. Sci. U.S.A., 86:3050.

Scudiero, D. A., Meyer, S. A., Clatterbuck, B. E., Tarone, R. E., and Robbins, J. H., 1981, Hypersensitivity to

N-methyl-N'-nitro-N-nitrosoguanidine in fibroblasts from patients with Huntington's disease, familial dysautonomia and other primary neuronal degenerations, Proc. Nat. Acad. Sci. U.S.A., 78:6451.

Seal, G., Brech, K., Karp, S. J., Cool, B. L., and Sirover, M. A., 1988, Immunological lesions in human uracil DNA glycosylase: Association with Bloom syndrome, Proc. Nat. Acad. Sci. U.S.A., 85:2339.

Setlow, R.B., 1978, Repair deficient human disorders and cancer, Nature., 271:713.

Setlow, R. B., 1983, Variations in DNA repair among humans, in: "Human Carcinogenesis", Academic Press, New York, 231.

Smith, K. A., and Cantrell, D. A., 1985, Interleukin 2 regulates its own receptors, Proc. Nat. Acad. Sci. U.S.A., 82:864.

Teebor, G. W., and Brent, T. P., 1981, Chapter 16: Measurement of alkali-labile sites, in: "DNA Repair: A Laboratory Manual of Research Procedures", E. C. Friedberg, and P. C. Hanawalt, eds., Vol. 1A, Marcel Dekker,Inc., New York, 203.

Van Duin, M., de Wit, J., Odijk,H., Westerveid, A., Yasni, A., Koken, M. H. M., Hoeijamakers, J. H. H., and Bootsma, D., 1986, Molecular characterization of the human excision repair gene ERCC-1: cDNA cloning and amino acid homology with the yeast DNA repair gene RAD10, Cell., 44:913.

van Zeeland, A. A., Mayne, L., and Mullenders, L. H. F., 1988, Repair of specific genes in human cells, J. Cell. Biochem., suppl. 12A:302.

Vollberg, T. M., Seal, G., and Sirover, M. A., 1987, Monoclonal antibodies detect conformational abnormality of uracil DNA glycosylase in Bloom syndrome cells, Carcinogenesis, 8:1725.

Waldstein, E. A., Cao, E.-H., and Setlow, R. B., 1982, Direct assay for O^6-methylguanine-acceptor protein in cell extracts, Anal. Biochem., 126:268.

Walker, I. G. and Ewart, D. F., 1973, The nature of single-strand breaks in DNA following treatment of L-cells with methylating agents, Mutation Res., 19:331.

Weber, C. A., Salazar, E. P., Stewart, S. A., and Thompson, L. H., 1988, Molecular cloning and biological characterization of a human gene, ERCC2, that corrects the nucleotide excision repair defect in CHO UV5 cells, Mol Cell Biol., 8:1137.

Weichselbaum, R. R., Nove, J., and Little, J. B., 1980, X-ray sensitivity of fifty-three human diploid fibroblast cell strains from patients with characterized genetic disorders, Cancer Res., 40:920.

Willis, A. E., and Lindahl, T., 1987, DNA ligase I deficiency in Bloom's syndrome, Nature, 325:355-357.

Yang, J., Masters, J., and Attardi, G., 1984, Human dihydrofolate reductase gene organization, J. Mol. Biol., 176:169.

Yarosh, D. B., Foote, R. S., Mitra, S., and Day, R. S., III, 1983, Repair of O^6-methylguanine in DNA by demethylation is lacking in Mer⁻ human tumor cell strains, Carcinogenesis, 4:199.

PERIPHERAL BLOOD LEUKOCYTES AS A SURROGATE MARKER

FOR CISPLATIN DRUG RESISTANCE: STUDIES OF ADDUCT

LEVELS AND THE REPAIR GENE ERCC1

Ricardo J. Parker[1], Miriam C. Poirier[2],
Freida Bostick-Bruton[1], Justine Vionnet[1],
Vilhelm A. Bohr[1], and Eddie Reed[1,3]

[1]Division of Cancer Treatment
[2]Division of Cancer Etiology
National Cancer Institute
Bethesda, Maryland 20892

INTRODUCTION

Cisplatin and its analogs are potent chemotherapeutic agents in the treatment of ovarian cancer, testicular cancer, and other malignancies. Studies by this group have shown that the level of platinum-DNA adduct formed in leukocyte DNA is directly related to disease response in ovarian cancer (Reed et al,1987) and testicular cancer (Reed et al,1988a), and that the level of adduct attained is influenced by the persistence of the adduct in leukocyte precursors in some patients for no less than 28 days (Reed et al,1986). Because this persistence has been observed in some patients but not in others (Reed et al,1986), we have been interested in the study of those factors that may influence persistence, and whether these factors are directly related to clinical parameters and/or subcellular parameters of cisplatin drug resistance. We have assessed the relative contribution of clinical parameters to disease response in a cohort of patients with ovarian cancer, and we compare those data to platinum-DNA adduct measurements in leukocyte DNA from these same individuals. We also discuss early studies of the possible contribution of the human DNA repair gene, ERCC1, to platinum drug resistance, as assessed by evaluation of peripheral blood leukocytes of a small cohort of ovarian cancer patients.

MATERIALS AND METHODS

In Vitro Cell Studies of Cisplatin Sensitivity

Cell lines used in this study have been described in detail elsewhere (Westerveld et al,1984; van Duin et al,1986; Hoeijmakers,1987). The 43-3B cell line is a Chinese hamster

---

[3]To whom correspondence should be addressed.

DNA Damage and Repair in Human Tissues
Edited by B. M. Sutherland and A. D. Woodhead
Plenum Press, New York, 1990

251

ovary (CHO) cell line which is UV-repair deficient and is of complementation group 1. We refer to this cell line as ERCC1(-). The 83-G5 cell line is a subline of the 43-3B cell line which contains a stable transfection of the human excision nuclease ERCC1. We refer to this cell line as ERCC1(+).

Sensitivity to cisplatin was assessed in colony growth assays using six well-plates, each well 35 mm in diameter. Cells were plated at 500 cells per well, and cisplatin treatments were preformed as 1-hour drug exposures on the day after plating. Cisplatin was initially dissolved in sterile phosphate buffered saline (PBS) at 1 mg per ml, and dilutions from this 1 mg per ml solution were made into media to obtain the desired concentration. Drug-containing media was placed onto cells for 1 hour, after which the media was aspirated, the plate was rinsed with PBS and fresh media was added to the wells. Cells were allowed to grow for 7 to 10 days, at which time colonies were stained with a methylene blue solution of 0.167 gm percent in absolute methanol. Visible colonies were counted by hand. Drug treatments were done in triplicate at each dose in each experiment. The value obtained in wells, where no drug was added, was assigned the value of 100% growth.

Measurement of Platinum in Cellular DNA

To assess the ability of these CHO cells to remove platinum from cellular DNA, cells were plated in 150 cc^3 flasks, and were allowed to reach 50 to 80 percent confluence with changes of fresh media twice weekly. Cells were then labeled with ^{3}H-thymidine, using media with a ^{3}H-thymidine concentration of 0.1 uCuries per ml. Cells were labeled with ^{3}H overnight, after which fresh media was placed onto the cells and incubation was again carried out overnight. At this time, cells were exposed to cisplatin drug concentrations for 1 hour at their respective IC50s, as was assessed by colony formation. The IC50 for the ERCC1(-) cell line was 0.75 uM; and for the ERCC1(+) cell line, 4.0 uM. After ^{3}H labelling, an aliquot of cells were harvested before drug treatment (time zero). Following a 1 hour exposure, cells were harvested at the following times: 1 hour (immediately at the end of the cisplatin exposure); 4 hours; 8 hours; and 24 hours. At each time, media was removed, cells were pelleted, and were stored at -20°C until DNA isolation.

DNA was isolated on cesium chloride density gradients, yielding DNA which was 99.6% free of contamination (Flamm et al,1969). This DNA was dialyzed against doubly distilled water for four exchanges over an approximate 36 hours. DNA was then measured by absorbance at 260 nanometers. ^{3}H-Thymidine content was assessed by liquid scintillation counting and platinum content was assessed by atomic absorption spectroscopy (Reed et al,1988b). The platinum content for cellular DNA at each time point was corrected for DNA replication based on the original ^{3}H-thymidine content of the DNA of cells studied at time zero.

RNA Slot Blotting and RNA Gel Electrophoresis

Slot blotting of RNA from both CHO cell lines, and human from leukocytes was done according to the method of

Schleicher and Schuell, Keene, NH (Fairchild et al, 1987). In our studies, all slot blotting was done with 1 ug, 5 ug, and 25 ug in sequential horizontal wells for each specimen. RNA was isolated from CHO cell lines using the guanidine isothiocyanate method, as described by Davis and colleagues (1986). RNA used in these studies was not poly-A selected. RNA gel electrophoresis was performed by the method described by Davis and colleagues (1986). The cDNA probe for ERCC1 has been described in detail elsewhere (van Duin et al,1986); the probe for actin was purchased from Oncor Co., Gaithersburg, Maryland.

Patients Studied, Specimens Collected, and ELISA

Patients were treated on approved experimental treatment protocols in the Medicine Branch of the National Cancer Institute, and received "high dose cisplatin" (Ozols et al,1985), or "high dose carboplatin" (Ozols et al,1987), or high-dose carboplatin with recombinant granulocyte-macrophage colony stimulating factor (rGM-CSF) (protocol on file,Clinical Oncology Program,National Cancer Institute,Bethesda,Maryland 20892). The medical records of these individuals were reviewed for analysis of any clinical variables that may influence response to therapy. Blood was obtained by venipuncture on the morning following the completion of platinum drug infusion, white blood cells (wbc's) were separated by centrifugation, and DNA and RNA was isolated using cesium chloride density gradient centrifugation (Flamm et al,1969). DNAs were used for measurements of platinum-DNA adduct levels, which were done by enzyme-linked immunosorbent assay (ELISA), and are expressed as attomoles of adduct per microgram of DNA (Reed et al,1987). RNAs from wbc's of six patients were used for probing for the ERCC1 and actin genes.

Statistical Methods

For each patient who received high dose cisplatin or high dose carboplatin, one or more cycles of therapy were studied to assess the level of adduct formed in DNA of wbc's. As reported previously, the peak adduct level observed during the course of therapy was used for statistical analysis (Reed,et al,1987). Univariate analyses were performed using both the Wilcoxon two-sample statistic to evaluate differences in continuous variable, and the Fisher exact test to compare proportions of patients in two groups possessing categorized characteristics (Conover, 1980).

RESULTS

Clinical Studies of Adduct Levels

The patient group studied for platinum-DNA adduct level is a subset of two studies that have been previously reported (Ozols et al,1985; Ozols et al,1987), and includes all patients from these original reports. In this group, twelve patients received high-dose cisplatin as single-agent salvage therapy for relapsed or progressive ovarian carcinoma (Ozols et al,1985) and twelve other ovarian cancer patients received high-dose carboplatin as single-agent salvage therapy (Ozols et al,1987). All individuals had primarily failed or relapsed from combination chemotherapy. There were eight patients who

Table 1. Univariate Analysis of Prognostic Variables in 24 Ovarian Cancer Patients Receiving Single Agent Cisplatin or Carboplatin Therapy

Continuous Variables	Mean + S.E.M.		p Value of Relation to Disease Response
	Responders	Non-Responders	
Leukocyte DNA Adduct Level (amol/ug DNA)	227 ± 33	79 ± 25	0.0058
Karnofsky Status	90 ± 5	85 ± 3	0.125
Total Previous Platinum Dose (mg per m^2)	444 ± 124	598 ± 80	0.358
Age (years)	50 ± 5	54 ± 3	0.374

Dichotomous Variables	Proportion of Total Number		
	Responders	Non-Responders	
Stage 3 Disease	7/8	9/16	0.189
Response to Previous Therapy	7/8	10/16	0.352
Disease <2 cm	3/8	4/16	0.647

experienced an objective response to therapy, and sixteen who did not, resulting in a 33% response rate. The median adduct level in wbc DNA in responders was 227 attomoles of adduct per ug of DNA. In non-responders, the median adduct level was 79 attomoles per ug DNA. There were seven patients who did not form measurable levels of adduct at any time during treatment and all failed therapy.

A number of variables have been reported to be associated with disease response in ovarian cancer (Reed et al,1988c). The contribution of these previously identified prognostic variables to disease response in this cohort was determined by univariate analysis. Data for each of the variables listed above (Table 1) were obtained by review of the medical records or by pathologic review of the original diagnostic material which established the diagnosis of ovarian cancer. For each of these variables a univariate analysis was performed, with the results shown in the table. As shown, adduct level in leukocyte DNA is the only variable related to disease response to a statistically significant degree, with a two-sided p value of 0.0058. Weak trends towards significance are shown for Karnofsky status (an objective assessment of patient performance status), and stage 3 disease versus stage 4. Minor associations are observed for the response to previous therapy, total previous platinum dose, and age. There was no relationship between adduct level and bulk of disease. Pathologic material was formally reviewed for histologic type on nineteen patients in this cohort, and for histologic grade on twelve patients. There was no relationship between histology and disease response in this cohort (data not shown).

Peak adduct level in leukocyte DNA was compared to duration of disease response in those individuals who responded to platinum therapy. These data are summarized in Table 2.

Table 2. The Relationship Between Peak Adduct Level and the Duration of Disease Response in Eight Patients who responded To Single Agent Therapy

Patient#	Therapy	Peak Leukocyte DNA Adduct Level	Disease Type	Response Duration (months)
1	Carboplatin	357	PR[a]	4
2	Carboplatin	304	PR	13
3	Carboplatin	300	PR	8
4	Carboplatin	242	PR	7
5	Cisplatin	210	CR[b]	9
6	Cisplatin	188	PR	3.5
7	Cisplatin	127	PR	19
8	Cisplatin	89	PR	14

[a]PR = partial response to therapy; i.e., a greater than 50% reduction in tumor mass.
[b]CR = complete response to therapy; eradication of all demonstrable tumor.

Table 3. Cisplatin Induced Cytotoxicity in Two Chinese Hamster Ovary Cell Lines In Vitro as Measured by Colony Formation

Level of Cisplatin Cytotoxicity	ERCC1 (+)	ERCC1 (-)	Fold Difference
IC20	1 uM	0.5 uM	2 fold
IC50	4 uM	0.75 uM	5 fold
IC90	10 uM	2.0 uM	5 fold

In this subset of eight patients (1 through 4 treated with carboplatin, 5 through 8 with cisplatin), adduct level was not associated with the duration of disease response. Of interest, the highest levels of wbc DNA adduct observed among the eight responders were in the carboplatin-treated patients.

For the total twenty-four patient cohort, the difference between adduct levels in the two treatment groups is substantial but not statistically significant, with the mean and median adduct levels of 93 and 108 amol/ug DNA, respectively, for cisplatin-treated patients, and 164 and 176 amol/ug DNA, respectively, for carboplatin-treated patients.

In Vitro Studies of ERCC1

Since peak adduct level is related to the occurence of disease response but not to the duration of disease response, we began to consider what factors may influence the duration of disease response to platinum-based therapy. In vitro, DNA repair is an important component of cisplatin drug resistance (Reed,1989), and we began to investigate the possible role of the human DNA repair gene ERCC1 in conferring resistance to cisplatin.

Initial studies were in Chinese hamster ovary (CHO) cells of UV-repair deficient complementation group 1, with and without the stable transfection of ERCC1. These cell lines have been described in detail elsewhere (Westerveld et al,198-4; van Duin et al,1986; Hoeijmakers,1987). Cellular sensitivity/resistance to cisplatin was assessed by colony formation, which determines a cell's ability to undergo multiple doublings. These data are shown in Table 3. For the ERCC1(-) cell line, 20 percent cell kill occurs at 0.5 uM, 50 percent cell kill at 0.75 uM, and 90 percent cell kill at 2.0 uM. For the ERCC1(+) cell line, the respective drug exposures are: 20% cell kill, 1.0 uM; 50% cell kill, 4.0 uM; and 90% cell kill, 10.0 uM. In comparing the drug exposures associated with 50% cell kill (the IC50) and 90% cell kill (the IC90), the ERCC(+) cell line is five-fold more resistant to cisplatin than the ERCC1(-) cell line.

Table 4.   Total Cisplatin-DNA Adduct Levels (by AAS) in Two Chinese Hamster Ovary Cell Lines After Treatment of the Cells at Their Respective IC50s

	ERCC1 (+) Cells	ERCC1 (-) Cells
Peak Adduct Level Attained	0.8 + 0.2	0.4 + 0.16
Adduct Level 24 Hrs After Drug Exposure	0.42 + 0.1	0.4 + 0.1
Percent of Total Adduct Load Removed:	48	None

To assess the manner in which the cell lines handle biologically important concentrations of cisplatin, we examined the formation and removal of cisplatin-DNA adduct in cellular DNA following IC50 drug doses to the respective cell lines. These data are summarized in Table 4. In the ERCC1(-) cell line, 0.4 pgm of platinum per ug of DNA had formed following the one-hour exposure of 0.75 uM. This level of adduct did not change during 24 hours. In the ERCC1(+) cell line, 0.8 pgm/ug DNA of adduct formed as a result of the one-hour exposure at its IC50 of 4.0 uM. By 24 hours, this value had been reduced to 0.4 pg/ug DNA of adduct. Thus, when treated at their respective IC50s, both cell lines retained the same amount of DNA-bound drug at 24 hours. In the resistant cell line, there was substantial removal of cisplatin from cellular DNA in the first 24 hours after drug exposure (48 percent of total platinum-DNA load), and this was not seen in the sensitive cell line.

Early Clinical Studies of ERCC1

We have also conducted studies to begin to assess whether ERCC1 may have clinical relevance to cisplatin drug resistance. Initial studies are shown in Fig. 1. RNA was isolated from patient's leukocytes; prepared for slot blotting as described above; and probed for actin to assess relative RNA integrity; and probed for ERCC1. In five of the patients studied (patients 1 through 5), ERCC1 was expressed to variable degrees. RNAs have not been studied at later times in these five patients. In one patient (patient # 6), leukocyte RNA was obtained before (sample 6,a) and after (sample 6,b) three cycles of chemotherapy with carboplatin and rGM-CSF. As shown, actin expression was approximately the same for samples 6,a and 6,b; however, ERCC1 expression was four-fold greater in sample 6,b than in sample 6,a. Clinically, this patient initially had a dramatic partial response to therapy (over 80% reduction in tumor bulk) which stabilized. After stabilization,the patient was removed from carboplatin/rGM-CSF therapy and given other non-cross resistant protocol therapy.

DISCUSSION

Clinical studies of platinum-DNA adduct formation demonstrate that the level of adduct formed in a patient's peripheral blood leukocytes is directly related to disease response, but does not appear to be related to the duration of response. These data suggested to us that other factors may play a role in determining response to platinum-based chemotherapy. Extrapolation from in vitro studies led us to investigate the possible role of the human DNA repair gene ERCC1 in clinical platinum drug resistance.

In Chinese hamster ovary cells of complementation group I, the human excision nuclease ERCC1 confers five-fold resistance to cisplatin and the ability to remove cisplatin from cellular DNA. This is similar to that seen in these cell lines with respect to sensitivity to UV irradiation and repair of UV dimers (Bohr et al,1988; Hoeijmakers 1987; van Duin et al,1986; and Westerveld et al,1984). In RNA isolated from the leukocytes of six patients, ERCC1 is expressed to variable degrees, and in one patient, enhanced expression was seen after receiving three cycles of carboplatin and rGM-CSF therapy. This enhanced expression of ERCC1 was associated with the development of clinical resistance to carboplatin. These data suggest that ERCC1 should be investigated further with respect to a possible causal association with platinum drug resistance in human malignancies.

Clinical studies of platinum-DNA adduct formation also suggest that DNA repair may be important in clinical resis-

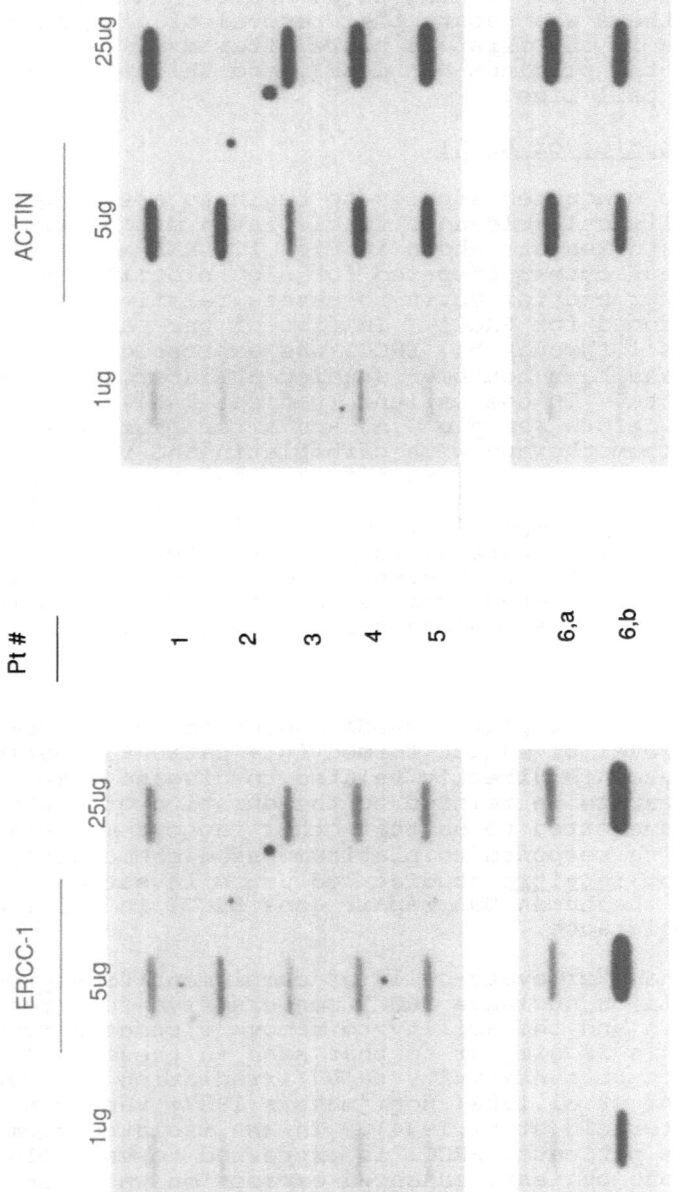

Fig. 1. Slot blot analyses of RNA (not polyA selected) from leukocytes of six ovarian cancer patients treated with carboplatin and rGM-CSF. The left part of the figure is the probe for ERCC1; the right part of the figure is the probe for actin. Patients 1 through 5 were assessed only once for gene expression. Patient 6 was assessed before (6,a) and after (6,b) three cycles of chemotherapy.

tance to cisplatin. When the kinetics of adduct formation was studied in patients with testicular and ovarian cancer, it was observed that cisplatin-DNA adduct accumulated in blood cell DNA of some patients with sequential monthly cycles of therapy, suggesting that adduct persisted on cellular DNA in some individuals for more than 28 days and contributed to total DNA adduct level (Reed et al,1986). Since DNA adduct level is directly related to disease response in these two diseases (Reed et al,1988a; and Reed et al,1987), this suggests that the relative ability to repair cisplatin-DNA lesions may be inversely related to adduct level and therefore, disease response. The fact that one patient in the current study revealed increased levels of expression of ERCC1 after three cycles of carboplatin and rGM-CSF therapy, and concurrently experienced clinical resistance to this treatment, supports the contention that DNA repair capability may influence disease response to chemotherapy.

In studies attempting to define what genes may be operative in conferring resistance to cisplatin, several genes associated with the DNA repair process have been reported to show enhanced expression in vitro. Kraker and Moore (1988) have shown increases in DNA polymerase beta in P388 murine leukemia cell lines. Scanlon and colleagues have shown increases in expression of thymidylate synthase and dihydrofolate reductase in human ovarian cancer cells resistant to cisplatin (Lu et al,1988; and Scanlon et al,1988).

ERCC1 is a human excision repair gene that confers resistance to cisplatin in UV repair deficient CHO cells of complementation group 1. Data presented also suggests that ERCC1 may play a role in cisplatin drug resistance in clinical settings. The study of the evolution of cisplatin drug resistance in human cancer tissue is limited by the inability to obtain repeated biopsies of an internal tumor mass. It is now clear that peripheral blood leukocytes can provide valuable information regarding clinical resistance to cisplatin, and may help establish the role(s) of selected genes in the evolution of platinum drug resistance.

REFERENCES

Bohr, V.A., Chu, E.H.Y., van Duin, M., Hanawalt, P.C., and Okumoto, D.S., 1988, Human repair gene restores normal pattern of preferential DNA repair in repair defective CHO cells, Nucleic Acids Res, 16:7397.

Conover, W.J., 1980, "Practical Non-Parametric Statistics," 2nd ed. Johns Wiley and Sons, New York.

Davis, L.G., Dibner, M.D., and Battey, J.F., 1986, "Basic Methods in Molecular Biology," Elsevier, New York.

Fairchild, C.R., Ivy, S.P., Rushmore, T., Lee, G., Koop, Goldsmith, M.E., Myers, C.E., Farber, E., and Cowan, K.H., 1987, Carcinogen induced mdr expression is associated with xenobiotic resistance in rat preneoplastic liver nodules and hepatocellular carcinomas. Proc. Natl. Acad. Sci. USA, 84:7701.

Flamm, W.H., Birnsteil, M.L., and Walter, P.M.B., 1969, in:
"Subcellular Components: Preparation and Fractiona-
tion," G. Birnie and S.M. Fox, eds, Butterworth and
Co., Ltd., London.

Hoeijmakers, J.H.J., 1987, Characterization of genes and
proteins involved in excision repair of human cells,
J Cell Sci (Suppl 6), 111.

Kraker, A.J., and Moore, C.W., 1988, Elevated DNA
polymerase beta activity in a cis-diamminedichloro-
platinum(II) resistant P388 murine leukemia cell line,
Cancer Letters, 38:307.

Lu, Y., Han, J., and Scanlon, K.J., 1988, Biochemical and
molecular properties of cisplatin-resistant A2780
cells grown in folinic acid, J Biol Chem, 263:4891.

Ozols, R.F., Ostchega, Y., Myers C.E., and Young, R.C.,
1985, High dose cisplatin in hypertonic saline in
refractory ovarian cancer patients, J Clin Oncol,
3:1246.

Ozols, R.F., Ostchega, Y., Curt, G.A., and Young, R.C.,
1987, High dose carboplatin in refractory ovarian
cancer patients, J Clin Oncol, 5:197.

Reed, E., 1989, Cisplatin. in "Cancer Chemotherapy and Biolog-
ical Response Modifiers Annual - Volume 11," H.M.
Pinedo, B.A Chabner, and D.L. Longo, eds, Elsevier
Science Publishers B.V., Amsterdam, in press.

Reed, E., Yuspa, S.H., Zwelling, L.A., Ozols, R.F., and
Poirier, M.C., 1986, Quantitation of cisplatin-DNA
intrastrand adducts in testicular and ovarian cancer
patients receiving cisplatin chemotherapy, J. Clin.
Invest., 77:545.

Reed, E., Ozols, R.F., Tarone, R., Yuspa, S.H., Poirier,
M.C., 1987, Platinum-DNA adducts in leukocyte DNA
correlate with disease response in ovarian cancer
patients receiving platinum-based chemotherapy, Proc.
Natl. Acad. Sci. USA, 84:5024.

Reed, E., Ozols, R.F., Tarone, R., Yuspa, S.H., Poirier,
M.C., 1988a, The measurement of cisplatin-DNA adduct
levels in testicular cancer patients, Carcinogenesis,
9:1909.

Reed, E., Sauerhoff, S., and Poirier, M.C., 1988b,
Quantitation of platinum-DNA binding in human tissues
following therapeutic levels of drug exposure -- A
novel use of graphite furnace spectrometry, Atomic
Spectroscopy, 9:93.

Reed, E., Poirier, M.C., Young, R.C., Ozols, R.F., 1988c,
High dose cisplatin in hypertonic saline: Toxicity
versus therapeutic benefit. in: "Organ Directed
Toxicities of Anti-Cancer Drugs," H.P. Hacker,
J.S. Lazo, and T.R. Tritton, eds., Martinus Nijhoff
Publishers, Boston.

260

Scanlon, K.J., and Kashani-Sabet, M., 1988, Elevated
    expression of thymidylate synthase cycle genes in
    cisplatin-resistant human ovarian carcinoma A2780
    cells, Proc Natl Acad Sci USA, 85:650.

Van Duin, M., de Wit, J., Odijk, H., Westerveld, A., Yasui,
    A., Koken, M.H.M., Hoeijmakers, J.H.J., and Bootsma,
    D., 1986, Molecular characterization of the human
    excision repair gene ERCC-1: cDNA cloning and amino
    acid homology with the yeast DNA repair gene RAD10,
    Cell, 44:913.

Westerveld, A., Hoeijmakers, J.H.J., van Duin, M., de Wit,
    J., Odijk, H., Pastink, A., Wood, R.D., and Bootsma,
    D., 1984, Molecular cloning of a human DNA repair
    gene, Nature, 310:425.

FACTORS WHICH AFFECT DNA REPAIR IN HUMAN LYMPHOCYTES

L. L. Larcom, M. E. Smith and T. E. Morris

Departments of Microbiology and of Physics and Astronomy
Clemson University,
Clemson, SC 29634-1911

INTRODUCTION

The realization that for most cancers the initiating event is a somatic mutation led naturally to the hypothesis that susceptibility to cancer could be inversely correlated with the ability to repair genetic damage. This possibility is supported by the observation that for some types of cancer susceptibility seems to be inherited. To evaluate such a hypothesis, it is necessary to have available a technique for measuring in vivo repair capacity in humans. It has been demonstrated clearly that carcinogenesis is a multistage phenomenon, and that the possibility of developing a neoplasm depends not only on exposure to a physical or chemical carcinogen, but also on physiological and metabolic parameters characteristic of each individual. Hormone levels, various components of the diet, and psychological stress are factors for which correlations with tumor development have been shown; but which are not DNA damaging agents. The complexity of the carcinogenic process and the extremely large number of parameters which could influence its progression make elucidation of this process by in vitro systems extremely difficult. The mechanisms of genetic damage by particular carcinogens and cellular repair responses to this damage can be elucidated with in vitro cell culture (Sutherland et al., 1980). However, factors which affect the amount of damage produced by a particular carcinogen and the efficiency with which this damage is repaired in a particular individual cannot be determined with standard in vitro methods or by studying isolated cells. Our aim is to determine how serum factors can influence the repair of DNA damage and the extent to which these factors vary from one individual to another. The ultimate goal is to design an in vitro system which will mimic as closely as possible the in vivo genetic repair responses of individuals. Such a system could be used to evaluate the hypothesis that efficient DNA repair capacity protects an organism from cancer.

Lymphocytes are an excellent cell type to use for such studies for several reasons:
1) These cells can be isolated and subjected to damage within an hour after they have been removed from the donor. This avoids changes which routinely occur when cells are cultured for several generations in artifical medium.

DNA Damage and Repair in Human Tissues
Edited by B. M. Sutherland and A. D. Woodhead
Plenum Press, New York, 1990

2) They can be cultured in their autologous plasma during the
assay. This contains the complement of hormones, growth factors and
biological response modifiers (BRM's) characteristic of the individual
being tested. It is not possible to mimic the effects of these factors
by performing assays in animal sera, pooled human serum, or serum-free
medium.
3) Lymphocytes can be cultured in liquid suspension. This avoids
artifacts which can result from attachment to an artificial substrate.
4) Over 98% of peripheral blood lymphocytes (PBL's) are in G_0 phase
(Connor and Norman, 1971; Pero and Ostlund, 1980).
5) They can be stimulated to divide with an antigen or lectin,
allowing one also to study DNA replication and how it is affected by
environmental changes (Maluish and Strong, 1986).

We have used PBL's to determine whether serum factors can affect
cellular responses to mutagenic damage or mitogenic stimulation and to
evaluate the effects of environmental changes on genetic repair and
immunocompetence.

METHODS

Experimental Methods

DNA Repair. Lymphocytes were isolated from approximately 14 ml of
peripheral blood anticoagulated with heparin. Whole blood was layered
over polysucrose-sodium diatriazoate gradients. These were centrifuged at 400 g or 30 min. The top layer consisted of undiluted plasma.
This was collected and saved to supplement the culture medium. The cells
were collected, washed, centrifuged, and resuspended in phosphate-
buffered saline (PBS). They were then adjusted to a concentration of
$2x10^6$/ml and divided into aliquots. Each aliquot was subjected to a
different fluence of UVC radiation from a GE 15T8 germicidal lamp having
a sharp maximum in intensity at 254 nm. The cells from each aliquot were
centrifuged and resuspended in RPMI 1640 culture medium containing 15%
serum. Hydroxyurea was added to a final concentration of 4mM to shut
down replicative synthesis in the small fraction of cells not in G_0
phase. Tritium-labeled thymidine was added to a concentration of $5\mu Ci$/ml
and the aliquots were incubated for 4 h at 37°C in an atmosphere of 5%
CO_2. The cells were then lysed and the DNA was collected on nitrocellulose filters (Smith et al., 1985). The amount of radioactivity incorporated into the DNA of each aliquot was measured by scintillation
analysis. A typical dose-response curve is given in Fig 1.

Lymphocyte Proliferation. The cells were isolated as described
above and suspended in RPMI culture medium supplemented with 15% serum.
The cell concentration was adjusted to 2×10^6/ml and phytohemagglutinin
(PHA) was added to a concentration of 7.5 μg/ml. Cultures were incubated
at 37°C in an atmosphere of 5% CO_2 for 48 h. The cells were then
collected by centrifugation and resuspended in medium supplemented with
15% serum, but without PHA. Radioactive dThd was added to a concentration of $5\mu Ci$/ml and the samples were incubated an additional 4h. The
cells were lysed and the amount of radioactivity incorporated
into the DNA was determined (Larcom and Smith, 1988).

Analysis

The Early Assay. In the first experiments, the measure of the
amount of repair performed was the amount of radioactivity incorporated
at saturating UV fluences. This assay is complicated by two factors:

i) Different sera contain different amounts of endogenous dThd which will compete with the radioactive label.

ii) Lymphocytes produce thymidine phosphorylase which will degrade the ^{3}H-dThd and prevent its incorporation into newly synthesized DNA or repair patches (Bodycote and Wolff, 1986). Both endogenous dThd concentrations and thymidine phosphorylase activities differ from sample to sample. Therefore, to accurately compare the DNA repair capacities or mitogenic potentials of cells from different individuals (or of the same individual at different times) it is necessary to remove these effects.

The Revised Assay. We assumed that the incorporation of ^{3}H-dThd into DNA can be described by the Michaelis-Menten formalism with dThd as a substrate. The results of Connor and Norman (1971) indicate that this is a good approximation for DNA repair. Our results support the assumption for the DNA repair and cell proliferation assays. The Michaelis-Menten expression for such a process is:

$$\frac{1}{C} = m\,\frac{1}{T} + b \qquad (1)$$

where C is the number of moles of dThd incorporated and T is the total concentration of dThd. The intercept b is the reciprocal of the maximum number of moles of dThd that could be incorporated into the DNA during a fixed incubation period.   This is the parameter which should be used to

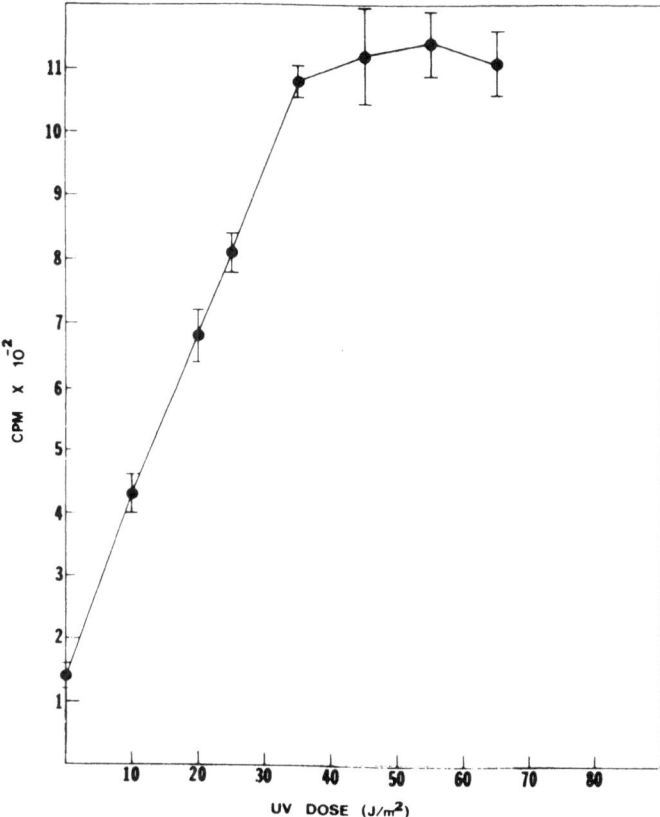

Fig 1.   Dose-response curve for unscheduled DNA synthesis in lymphocytes irradiated with UVC and cultured in 15% FBS.

265

characterize the DNA repair capacity or the proliferative capacity of the cells. The total concentration of dThd in the medium is not known. However, if a culture of cells is divided into several aliquots and a different amount of non-radioactive dThd is added to each, the parameter b can be determined. If μ is the ratio of the concentration of unlabeled-to-labeled dThd added in a particular aliquot and σ is the ratio of the concentration of endogenous dThd in the serum (an unknown quantity) to the concentration of ^{3}H-dThd, equation (1) can be transformed to (Larcom and Smith, 1988):

$$\frac{1}{C*} = \frac{M}{T*} + b(1 + \mu) + b\sigma \qquad (2)$$

Here C^* is the amount of radioactively-labeled dThd incorporated during a fixed incubation time and T^* is the concentration of <u>labeled</u> dThd - a known value. A plot of $1/C^*$ versus $(\mu+1)$ should be linear with slope b.

In the lymphocyte proliferation assay, each culture was divided into six aliquots and the same amount of ^{3}H-dThd was added to each. A different amount of dThd was added to each aliquot so that the ratios of unlabeled-to-labeled dThd (μ of equation (2)) were 0,2,4,6,8 and 10. A plot of $1/C^*$ versus μ is given in Fig 2. The slope of the line is b. The reciprocal of b is the maximum amount of label which could be

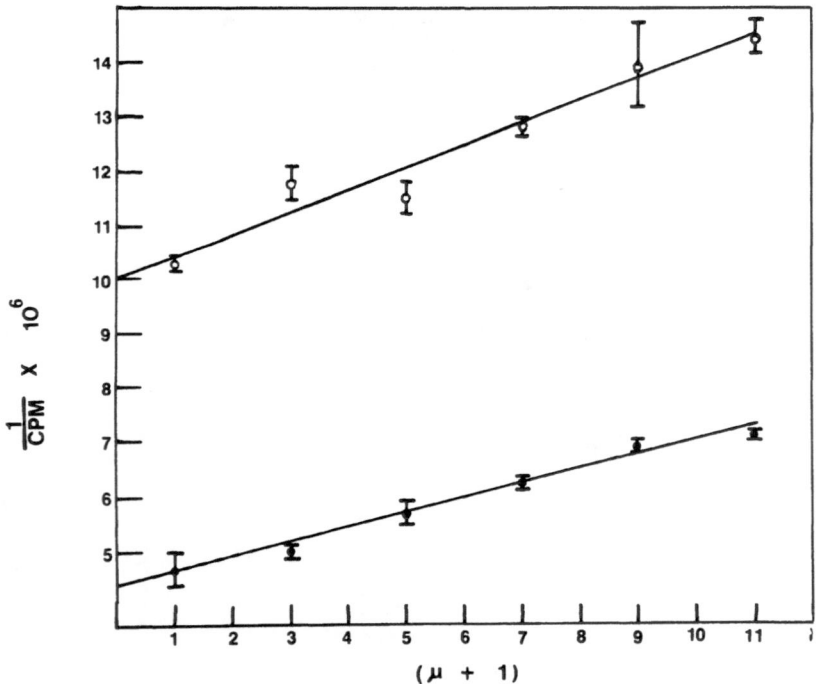

Fig 2. Incorporation of dThd as a function of dThd concentration for lymphocytes stimulated with PHA in medium containing 15% FBS (top line) or 15% autologous plasma (bottom line).

incorporated in the absence of competing serum dThd and of degradation of the label by phosphorylases. We designate this C_m.

To measure DNA repair, it is necessary to consider two substrates-dThd and the lesions to be repaired. For each DNA sample exposed to a particular UV fluence, a plot of $1/C^*$ versus $(\mu+1)$ must be constructed. A family of such plots is given in Fig 3. For a sample exposed to a

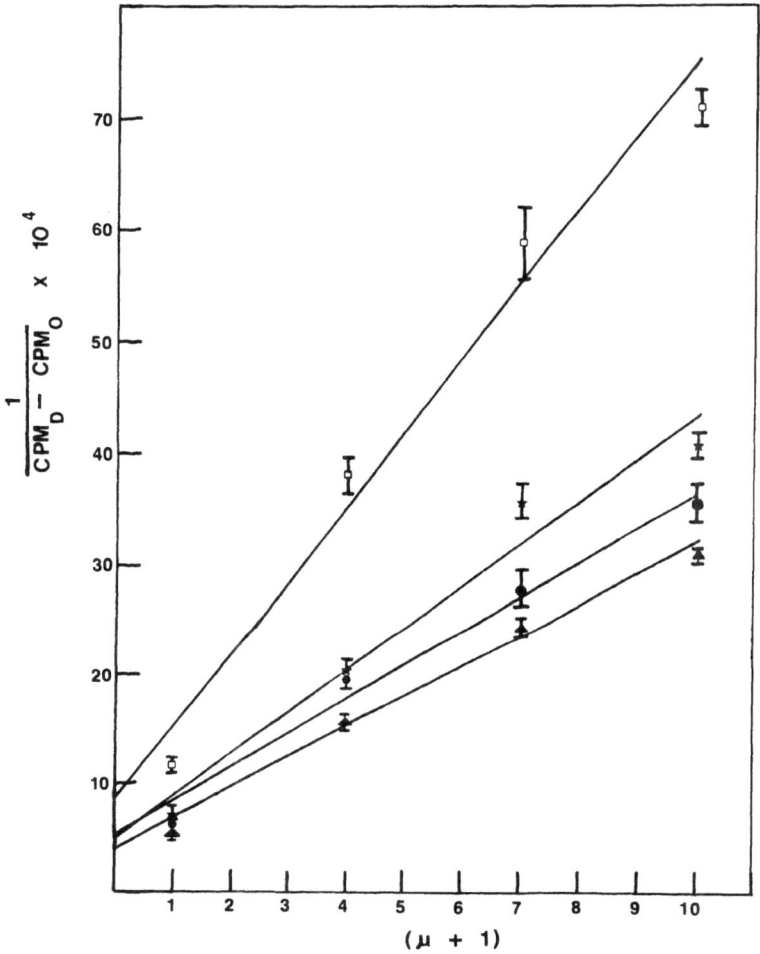

Fig 3. Incorporation of dThd by UVC-damaged resting lymphocytes as a function of dThd concentration. Each line represents cells irradiated with a different fluence: □,10; *,20; ●,30; ▲,40 J/m².

particular fluence, the slope of the line which best fits the data is b - the reciprocal of the maximum amount of ^{3}H-dThd which could be incorporated during UDS repair of DNA exposed to that particular fluence of UVC. If one assumes that the concentration of lesions in the DNA is proportional to the fluence, the DNA repair capacity can be determined by plotting these values of b versus the reciprocal of the UV fluence (Larcom and Smith, 1988). This plot is shown for the data of Fig 3 in Fig 4. The intercept is the reciprocal of the total amount of label which could be incorporated into the DNA at infinite dose in the absence of endogenous serum thymidine, and of thymidine degradation by cellular enzymes. We designate this C_m. It is the parameter which should be used to compare the repair capacities of different samples.

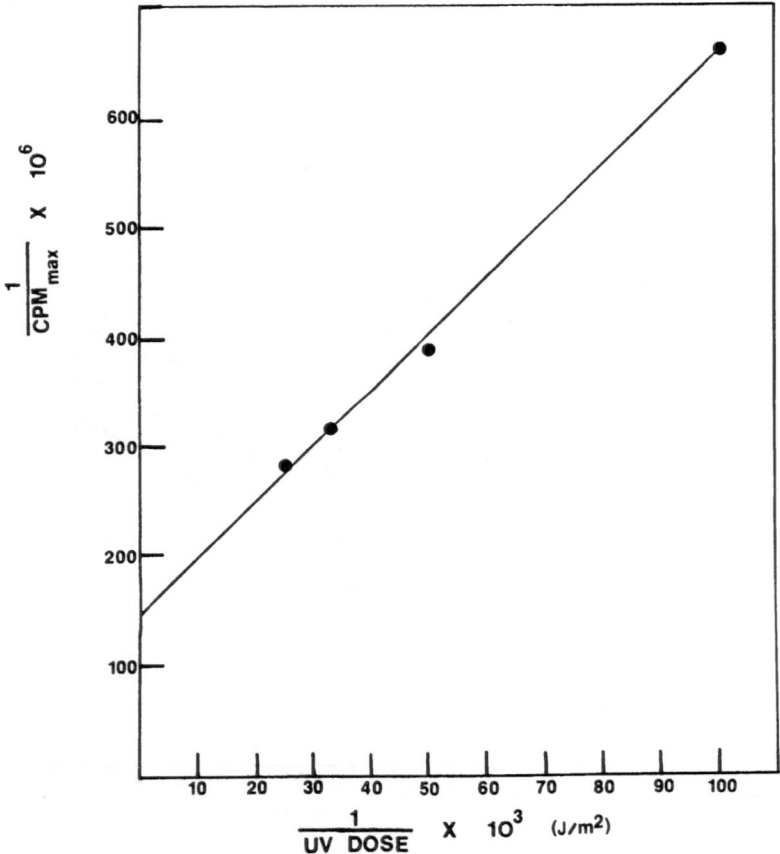

Fig 4. Maximum dThd incorporated corrected for endogenous serum dThd as a function of fluence.

RESULTS

Serum Effects

DNA Repair. To assess the possibility that serum factors might affect DNA repair capacity, UVC-damaged cells were allowed to perform repair in serum. The cells from a particular donor were irradiated in PBS and separated into three fractions, which were centrifuged. The cells from one fraction were resuspended in medium supplemented with 15% autologous plasma; those from the second, in medium supplemented with 15% FBS; and those from the third, in unsupplemented medium. These were allowed to perform UDS for 4 h and the amount of ^{3}H-dThd incorporated into the DNA was determined. In these experiments, the measure of the amount of repair performed was the cpm incorporated above background at saturating UV doses. UDS repair curves for cells from one donor are given in Fig 5. To minimize the effects of the complicating factors discussed above, the fractional increase in cpm over that incorporated by undamaged cells was calculated:

$$R = \frac{cpm_f - cpm_o}{cpm_o} \qquad (3)$$

where cpm_f is the cpm incorporated at fluence f and cpm_o is the cpm incorporated by undamaged cells. This ratio was used to characterize the repair capacity of cells in a particular environment and to compare the amounts of repair performed by cells in the three fractions.

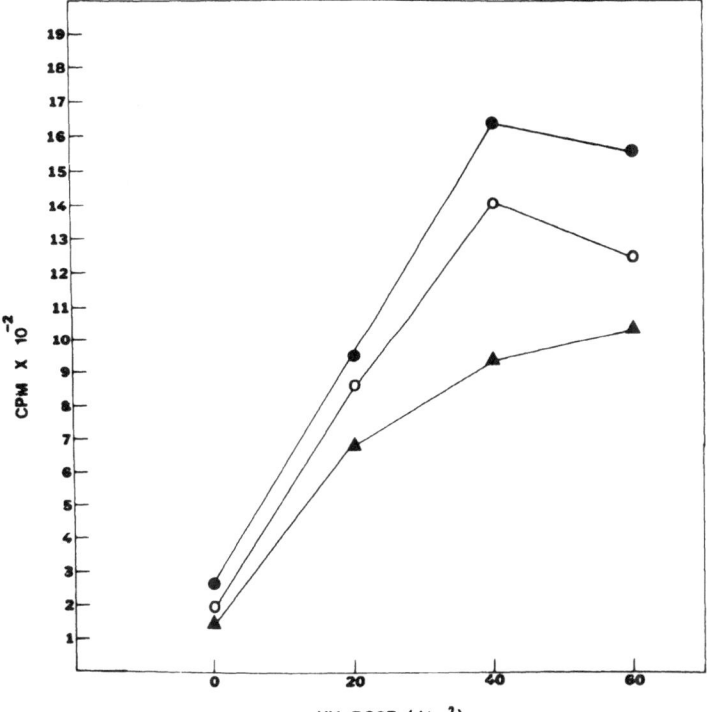

Fig 5. Dose-response curves for UVC-damaged cells
incubated in: (●), medium supplemented with
their autologous plasma; (o), unsupplemented
medium or (▲), medium supplemented with FBS.

Table 1. Average Repair Capacity for UVC-Damaged Lymphocytes from 10
Donors in Three Different Media.

Dose (J/m^2)	Medium	R[a]	FD[b] ($\times 10^3$)
20	Autologous plasma	5.5	170
	FBS	4.1	160
	No Serum	4.4	120
40	Autologous plasma	7.9	190
	FBS	5.7	150
	No Serum	6.0	150
60	Autologous plasma	8.7	200
	FBS	6.0	200
	No Serum	6.1	140

[a]See equation 13 in the text.
[b]FD is the fractional deviation, defined as the standard error of
the mean divided by the mean.

For every donor, the cells performed more repair in medium
supplemented with their autologous plasma than in the other two media.
The average R values for 10 donors are given in Table 1. For 70% of the
donors tested, the difference between the R values obtained in
autologous plasma and in FBS could be obtained by random experimental
error with a probability of only 0.01 or less (Smith et al., 1985).

Cell Proliferation. Serum used to supplement the culture medium
was also found to affect the proliferative capacity of human
lymphocytes. Freshly isolated PBL's were stimulated with PHA and
cultured for 48 h in RPMI 1640 medium supplemented with either 15%
autologous plasma or 15% FBS. The cells from each culture were then
collected, resuspended in the same medium and separated into aliquots
containing different ratios of unlabeled-to-labled dThd. Typical
results are given in Fig 2. For every donor studied, the lymphocyte
proliferation response was greater in autologous plasma than in FBS.
Results are given in Table 2. Cells cultured in autologous plasma
performed almost twice as much DNA synthesis as those cultured in FBS
(Larcom and Smith, 1988).

Variability Among Donors

DNA Repair. Before the revised assay had been devised, the
variability in repair capacity was measured among 19 individuals using
the parameter R as the measure of repair capacity. In both medium
supplemented with FBS and in unsupplemented medium, there was a large
variation in repair capacity among the samples studied (Fig 6). The
results are summarized in Table 3. The fractional deviation for cells
allowed to perform repair in FBS-supplemented medium was twice as great
as for those in unsupplemented medium. The range of R values for these
samples was much greater than for samples taken from the same individual
on four consecutive weeks, as indicated in Fig 7 (Smith et al.,
1985).

DNA repair capacities were measured for lymphocytes from eleven donors with the revised assay (Larcom and Smith, 1988). The cells were cultured in medium supplemented with their autologous plasma and assayed for repair capacity in aliquots containing different ratios of labeled-to-unlabeled dThd as indicated in Fig 3 and Fig 4. The results are given in Table 4. There was only 4% deviation among samples from the seven healthy donors. It is not yet clear whether this amount of variability is indicative of the healthy population as a whole, or resulted from the limited sample size. All of these donors were college students between 20 and 30 years of age. Earlier studies have reported much greater amounts of variability in repair capacity, but artifacts resulting from variations in dThd concentration, thymidine degradation and changes in the cells during _in vitro_ culturing probably contributed the results. The average value of C_m found for mononucleosis patients was only half as great as for healthy donors. Higher repair capacity during pregnancy remains to be verified.

Cell Proliferation. Values of C_m for PHA-stimulated cells from nine donors are given in Table 2 (Larcom and Smith, 1988). The values of C_m for donors 8 and 9 are much higher than for donors 1-7. Donor 9 was found to have mononucleosis. It is possible that donor 8 also had an unrecognized infection which caused lymphocyte stimulation. Therefore, mean C_m values were calculated for all samples and for samples from donors 1-7. When the first seven samples were used, the fractional deviation in C_m for cells cultured in FBS was found to be 6%. The FBS

Table 2. Lymphocyte proliferation.

Donor	Serum Autologous: $C_{m,A}(X\ 10^{-3})$	FBS: $C_{m,F}(X10^{-3})$	$C_{m,A}/C_{m,F}$ [a]
1	269	139	1.94
2	256	115	2.23
3	307	133	2.32
4	226	100	2.27
5	102	98	1.04
6	174	98	1.77
7	167	103	1.62
8	664	318	2.09
9 [b]	658	379	1.73
1-7 $C_m(X10^{-3})$ [c]	214 ± 27	112 ± 6	1.88 ± 0.17
FD [d]	0.120	0.058	0.092
1-9 $C_m(X10^{-3})$ [c]	314 ± 69	165 ± 35	1.89 ± 0.14
FD [d]	0.220	0.210	0.072

C_m in counts per minute per 10^6 cells as determined from a plot of $(C*)^{-1}$ vs. $(\mu+1)$. $C_{m,A}$ is C_m for cells stimulated in autogolous serum; $C_{m,F}$ is C_m for cells stimulated in FBS.

[a]Ratio of C_m measured in autologous serum to C_m measured in FBS.
[b]This donor had mononucleosis.
[c]Mean value of C_m ± standard error of mean.
[d]Standard error of mean divided by mean.

used in all of these experiments was from the same bottle. Therefore, any variation found for cells cultured in the FBS-supplemented medium should represent variability in the cells themselves. The fractional deviation for cells cultured in their autologous plasma was found to be twice as great as when those same cells were cultured in FBS. This additional variability must have resulted from differences in serum factors from one individual to another. This finding adds further support to the hypothesis that serum factors can have a significant effect on cellular responses, in this case mitogen-induced proliferation.

NUV Irradiation. The effects of in vivo NUV exposure on DNA repair capacity and cell proliferation were examined with the assays described above. College students intending to tan in commercial tanning salons were asked to donate blood immediately before tanning and again 24 h afterwards. For every subject studied, tanning caused a decrease in repair of UVC-induced lesions (Smith, 1987).

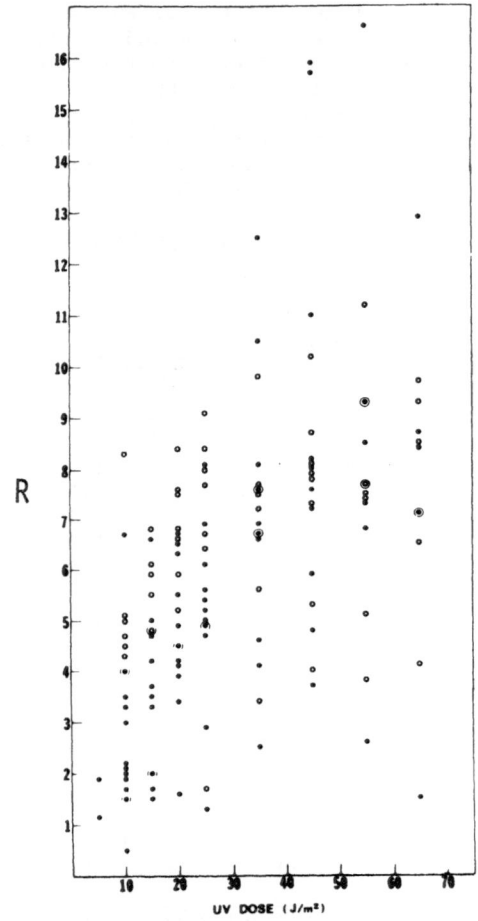

Fig 6. DNA repair synthesis in UVC-irradiated lympho-cytes allowed to perform repair in medium supple-mented with FBS (●, 12 donors) or unsupplemented medium (o, 7 donors).

272

Table 3. Average Repair Capacity and Variability in Repair Capacity for
UVC-Damaged Human Lymphocytes.

Dose (J/m^2)	Medium			
	RPMI + FBS		RPMI - No Serum	
	R	FD(X10^3)	R	FD(X10^3)
45	8.8	151	7.9	71
55	8.5	219	8.0	89
65	7.7	237	7.8	121

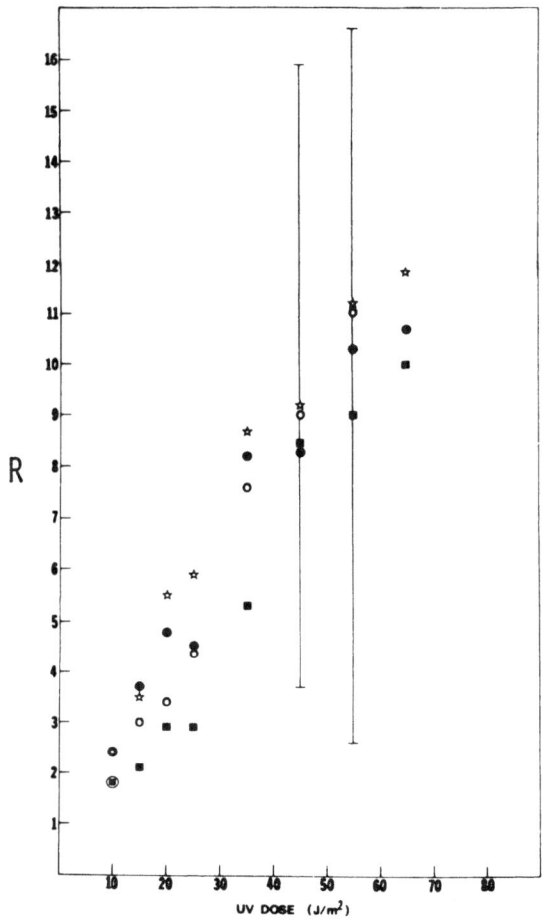

R

Fig 7. DNA repair synthesis in
irradiated lymphocytes collected
from the same individual on 4
consecutive weeks and allowed to
perform repair in FBS-supplemented
medium. Bars represent the range
of repair values for different
individuals from Fig 6.

Table 4. Repair of UV Radiation Damage.

Donor	$C_m^*(\times 10^{-3})$
1	12.3
2	11.2
3	13.2
4	13.6
5	15.0
6	12.9
7	10.0
8[a]	5.3
9[a]	6.9
10[a]	6.1
11[b]	24.3

Condition of donor	No.[c]	$C_m{'}^d(\times 10^{-3})$	Fractional deviation[e]
Healthy	7	13.0 ± 0.5	0.04
Mononucleosis	3	6.1 ± 0.4	0.07
Pregnant	1	4.3	--

[*] $C_m{'}$ in counts per minute per 10^6 cells as determined from a plot of $(C_m)^{-1}$ vs. D^{-1}.

[a]This donor had mononucleosis.
[b]This donor was pregnant.
[c]No. of donors in each category.
[d]Mean value of $C_m{'}$ (in counts per minute) ± standard error of mean.
[e]Standard error of mean divided by mean.

Likewise, for every subject studied, the amount of PHA-induced proliferation performed by cells collected 24 h after tanning was significantly lower than that performed by cells drawn before the donor
was exposed to NUV (Morris, 1989). The results are given in Table 5
(Larcom et al., 1989). Two different tanning salons were used. These
differed in the amount of UVB emitted, but we were unable to obtain
detailed emission spectra for the lamps used. Tanning system 1 had a
significantly greater effect than system 2 on DNA repair capacity and a
somewhat larger effect on proliferation. System 1 is reported to have a
higher fraction of its total emission in the UVB range (Gies et al.,
1986).

DISCUSSION

In human cells, serum factors have significant effects on both DNA
repair capacity and the ability to perform mitogen-stimulated DNA
synthesis. Therefore, to determine the DNA repair capacity of a
particular individual, the assay should be performed in autologous
plasma. Only this contains the complement of biological response
modifiers specific to that individual. A revised assay was used to
remove artifacts which complicate the previously used unscheduled DNA
synthesis assay. The variability observed with this revised assay was
much smaller than that obtained with the earlier assay. It remains to be
determined whether this was because the sample size was small and
composed of only college students. Using the revised assay, it was

Table 5. Suppression of DNA Repair and Cell Proliferation By NUV.

Tanning System	DNA Repair % Suppression	Range	No. Samples	Proliferation % Suppression	Range	No. Samples
1	39	23-56	7	48	24-68	4
2	10	8-11	5	30	8-58	5

demonstrated that exposure in NUV tanning salons produces suppression of DNA repair capacity and of DNA synthesis in response to mitogen stimulation. The latter effect is indicative of decreased immunocompetence. The suppression of natural killer cell activity by exposure in tanning salons has also been observed by Hersey et al., (1983, 1988).

ACKNOWLEDGEMENT

We thank Elsevier Scientific Publishers Ireland, Ltd. for permission to reproduce Fig 1, Fig 5, Fig 6, and Fig 7 from Chemico-Biological Interactions.

REFERENCES

Bodycote, J., and Wolff, S., 1986, Metabolic breakdown of ^{3}H-thymidine and the inability to measure lymphocyte proliferation by incorporation of radioactivity, Proc. Natl. Acad. Sci. USA, 83: 4749.

Conner, W. G. and Norman, A., 1971, Unscheduled DNA synthesis in human leukocytes, Mutat. Res., 13: 393.

Gies, H. P., Roy, C. R., and Elliott, G., 1986, Artificial suntanning: Spectral irradiance and hazard evaluation of ultraviolet sources, Health Physics, 50:691.

Hersey, P., Hasic, E., Edwards, A., Bradley, M., Harhan, G. and M[c]Carthy, W. H., 1983, Immunological effects of solarium exposure, Lancet, 1: 545.

Hersey, P., M[c]Donald, M., Henderson, C., Schibeci, S., D' Alessandro, G., Pryor, M. and Wilkinson, F. J., 1988, Suppression of natural killer cell activity in humans by radiation from solarium lamps depleted of UVB, J. Invest. Dermatol., 90: 305.

Larcom, L. L. and Smith, M. E., 1988, Quantitative assay for evaluating immunocompetence and DNA repair capacity, J. Natl. Cancer Inst., 80: 1112.

Larcom, L. L., Morris, T. and Smith, M. E., 1989, Suppression of DNA repair and immunocompetence by exposure in commercial tanning salons, Photochem. Photobiol., 49: 24S.

Maluish, A. E. and Strong, D. M., 1986, Lymphocyte proliferation, in "Manual of Clinical Immunology," N. R. Rose, H. Friedman and J. L. Fahey, eds., Am. Soc. Microbiol., Washington, DC.

Morris, T. E., 1989, "Changes in Immunocompetence Levels of Individuals Exposed in Tanning Beds and of Cancer Patients Undergoing Therapy," Ph.D. Dissertation, Clemson University, Clemson, SC.

Pero, R. W. and Ostlund, C., 1980, Direct comparison, in human lymphocytes, of the inter-individual variations in unscheduled DNA synthesis induced by N-acetoxy-2-acetyl-aminofluorene and ultraviolet radiation, Mutat. Res., 73:349.

Smith, M. E., 1987, "The Effects of Serum on DNA Repair and Replication: Development of a Quantitative Thymidine Incorporation Assay for Inter-Individual Comparisons of Immunocompetence and DNA Repair Capacity," Ph.D. Dissertation, Clemson University, Clemson, SC.

Smith, M. E., Larcom, L. L., and Freeman, S. E., 1985, Serum effects on DNA repair in human cells, Chem.-Biol. Interactions, 54: 325.

Sutherland, B. M. Cimino, J. S. and Delihas, N., 1980, Ultraviolet light-induced transformation of human cells to anchorage-independent growth, Cancer Res., 40: 1934.

METHYL TRANSFERASE ACTIVITY IN SECONDARY LEUKEMIA

Bernard Strauss, Daphna Sagher, Theodore Karrison,
Jeffrey Schwartz, Richard Larson, and Stephanie Williams

Departments of Molecular Genetics and Cell Biology,
Medicine and Radiation and Cellular Oncology, The
University of Chicago, Chicago, IL 60637

During a typical course of treatment for Hodgkin's disease or non-Hodgkin's lymphoma with MOPP, individuals receive approximately 1400 mg/m^2 of procarbazine over a period of 14 days (DeVita et al., 1970). Procarbazine is metabolized and one of its products is a methylating ion which produces O-alkylation products including O^6-methylguanine (Wiestler et al., 1984). Most organisms have a protein which removes O^6-methylguanine in a stoichiometric manner (Samson and Cairns, 1977; Pegg, 1983). In bacteria, this protein is adaptive so that exposure to methylating agents increases the amount of O^6-alkylguanine DNA alkyltransferase (AGT) over a hundred-fold in less than a cell generation (Lindahl and Sedgwick, 1988). It is still not clear whether the formation of protein responds adaptively to methylation damage in mammals. In rats there does seem to be a non-specific response of AGT production to damage (Pegg, 1983). If there is such an effect in humans, the effect is not rapid. As with other repair processes, the AGT content of peripheral blood lymphocytes (PBLs) from individuals varies (Waldstein et al., 1982; Sagher et al., 1988). If this variation were idiosyncratic and persisted, then individual response to procarbazine might be an etiologic factor in the development of secondary cancer. One might suppose, for example, that methylation lesions remained unrepaired in individuals with low AGT activity and that, as a result, mutations leading to secondary malignancy occurred during cell replication.

Therefore, we decided to test this hypothesis, insofar as possible in the absence of long-term prospective studies. Our plan was to establish that AGT level was indeed idiosyncratic, to assay AGT activity in individuals with Hodgkin's disease (HD) and non-Hodgkin's lymphoma (NHL) before, during, and after treatment, and to assay the AGT activity in individuals with acute myeloid leukemia (AML) both de novo and in those AML patients with a history of therapy for prior malignancy (t-AML). At the time we assumed that AML is a single disease, so that de novo AML values are controls for the t-AML series. We decided to assay AGT activity in PBLs because of the availability of these cells. The activity in PBLs has been shown to be higher but proportional to that of the myeloid precursors in bone marrow, the stem cells which, presumably, suffer the mutagenic damage (Gerson et al., 1985). We supposed that the level of AGT in PBLs reflects that of the target cells.

DNA Damage and Repair in Human Tissues
Edited by B. M. Sutherland and A. D. Woodhead
Plenum Press, New York, 1990

277

Our assay for AGT activity measures the transfer of radioactivity in the methyl group (CH_3) of O^6-methylguanine from (hot acid soluble) nucleic acid to (hot acid insoluble) protein (Myrnes et al., 1984). Cell extracts were made and stored in liquid N_2 for assay. We carried out a series of experiments to determine the reliability of the assay, and the variability of the activity among individuals and within the same individual on repeated samplings. The assay itself is stable and repeatable; aliquots of the same sample analyzed at different times gave values with an intra-assay coefficient of variation of about 10%.

We followed the AGT activity in blood from five individuals over about a year. The values of samples drawn three times during one week showed little intra-individual variability (14% of the contribution to the total variation), whereas differences between individuals contributed 73% to the total variance. When these five individuals were followed over eight months, with some individuals followed for a year (Fig. 1), there was increased intra-individual variability but the interindividual variability was still the dominant factor. An estimate of the components of variability showed 64% was due to the variation between subjects, 25% due to the variation between repeated samples from the same subject, and 12% due to the variation between different aliquots of the same sample. We conclude that there is a characteristic individual value for AGT activity.

We analyzed PBLs from 181 individuals in six groups (Table 1; Fig. 2): 1. AML de novo. Lymphocytes are taken from patients with less than 10% blasts in the circulating blood; 2. Therapy-related AML; 3. Previously untreated Hodgkin's patients (HD); previously untreated non-Hodgkin's lymphoma (NHL); 4. HD, NHL patients receiving therapy: P, receiving MOPP and/or ABVD; R, receiving radiotherapy; O, receiving other chemotherapy; 5. HD, NHL patients in remission, > 3 months off therapy; and 6. Normal controls (Sagher et al., 1988).

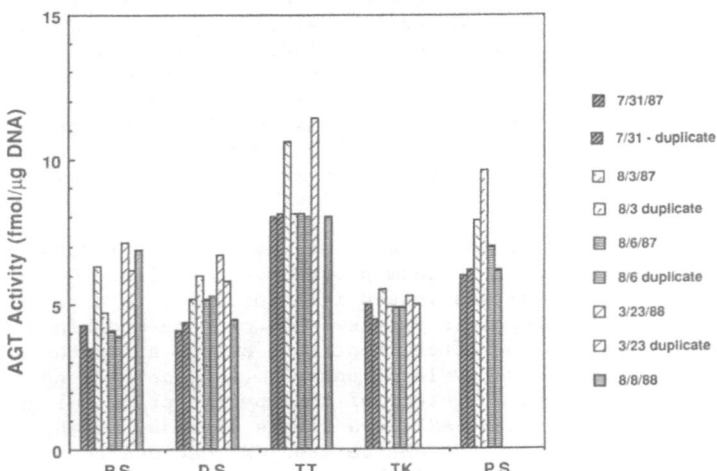

Fig. 1.   AGT activity in the PBLs of individuals assayed several times over the course of a year. Duplicate, blinded assays are given the same symbols. (Taken from Sagher et al., 1989 with permission.)

Table 1. O^6-Alkylguanine DNA Alkyltransferase in PBLs

	Group	N	Mean	±S.E.
(1)	A-AML de novo	6	7.78	1.72
	B-AML in remission	12*	6.90	1.07
(2)	A-t-AML	11	4.30	0.58
	B-t-AML in remission	2	4.35	2.45
(3)	HD/NHL Untreated	25	4.97	0.42
	HD "	14	5.59	0.53
	NHL "	11	4.19	0.61
(4)	HD/NHL - P	17	3.88	0.44
	HD - P	14	4.03	0.52
	NHL - P	3	3.13	0.58
	HD - R	5	4.40	1.07
	HD/NHL - O	26	5.65	0.72
	HD - O	11	6.09	1.08
	NHL - O	15	5.33	0.99
(5)	HD/NHL in remission	75	5.51	0.33
	HD "	51	5.97	0.40
	NHL "	24	4.53	0.56
(6)	Controls	34	7.05	0.36

Values for each individual were first averaged over all samples taken.
N is the number of individuals whose average value was used to calculate
the group mean.
*One outlying value of 29.9 excluded (see Fig. 2). If this value is
included, the mean and SE increase to 8.67 ± 2.02 (Sagher et al., 1988).

The mean AGT activity of PBLs in each of the HD-NHL patient groups
3, 4P, and 5 was significantly lower ($P<0.05$) than that from normal
individuals (Table 1, Fig. 2). Patients treated with regimens including
procarbazine or dacarbazine had the lowest activity, although the mean
value was not significantly different from that measured for HD-NHL patients treated with other agents. The means for the AML de novo patients
were not significantly different from the control mean. However, the mean
value for the AML de novo patients (pooled 1A + 1B) was significantly
different from the mean value for the t-AML patients [7.19 ± 0.89 versus
4.38 ± 0.53, P = 0.012 by two-sample t test] as would be expected by the
hypothesis. The de novo AML data suggest that low AGT activity is not
a general effect of ill health nor a consequence of a myeloid leukemia.

We eliminated age, sex, alcohol use, and smoking differences as an
explanation of our observations. B lymphocytes have about 70% of the AGT
activity of T lymphocytes (Gerson et al., 1985) and it might be supposed
that the observed differences between HD and NHL patients and normal controls are related to their distribution of B and T cells. However, the
percent of peripheral blood B lymphocytes in normal, NHL, HD, and HD

in remission is reported as 10.8, 15.5, 11.2, and 15.7 respectively (Herrmann et al., 1983) which is not sufficient variation to account for the differences we observed.

We originally supposed that treatment with procarbazine would result in considerable reduction in AGT activity. In fact, our analyses of a group of patients throughout several cycles of treatment failed to demonstrate a drastic effect on AGT levels either by analysis of group means (Table 1), or by sequential analysis of PBLs from individual patients. In some patients we saw a pattern of random increases and declines, not unlike the pattern seen in normal subjects (Fig. 1). In other patients we saw a more dramatic decline, but only after several courses of treatment (Fig. 3). We do not think the lack of a drastic lowering is due to the rapid regeneration of AGT, since resting lymphocytes do not appear to restore such activity even after extended periods. However, it can be calculated on the basis of the data of Wiestler et al. (1984) that at the dose of procarbazine administered during a single course of therapy only about 5,000 O^6-MeG residues per cell should be produced. According to our measurements, each average PBL [AGT level 6 fmol/μg DNA] should have about 20,000 AGT molecules so that, at most, one should expect a 25% lowering during one course of treatment of individuals with average AGT levels.

As part of a study on the etiology of secondary leukemia we had the opportunity to develop Epstein Barr virus transformed lymphoblastoid cell lines (LCLs) from patients and normal individuals. We analyzed these lines for AGT activity and compared the values with those of the lymphocytes from which they were derived. The samples analyzed belong to four of the groups reported above (Table 1: Groups 3, 4, 5 and 6). We correlated AGT activity in the PBLs with the first line derived from each

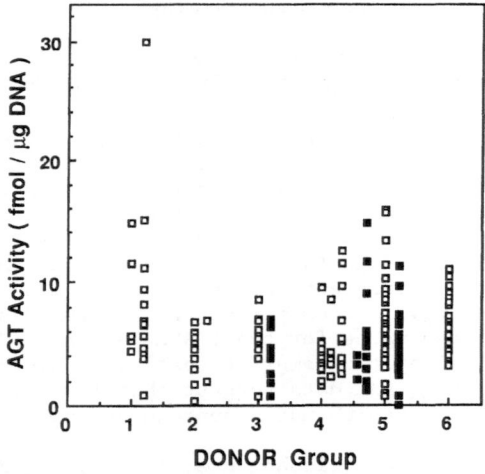

Fig. 2. Group designations as in Table 1. In groups 1 and 2, the left column indicates patients at diagnosis and the right column, patients in remission. In groups 3, 4, and 5, open squares are HD, closed squares are NHL. Group 4 (HD) includes patients receiving procarbazine (left), radiation (center), and other treatment (right). The outlying value at 29.9 fmol/μg was excluded from the calculations in Table 1 (Sagher et al., 1988).

Table 2. Correlation of AGT Activity in PBLs and in Lymphoblastoid Lines

Group	Description	n	r	p value
3	HD/NHL untreated	12	0.407	0.190
4P	HD/NHL treated procarb.	16	-0.225	0.403
4	HD/NHL treated all sets[a]	26	0.281	0.164
5	HD/NHL remission	50	0.270	0.058
6	CONTROL subjects	24	0.742	<0.001

[a]Includes individuals treated with radiation or other chemotherapeutic agents in addition to those treated with a regimen including procarbazine.

Note: The sum of the individuals listed in this table does not equal the total number of individuals enrolled in this study since only individuals for whom AGT values are available in both PBLs and lines are included.

sample. There is a statistically significant correlation between these two values for the normal control group (Table 2, Fig 4). However, there is a little correlation between lines and the lymphocytes from which they were derived for individuals in remission or under treatment, especially with a regimen including procarbazine (Table 3, Fig. 5). There was only a fair correlation between lines and PBLs among HD/NHL patients prior to treatment. In contrast, when we compared the AGT activity in two lines from the same blood sample of an individual, the correlation was not only significant in controls but also for patients in remission or under treatment and nearly significant for the small number of HD/NHL patients studied before treatment (Table 3).

The average AGT activity of lines derived from normal controls is usually higher than their PBL progenitors (Fig. 4). However, we have isolated a number of lines with lower AGT activity from treated patients and those in remission (Fig. 5): only one such case of a low line was seen in cultures from normal individuals.

Since B cells have about 70% of the AGT activity of T cells, and assuming that the B cells which are transformed by EBV in the normal PBL population also have this (average) activity, the correlation between normal PBL and lymphoblastoid AGT activity suggests that the AGT activity of the B lymphocytes is controlled by a mechanism which survives transformation by EBV virus. The highly significant positive correlation found in all groups between the AGT activities of different lymphoblastoid lines derived from the same PBL sample argues against random values for transformed lymphocytes. Therefore, it is necessary to account for the lack of a relationship between the AGT activity of PBLs and of lines derived from individuals with malignancy and, particularly, from treated individuals. One interpretation of our results is that B cells from the HD/NHL patients which can be transformed by EBV are no longer representative of the overall PBL cell population, and that this distortion is accentuated in the cells of individuals being treated for, or in remission for malignancy. One example of a possible hypothesis is that the lymphocyte population of an individual is heterogeneous with respect to its AGT activity with a distribution around a characteristic value. As a result of malignancy and/or treatment only a subset of the population of peripheral B lymphocytes can be transformed by EBV. This subgroup no longer reflects the AGT activity of the overall lymphocyte population (Fig. 6).

Table 3. Correlation of AGT Activity in Two Cell Lines Transformed From
Aliquots of the Same PBL Sample

Group	Description	n	r	p value
3	HD/NHL: untreated	7	0.73	0.062
4P	HD/NHL: treated-procarbazine	10	0.821	0.004
4	HD/NHL: total treated[a]	15	0.93	<0.001
5	HD/NHL: remission	34	0.852	<0.001
6	Control subjects	19	0.586	0.008

[a]Includes individuals treated by radiation or other chemotherapeutic
agents in addition to those treated with a regimen including
procarbazine.

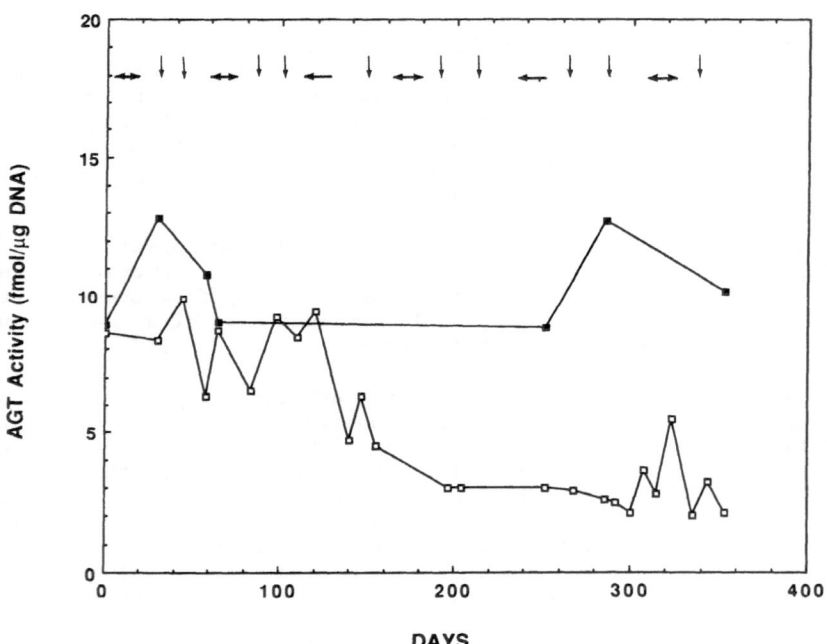

DAYS

Fig. 3. AGT Activity in PBLs and in the EBV transformed lines derived
from them in a patient on MOPP/ABVD therapy including procarbazine and dacarbazine. Horizontal lines indicate the duration
of procarbazine treatments. Vertical arrows show the times at
which dacarbazine was administered. Open symbols, AGT activity
in PBLs. Closed symbols, AGT activity in lymphoblastoid lines
derived from the PBL samples (Sagher et al., 1989).

This hypothesis of heterogeneity of lymphocytes both as to AGT activity and transformability accounts for a number of our observations. In some of the patients enrolled in this study and in whom there was a decline of AGT activity during long periods of treatment, the activity of the corresponding lymphoblastoid lines did not follow the decrease in AGT activity observed in the PBLs, but rather remained at a high level (Fig. 3). The low level of AGT activity in the lymphocytes of such individuals might reflect inactivation in non-replicating PBLs due to the treatment with regeneration in the proliferating lymphocytes. However, since lowered PBL activity of AGT is not seen in the PBLs of all patients, the high lymphoblastoid line activity might reflect the presence of a subset of transformable PBLs with higher AGT activity. More convincing is our experience with the continued cultivation of lymphoblastoid lines. We kept a group of lines in culture for over a year and assayed them several times during this extended period. In order to assess the variability in the activity of the cultures we calculated the coefficient of variation for each culture. Cultures for which this value was 25% or less were classified as having "no change" in AGT, since the average coefficient of variation for multiple lines from the same PBL sample is 23.2%. Using this criterion, 15 of 21 lines showed great variability in their AGT activity. Approximately a year to two years after being established, 10 lines were lower than the the original culture, and 5 were higher, while 6 remained relatively unchanged. Changes were still occurring in some of the lines after long periods in culture, although others remained stable. This observation is what might be expected from an initial heterogeneous population upon which selection, not involving AGT activity, operates (Migeon et al., 1988). Even after long periods in culture very few of our lines are completely devoid of detectable AGT activity, suggesting that continued growth of transformed cells does not, by itself, select lines with zero AGT activity.

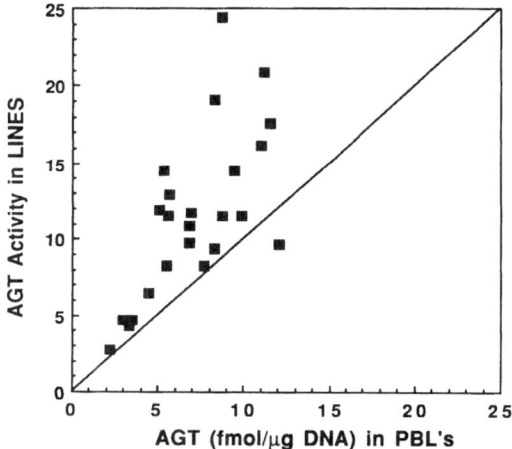

Fig. 4. Relationship between PBL activity in lymphoblastoid lines and in the PBLs of the healthy control individuals from which the lines were derived. The 45° line indicates positions of hypothetical equal AGT activity in PBLs and lymphoblast cultures and is not a regression line (Sagher et al., 1989).

283

The availability of lymphoblastoid cell lines (LCLs) with stable, but different, AGT activities has made it possible to determine the relationship between this activity and sensitivity to the effect of a number of alkylating agents in producing sister chromatid exchanges (SCEs). Schwartz et al. (1989a) used PBLs obtained from AML de novo, t-AML, primary malignancy, and a control unexposed healthy group to determine the sensitivity to SCEs as a result of treatment of lymphocyte cultures with either mitomycin-C or N-methyl-N'-nitro-N-nitrosoguanidine (MNNG). Baseline and induced frequencies of SCEs were determined by stimulating cultures with phytohemagglutinin and then, after 24 hours, treating with either mitomycin or MNNG and adding bromodeoxyuridine to the cultures. These studies failed to detect any correlation between SCE induction by MNNG and the endogenous level of AGT in the PBLs at two MNNG concentrations. AGT activity in the lymphocytes studied ranged from under 3 fmol/μg DNA to 15 fmol/μg DNA.

In studies using LCLs, Schwartz et al. (1989b) took five recently prepared LCLs and determined their sensitivity to SCE induction by MNNG, methyl methanesulfonate (MMS), and 1,3-bis (2-chloroethyl)-1-nitrosourea (BCNU). The LCLs ranged in AGT activity from 2.4 to 13.2 fm/μgDNA: the line with the highest activity derived from a HD patient being treated with procarbazine, and the other lines came from groups 1, 3, 5, and 6 (Table 2). Of the five cell lines, the cell line with highest AGT was the most sensitive to MNNG-induced SCE formation (Fig. 7). Even after taking into account the different overall alkylation by MNNG of the different lines, no relationship between overall alkylation and sensitivity to MNNG-induced SCE formation was noted. In contrast, there was a correlation between AGT activity and BCNU-sensitivity to SCE induction: cell lines with low AGT activities were more sensitive to the bifunctional agent than cells with higher activities. These data imply that SCE induction by monofunctional alkylating agents, or at least by MNNG, is not simply due to reaction at the O^6-position of guanine.

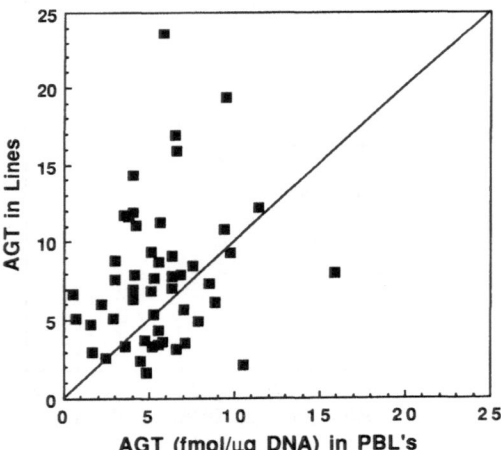

Fig. 5. AGT activity in PBLs and in EBV-transformed lines from individuals in remission after treatment for malignancy. The 45° line indicates positions of hypothetical equal AGT activity in PBLs and lymphoblast cultures and is not a regression line (Sagher et al., 1989).

We suppose that all of the lines we have obtained come from "normal" PBLs and were not derived from tumor cells since the PBL samples we use do not contain lymphoma cells. Nonetheless, it is certainly possible that the PBL population in HD and NHL patients differs from the premalignancy population in the same individuals. The lymphocytes might differ in response to growth factors (Gordon et al., 1985), in the type of immunoglobin produced (Miyawaki et al., 1988) or in other characteristics. The lower AGT values in the lymphocytes of such patients might be a consequence of some of these differences, e.g., the response of the subpopulations to growth factors circulating in the serum of individuals with malignancy. The difference in AGT activity in PBLs (Table 2) could be an effect secondary to some other process (e.g. differential growth factor stimulation) acting on the subpopulations of lymphocytes. This hypothesis accounts for some of the other reports of variations in alkyl transferase activity. Harris et al. (1982), Lawley et al. (1988), and Colaço et al. (1988) have reported differences in the ability of PBLs from individuals with immunodeficiency disease to remove O^6-alkylguanine as compared to healthy controls and patients with other disorders. Selection operating on PBL populations in individuals with some, but not all, diseases may result in low AGT activity for still unknown reasons. Our observation of differences in AGT activity between ANLL de novo and t-ANLL may be yet another indication of the heterogeneity of this disease (Ferraris et al., 1985; Gerhartz et al., 1989).

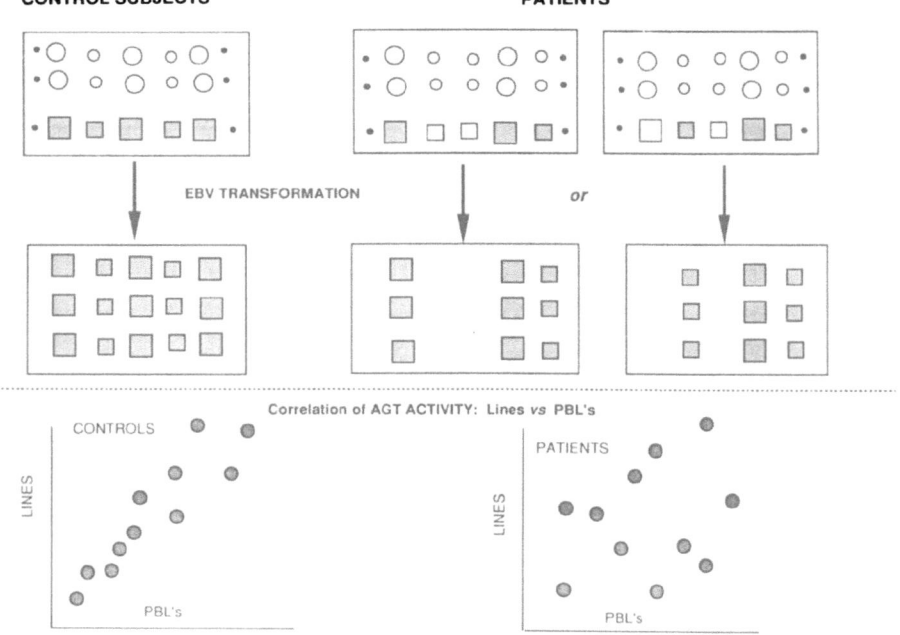

Fig. 6. Schematic representation of the difference in EBV-transformable cell populations in control subjects and in HD/NHL: patients. Open circles represent T lymphocytes. Squares represent B cells. Filled squares indicate cells transformable by Epstein Barr virus. Larger figures (circles or squares) indicate higher AGT values. Small dots indicate the portion of the population not shown in the figure. The lower portion of the cartoon is a representation of the data in Figs. 4 and 5 (Sagher et al., 1989).

Patients refractory to other treatments for cancer are now given "high dose chemotherapy" in which bone marrow is removed and stored, the individual is then treated with high levels of alkylating agents, after which the autologous bone marrow is transplanted (Philip et al., 1987). One of the major chemical constituents of such high dose chemotherapy is the chloroethylating nitrosourea, BCNU (Carmustine). Since the initial target for this compound is the O^6 position of guanine (Eisenbrand et al., 1986) and since the initial adduct is a substrate for AGT, we assayed AGT activity in PBLs from these patients. A typical course of therapy involves three treatments with 100 mg/m^2 of drug two days apart. When possible, we assayed patients both immediately before, and two hours after, receiving drugs. Our results (Fig. 8) indicated an erratic pattern of AGT activities following drug administration. In some cases there was little or no change (JF, JW). Other cases showed a dramatic lowering in AGT activity (EG, MR). Yet other individuals displayed an increase in AGT activity (PC, CK) at least for some of the determinations. It can be calculated that no change in AGT activity should have been expected. The dose given, if uniformly distributed, would yield a maximum BCNU concentration of 10 μM. BCNU is a direct acting alkylating agent and Brent (1986) has shown that it requires a concentration of 2 to 3 mM BCNU to react with DNA and produce a 50% lowering of AGT activity. We suppose that the drastic shifts in AGT activity observed in this study must be the result of changes of a major portion of the PBL population and recruitment of a new population with differing AGT value. This explanation can also account for the swings in AGT activity in one of the patients followed over a long period of MOPP therapy (Fig. 3).

Notwithstanding their easy availability, the PBLs are, therefore, an inadequate population to use for the test of our hypothesis. The statistical results are clear enough in indicating the probability of characteristic individual AGT values and a trend for depletion of AGT activity on treatment with procarbazine. However, the conclusion of a heterogeneity in the PBL population and the possibility of rapid shifts in this population, possibly as the result of trauma, with consequent

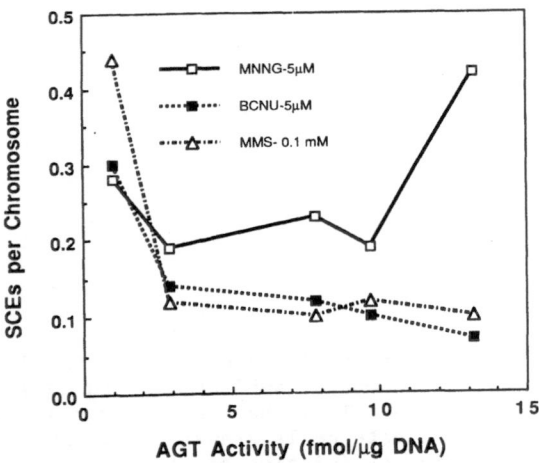

Fig. 7. Relationship between SCE induction and AGT activity in five cell lines after treatment with MNNG, BCNU, or MMS. Data from Schwartz et al. (1989).

changes in AGT protein level make it difficult to draw conclusions about the meaning of small, albeit significant differences. At the same time, the conclusion of PBL heterogeneity implies that individuals with low average AGT activity should have subpopulations with almost no AGT activity, highly susceptible to procarbazine.

The data reinforce the concept that there must be regulatory mechanisms which can set the AGT level of a cell at any one of a series of possible values. The correlation between PBL and lymphoblastoid AGT values for cells from normal individuals and the maintenance of different values for long periods of time indicate this to be the case. This is hardly a surprising conclusion. The conclusion that different cell types, even within the same organ, may have different AGT values is well established (Pegg and Dolan, 1987). It would appear that a great deal will be learned when a cloned structural gene is available for the study of regulatory elements.

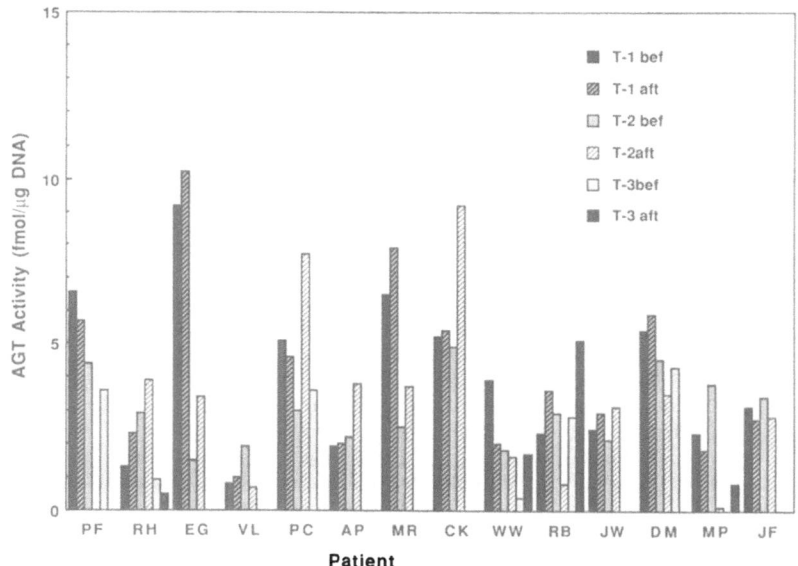

Fig. 8. AGT activity in the PBLs of patients undergoing high dose chemotherapy. Patients received three treatments (T1, T2, T3) at two day intervals. Blood was collected either immediately before (bef) or two hours after (aft) treatment.

ACKNOWLEDGEMENT

The work reported in this paper was supported by funds provided by a Program Project grant from the National Cancer Institute (PO1 CA 40046).

REFERENCES

Brent, T., 1986, Inactivation of purified O^6-alkylguanine-DNA-alkyltransferase by alkylating agents or alkylated DNA, Cancer Res., 46:2320.
Colaço, C., Harris, G., Lawley, P., Lydyard, P., and Roitt, I., 1988, Deficient repair of O^6-methylguanine in lymphocytes from rheumatoid arthritis families may be an acquired defect. Clin. Exp. Immunol., 72:15.

DeVita, V., Serpick, A., and Carbone, P., 1970, Combination chemotherapy in the treatment of advanced Hodgkin's disease, Ann. Intern Med., 73:881.

Eisenbrand, G., Muller, N., Denkel, E., and Sterzel, W., 1986, DNA adducts and DNA damage by antineoplastic and carcinogenic N-nitroso compounds, J. Cancer Res. Clin. Oncol., 112:196.

Ferraris, A., Raskind, W., Bjornson, B., Jacobson, R., Singer, J., and Fialkow, P., 1985, Heterogeneity of B cell involvement in acute nonlymphocytic leukemia, Blood, 66:342.

Gerhartz, H., Bartram, C., Raghavacher, A., Schmetzer, H., Clemm, C., Wilmanns, W., and Thiel, E., 1989, Spontaneous Epstein-Barr virus transformed B-cell line sharing the identical immunoglobulin gene rearrangement with acute myeloid leukemia, Blood, 73:684.

Gerson, S., Miller, K., and Berger, N., 1985, O^6-alkylguanine DNA alkyltransferase in human myeloid cells, J. Clin. Invest., 76:2106.

Gordon, J., Åman, P., Rosen, A., Ernberg, I., Ehlin-Henriksson, B., and Klein, G., 1985, Capacity of B-lymphocytic lines of diverse tumor origin to produce and respond to B-cell growth factors: a progression model for B-cell lymphomagenesis, Int. J. Cancer, 35:251.

Harris, G., Lawley, P., Asbery, L., Denman, A., and Hylton, W., 1982, Defective repair of O^6-methylguanine in autoimmune diseases, Lancet, 2:952.

Herrmann, F., Sieber, G., Jauer. B., Lochner, A., Komischke, B., and Ruhl, H., 1983, Evaluation of the circulating and splenic lymphocyte subpopulations in patients with non-Hodgkin's lymphomas and Hodgkin's disease using monoclonal antibodies, Blut, 47:41.

Lawley, P., Topper, R., Denman, A., Hylton, W., Hill, I., and Harris, G., 1988, Increased sensitivity of lymphocytes from patients with systemic autoimmune diseases to DNA alkylation by the methylating carcinogen N-methyl-N-nitrosourea, Ann. Rheumatic Dis., 47:445.

Lindahl, T., and Sedgwick, B., 1988, Regulation and expression of the adaptive response to alkylating agents, Ann. Rev. Biochem., 57:133.

Migeon, B., Axelman, J., and Stetten, G., 1988, Clonal evolution in human lymphoblast cultures, Am. J. Human Genet., 42:742.

Myrnes, B., Norstrund, K., Giercksky, K., Sjuueskog, C., and Krokan, H., 1984, A simplified assay for O^6-methylguanine-DNA-methyltransferase activity and its application to human neoplastic and non-neoplastic tissues, Carcinogenesis, 5:1061.

Miyawaki, T., Kubagawa, H., Butler, J., and Cooper, M., 1988, Ig isotypes produced by EBV-transformed B cells as a function of age and tissue distribution, J. Immunol., 140:3887.

Pegg, A., 1983, Alkylation and subsequent repair of DNA after exposure to dimethylnitrosamine and related carcinogens, Rev. Biochem. Toxicol., 5:83.

Pegg, A., and Dolan, M., 1987, Properties and assay of mammalian O^6-alkylguanine-DNA alkyltransferase, Pharmac. Ther., 34:167.

Philip, T., Armitage, J., Spitzer, G., Chauvin, F., Jagannath, S., Cahn, J., Colombat, P., Goldstone, A., Gorin, N., Flesh, M. et al., 1987, High-dose therapy and autologous bone marrow transplantation after failure of conventional chemotherapy in adults with intermediate-grade or high-grade non-Hodgkin's lymphoma, N. Engl. J. Med., 316:1493.

Sagher, D., Karrison, T., Schwartz, J., Larson, R., Meier, P., and Strauss, B., 1988, Low O^6-alkylguanine DNA alkyltransferase activity in the peripheral blood lymphocytes of patients with therapy-related acute nonlymphocytic leukemia, Cancer Res., 48:3084.

Sagher, D., Karrison, T., Schwartz, J., Larson, R., and Strauss, B., 1989, Heterogeneity of the O^6-alkylguanine DNA alkyltransferase (AGT) activity in peripheral blood lymphocytes (PBLs): Relationship between the activity of lymphocytes and of lymphoblastoid lines in normal controls and in patients with Hodgkin's disease or non-Hodgkin's lymphoma, Cancer Res., 49:5339.

Samson, L., and Cairns, J., 1977, A new pathway for DNA repair in E. coli, Nature, 267:281.

Schwartz, J., Karrison, T., LeBeau, M., Larson, R., Sagher, D., Strauss, B., Rowley, J., and Weichselbaum, R., 1989a, Chromosomal sensitivity of lymphocytes from individuals with therapy-related acute nonlymphocytic leukemia, Mutation Res., 216:119.

Schwartz, J., Turkula, T., Sagher, D., and Strauss, B., 1989b, Relationship between O^6-alkyltransferase activity and sensitivity to alkylation-induced sister chromatid exchanges in human lymphoblastoid cell lines, Carcinogenesis, 10:681.

Waldstein, E., Cao, E., Bender, M., and Setlow, R., 1982, Abilities of extracts of human lymphocytes to remove O^6-methylguanine from DNA, Mutation Res., 95:406.

Wiestler, O., Kleihues, P., Rice, J., and Ivankovic, S., 1984, DNA methylation in maternal, fetal and neonatal rat tissues following perinatal administration of procarbazine, J. Cancer Res. Clin. Oncol., 108:56.

THE SINGLE CELL GEL ASSAY: A SENSITIVE TECHNIQUE FOR EVALUATING

INTERCELLULAR DIFFERENCES IN DNA DAMAGE AND REPAIR

R.R. Tice*, P.W. Andrews* and N.P. Singh**

*Integrated Laboratory Systems, P.O. Box 13501, Research
Triangle Park, NC 27709, and **Biology Dept., Eastern
Washington University, Cheney, WA 99004

INTRODUCTION

While providing information at the level of the individual cell,
cytogenetic techniques for evaluating DNA damage or repair are, by their
very nature, largely limited to proliferating cell populations.
Furthermore, these techniques require the processing of DNA damage into
microscopically visible lesions. Biochemical techniques, such as alkaline
elution and nucleoid sedimentation, circumvent these difficulties in that
DNA damage can be evaluated directly in almost any cell population.
However, the resulting data do not provide any information about the
distribution of damage or repair among individual cells. Since the effects
of genotoxic agents are often tissue and cell-type specific, techniques
which can directly detect DNA damage in individual cells are needed.
Rydberg and Johanson (1978) were the first to directly quantitate DNA
damage in individual cells by lysing cells embedded in agarose on slides
under mild alkali conditions to allow the partial unwinding of DNA. After
neutralization, the cells are stained with acridine orange and the extent
of DNA damage quantitated by measuring the ratio of green (indicating
double-stranded DNA) to red (indicating single-stranded DNA) fluorescence
using a photometer. To improve the sensitivity for detecting DNA damage in
isolated cells, Ostling and Johanson (1984) developed a microgel
electrophoresis technique, in which cells are embedded in agarose gel on
microscope slides, lysed by detergents and high salt and then
electrophoresed under neutral conditions. Cells with increased DNA damage
display increased migration of DNA from the nucleus towards the anode. The
migrating DNA is quantitated by staining with ethidium bromide and
measuring the intensity of fluorescence at two fixed positions within the
migration pattern using a microscope photometer. However, this technique
permits the detection of double-stranded DNA breaks only and the presence
of RNA can lead to potential artifacts. Since many agents induce from 5-
to 2000-fold more single-stranded breaks than double-stranded ones, and
because many agents preferentially induce alkali-labile damage, neutral
conditions are clearly not as sensitive as alkaline conditions in detecting
DNA damage.

Recently, we introduced an electrophoretic technique capable of
detecting DNA single-strand breaks and alkali labile sites in individual
cells (Singh et al., 1988). Eukaryote cells are embedded in an agarose gel
on a microscope slide, lysed by detergents and high salt at pH 10, and then

DNA Damage and Repair in Human Tissues
Edited by B. M. Sutherland and A. D. Woodhead
Plenum Press, New York, 1990

electrophoresed for a short time under alkaline conditions. Cells with increased DNA damage display increased migration of the DNA from the nucleus towards the anode. The importance of this technique lies in its ability to detect intercellular differences in DNA damage and repair in virtually any eukaryote cell population, and in its requirement for extremely small cell samples (from 1 to 10,000 cells). Here, we describe the utility of this technique, summarizing the results of a variety of in vitro and in vivo experiments to evaluate DNA damage and repair in human and nonhuman cells.

THE SINGLE CELL GEL (SCG) TECHNIQUE

The basic technique is described in detail in Singh et al. (1988). Briefly, up to 500,000 cells are mixed with 0.5% low-melting agarose at 37^0C and then placed on a fully frosted microscope slide coated with 0.5% agarose. After the agarose has solidified, an additional layer of agarose is added. After solidification of the agarose covering, the slides are immersed in a lysing solution (1% sodium sarcosinate, 2.5 M NaCl, 100 mM Na_2EDTA, 10 mM Tris, pH 10, and 1% Triton X-100, added fresh) for 1 hour to lyse the cells and to permit DNA unfolding. The slides are then removed from the lysing solution and placed on a horizontal gel electrophoresis unit. The unit is filled with fresh electrophoretic buffer (1 mM Na_2EDTA and 300 mM NaOH; pH ~13) and the slides are allowed to sit in this high pH buffer for 20 minutes to allow the DNA to unwind before electrophoresis. Depending on the basal level of DNA damage in the target cell population, electrophoresis is conducted for from 10 to 40 minutes at 25 volts. These steps are conducted under yellow light or in the dark to prevent additional DNA damage. After electrophoresis, the slides are washed with 0.4 M Tris, pH 7.5, to remove alkali and detergents. The slides are then stained with ethidium bromide (10 ugm/ml) in distilled water. Observations are made at 250x magnification using a fluorescent microscope equipped with an excitation filter of 515-560 nm and a barrier filter of 590 nm. In some studies, cells were photographed using Kodak 35 mm Tri-X black and white film, the negatives developed and migration lengths for 20 to 25 randomly selected cells measured with a millimeter ruler. In other studies, images of 25 randomly selected cells were analyzed for migration length using a Cambridge Instruments Quantimet 520 image analyzer. The mean DNA migrations lengths, as well as the distribution of damage among cells, were statistically evaluated using appropriate parametric or nonparametric statistics, with an alpha level of 0.05.

X-RAY AND HYDROGEN PEROXIDE INDUCED DNA DAMAGE IN HUMAN PERIPHERAL BLOOD LYMPHOCYTES

The first formal experiments with the SCG technique involved an evaluation of the ability of x-rays and hydrogen peroxide to induce DNA damage under conditions in which repair was prevented (Singh et al., 1988). Briefly, lymphocytes were separated from human whole blood utilizing Ficoll hypaque, washed in RPMI-1640 and suspended in calcium-magnesium free, phosphate-buffered saline (PBS). Before treatment, lymphocytes were embedded in agarose on microscope slides. For x-irradiation, a Phillips Model MG 300 x-ray machine (Ridge Instrument Company, Inc., Tucker, GA) was used at a dose rate of 200 rads/min. For the hydrogen peroxide experiments, human lymphocytes were treated at concentrations of 9.1 to 291 uM. To prevent repair of x-ray and hydrogen peroxide induced DNA damage, the cells were irradiated or treated at 4^0C. The effect of dose on the length of the DNA migration was analyzed using a one-tailed trend test, with the alpha level set at 0.05. To determine the lowest dose at which a significant increase in the length of migration occurred, multiple pairwise comparisons were conducted between the control data and each dose using a student's t test.

Table 1. DNA Migration in Human PBL Irradiated with
X-Rays or Treated with Hydrogen Peroxide

X-Rays			Hydrogen Peroxide		
Dose	Migration		Dose	Migration	
(rads)	mean	sd	(uM)	mean	sd
0	3.7	1.10	0	2.7	1.08
25	5.3	1.19*	9.1	3.9	1.30*
50	12.4	4.69*	36.4	6.0	1.48*
100	23.3	3.27*	145	6.4	2.47*
200	29.6	2.99*	291	7.3	1.79*

25 cells were scored per sample; data presented in mm.

*Significantly different from control data at P<0.05,
using a one-tailed students t test.

A significant increase (P<0.001) in the length of DNA migration was
observed in human lymphocytes exposed to ionizing radiation beginning at 25
rads (Table 1). Under the electrophoretic conditions used, no migration of
DNA occurred among the majority of the control cells and an approximately
linear increase in the length of DNA migration was observed for doses
between 25 and 100 rads (correlation coefficient r = 0.92). At 200 rads,
the length of migration appeared to plateau, while the extent of DNA damage
in cells exposed to greater doses was too great to permit an accurate
measurement. At each dose of radiation, a relatively homogeneous response
in the extent of DNA migration among cells was observed (Singh et al.,
1988).

Exposure to hydrogen peroxide at concentrations between 9.1 and 291 uM
also induced a significant increase in the migration of DNA (P<0.001)
(Table 1). The extent of migration plateaued at hydrogen peroxide
concentrations above 36.4 uM. However, in contrast to the relatively
homogeneous DNA migration patterns observed for lymphocytes exposed to x-
rays, extensive differences in the length of DNA migration, and thus in the
extent of DNA damage, were observed among the treated cells (Singh et al.,
1988). There are several explanations possible for the greater
heterogeneity in DNA damage following treatment with hydrogen peroxide.
Individual cells may vary in their permeability to hydrogen peroxide, their
radical scavenging capabilities, the accessibility of DNA to the damaging
species and other mechanisms which either enhance or diminish the effects
of hydrogen peroxide. Whatever the mechanism for the increased cellular
heterogeneity, these data demonstrate the usefulness of examining DNA
damage in individual cells.

REPAIR KINETICS FOR X-RAY INDUCED DNA DAMAGE IN HUMAN PERIPHERAL BLOOD
LYMPHOCYTES

To explore the utility of the SCG assay for evaluating DNA repair
kinetics, human peripheral blood lymphoctes, isolated as described earlier,
were exposed to 200 rads of x-rays and incubated in complete RPMI 1640
medium at 37°C for from 15 to 120 minutes (Singh et al., 1988). The
majority of the repair occurred within the first 15 minutes, followed by a
slower, second component that was essentially complete by the end of the
120-minute incubation (Figure 1). However, even at 120 minutes, there were
small populations of cells with significant migration patterns (Singh et
al., 1988).

Based on these data, it was decided to evaluate the effect of donor age on the repair of x-ray induced DNA damage in peripheral blood lymphocytes. Peripheral blood was obtained from healthy, nonsmoking, normotensive Caucasian members of the Baltimore Longitudinal Study on Aging, sponsored by the National Institute on Aging (Singh et al., 1990). Twenty-three men (aged 28 to 91 years) and 8 women (aged 25 to 80 years), free from overt pathology and medication known to cause DNA damage, were selected to participate in the study. For x-irradiation, Ficoll hypaque isolated lymphocytes were exposed, on ice, to 200 rads of x-rays as described in Singh et al. (1988). Immediately before (time 0 control) and immediately after irradiation (time 0 exposed), cells samples were processed for DNA migration analysis. Some cells were incubated at 37°C as described earlier and cell samples collected at 15, 30, 60 and 120 minutes after irradiation to evaluate repair kinetics. Cell viability was assessed by trypan blue exclusion at each time point of the study, and was found to be >98%. Male and female data were combined in this study since sex-dependent differences in response were not detected. The effect of age on mean DNA migration prior to irradiation and at various times after irradiation was analyzed, using least squares regression analysis. To compare the effects of age, irradiation, and repair time on the intercellular distribution of DNA migration patterns within an individual, the dispersion coefficient H, which is the ratio of the variance to the mean, was calculated and analyzed using least squares regression analysis (Singh et al., 1990).

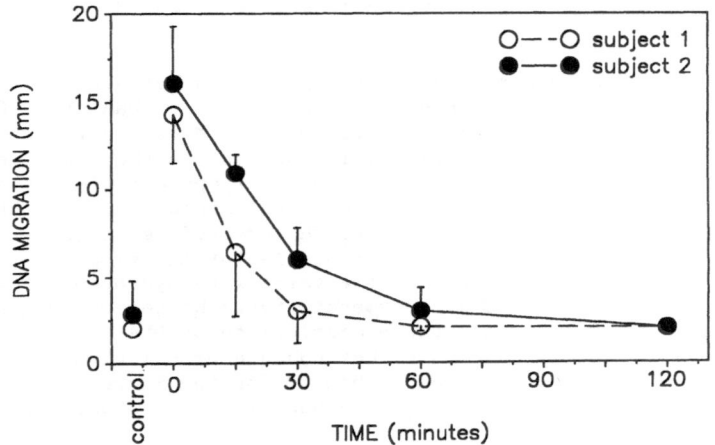

Fig. 1. Repair kinetics for x-ray induced (200 rads) DNA damage in human peripheral blood lymphocytes obtained from two individuals.

In this study, the mean basal levels of DNA damage remained unaltered (Fig. 2, panel labeled CONTROL) as a function of the subject's age. Immediately following irradiation, and before significant repair could occur (Fig. 2, panel labeled 0 MIN), a highly significant (P<0.0001) age-related increase in DNA damage was detected. As damage was repaired

increased dispersion (Fig. 3). This increase in dispersion was due to the presence of a small number of lymphocytes with extended DNA migration patterns, indicating deficient DNA repair competency in these cells. These few, heavily damaged cells have little effect on the mean frequency of DNA migration but a large effect on the dispersion.

Two aspects of these results are of considerable interest. First, the age-related increase in DNA damage induced in peripheral blood lymphocytes by x-radiation is a novel observation. Second, despite an apparent normal rate of DNA repair among the majority of lymphocytes from all subjects, a (panels labeled 15, 30, 60 MIN), this age-related increase disappeared. By 120 minutes after irradiation, the mean DNA migration patterns for cells obtained from young and old subjects were not different from each other and were equal to that of non-irradiated cells. However, an analysis of the dispersion of DNA migration patterns among cells revealed at 120 minutes an age-dependent increase in the number of individuals with subset of repair deficient cells are present, the frequency of which is increased among older individuals. The presence of these cells would not be identified by techniques based on pooled cell samples.

It is unlikely that the age-related increase in DNA damage following x-irradiation is due to a decreased level of DNA repair in the cells from older individuals. Irradiated cells were kept on ice and, in all subjects,

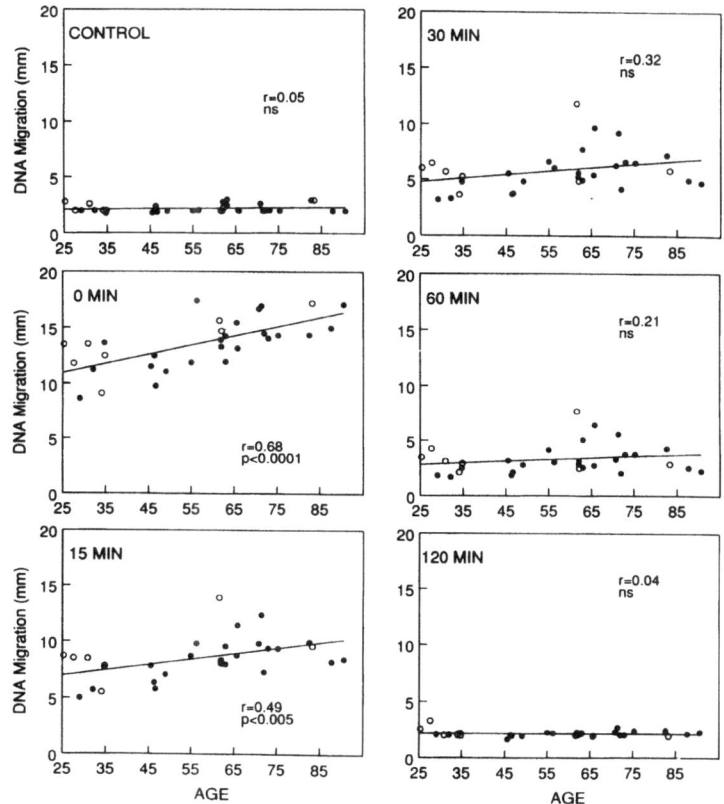

Fig. 2. Effect of donor age on repair kinetics for x-ray induced (200 rads) DNA damage in lymphocytes. Data presented as mean migration lengths in mm. Reprinted with permission of Mutation Research.

regardless of age, DNA repair is essentially complete in about the same period. Another possible explanation is that cells from older individuals have lower levels of factors, such as free radical scavengers, which protect DNA from the effects of x-irradiation. This possibility was tested by comparing the DNA migration patterns for lymphocytes from three young (ages 41-44) and three old (ages 71-73) subjects irradiated prior to lysis or irradiated after lysis (Singh et al., 1990). If intracellular factors were responsible for the age-dependent increase in x-ray induced DNA damage, then the lysis of cells prior to irradiation should remove the age-dependent relationship. However, lysis prior to irradiation resulted in an increased level of DNA damage, the magnitude of which was independent of donor age (Singh et al., 1990). Whether or not the increased levels of DNA damage reflects an age-dependent alteration in DNA conformation remains to be investigated.

UV-INDUCED DNA DAMAGE IN HUMAN PERIPHERAL BLOOD LYMPHOCYTES

To evaluate the ability of the SCG assay to identify cells in the process of excision repair, a pilot experiment was conducted in which human lymphocytes were exposed to ultraviolet (UV) light. Peripheral blood lymphocytes were isolated from whole blood and resuspended in calcium-magnesium free PBS as described earlier, exposed to 6 and 24 J/m^2 UV at a rate of 20 J/m^2/min, and then incubated at 37°C for up to 6 hours. At

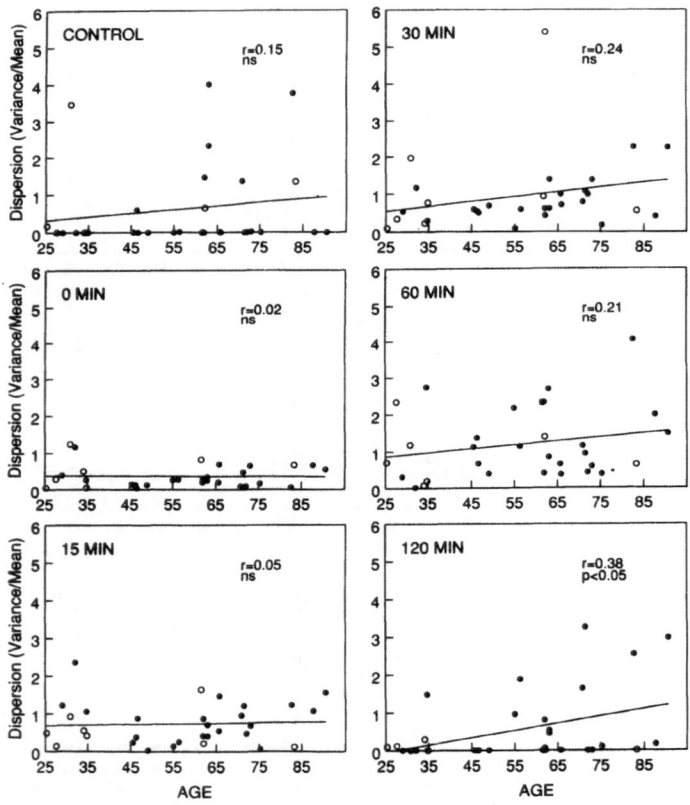

Fig. 3. Effect of age on repair of kinetics for x-ray induced (200 rads) DNA damage in lymphocytes. Data presented as the dispersion of DNA migration patterns among cells within an individual. Reprinted with permission of Mutation Research.

various times, samples of the cell population were processed in the SCG assay and DNA migration lengths determined on 25 cells using photographic negatives as described. Exposure to UV does not result directly in the formation of DNA SSB or alkali-labile sites. However, during the excision repair of UV-induced damage, transitory strand breaks occur, the presence of which can be identified in the SCG assay. The resulting mean DNA migration data is presented in Figure 4, while the histograms of individual cell responses at selected sample times are presented in Figure 5. The extent of repair at any single sample time, as well as the length of time over which repair occurred was greater for cells exposed to 24 J/m². Even at 6 hours, when excision repair had ceased in cells exposed to 6 J/m², some cells exposed to the higher UV dose still exhibited considerable evidence of repair. This experiment demonstrates the feasibility of evaluating DNA repair in cells exposed to agents which do not induce SSB or alkali-labile sites directly.

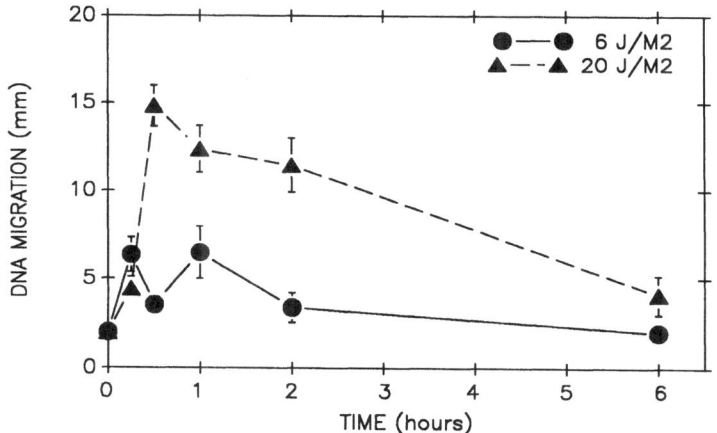

Fig. 4. Repair kinetics for UV-induced DNA damage in human peripheral blood lymphocytes. Data presented as the mean plus standard deviation.

CHEMICALLY-INDUCED DNA DAMAGE IN VIVO IN MICE

One of the main advantages of the SCG assay is its requirement for extremely small cell samples (i.e., from a few to a few thousand cells). This advantage makes this assay extremely useful in studies where only small numbers of cells are available. One such area of research involves the evaluation of organ-specific levels of DNA damage induced in vivo in animal models of carcinogenesis. In a series of pilot studies to explore the applicability of this technique for examining the kinetics of DNA damage induced in vivo in various organs/tissues, mice were treated by gavage with acrylamide (ACR), trichlorethylene (TCE) or dimethylbenz-anthracene (DMBA) and blood, brain, liver and spleen cells evaluated for DNA damage (Andrews et al., 1989). Briefly, male B6C3F1 mice (9 - 13 weeks of age, 25 to 32 gm in body weight, 4 mice per group) were gavaged with 100 mg/kg ACR in PBS, with 1000 mg/kg TCE in PBS, or with 100 mg/kg DMBA in corn oil. At 4 and 24 hours after treatment, groups of mice were killed by over etherization, and samples of the various organs and blood removed from each mouse and stored on ice in Hanks buffer. The liver and brain samples were minced and exposed to collagenase, the brain was minced only, while the lymphocytes were isolated from blood using Ficoll hypaque centrifugation. Samples of the single cell suspensions were electrophoresed for 15 minutes, stained with ethidium bromide and evaluated for DNA migration lengths using the Quantimet 520 image analyzer.

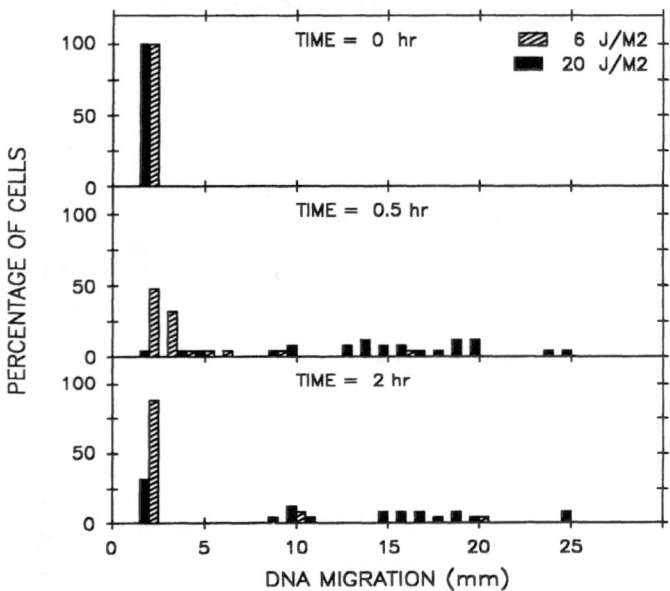

Fig. 5. Distribution of DNA migration among human peripheral blood lymphocytes exposed to UV light and evaluated immediately after exposure and at 0.5 and 2 hours later. 25 cells analyzed per sample.

Four hours after treatment with ACR, cells from all four organs/tissues exhibited a significant increase in DNA migration, with liver cells exhibiting the greatest response (Fig. 6). To account for tissue specific differences in migration patterns, the data are presented as the percentage of change in mean migration between the control and treated groups. By 24 hours after treatment, only the PBL still exhibited an increased level of damage. An analysis of the distribution of damage at 24 hours after treatment indicated that only a small proportion of PBL were affected. None of the cells obtained from organs/tissues sampled four hours after treatment with DMBA exhibited an increase in DNA migration. However, at 24 hrs after treatment, cells from all but one organ/tissue (brain) exhibited a significant increase in DNA migration, with spleen cells exhibiting the

greatest response. Four hours after treatment with TCE, cells from all 4
organs/tissues exhibited a significant increase in DNA migration, with
spleen cells exhibiting the greatest response. By 24 hours after
treatment, all tissues exhibited DNA migration patterns not significantly
different from control animals. These experiments demonstrate the utility
of the SCG assay for in vivo studies and, not unexpectedly, that the
induction and persistence of DNA damage in vivo is chemical-specific and
both organ- and temporally-dependent. Although not examined in this
particular study, other tissues such as bone marrow, lung and gonads are
equally amenable to analysis.

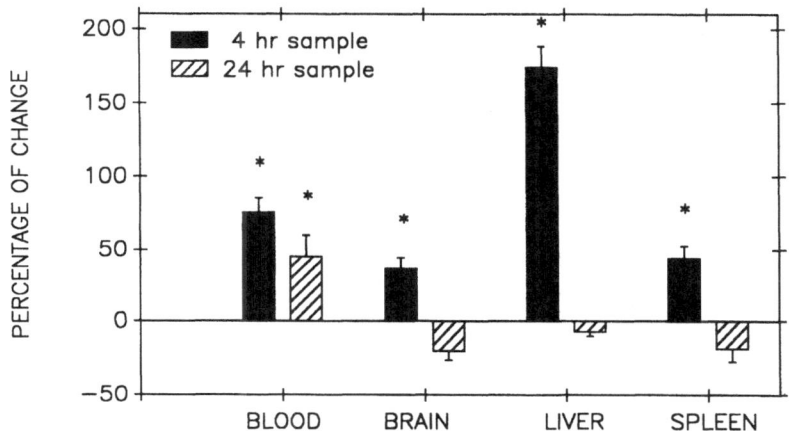

Fig. 6.   Organ and sample time-dependent induction of
          DNA damage by ACR (100 mg/kg) in male B6C3F1
          mice. Data presented as the mean percentage
          of change (and standard error of the mean)
          between control and treated groups (N = 4).
          * = P < 0.05.

IN VIVO DNA DAMAGE IN HUMAN PBL

     An obvious use for this assay is in the biomonitoring of humans for
possible exposure to genotoxic agents. Since the assay can be conducted
using the number of leukocytes present in 5 to 10 uL of blood, the amount
of blood generally available from a finger prick is more than sufficient
for most studies. While considerable more research must be conducted to
determine the sensitivity of the assay for various types of DNA damage, it
was felt useful to evaluate the applicability of this technique to sampling
humans outside the laboratory. Due to the lack of areadily available human
population in which to make a properly controlled study, the effects of a 5
Km road race on DNA migration patterns in PBL was selected for initial
study. Three nonsmoking males who were recreational joggers, ranging in
age from 28 to 42 years, volunteered for the study. 10 uL of blood was
obtained by finger prick from each runner within 15 minutes of the start of
the race, and at 5 minutes after each runner completed the 5 Km course.
The blood was added to RPMI 1640 containing 10% fetal calf serum and kept
cold until processed back in the laboratory (approximately 1 hour). PBL
were isolated by Ficoll hypaque centrifugation, electrophoresed using the

Table 2. DNA Migration in PBL Sampled from Three
          Participants in a 5 Km Road Race

	Race Start		Race Finish	
Runner	mean	sd	mean	sd
1	98.3	20.13	102.8	21.48
2	111.4	38.16	176.4*	48.96
3	119.6	22.79	120.0	29.53

25 cells were scored per sample, data presented
  in pixels
*Significantly different from control data at
  $P<0.05$.

SCG assay and 25 cells from each sample analyzed for DNA migration using an
image analyzer. The mean DNA migration data are presented in Table 2. For
two of the runners, the migration patterns were not significantly different
between the two samples. For the third runner, the distribution of
migration length for PBL sampled after the race was shifted to greater
lengths. While the significance of these data are unclear, the experiment
demonstrated that small blood samples could be easily obtained outside of
the laboratory and evaluated for DNA damage using the SCG assay.

CONCLUSION

     The results of a series of studies conducted to evaluate the
sensitivity and utility of the SCG assay for detecting DNA damage induced
in a variety of cell types by a variety of physical and chemical agents
have been presented. These studies demonstrate the sensitivity pf the
technique for identifying the presence of DNA damage among a variety of
cell types and the importance of data collected on a cell by cell basis.
Since these early studies, additional data has been collected on other cell
types, including sperm, and several technical advances have been made
which have helped greatly to control the extent of experiment to experiment
variability observed especially in in vivo experi- ments. The advantages
of this technique include its apparent sensitivity for detecting DNA
damage, the fact that the data are collected on an individual cell basis,
that extremely small cell samples are required and that virtually any
eukaryote cell population is amenable to analysis. The disadvantages
include the necessity for single cell suspensions, and the fact that small
cell samples may not be representative of the total cell population. We
anticipate that this technique will play an increasingly important role in
future studies to evaluate DNA damage in humans, organ-specific levels of
damage in animals exposed to potential carcinogens, in reproductive and
teratological studies, and in studies to examine the basic mechanisms of
DNA damage and repair.

ACKNOWLEDGEMENTS

     This research was supported by the National Institute on Aging and by
EPA contract 68-68-0069. Although portions of the research described in
this article have been supported by the U.S EPA, it has not been subjected
to Agency review and therefore does not necessarily reflect the views of
the Agency and no official endorsement should be inferred.

REFERENCES

Andrews, P.W., Tice, R.R., Nauman, C.H. (1989) The single cell gel (SCG) assay: A new tool for detecting organ-specific levels of DNA damage induced by genotoxic agents. Environ. Molec. Mutagen. 14(S15):10.

Ostling, O., and Johanson, K.J. (1984) Microelectrophoretic study of radiation-induced DNA damages in individual mammalian cells. Biochem. Biophys. Res. Commun. 123:291-298.

Rydberg, B., and Johanson, K.J. (1978) in: DNA Repair Mechanism (Hanawalt, P.C., and Friedberg, E.C., eds) pp 465-468, Academic Press, New York

Singh, N.P., McCoy, M.T., Tice, R.R. and Schneider, E.L. (1988) A simple technique for quantitation of low levels of DNA damage in individual cells. Exp. Cell Res. 175:184-191.

Singh, N.P., Danner, D.B., Tice, R.R., McCoy, M.T., Collins, G.D., and Schneider, E.L. (1989) Abundant alkali-labile sites in human and mouse sperm DNA. Exp. Cell Res., in press.

Singh, N.P., Danner, D.B., Tice, R.R., Brant, L., and Schneider, E.L. (1990) DNA damage and repair with age in individual human lymphocytes. Mutat. Res., in press.

CYTOGENETIC INVESTIGATIONS OF DNA DAMAGE IN AGING:

A TWIN STUDY

Betsy Hirsch

Department of Laboratory Medicine & Pathology
University of Minnesota
Minneapolis, Minnesota

INTRODUCTION

Increased induction and accumulation of DNA damage remain central concepts to many of the biological theories of aging (Gensler and Bernstein, 1981; Kirkwood, 1989). Cytogenetic techniques, which offer the ability to evaluate damage across the entire genome at the single cell level, have been utilized by numerous investigators to determine whether or not there is evidence of increased DNA damage with increasing in-vivo age. The data from these different laboratories have not yielded a consensus conclusion regarding age effects for sister chromatid exchange (SCE) or chromosomal aberration rates (Schneider, 1985; Tice and Setlow, 1985). What they have, however, clearly documented are the marked individual differences within age groups and the significant overlap in responses between age groups. Such individual variation argues for aging studies aimed not merely at classifying average aging effects, but those which also aim to understand and investigate the factors contributing to variability in aged populations.

The twin study design provides a unique paradigm for evaluating the contribution of genetic and environmental factors to the observed interindividual variability in cytogenetic damage in the aged. The classic twin method, first proposed by Galton in 1876, is based upon the comparison of pairs of identical or monozygotic (MZ) twins to pairs of fraternal or dizygotic (DZ) twins. MZ twins share 100% of their genes by descent, while DZ twins share on the average, 50% of their genes. Thus, if a trait is largely influenced by genetic factors, the within pair similarity of MZ twins will be significantly greater than that of DZ twins. The twin study method has been utilized to demonstrate that genetic factors significantly influence such varied traits as pulmonary capacity (Lewiter et al., 1984), serum cholesterol levels (Berg, 1981), risk for schizophrenia (Gottesman and Shields, 1977) and the cytogenetic visualization of nucleolus organizing region activity (Zakharov et al., 1982).

DNA Damage and Repair in Human Tissues
Edited by B. M. Sutherland and A. D. Woodhead
Plenum Press, New York, 1990

303

In addition to permitting evaluation of genetic influences, the twin study method can be modified to evaluate the importance of specific environmental or lifestyle factors. This modification of the classical twin method involves the comparison of MZ twin pairs discordant for a specified environmental factor to MZ twin pairs concordant for the factor. As any difference between MZ twins must be environmental in origin, correlating MZ twin differences with differences in environmental exposure provides a powerful test for environmental etiology. For example, one lifestyle factor which has been well documented to influence SCE rates is smoking status. It has generally taken large population studies to document this effect. Utilizing the discordant MZ twin method, one can demonstrate the importance of smoking on SCE frequencies with a much smaller cohort. In a small pilot study, our analyses of MZ pairs in which both twins were concordant for nonsmoking status showed an average intrapair difference of 0.13 SCE. Similarly, the average intrapair difference for MZ twin pairs in which one twin was an exsmoker and the other a nonsmoker was -0.27 SCE. In contrast, in MZ twin pairs discordant for current smoking status, the twin who smoked had, on average, 1.4 more SCEs per cell than his/her nonsmoking cotwin, implicating current smoking status as a significant factor affecting baseline SCE rates, one to be pursued in more depth in the full scale study.

Thus, using a twin study paradigm, a researcher can evaluate and estimate genetic as well as environmental influences.

MINNESOTA TWIN STUDY OF NORMAL AGING

The data reported on the following pages represent the findings, to date, of our ongoing twin study. The cytogenetic investigations represent one component of the Minnesota Twin Study of Normal Aging, a cross-sectional twin study involving evaluation of selected psychological, medical, and biological variables.

All of the twin pairs included in this study have been ascertained from birth records maintained by the State of Minnesota. So far, approximately 200,000 births from 15 different birth years have been reviewed, and approximately 287 pairs have been successfully traced and have survived intact into adulthood. Of these, 60% have agreed to participate in the study. As these twin pairs are identified from birth records and thus are, in effect, randomly sampled, they comprise a representative and heterogeneous group of individuals, an important concern for gerontological studies.

Cytogenetic Methods

Lymphocyte cultures were initiated using standard microculture techniques. For each culture an aliquot of .3 ml heparinized whole blood is dispensed into 5 ml of complete media containing 80% RPMI 1640 (GIBCO), 18% fetal calf serum (HyClone), 2% penicillin-streptomycin, (GIBCO) and 1% L-glutamine (GIBCO). Those cultures evaluated for SCE and replication index contained BrdU at a final concentration of 25uM which was added at the time of culture initiation.

Table 1. Effect of Age on Replication Index

Age Group (N)[a]	48 hrs[b]	Mean (±se) at 68 hrs[c]	76 hrs[d]	96 hrs[e]
25-39 (14-54)	1.08(±.02)	2.13(±.06)	2.49(±.05)	2.78(±.02)
60-69 (42-57)	1.05(±.01)	1.75(±.04)	2.09(±.04)	2.59(±.03)
70-85 (27-34)	1.05(±.01)	1.73(±.05)	2.07(±.05)	2.61(±.03)

[a] Not all subjects were able to be evaluated at all time points; the range for the no. of subjects in each age group is presented.
[b] $F(2, 82) = 2.1$; $p > .10$
[c] $F(2,101) = 11.1$; $p < .001$
[d] $F(2,101) = 11.5$; $p < .001$
[e] $F(2, 75) = 4.5$; $p < .05$

Chromosomes were harvested and slides prepared according to standard cytogenetic procedures.

Effect of Age on Replication Index

Calculation of replication index (RI) is based on the evaluation of the differential staining patterns of cells which have undergone one, two, or three or more cell divisions in the presence of BrdU (Tice et al., 1976). Twin samples were incubated for four different culture durations: 48, 68, 76,and 96 hours. At each time point, 100 cells were evaluated (50 from each of two replicate cultures). RI was calculated as M1 + 2*(M2) + 3*(M3)/(M1 + M2 + M3) where M1, M2, and M3 represent the number of cells having undergone 1, 2, or 3 or more cell divisions, respectively. As illustrated in Table 1, there is a significant age effect, with twins aged 60 years and older showing significantly decreased RI compared to twins aged 25-40 years. The most informative time points were 68 and 76 hours. (At 48 hours, almost all cells sampled from all individuals had undergone only a single division). This age effect for RI, which represents, in part, a decreased responsiveness to phytohemagglutinin, is in accord with the documented findings of numerous other laboratories (for example, see Tice et al., 1979; Murasko et al., 1987).

Interestingly, the genetic analyses showed moderate genetic effects for RI at 68, 76, and 96 hours, with corresponding heritabilities of .380 (± .288), .292 (± .305), and .285 (± .461) respectively. Thus, genetic factors appear to be accounting for approximately 30% of the observed interindividual variation in RI. Given the relatively small size of the sample, these heritability estimates should be interpreted with caution. Nonetheless, if these estimates hold over the additional projected sample of 100 twin pairs, they would have important implications for studies of immune function and aging. In addition to age and genetic effects, analyses of the environmental questionnaire and clinical laboratory data enabled the identification of other factors contributing to individual differences in RI. Differential

Table 2. Effect of Age on Baseline SCE Rates

Age Group years	N	Mean	SCE	C of V[a]
25-40	77	7.56	0.15	0.39
50-60[b]	32	7.61	0.24	0.45
61-69	54	7.93	0.21	0.45
70-85	30	7.91	0.26	0.45

[a] C of V represents the average coefficient of variation (sd/mean)
[b] The 32 subjects in the 50-60 yr. age group were singletons.

blood counts showed that the absolute lymphocyte count and the % lymphocytes were both significantly negatively correlated with RI. (For example, at the 68 hr timepoint, for absolute lymphocyte count, r= -.26, p<.05; and for % lymphocytes, r= -.35, p<.01). Smoking status and lifetime pack years were also negatively correlated to RI. At the 68 hr. timepoint, for lifetime pack years, r= -.29, p<.01 with current and lifetime heavy smokers having decreased RI relative to non-and light smokers. A similar smoking effect on RI was recently reported by Anderson et al (1988) in their large control population study in the United Kingdom.

Baseline Sister Chromatid Exchange Rates

Baseline SCE rates were determined for 161 twins and an additional 32 singletons (nontwins). SCE rates were based on the scoring of 50 second division metaphase cells (including, whenever possible, 25 cells from each of two replicate cultures). As shown in Table 2, there was no significant age effect for baseline SCE rates over the age range of 25 to 85 years [F(3,184)=0.99; p>.25]. Furthermore, comparison of the coefficients of variation showed no significant age effects, affording no evidence that the older and younger subjects differed with respect to intraindividual (i.e. cell to cell) variability.

Listed in Table 3 are some of the more recently published studies which have addressed the issue of age effects and SCE. As can be readily seen, these investigations differ with respect to the extensiveness of the age ranges studied and the number of subjects evaluated, two factors that influence the potential for demonstrating age effects. In the larger control population studies of Soper et al (1984), Sarto et al (1985) and Husum et al (1986), significant age effects were reported, yet the magnitude of these effects varied considerably. The age effect was small in both the Husum et al and the Soper et al studies (accounting for 0.8% of the total interindividual variation in SCE rates in the latter), whereas for the Sarto et al investigation, age accounted for 18% of the variation. In

Table 3. Studies of Peripheral Blood Lymphocyte SCE Rates
          and In-Vivo Aging[a]

Mean Reference	Age Range[b] (years)	N	Increase in SCE rate with Age?
Schmidt & Sanger '81	0-85	26	–
Goh '81	24-85	45	+
Soper et al '84	18-66	479	+
Das et al '85	1-75	24	+
Sarto et al '85	16-70	88	+
Dutkowski et al '85	23-78	16	+
Nagaya & Toriumi '86	33-58	46	–
Dewdney et al '86	15-54	106	–
Husum et al '86	19-85	553	+
Bender et al '88,'89	1-84	493	–
Present study	25-85	188	–

[a] Only studies including comparisons of early, middle, and/or
    late adulthood are listed. (Studies of newborns vs. adults
    are not included).
[b] Age ranges represent the highest and lowest ages of subjects
    included in these studies; these do not imply continuous or
    equal sampling of all ages included within the ranges.

the present study, age accounted for less than 1% of the
interindividual variance.

    Other factors contributing to individual differences in
baseline SCE in our twin study are depicted in Figure 1. Age
and sex combined, contributed approximately 1% of the total
variance. Similarly, genetic factors were not found to be
significant; the heritability estimate for mean SCE rate was
.046 (±.379). In contrast, smoking and differential blood

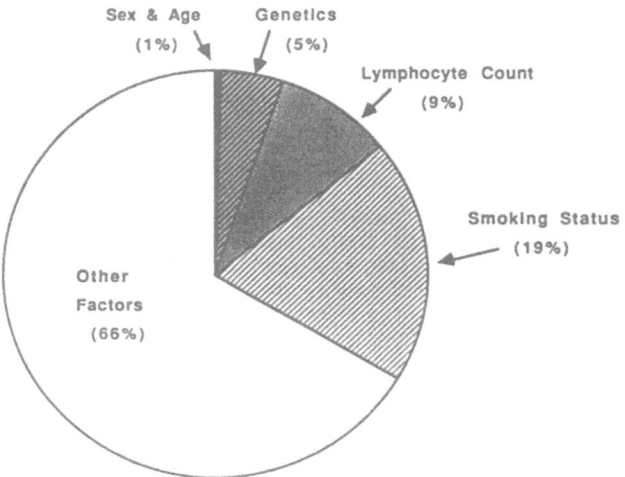

Fig. 1. Decomposition of the interindividual variance in
         baseline SCE

Table 4. Stable Chromosomal Rearrangements as a
          Function of Donor Age

Age Group	(N)	Mean % ($\pm$se) of cells with stable rearrangements[a]
25-40 years	(25)	.44 (.87)
45-60 years	(27)	.86 (1.01)
61-85 years	(26)	2.44 (3.14)

[a] the common 7/14 rearrangements described in the text were
    excluded from this tabulation.

count measures accounted for larger and significant portions of
the variance. Mean SCE rate was found to correlate .28 (p=.02)
and .30 (p=.01) with subjects' total white blood counts and
absolute lymphocyte counts, respectively. The former is in
good agreement with the results of the Bender et al study
(1988) in which a correlation of .32 was reported for total
white blood count and mean SCE rate.

Smoking remains as the single environmental/lifestyle factor
accounting for the largest portion (19%) of the observed
variance. Currents smokers had a mean SCE rate of 9.54
(sd=1.95) compared to 7.82 for ex-smokers (sd=1.38) and 7.56
(sd=1.06) for nonsmokers.

As illustrated in Figure 1, 66% of the variance still
remains unaccounted for. Additional analyses of environmental,
lifestyle, medical, and clinical laboratory findings using the
discordant MZ twin method are in progress to identify and
evaluate other factors affecting baseline SCE.

Chromosomal Rearrangements

Chromosomal aberrations have generally been divided into two
classes: unstable and stable (Carrano and Natarajan, 1988).
The former include aberrations such as rings, dicentrics,
acentric fragments, and radial figures, which would not be
expected to persist through successive cell divisions after
their formation. In contrast are the stable rearrangements,
including such aberrations as translocations and inversions
which can persist through many cell generations. From the
earlier studies of individuals accidentally or therapeutically
exposed to X-rays, it has been shown that stable rearrangements
can persist in-vivo in peripheral blood lymphocytes for years
after their induction (Ohtaki et al., 1982; Buckton et al.,
1987). Similarly, it has been shown that patients treated with
radiation followed by maintenance chemotherapy will manifest
elevated frequencies of stable chromosomal rearrangements in
their peripheral blood years after the cessation of therapy
(Robison et al., 1982). Thus, for addressing the question of
whether or not in-vivo aging is accompanied by an increase in
chromosomal aberrations, the enumeration of the frequencies of
stable rearrangements would appear most valuable, as these

provide a means for measuring an accumulation of lesions over long periods of time. Despite this fact, although numerous studies of unstable chromosomal rearrangements in aging have been conducted (for review, see Tice and Setlow, 1985), there are, to date, no large published studies of G-banded chromosomes in the aged, which would permit all types of stable rearrangements to be evaluated.

In the present study, stable chromosomal rearrangements are evaluated in G-banded metaphase cells harvested at 72 hours. Slides are G-banded with Wright stain using a modification of the method of Sanchez et al (1973). For each subject, 100 G-banded metaphase cells are completely analyzed (i.e. karyotyped under the microscope). All aberrations are described according to the ISCN 1985. All breakpoints involved in these aberrations are checked against Human Gene Mapping 9 (1987) to determine if they represent rare heritable or common fragile sites. (For comparison, chromosomal aberrations including unstable rearrangements are also scored in 48 hr. cultures; these data will be described elsewhere).

In addition to determining whether or not there is an overall increase in the frequency of stable chromosomal rearrangements in the aged, it is also of interest to determine whether or not there are any specific recurring abnormalities. Certain rearrangements have been well documented to recur in phytohemagglutin-stimulated peripheral blood lymphocytes. These include a paracentric inversion of chromosome #14 [inv (14)(q11q32)] and reciprocal translocations involving chromosomes #7 and #14 [e.g. t(7;14)(p13;q11)] (Welch and Lee, 1975; Zech and Haglund, 1978; Petersson and Mitelman, 1985; and Tawn, 1988). These specific rearrangements involve breakpoints in G-bands where the T-cell antigen receptor genes have been mapped, and it has recently been suggested that these rearrangements represent the physical correlates of human chimeric antigen receptor genes (Tycko et al, 1989). Thus, in enumerating stable rearrangements, these 7/14 abnormalities were tabulated separately.

As shown in Table 4, stable chromosomal rearrangements clearly increase with age over the range of 25 to 85 years. Among the 25-40 year olds, 24% of individuals had one or more cells with such structural aberrations, among the 45-60 year olds, 50%, and within the 61-85 year olds, 80.8%. A Chi-Square analysis of these proportions yielded a X^2 on 2 degrees of freedom of 16.6 (p<.001).

The karyotypic abnormalities detected were different in each cell; no clonal abnormality within an individual or specific recurring abnormality between individuals was found. Future investigations will include examination of the distribution of breakpoints involved in these rearrangements, and of the genetic and environmental factors contributing to the observed interindividual variability within age groups.

4NQO- Induced SCE Rates

One of the primary objectives of the twin study was to determine not only whether baseline levels of chromosomal damage were increased in the aged, but also whether or not

Table 5.   4NQO Induced SCE Rates as a Function of Donor Age

Age Group	N	Mean SCE (±se)
25-40 years	(51)	16.61 (±0.34)
61-85 years	(40)	18.41 (±0.50)

t=5.27 (df=89), p<.001

there was increased damage after <u>in-vitro</u> mutagen treatments as a function of age. Such increased sensitivity could result from a number of different factors including alteration of chromatin structure with age, decreased DNA repair efficacy, or alteration in drug metabolism. In order to determine whether or not there is differential sensitivity of aged cells to different types of DNA damaging agents, four mutagen treatments (X-ray, MMC, 4NQO, and MNNG) are being evaluated. As an example, some of the relevant data on 4NQO-induced SCE are presented below.

As can be seen in Table 5, there is a significant increase in the mean frequency of 4NQO-induced SCE in the lymphocytes of twins aged 61-85 years compared to those in the 25-40 year age group. Thus, it appears that cells from aged individuals are more sensitive to the DNA-damaging effects of 4NQO than are cells from younger individuals. Future experiments will determine whether or not this elevation reflects either increased levels of damage initially induced or decreased levels of repair.

To date, the genetic analyses have been limited to the younger twin group. As depicted in Figure 2, unlike baseline SCE, genetic factors account for the major portion of the variance in 4NQO-induced SCE. Such data help direct future investigations aimed at understanding the mechanisms underlying SCE induction, by arguing for in-depth study of factors also likely to be under genetic control.

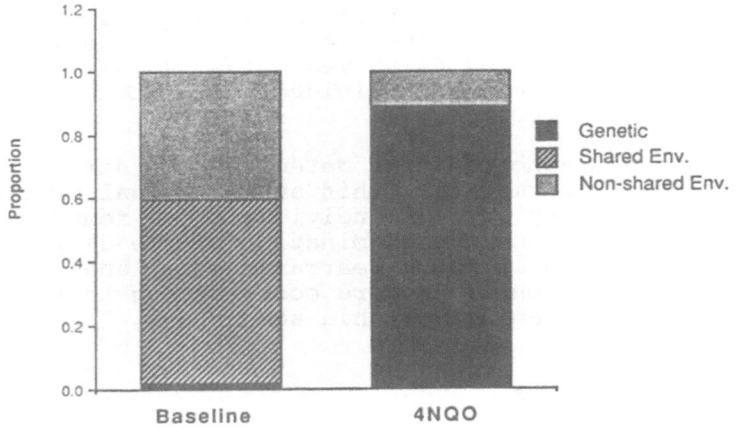

Fig. 2.   Proportions of variance in mean SCE rates accounted for by genetic and environmental factors

CONCLUSIONS

The twin study method has provided a unique paradigm for investigating the effects of genetic and nongenetic factors on aging processes and on the induction and accumulation of chromosomal damage. The cytogenetic measures of replication index, sister chromatid exchange, and chromosomal rearrangement differ markedly in both their relationships to _in-vivo_ aging and to genetic and specific nongenetic (e.g.environmental / lifestyle) factors. The twin analyses have served not only to identify these salient characteristics but also to help direct future investigations aimed at gaining further understanding of individual differences in aging and of mechanisms giving rise to chromosomal damage.

Anderson, D., Jenkinson, P. C., Dewdney, R. S., Francis, A. J., Godbert, P., and Butterworth, K. R., 1988, Chromosome aberrations, mitogen-induced blastogenesis and proliferative rate index in peripheral lymphocytes from 106 control individuals of the U.K. population, _Mutation Research_, 204:407.

Berg, K., 1981, Twin research in coronary heart disease, _in_: "Twin Research 3: Epidemiological and Clinical Studies," Alan Liss Inc., N.Y.

Bender, M. A., Preston, R. J., Leonard, R. C., Pyatt, B. E., Gooch, P. C., and Shelby, M. D., 1988, Chromosomal aberrations and sister-chromatid exchange frequencies in peripheral blood lymphocytes of a large human population sample, _Mutation Research_, 204:421.

Bender, M. A., Preston, R. J., Leonard, R. C., Pyatt, B. E., and Gooch, P. C., 1989, Chromosomal aberrations and sister chromatid exchange frequencies in peripheral blood lymphocytes of a large human population sample. II. Extension of age range, _Mutation Research_, 212:149.

Buckton, K. E., Hamilton, G. E., Paton, L., and Langlands, A. O., 1978, Chromosome aberrations in irradiated ankylosing spondylitis patients, _in_: "Mutagen-Induced Chromosome Damage in Man, H. J. Evans, and D. C. Lloyd, eds., Yale University Press, New Haven.

Carrano, A. V., and Natarajan, A. T., 1988, ICPEMC Publication No. 14. Considerations for population monitoring using cytogenetic techniques, _Mutation Research_, 204:379.

Das, B. C., Rani, R., Mitra, A. B., and Luthra, U. K., 1985, Baseline frequency of sister-chromatid exchanges (SCE) in newborn lymphocytes and its relationship to in-vivo aging in humans, _Mutation Research_, 144:85.

Dewdney, R. S., Lovell, D. P., Jenkinson, P. C., and Anderson, D., 1986, Variation in sister-chromatid exchange among 106 members of the general U.K. population, _Mutation Research_, 171:43.

Dutkowski, R. T., Lesh, R., Staiano-Coico, L., Thaler, H., Darlington, G. J., and Weksler, M. E., 1985, Increased chromosomal instability in lymphocytes from elderly humans, _Mutation Research_, 149:505.

Gensler, H. L., and Bernstein, H., 1981, DNA damage as the primary cause of aging, _The Quarterly Review of Biology_, 56:279.

Goh, K., 1981, Sister-chromatid-exchange in the aging population, _Journal of Medicine_, 12:195.

Gottesman, I. I., and Shields, J., 1977, Twin studies and schizophrenia, a decade later, in: "Contributions to the Psychopathology of Schizophrenia", B.A. Maher, ed., Academic Press, N.Y.

Husum, B., Wulf, H. C., and Niebuhr, E., 1986, Sister chromatid exchange frequency correlates with age, sex and cigarette smoking in a 5-year material of 553 healthy adults, Hereditas, 105:17.

Human Gene Mapping 9: Paris Conference (1987) Ninth International Workshop on Human Gene Mapping. Cytogenetics and Cell Genetics, 49:Nos. 1-4.

ISCN 1985: An International System for Human Cytogenetic Nomenclature, S. Karger, Basel and New York.

Kirkwood, T. B. L., 1989, DNA, mutations, and aging, Mutation Research, 219:1.

Lewiter, F. I., Tager, I. B., McGue, M., Tishler, P. V., and Speizer, F. E., 1984, Genetic and environmental determinants of level of pulmonary functioning, American Journal of Epidemiology, 120:518.

Murasko, D. M., Weiner, P., and Kaye, D., 1987, Decline in mitogen induced proliferation of lymphocytes with increasing age, Clinical and Experimental Immunology, 70:440.

Nagaya, T., and Toriumi, H., 1986, Spontaneous and induced sister chromatid exchanges in lymphocytes of healthy persons, Environmental Research, 40:181.

Ohtaki, K., Shimba, H., Awa, A. A., and Sofuni, T., 1982, Comparison of type and frequency of chromosome aberrations by conventional and G-staining methods in Hiroshima atomic bomb survivors, Journal of Radiation Research, 23:441.

Petersson, H., and Mitelman, F., 1985, Nonrandom de novo chromosome aberrations in human lymphocytes and amniotic cells, Hereditas, 102:33.

Robison, L. L., Arthur, D. C., Ball, D. W., Danzl, T. J., and Nesbit, M. E., 1982, Cytogenetic studies of long-term survivors of childhood acute lymphoblastic leukemia, Cancer Research, 42:4289.

Sanchez, O., Escobar, J. I., Yunis, J. J., 1973, A simple G-banding technique, Lancet, I:7823:269.

Sarto, F., Faccioli, M. C., Cominato, I., and Levis, A. G., 1985, Aging and smoking increase the frequency of sister-chromatid exchanges (SCE) in man, Mutation Research, 144:183.

Schmidt, M. A., and Sanger, W. G., 1981, Sister chromatid exchange in aged human lymphocytes. A brief note; Mechanisms of Aging and Development, 16:67.

Schneider, E. L., 1985, Cytogenetics of aging, in: "Handbook of the Biology of Aging. 2nd Edition", C. E. Finch, and E. D. Schneider, eds., Van Nostrand Reinhold, N.Y.

Soper, K. A., Stolley, P. D., Galloway, S. M., Smith, J. G., Nochols, W. W., and Wolman, S. R., 1984, Sister-chromatid exchange (SCE) report on control subjects in a study of occupationally exposed workers, Mutation Research, 129:77.

Tawn, E. J., 1988, The non-random occurrence of exchanges involving chromosomes 7 and 14 in human lymphocytes: A prospective study of control individuals, Mutation Research, 199:215.

Tice, R., Thorne, P., and Schneider, E. L., 1979, BISACK analysis of the phytohaemagglutinin-induced proliferation of human peripheral lymphocytes, Cell Tissue Kinetics, 12:1.

Tice, R. R., and Setlow, R. B., 1985, DNA repair and replication in aging organisms and cells, in: "Handbook of the Biology of Aging. 2nd Edition", C. E. Finch, and E. L. Schneider, eds., Van Nostrand Reinhold, N.Y.

Tice, R. R., Schneider, E. L., Kram, D., and Thorne, P., 1979, Cytokinetic analysis of the impaired proliferative response of peripheral lymphocytes from aged humans to phytohemagglutinin, Journal of Experimental Medicine, 00:1029.

Tycko, B., Palmer, J. D., and Sklar, J., 1989, T-cell receptor gene trans-rearrangements: Chimeric γ-δ genes in normal lymphoid tissues, Science, 245:1242.

Welch, J. P., and Lee, C. L. Y., 1975, Non-random occurrence of 7-14 translocations in human lymphocyte cultures, Nature, 255:241.

Zakharov, A. F., Davudov, A. Z., Benjush, V. A., and Egolina, N. A., 1982, Genetic determination of NOR activity in human lymphocytes from twins, Human Genetics, 60:24.

STUDIES OF DNA ALTERATIONS IN IN VIVO SOMATIC CELL MUTATIONS IN HUMANS

Richard J. Albertini, Janice A. Nicklas
and J. Patrick O'Neill

VRCC-Genetics Laboratory, University of Vermont
32 N. Prospect St., Burlington, VT, 05401

INTRODUCTION

Gene mutations that arise in vivo in humans are now amenable to study. One method involves the direct cloning in vitro of T-lymphocytes that have undergone mutations in vivo of the X-chromosomal gene for hypoxanthine-guanine phosphoribosyltransferase (hprt) (Albertini et al., 1982; Morley et al., 1983, O'Neill et al., 1987; O'Neill et al., 1989). This method, called the T-cell cloning assay, permits recovery of the mutant clones for further characterization. Therefore, in addition to quantitating in vivo mutant frequencies, "mutational spectra" can be defined, at least for hprt. This paper summarizes results of recent studies in our laboratory that have characterized in vivo hprt T-cell mutations for normal young adults, normal newborns, and individuals exposed to total body ionizing irradiations delivered by internal gamma emitters.

METHOD OF T-CELL CLONING ASSAY

The method of assay has been described in detail elsewhere (Albertini et al., 1982; O'Neill et al., 1987; O'Neill et al., 1989). Briefly, it involves obtaining a sample of blood, usually 30 to 60 ml., in a heparinized container. The mononuclear cell (MNC) fraction, which contains the T-lymphocytes, is separated by density gradient centrifugation. This fraction is removed by Pasteur pipette, washed, suspended in appropriate medium, and the MNC are counted. At this point, the cells may be cryopreserved in dimethyl sulfoxide (DMSO) and stored in liquid nitrogen for later study, or assayed directly.

Assay involves "activating" the T-cells by stimulating with a polyclonal activator such as phytohemagglutinin (PHA). This serves to induce the T-cells to express surface interleukin-2 (IL-2) receptors. Activation is for approximately 40 hours only, so that cell division does not occur, and hprt mutations are not induced in vitro. (More recent assays have incorporated this "activation" step directly in the assay procedure itself, which gives equivalent results if PHA is incorporated in the culture medium and a sufficiently potent source of IL-2 is used.) Following this, the activated cells are washed, counted, and appropriately diluted for inoculation into the microtiter wells used in the assay.

DNA Damage and Repair in Human Tissues
Edited by B. M. Sutherland and A. D. Woodhead
Plenum Press, New York, 1990

315

The cloning assay requires that T-cells be cultured in appropriate medium (RPMI medium containing medium HL-1 (Ventrex) at 20% final v:v), supplemented by fetal calf serum, usually at 5-10% and a source of IL-2 at optimum concentration determined by experiment. (We currently use the supernatant obtained after ex vivo activation of "lymphokine-activated killer" (LAK) cells in a tumor immunotherapy program as a source of IL-2.) In addition, cloning and culture of T-lymphocytes in vitro require an X-irradiated feeder cell. We use an hprt deficient B-lymphoblastoid line (TK-6) given 8000 rad gamma irradiation at 5×10^3 per microtiter well.

Microtiter cells are inoculated with one, two, five, or ten activated test MNC in 0.2 ml volumes, containing the above constituents, in the absence of 6-thioguanine (TG), or 10^4 or 2×10^4 activated MNC in 10^{-5} M TG. TG serves to select the TG resistant hprt deficient T-cells. One or more 96-well micro-titer plate is inoculated at each MNC density in the absence of TG, and five to ten plates are inoculated at the higher cell densities in TG.

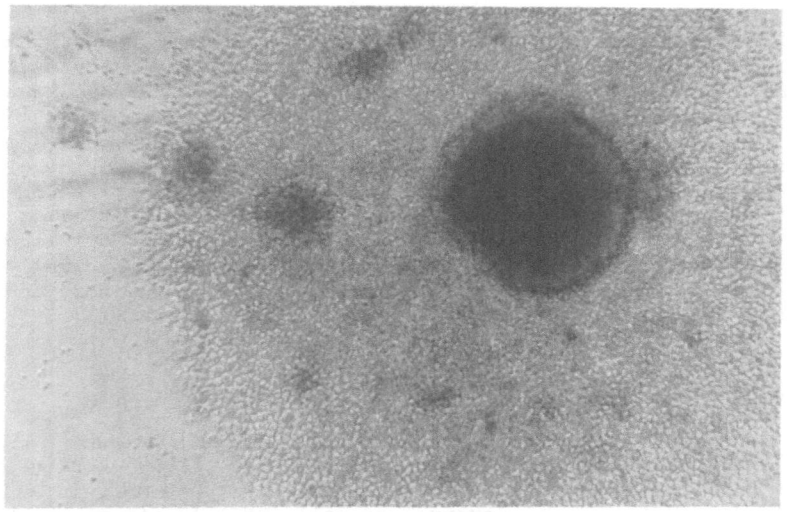

Fig. 1. Photograph of a growing T-cell clone in the well of a 96-well plate.

Plates are cultured from 8 to 14 days, and wells are scored for growing clones by microscopic inspection. Cloning efficiencies (CE) in the absence or presence of TG are calculated from the Poisson relationship; $P_o = e^{-x}$, where "x" is the average number of growing cells per well. "x", divided by the inoculum size, yields the CE. The mutant frequency (Mf) is ratio of the CE in TG to the CE without TG.

"Positive" wells have from 2×10^4 to 10^5 growing cells (Fig. 1). These are picked, transferred to larger culture vessels containing the above constituents, and propagated by successive sub-culturing to populations of sufficient size for characterizations.

316

QUANTITATIVE RESULTS AND PHENOTYPING

In a recent study, cumulative Mf values (mean ± SD) for 115 assays of 27 individuals, ages ~ 20-35 years, were 6.5 (± 4.8) x 10^{-6} (Albertini et al., 1988). Most normal young adults have "background" Mf values between 10^{-5} and 10^{-6}. There is an age effect however, with progressive elevations in "background" Mf values with advancing age. This has been most clearly shown by Cole et al (Cole et al., 1988). Our finding in 84 individuals, ages 33 to 80 years, in a twin study of a mean value (± SD) of 16.0 (± 9.2) x 10^{-6} agrees with this. By contrast, "background" Mf values in newborn placental-cord blood samples, reflecting mutations arising in vivo in the fetus, are 10-fold lower (McGinniss et al., 1989a). Assays of 45 newborns yielded a mean (± SD) Mf value of 0.6 (± 0.4) x 10^{-6}. Individuals exposed to a variety of mutagens show elevated Mf values. For example, adult cancer patients receiving total body ionizing irradiation from an internal emitter (radioimmunoglobulin therapy) show decidedly elevated hprt T-cell Mf values, as compared to controls.

Mutant isolates from normal adults and newborns have been characterized at the phenotypic level. Whenever tested, the TG resistant T-cells isolated from blood have maintained their resistance in vitro in the absence of selection (Albertini et al., 1982; McGinniss et al., 1989a). Also, whenever studied, the TG resistant T-cells isolated have been deficient in HPRT enzyme activity (Albertini et al., 1982; McGinniss et al., 1989a). Most of the mutant (and wild type) T-cell clones recovered from cloning assays have been of the helper/inducer (CD4) phenotype, although some cytotoxic/suppressor (CD8) clones have been isolated (Albertini et al., 1982, 1985; Nicklas et al., 1988). This seems to indicate that the conditions of cloning that we use favor growth of the CD4 cells.

MOLECULAR ANALYSES OF hprt MUTANT T-CELL CLONES

General Scheme for Studying T-Cell Isolates

T-cell clones growing in microtiter wells containing TG are subcultured to larger culture vessels. Cells are then progressively subcultured in medium containing serum, PHA, a source of IL-2 and X-irradiated feeder cells. TG is included for the first subculture only. Cells are grown to 2 x 10^7 to 10^8, and either studied directly, or cryopreserved in liquid nitrogen for later analyses.

All studies begin with Southern blot analysis. DNA is extracted by standard methods, digested with restriction enzymes (usually Pst I, Hind III and/or Bam HI), electrophoresed on agarose gels to size separate DNA fragments, and transferred to nitrocellulose filters. Filters are hybridized initially with full or partial length hprt probes. After reading of blots, the radioactivity is removed by appropriate washing, and the filters are rehybridized with T-cell receptor (TCR) gene probes. This may be repeated several times if it is necessary to study the rearrangement patterns of several TCR genes. Figure 2 shows the same filter after successive hybridizations, first with a hprt probe, then with TCR β gene probe.

The Southern blot analyses identify those mutant isolates in which gross structural alterations of hprt have occurred. Further study of the remainder involves extraction of mRNA, synthesis of mutant hprt cDNA, the polymerase chain reaction for amplification, and sequencing. These studies are being done on mutants isolated in our laboratory by L. Recio and T. R. Skopek of CIIT, Research Triangle Park, N.C.

The results of these studies provide information regarding the molecular basis of the <u>hprt</u> mutations, and the TCR gene rearrangement patterns that are found in all of the mutant isolates. As described below, this allows inferences to be made regarding the frequencies of <u>in vivo</u> mutational events that gave rise to the mutants, and the differentiation stage of T-cells at which <u>hprt</u> mutation is likely to occur.

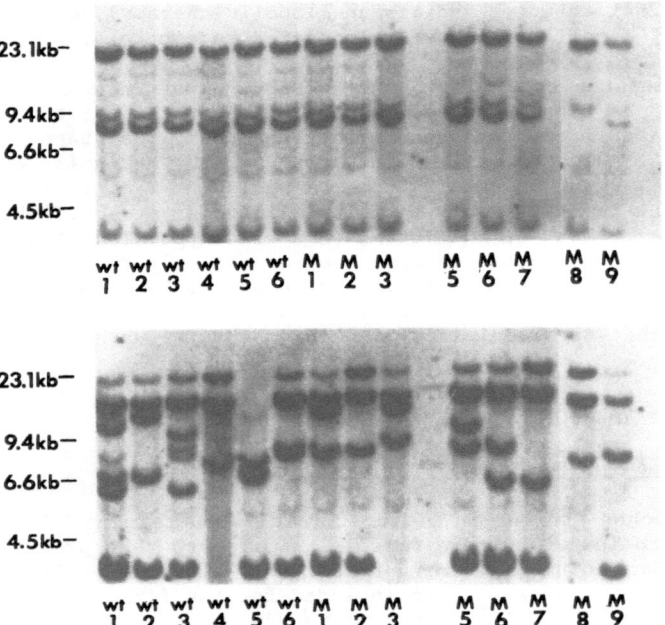

Fig. 2. HindIII Southern blots of 6 wild type and 9 <u>hprt</u> mutant clones. (top) <u>hprt</u> probe. Mutant 7 shows a new fragment of 7.4kb and mutant 8 has a deletion of the exon 2+3 fragment (7.0kb). (bottom) Same filter using a T-cell receptor β gene probe. This demonstrates a variety of TCR gene rearrangement patterns.

An attempt is made in any large cloning assay to isolate, propagate and characterize as many <u>hprt</u> mutant clones as possible. Approximately 50% of the clones can be successfully carried to the numbers needed for these studies. A large number of wild-type clones is also studied for comparisons.

hprt Changes in T-Cell Mutants

Approximately 15% of the _hprt_ mutant isolates from normal young adults show gross structural alterations of the gene as detected on the Southern blots (Albertini et al., 1985, Nicklas et al., 1987, 1989a). These alterations consist of simple deletions and more complex rearrangements. Sequence studies of the remaining 85% of mutants are revealing a variety of changes, including base substitutions (transitions and transversions), single base loses and gains, microdeletions, frameshifts, and apparent splice site mutations with exon losses in the cDNA (but not in the genomic DNA as revealed on Southern blots) (Nicklas et al., 1988b).

Analyses of the mutant isolates from new-born placental cord blood samples have revealed a strikingly different pattern of _in vivo_ _hprt_ mutations (McGinniss et al., 1989b). These isolates reflect _in vivo_ mutations that occurred during fetal development. Southern blot analyses show that 85% of mutants have structural alterations of _hprt_ (compared to 15% for adults). Furthermore, these structural alterations show a predelection for deletions involving exons 2 and 3. We have not yet begun sequence analyses for the remaining 15% of mutant isolates from cord blood.

"Induced" _in vivo_ _hprt_ mutations in T-lymphocytes are also being studied by these methods. Analyses of the T-cell mutants recovered from radioimmunotherapy patients by Southern blots show that approximately 35% have structural alterations of _hprt_.

TCR Gene Rearrangement Patterns in T-Cell Mutants

The above paragraphs give a description of the _hprt_ changes at the DNA level that occur in populations of T-cell mutants. This information may be used for describing _in vivo_ _hprt_ mutational spectra for "background" and "induced" mutations. However, a mutational spectrum is a description of the frequencies of specific mutations (defined as specific molecular changes) in a population of mutations. In order to use the above data for such a description, the number of mutations represented by the population of mutants must be known. Estimating the number of mutations is accomplished by characterizing the TCR gene rearrangement patterns in the mutants as markers of their _in vivo_ clonal independence. In addition to quantifying mutational events, this analysis allows definition of the _in vivo_ T-cell differentiation stage at which the _hprt_ mutational events most likely occurred.

Rationale For Using TCR Gene Rearrangement Patterns. One characteristic of the _in vivo_ T-lymphocyte population is its enormous heterogeneity. This heterogeneity has many levels, but, at the extreme, it is seen in the specific antigen reactivity of T-cells. Vast numbers of different molecular moieties can be recognized as "foreign" by the T-cell system. Each foreign molecular moiety is recognized by a specific T-cell, or clone of T-cells. Recognition is through a specific antigen receptor, called the T-cell receptor (TCR) on the cell's surface.

The human TCR is a dimeric protein composed of alpha and beta chains, or gamma and delta chains. This dimeric protein is structurally unique for each antigen reactive cell or clone of cells. Diversity is generated at the somatic level.

The TCRs are encoded by TCR genes. There are two TCR genes on chromosome 7, i.e. β and γ and two TCR genes on chromosome 14, i.e. α and delta. TCR genes, like those for immunoglobulins, contain constant (C), variable (V), diversity (D) and joining (J) segments which undergo DNA rearrangement during T-cell differentiation in the thymus to generate the diversity seen in the T-cell repertoire, i.e. ~ 10^7 different TCRs. TCR gene rearrangements occur in the thymus during the functional life of that organ, i.e. during fetal life, childhood, and adolescence, after which the organ regresses. Once rearranged, the unique TCR gene rearrangement pattern marks the T-cell and its clonal descendants. TCR gene patterns are easily observed on Southern blots.

This vast heterogeneity of TCR gene patterns can be used to define the in vivo independence of hprt mutant isolates, and the differentiation stage in vivo at which the mutations occurred, by comparing the TCR gene rearrangement pattern and the hprt molecular change of each mutant (and wild type) isolate with those of all other isolates from the same individual.

The analysis is as follows. If two or more isolates share the same TCR gene rearrangement pattern, they are descendants of the same mature, post-thymic T-cell precursor. If, in addition, these two or more isolates are mutants, and show the identical change at hprt, they are "sibling" non-independent mutants that derived from the same in vivo mutational event. These two or more mutants therefore, represent only one mutation. On the other hand, these two or more isolates that share the same TCR gene rearrangement pattern may, if they are mutants, show different changes at hprt. They then represent two or more independent in vivo hprt mutations that occurred in the same post-thymic T-cell clone, the number determined from the number of different hprt changes. Also, this pattern of TCR and hprt alterations in a group of isolates localizes the in vivo mutational event to post-thymic cells, i.e. to cells after their TCR gene rearrangement has occurred.

Another possible combination of TCR gene rearrangement pattern and hprt change in mutants is that two or more isolates differ by both their TCR gene rearrangement patterns and their hprt alterations. This occurrence indicates that each mutant represents an independent mutational event, probably occurring in an independent in vivo post-thymic clone, with the number of in vivo mutations being equivalent to the number of mutants. Finally, the TCR gene rearrangement patterns of two or more mutant isolates may be different, but their hprt change identical. This pattern can signify pre- or intra-thymic in vivo mutation where the hprt event occurred in a cell before it had undergone maturation and TCR gene rearrangement. All of the mutants in such a group have derived from one in vivo mutation. However, this particular combined TCR gene-hprt pattern can have another interpretation. The in vivo hprt mutations could be occurring independently in post-thymic T-cells, but the specific hprt change could represent a "hot-spot". Such repetitive mutations, describing a "hot-spot" for specific change, might be expected if due to a specific environmental mutagen, i.e. a chemical.

The alternative interpretations of the combined TCR gene-hprt pattern just discussed, i.e. different TCR gene rearrangements in a group of mutants showing the same hprt change, can be resolved if hprt mutational changes are compared among individuals. True mutational "hot-spots" should be observed in many individuals, where pre- or intra-thymic hprt mutational events should be different in different individuals.

In Vivo Differentiation Stage for hprt Mutation. Because interpretation of combined TCR gene-hprt patterns requires knowledge of the differentiation stage at which in vivo mutational events occur, this is considered first. In normal young adults, there are frequent examples of two or more mutant isolates from the same individual showing different mutational changes at hprt, but the same TCR gene rearrangement pattern

320

(Nicklas et al., 1989a). This clearly indicates post-thymic mutation. Furthermore, there are examples of two or more isolates consisting of a wild type and one or more mutants that show identical TCR gene rearrangement patterns. This too supports the thesis of post-thymic hprt mutation in adults by demonstrating the isolation of two classes of cells, based on their hprt genotypes, from the same in vivo post-thymic T-cell clone, i.e., those that have, and those that have not undergone mutation of hprt. In adults then, post-thymic mutation at hprt is the norm.

The hprt mutant isolates obtained from newborn placental-cord blood show the contrasting pattern (McGinniss et al., 1989b). Here, we have frequent instances of two or more mutants sharing their hprt mutational change, but differing by their TCR gene rearrangement pattern. The specific hprt change however, often differs from newborn to newborn, indicating that these "background" mutations in the fetus are not arising in "hot-spots". This combined TCR gene-hprt pattern is characteristic for newborns, indicating that pre-thymic (or intra-thymic) hprt mutations are common in the fetus.

Our data to date indicate that there are exceptions to both of the above generalizations regarding in vivo differentiation stage of hprt mutations. There are infrequent instances of combined TCR gene-hprt pattern in adults that are best explained by pre-thymic mutation (e.g. see below). Also, post-thymic mutations occur in the fetus as reflected in cord blood isolates. Nonetheless, the general conclusion is that post thymic hprt mutations are the usual mutations in adults, and pre-thymic mutations are frequent in the fetus.

In Vivo Clonality of hprt Mutants as Revealed by TCR Gene Patterns. Southern blot analysis using TCR gene probes has been accomplished for hundreds of wild type and hprt mutant isolates from normal adults, from adults with disease conditions associated with in vivo T-cell proliferation, from normal newborns, and from adults receiving total body ionizing radiations. These results are summarized here.

One remarkable observation in all of these studies is the enormous heterogeneity of TCR gene rearrangements within and between individuals. Essentially, each wild type isolate from a given individual has been unique among all of the wild type isolates from that person. That is, there has been no TCR gene pattern sharing among the wild type isolates from any individual. This result is in marked contrast to the findings for hprt mutant isolates, where TCR gene pattern sharing among mutants from an individual is not unusual. Clearly, the "background" mutants are drawn from a different, probably smaller, in vivo T-lymphocyte population than are the wild type isolates.

This fact is illustrated by a recently reported study of TCR gene rearrangements in 326 hprt mutant isolates from three normal young men (Nicklas et al., 1989a). Here, only 90% of the mutant isolates showed unique TCR gene patterns. Although hprt studies are not yet complete, our current results suggest that the 90% resulted from independent in vivo mutations in post-thymic T-cells, with one possible exception. The exception involves an hprt mutation that was due to an exon 2-3 deletion as seen in six separate mutant isolates from a single individual. (The same change that characterizes mutants from placental-cord blood samples.) Four of the six isolates share their TCR β and γ gene rearrangement patterns. By definition, these four are post-thymic hprt "sibling" mutants. The remaining two of the group share their TCR β gene pattern, which is different from that of the "foursome" just described. This pair, however, differ in their TCR γ gene pattern. The most conservative interpretation of this group of six mutants is that two in vivo hprt mutations were involved, at least one of which probably occurred pre- or intra-thymically.

The 10% of mutant isolates that showed a sharing of their TCR gene rearrangement patterns were mostly represented by pairs, although there were some triplets and quadruplets. In one of these three individuals, however, nine independent mutant isolates, obtained over several blood drawings, showed identical TCR gene rearrangement patterns. These isolates represent 10% of the mutants recovered from this individual. This clearly is a case of repetitive isolation of mutants deriving from the same in vivo mutational event, as evidenced by sequencing of the hprt gene in these mutants. The same hprt change is seen in all nine isolates. This in vivo mutant clone has persisted in this individual for more than two years.

If 90% of the hprt mutant isolates derive from independent in vivo hprt mutations, the error in estimating the frequencies of mutations from the frequencies of mutants is not great. This probably will be the case for normal young adults with essentially "normal mutant frequency values". However, such estimations must be made cautiously. This is best illustrated in the case of "outliers", i.e., individuals with high mutant frequency values without correspondingly elevated mutation frequencies.

Outliers. An apparently normal woman, 35 years of age, has shown a progressive rise in her hprt T-cell mutant frequency value over four years (Nicklas et al., 1988). This value has risen to ~ 700 x 10^{-6}. Several hundred of the mutant and wild type isolates from this individual have been studied at the molecular level (Nicklas et al., 1988). Approximately 99% of the mutant isolates share the identical TCR gene rearrangement pattern indicating that they arose in vivo in the same expanding T-lymphocyte clone. Clearly, in this otherwise normal woman, the extremely high mutant frequency does not correspond to a high mutation frequency. Any judgments concerning environmental genotoxicity, or attempts to define mutational spectrum, made without this realization, will be hopelessly confounded.

A cloning assay in a patient with the disease chronic active hepatitis, gave a mutant frequency value of 69.5 x 10^{-6}. The patient was taking the immunosuppressive drug azathioprine, which is metabolized in vivo to 6-mercaptopurine and will select for hprt deficient cells. Therefore, the elevated mutant frequency value is not unexpected. However, molecular analyses of three wild type and 32 hprt mutant isolates revealed that only 12 of the mutants had unique TCR gene rearrangement patterns. In addition, there were two pairs and one triplet, where two and three isolates, respectively, shared their TCR β and γ gene rearrangements. Of more significance, 13 of the 32 mutant isolates (~ 40%) shared the same TCR β and γ gene pattern. (Studies to date have been with Hind III digests only, but usually two TCR gene identity in patients with this disorder persist when the DNA is studied following digestion with a second restriction enzyme.)

A woman with ovarian cancer undergoing experimental IL-2/LAK intraperitoneal therapy was studied by cloning assay for hprt mutant T-lymphocytes in the leukopheresis cell population. The hprt T-cell mutant frequency value was > 50 x 10^{-6}. Five of 13 hprt mutant isolates studies showed identical TCR β and γ gene rearrangement patterns in both Hind III and Bam HI digests. Here again, ~ 38% of the hprt mutants arose in the same in vivo expanding post-thymic T-cell clone, and most likely represent "sibling" hprt mutants.

A patient with an early stage of the T-cell malignant condition known as mycosis fungoides was studied as a "positive control" for the normal woman presented first in this series of "outliers". The malignancy in this patient was thought to be confined to the skin. Nonetheless, the mutant frequency value determined by cloning assay was ~ 80 x 10^{-6}. Approximately 40% of the hprt mutant isolates studied showed the identical TCR gene rearrangement pattern, consistent with the presence of a large population of "sibling" post-thymic hprt mutants.

These four "outliers" represent a range of medical conditions, from "normal", to patients with autoimmune disorders, to patients with solid tumors, to patients with malignancies of the same cell type, i.e. the T-lymphocyte, that is studied in the cloning assay. Other examples could be presented, but this small sample of "outliers" illustrates certain features. First, one process that is occurring in all of these individuals is apparent in vivo clonal amplification of one or more T-lymphocyte clones. This must be achieved by unremitting cell division in one or more clones of post-thymic T-cells, a population of cells whose usual in vivo state is quiescence in an arrested G_0 stage. The patients have disorders known to be associated with in vivo T-cell proliferation. Second, a feature that these four "outliers" have in common is a high mutant frequency. Finally, the individual receiving the drug azathioprine illustrates the importance of in vivo selection, in this case positive selection for hprt mutant T-cells, in determining the frequency of these mutant cells and their in vivo clonality.

hprt Mutational Spectra for in vivo Arising T-Cell Mutants

Given the above information, hprt mutational spectra can be defined, at least for adults where the predominant stage of mutation is the post-thymic T-cell. As noted, for normal young adults with "normal" mutant frequency values, approximately 90% of the mutant isolates arise from independent in vivo hprt mutations. Therefore, the observation, given above, of 15% of "background" mutant isolates showing gross structural alterations of the hprt gene is approximately true also for the underlying "background" mutations, i.e. 15% of the mutations involve such changes in the gene. However, precise knowledge of the numbers of mutations represented by the material under study is important for defining where breakpoints occur and for allowing conclusions regarding breakpoint frequencies.

The hprt mutations can be subdivided into subgroups that do or do not show gross changes of hprt. (Information on mutations comes from the hprt molecular data obtained for the mutant isolates, "corrected" by the clonality data defined by TCR gene patterns.) A recently reported study analyzed the subgroup of hprt mutations in the three normal young men mentioned above that involved deletions in order to define their breakpoint distribution patterns (Nicklas et al., 1989a). Breakpoints may be designated as occurring in hprt introns, or in the 5' or 3' flanking regions for those deletions that extend beyond the gene. Table 1 gives these breakpoint distributions with the hprt gene being divided into three approximately equal sized pieces.

Figure 3 shows that these breakpoints are distributed evenly along the length of hprt, suggesting that there is no "hot-spot" for this type of mutation. Based on this even distribution and the total number of breaks that lie within the gene (25/55), the approximate size of deletions that extend into hprt flanking regions can be calculated. This calculation assumes that the frequency of extragenic breakage events per kb of DNA is equal to the frequency of intragenic breakage events, per kb of DNA.

Table 1. Distribution of deletion breakpoints in hprt mutations

Group	Intron number (size in kb)				
	5' flanking	1 (13.8 kb)	2+3 (15.0 kb)	4-8 (13.2 kb)	3' flanking
A adults (28 mutations)					
number	13	9	9	7	17
percent	24	16	16	13	31
B newborns (22 mutations)					
number	5	15	17	1	6
percent	11	34	39	2	14

    In this population of 28 hprt deletion mutations, there were 25
intragenic breakpoints, or 25 breakpoints in 43 kb of DNA. There were, in
addition, 13 breakpoints 5' to the gene and 17 breakpoints 3' to the gene,
indicating an average sized deletion of 22 kb in the 5' region of the gene
and 29 kb in the 3' region of the gene. (It could not be determined if
one breakpoint was in the 5' region of the gene, or 5' to hprt, so it was
eliminated from the analysis.) Therefore, X-chromosomal deletions of hprt
may involve at least 94 kb (43+22+29), and still be recovered as a viable
mutant. Quite large deletions of hprt can be recovered!

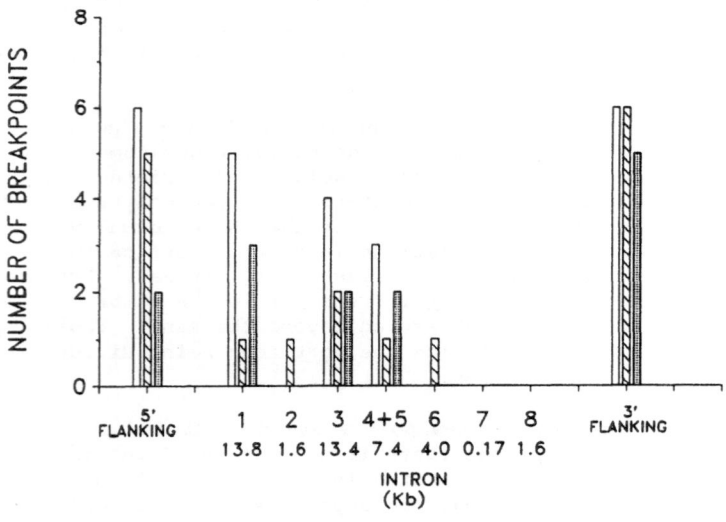

Fig. 3. Breakpoint distribution of deletion mutations from 3 normal
         male individuals D (open), E (hatched) and F (filled).

We are investigating the deletion size of hprt mutations that can be tolerated, and still result in a viable mutant for analysis. To this end, we are using a series of X-linked DNA probes for deletion mapping. We report elsewhere on initial studies using two anonymous X-chromosomal probes, DXS10 and DXS144, in Southern blot analyses to determine their co-deletion with hprt in deletion mutants. Figure 4 shows that two of five total hprt deletion mutations also lost the fragment that hybridizes with the DXS10 probe. In terms of genetic distance, the region between hprt and DXS10 has ranged up to 14 cM, indicating that large deletions of the human X-chromosome can be recovered as viable T-cell hprt mutants.

The spectrum for "background" in vivo hprt mutations involving "point mutations" is still being defined. As noted above, a wide variety of changes has been observed in mutant isolates from normal young adults. No other groups of individuals have yet been so studied. As for the gross structural alterations, no definite "hot-spots" have been observed for these "background" point mutations after corrections are made for clonality. However, at present this is a tentative judgment, and can only be made definitely as more isolates are studied.

A) probe DXS10

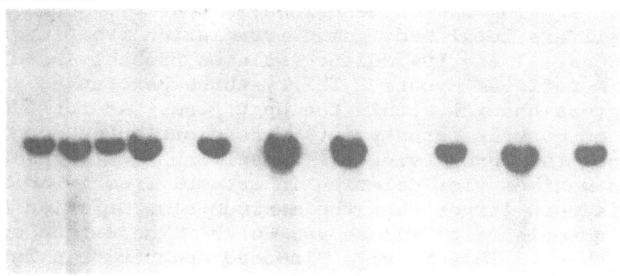

B) probe DXS144

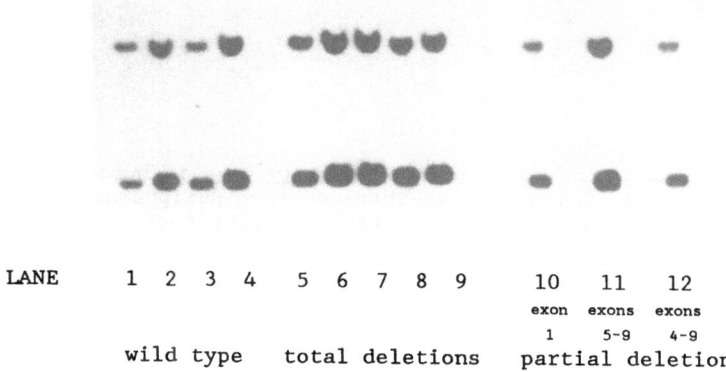

LANE	1 2 3 4	5 6 7 8 9	10	11	12
			exon	exons	exons
			1	5-9	4-9
	wild type	total deletions	partial deletions		

Fig. 4. Pst I Southern blot of 4 wild type, 5 total deletion and 3 partial deletion mutants using hprt gene linked probes. A) DXS10 probe. Two of the total deletion mutants (6 and 8) show loss of hybridization with the DXS10 probe indicating the hprt deletion extends through the DXS10 locus in these mutants. B) Same filter using the DXS144 probe. None of the mutants show loss of hybridization indicating that the hprt deletion does not extend to the DXS144 locus.

When the TCR gene rearrangement patterns of 41 hprt mutant isolates obtained from placental cord blood samples were analyzed, it was determined that 31 independent in vivo mutations had occurred (McGinniss et al., 1989b). Most of these were pre- or intra-thymic mutations. Twenty-six of the 31 independent in vivo mutations (85%) were characterized by structural alterations of hprt, of which 13 (50%) showed deletions of exons 2-3. These 13 deletions, plus an additional nine that involved other regions of the gene, give a total of 22 of the 26 mutations that were simple deletions. The distribution of breakpoints is shown in Table 1. As can be seen, 31 of the 44 breakpoints that were involved in these deletions were in intron 1 or intron 3. Of the 33 intragenic breakpoints observed in these mutations that arose in vivo in the human fetus, 31 (94%) occurred in these two introns. This is in sharp contrast to the even distribution of breakpoints along the length of the hprt gene that was seen in in vivo mutations arising in normal young adults. The "background" fetal hprt mutations that involve gross changes of the gene have a characteristic mutational spectrum that is clearly different from their adult counterparts. Sequence analyses of the remainder of the fetal hprt mutant isolates have not yet begun.

We have thus far analyzed 104 hprt mutant isolates from cancer patients undergoing radioimmunoglobulin therapy. As noted above, this therapy delivers total body gamma irradiation from internal emitters, i.e. radionuclides. These 104 mutant isolates probably resulted from 96 in vivo hprt mutational events. Thirty-three percent of these mutations involved gross changes within the hprt gene. As for the "background" mutations in normals, breakpoints were distributed evenly along the length of the gene, thus preserving the underlying "adult spectrum". The calculated maximum size deletion in mutants from irradiated patients, however, is much larger than the maximum size deletion in mutants from unexposed normals, i.e. 143 kb vs. 94 kb. The method of calculation is as described above. This in vivo "induced spectrum" is intermediate between the adult "background" spectrum and one generated by 300 rad external beam gamma irradiation of G_o human T-cells in vitro. These findings will be reported in detail elsewhere. Sequence studies have not yet been initiated.

CONCLUSIONS

Somatic cell gene mutations do arise in vivo in humans, and can be easily studied in T-lymphocytes obtained from peripheral and placental cord blood. Analyses of hprt mutations suggest that the "spontaneous" mutations arise preferentially in in vivo dividing T-cells. This is a minority population of the human T-cell population because most mature T-lymphocytes in vivo are in an arrested G_o stage. Although not described here, there is clear evidence that the hprt mutant T-cells are at a selective disadvantage in vivo, and that, on average, their life span is shorter than non-mutant cells (Strauss et al., 1974; Ammenheuser et al., 1988). This shortened life span coupled with the origin of mutants preferentially in dividing cells, suggest that the in vivo hprt mutant fraction of T-cells may represent cells that have recently undergone cell division. Use is being made of this to identify such cells, which may have immunological and other biological relevances. Also, T-cell division in vivo may predispose to "spontaneous" gene mutations, of which hprt mutation is simply a marker. The cell division attendant to hprt mutation may serve, furthermore, to amplify the resulting mutants. This then makes it necessary to correct mutant frequencies, as determined by cloning assays, for clonality, in order to define numbers of in vivo mutations.

In vivo somatic cell gene mutation, at least for the hprt gene in T-lymphocytes, appears to be much more complex than initially thought. However, recovery of the in vivo arising mutant clones permits their characterization at several levels. We have illustrated here characterization at the molecular level, which is permitting the description of in vivo mutational spectra. Studies of this sort should eventually give better insight into fundamental mechanisms of human in vivo gene mutation, and a better understanding of the maintenance of genetic integrity. Ultimately, this should permit more meaningful human mutagenicity monitoring using assays of in vivo gene mutation.

REFERENCES

Albertini, R. J., Castle, K. L., and Borcherding, W. R., 1982, T-cell cloning to detect the mutant 6-thioguanine-resistant lymphocytes present in human peripheral blood, Proc. Nat. Acad. Sci. U.S.A., 79:6617.

Albertini, R. J., and DeMars, R., 1974, Mosaicism of peripheral blood lymphocyte populations in females heterozygous for the Lesch-Nyhan mutation, Biochem. Genet., 11:397.

Albertini, R. J., O'Neill, J. P., Nicklas, J. A., Heintz, N. H., and Kelleher, P. C., 1985, Alterations of the hprt gene in human in vivo derived 6-thioguanine resistant T-lymphocytes, Nature, 316:369.

Albertini, R. J., Sullivan, L. S., Berman, J. K., Greene, C. J., Stewart, J. A., Silveira, J. M., and O'Neill, J. P., 1988, Mutagenicity monitoring in humans by autoradiographic assay for mutant T-lymphocytes, Mutation Res., 204:481.

Ammenheuser, M. M., Ward, J. B., Jr., Whorton, E. B., Jr., Killian, J. M., and Legator, M. S., 1988, Elevated frequencies of 6-thioguanine resistant lymphocytes in multiple sclerosis patients treated with cyclophosphamide: A prospective study, Mutation Res., 204:509.

McGinniss, M. J., Falta, M. T., Sullivan, L. S., and Albertini, R. J., 1989a, In vivo hprt mutant frequencies in T-cells of normal human newborns, Mutation Res., (in press).

McGinniss, M. J., Nicklas, J. A., and Albertini, R. J., 1989b, Molecular analyses of in vivo hprt mutations in human T-lymphocytes IV. Studies in newborns, Environ. and Molec. Mutagenesis, (in press).

Morley, A. A., Trainor, K. J., Seshadri, R., and Ryall, R. G., 1983, Measurement of in vivo mutations in human lymphocytes, Nature, 302:155.

Nicklas, J. A., Hunter, T. C., Sullivan, L. M., Berman, J. K., O'Neill, J. P., and Albertini, R. J., 1987, Molecular analyses of in vivo hprt mutations in human T-lymphocytes I. Studies of low frequency "spontaneous" mutants by Southern blots, Mutagenesis, 2:341.

Nicklas, J. A., O'Neill, J. P., Sullivan, L. M., Hunter, T. C., Allegretta, M., Chastenay, B. F., Libbus, B. L., and Albertini, R. J., 1988, Molecular analyses of in vivo hypoxanthine-guanine phosphoribosyltransferase mutations in human T-lymphocytes II. Demonstration of a clonal amplification of hprt mutant T-lymphocytes in vivo, Environ. and Molec. Mutagenesis, 12:271.

Nicklas, J. A., Hunter, T. C., O'Neill, J. P., and Albertini, R. J., 1989a, Molecular analyses of in vivo hprt mutations in human T-lymphocytes: III. Longitudinal study of hprt gene structural alterations and T-cell clonal origins, Mutation Res., (in press).

Nicklas, J. A., Hunter, T. C., O'Neill, J. P., Recio, L., Simpson, D., Skopek, T. R., and Albertini, R. J., 1989b, Molecular analysis of hprt mutations arising in vivo in human T-lymphocytes, Environ. and Molec. Mutagenesis, 14:142.

O'Neill, J. P., McGinniss, M. J., Berman, J. K., Sullivan, L. M., Nicklas, J. A., and Albertini, R. J., 1987, Refinement of a T-lymphocyte cloning assay to quantify the _in vivo_ thioguanine-resistant mutant frequency in humans, _Mutagenesis_, 2:87.

O'Neill, J. P., Sullivan, J. P., Booker, J. K., Pornelos, B. S., Falta, M. T., Greene, C. J., and Albertini, R. J., 1989, Longitudinal study of the _in vivo hprt_ mutant frequency in human T-lymphocytes as determined by a cell cloning assay, _Environ. and Molec. Mutagenesis_, 13:289.

Strauss, G. H., Allen, E. F., and Albertini, R. J., 1980, An enumerative assay of purine analogue resistant lymphocytes in women heterozygous for the Lesch-Nyhan mutation, _Biochem. Genet._, 18:529.

MECHANISMS OF INDUCTION OF SPECIFIC CHROMOSOMAL ALTERATIONS

R. Julian Preston

Biology Division
Oak Ridge National Laboratory*
Oak Ridge, TN 37831

INTRODUCTION

There has been a great deal of discussion in the past few years
on the mechanism of induction of chromosome aberrations by radiations
and chemical agents, and also how similar alterations might arise
"spontaneously." This is an important issue, and yet it is perhaps of
greater significance to determine how specific aberrations might be
induced, i.e., are they formed by the same mechanism as aberrations in
general or are they produced by a different process. Another way of
stating this is, are specific aberrations, such as those observed in
individuals with birth defects or those present in many tumors, a subset
of total aberrations that are observed because of a particular phenotype
that they, in part, elicit. This paper will address these various possibilities in the form of the development of a hypothesis, rather than by a
review of the published literature.

INDUCTION OF CHROMOSOME ABERRATIONS BY IONIZING RADIATIONS

In our laboratory we have studied the mechanisms by which ionizing
radiations induce chromosome aberrations by utilizing DNA repair/repli-
cation inhibitors. In our initial studies, we showed that if G_0 human
lymphocytes were X-irradiated and incubated with cytosine arabinoside
(ara-C), the frequencies of all chromosome-type aberrations were increased
compared to the frequencies in cells X-irradiated alone (Preston, 1980).
The inhibitory effects of ara-C were reversed by deoxycytidine. This
indicated that the repair of some or all X ray-induced DNA damages could be
inhibited by ara-C, and that on reversing the inhibition the repair of the
damage could be completed but in a more error-prone way than it would be in
the absence of ara-C treatment of additional significance was the fact that
the frequency of aberrations (most particularly dicentrics) increased with
increasing ara-C incubation times up to 3 h. This indicated that the
repair process that could be inhibited by ara-C was functioning for at

---

*Research sponsored by the Office of Health and Environmental Research,
 U. S. Department of Energy under contract DE-AC05-84OR21400 with the
 Martin Marietta Energy Systems, Inc.

DNA Damage and Repair in Human Tissues
Edited by B. M. Sutherland and A. D. Woodhead
Plenum Press, New York, 1990

329

least 3 h. and that at least some proportion of induced aberrations were produced by misrepair during this repair process. It was concluded, on the basis of these results, and the fact that we had also demonstrated that ara-C did not inhibit the repair of directly-induced double-strand breaks (dsb) (Hiss and Preston, 1977) that at the X ray dose used (2 Gy), a significant proportion of aberrations was produced by the misrepair during excision repair of base damages. In order to produce an interchange (and quite probably any aberration) it is necessary that two lesions will be repairing coincidentally in time, in order that misrepair can be one consequence, and that such lesions will also be in close proximity (within the rejoining distance). Additional studies supported this general conclusion. For example, if G_0 human lymphocytes were X-irradiated with doses of 0.5, 1, 2, or 3 Gy and again incubated with ara-C, the increase in aberration frequency with time of incubation in ara-C was greatest at the highest dose and decreased to the point where there was no apparent influence of ara-C on the frequency of X ray-induced aberrations at 0.5 Gy (Heartlein and Preston, 1985b). This can quite simply be interpreted as showing that the probability of there being coincidentally repairing base damages, that can be misrepaired to produce an aberration, is not linear with dose, and at low doses (less then 0.5 Gy) this probability is sufficiently low that no aberrations appear to be formed by the misrepair of base damages. At lower doses, therefore, it is most likely that aberrations are produced by the misrepair of directly induced dsb, a process that should not be inhibited by ara-C, as is borne out by our data. An extension of this interpretation is that the linear component of the X ray dose response curve for aberrations is the result of the misrepair of dsb, and that the dose-squared component is determined by two processes, a two-track induction of DNA damages leading to the aberration and the increase in rate of excision repair of base damages as the dose increases (Heartlein and Preston, 1985b). It should be added that ultimately the formation of an aberration requires a DNA double strand exchange; the hypothesis presented above suggests that such an exchange can occur by more than one process, or rather can be initiated by more than one type of induced DNA damage.

Studies on the induction of aberrations by fission neutrons lend further support to this hypothesis. When G_0 lymphocytes were irradiated with 0.3 Gy of fission neutrons and incubated with ara-C for 1, 2, or 3 h., there was no effect on aberration frequency compared to that induced by neutrons alone (Heartlein and Preston, 1985a, and unpublished data). The interpretation is that high-LET radiations, such as neutrons, induce a much higher proportion of dsb (or double strand gaps) than do low-LET radiations, and that for high-LET radiations the majority of aberrations are produced by the misrepair of these lesions. The linear dose-response curve would be predicted from the one-track induction of the dsb and the noninvolvement of dose-dependent repair kinetic.

It can be further concluded from the above studies that the relative effectiveness (RBE) of high- and low-LET radiations for the induction of aberrations for different cell types or for different species will be influenced by DNA content (dsb induction) and the rate of incision, the rate-limiting step for excision repair. Thus, the RBE would be expected to vary from one cell type to another within a species, and for the same cell type in different species. This conclusion is important in the estimation of risk to man from radiation exposure when extrapolation is made from data obtained in another species or in cell types different from those appropriate for risk estimation.

The spectrum of aberration breakpoints for low-LET radiations will be a reflection of the pattern of induced DNA damages, the probability of misrepair of dsb and base damages for different genomic sites, and the temporal pattern of DNA excision repair that allows for coincidentally repairing base damages. For high-LET radiations, the pattern of excision repair will not be influential. Therefore, the spectra of aberration breakpoints should be different for high- and low-LET radiations. There is as yet no adequate study that has addressed this issue, but it would seem to be of importance to do so. It can be argued that an excision repair process that produces coincidentally repairing lesions might be expected to result in the formation of some rather specific aberrations, whereas the repair of dsb might be expected to be more random. For chromatid-type aberrations there is a general localization of aberration breakpoints to light bands in G-banded chromosomes (Savage, 1977). "Active" genes are generally located in these light bands (Holmquist et al, 1982), and the initiation of excision repair has been shown to occur more rapidly in these regions, for ultraviolet radiation, chemical agents, and ionizing radiations (Bohr et al., 1986; Mellon et al., 1986; Patil et al., 1985).

INDUCTION OF CHROMOSOME ABERRATIONS BY CHEMICAL AGENTS

The chromosome aberrations induced by the majority of chemical agents appear to involve errors during DNA replication on a damaged template, i.e., irrespective of the cell stage treated chromatid-type aberrations are produced. This has led to the concept that the production of aberrations by chemicals is S-dependent. Our studies have led to a modification of this view, namely that the probability of an aberration being produced by S replication is much more likely than by misrepair of chemically induced DNA damage. If it is possible to increase the probability of misrepair, then chemically-induced aberrations might be expected to reflect an S-independent process. When G_1 human lymphocytes were treated with 4-Nitro-quinoline-N-oxide (4NQO) no aberrations were observed at metaphase. However, if the cells were treated with 4NQO and then incubated with ara-C for 6 hours, aberrations were produced, and these were of the chromosome-type, particularly dicentrics, exactly the same type as induced by X rays in G_1 cells (Preston and Gooch, 1981). This shows that if the probability of misrepair of 4NQO-induced DNA damage is increased by "accumulating" intermediates of excision repair by ara-C inhibition, then indeed aberrations can be formed by misrepair in G_1. The fact that much longer ara-C incubation times are required following 4NQO treatment than for X-irradiation, in order to observe an influence of ara-C on aberration frequency, suggests that the repair of ara-C inhibitible 4NQO-induced DNA damage is much slower than for X ray-induced base damages. This would explain why most chemical agents do not normally induce aberrations in G_1 cells, since the probability of there being coincidentally repairing lesions, that could be subject to misrepair, is very low, and the probability of misreplication is generally much higher, resulting in the apparent S-dependence.

It is interesting to note in this context that the DNA damages induced by X rays can interact with those induced by chemical agents during their repair. If G_1 lymphocytes were treated with 4NQO and X rays, the aberration frequency was the same as that induced by X rays alone. However, if the cells were incubated with ara-C between the two treatments, a much higher than additive frequency of aberrations was observed (Preston, 1982). A similar interaction was observed for bleomycin and X ray treatments, but as predicted, since bleomycin is a radiomimetic agent capable of inducing chromosome-type aberration in G_1, no ara-C treatment was necessary to obtain the interaction. Thus, a similarity of mechanism of induction of aberrations by X rays and chemicals, i.e., by misrepair, is not precluded; misrepair is simply a low probability event for chemically-induced DNA damages.

The fact that the aberrations induced by most chemical agents result from errors of DNA replication will mean that the location of breakpoints for such aberrations will be a reflection of the temporal pattern of DNA replication in the cell, i.e., aberrations (particularly interchanges) would be expected to involve coincidentally replicating genomic sites. This is contrast to the patterns predicted for ionizing-radiation induced aberrations.

THE DISTRIBUTIONS OF ABERRATIONS INDUCED BY MISREPAIR VS. MISREPLICATION

In order to test the idea that different patterns of aberrations within a cell would be produced by X rays and chemical agents, as a result of the different mechanisms of formation, we conducted a series of experiments with Chinese hamster, mouse cell hybrids (Winegar and Preston, unpublished data). The rationale was that interchanges that resulted from misrepair would be equally likely to occur between and among the two chromosome complements, whereas those being produced by misreplication would be intra-specific as a result of the increased likelihood of induced misreplication at coincidentally replicating regions occurring within either the mouse or hamster complements rather than between them. The approach was to treat G_2 or S phase cells with X rays or mitomycin C (MMC) and analyze interchanges with regard to whether they involved hamster/ hamster, mouse/mouse or hamster/mouse chromosomes. The frequency of deletions was used as a comparative measure of the relative sensitivities of the hamster and mouse chromosome sets. Three hybrid cells were utilized in which the proportion of mouse chromosomes was 0.27, 0.23, or 0.15. With X rays, the proportion of the total deletions that involved mouse chromosomes was identical to the proportion of the total hybrid chromosome complement contributed by mouse chromosomes. Similarly, the involvement of mouse chromosomes in interchange formation was proportional to their contribution to the hybrid complement. The frequency of mouse/hamster chromosome interchanges was equal to that calculated on the basis of random involvement. Thus, misrepair of X ray-induced DNA damage that resulted in aberration formation was random with regard to interspecific chromosomal involvement. Whether or not the aberration breakpoints were distributed randomly along the chromosomes was not assessed in this study. When S-phase cells were treated with MMC, a very different result was obtained. Deletions were induced in both hamster and mouse chromosomes, at relative frequencies expected on the basis of relative DNA contents, i.e., there was an equivalent sensitivity of two genomes to MMC-induced deletions. In contrast, all but one interchange involved only mouse chromosomes (the exception was a hamster/hamster interchange), and additionally these interchanges were located almost exclusively in the centromeric hetero- chromatin. Since the centromeric regions of mouse chromosomes contain highly repetitive DNA, and replicate late in the S-phase, it would be expected that misreplication in these regions would be a high probability event (Hayman, 1982). Thus, misreplication can lead to the production of a very specific set of aberrations. Whether or not such patterns are a general phenomenon, or restricted to a particular group of agents or cell types is not known, but can be quite readily tested.

INDUCTION OF CHROMOSOME ABERRATIONS BY RESTRICTION ENDONUCLEASES

Restriction enzymes produce defined double-strand cuts in DNA; they produce either blunt-end or cohesive-end cuts at a recognition site that is specific for each enzyme. Thus, the production of chromosome aberrations by such enzymes should provide a model system for determining if and how double-strand breaks can be converted into chromosome aberrations. Several groups have conducted studies on the induction of aberrations by restriction enzymes, and the results can be summarized as follows (Natarajan and Obe, 1984; Bryant, 1984, 1988; Obe et al., 1985; Winegar and Preston, 1988; Morgan et al., 1988). All restriction enzymes so far tested induce chromosome aberrations, irrespective of whether they produce blunt-end or cohesive-end cuts; aberrations are induced in all stages of the cell cycle, chromosome-type in G_1 and chromatid-type in S and G_2; and the frequency of aberrations is generally proportional to the calculated cutting frequency for a particular enzyme. This latter point is the subject of some debate. Bryant (1984,1988) determined that blunt-end cuts were much more efficiently converted into aberrations than were cohesive-end cuts, whereas Winegar and Preston (1988) demonstrated that calculated cutting frequency rather than cut-end structure determined aberration frequency. These different conclusions could be due to the fact that the methods of introducing restriction enzymes into cells were quite different (inactivated Sendai virus vs. osmolytic shock or electroporation). This still needs to be resolved. Suffice it to say that both general types of double-strand cut can be converted into aberrations.

It can be further concluded that directly-induced double-strand breaks can be converted into aberrations, a not unexpected observation. However, it does not allow for the conclusion that this is the only way by which aberrations are produced following X-irradiation, for example. If the only lesion introduced is a dsb, unlike the situation with X rays, then aberrations can only result from dsb misrepair. It should be noted from the data of Bryant (1988) that to produce similar aberration frequencies by restriction enzymes and X rays, considerably higher frequencies of restriction enzyme dsb are required than X ray-induced dsb. This could be interpreted as showing that enzyme induced dsb are less efficiently converted into aberrations, but it is much more likely that damage other than dsb can be converted into aberrations following X ray treatments. The data presented above have demonstrated that misrepair of base damages is a major contributor to X ray-induced aberrations.

Additional studies with restriction enzymes in our laboratory shed light on how X ray-induced dsb might be converted into aberrations (Winegar and Preston, unpublished data). Experiments were performed with pairs of enzymes that produced similar or different types of cut-end structures to determine which types of dsb could interact to produce aberrations. In summary, it was shown that blunt-end cuts produced by one enzyme could interact with blunt-end cuts produced by a second enzyme to give aberration frequencies that were significantly higher than the additive frequency from the two enzymes alone. Similarly, blunt-end cuts could interact with two-base overlap cohesive-end cuts to give greater than additivity. However, of particular interest, was the fact that four-base overlap cohesive-end cuts could not interact with any other cut-end structure (blunt or cohesive), although enzymes that produced such cohesive ends were themselves efficient inducers of aberrations. This observation suggests that in order for an aberration to be induced by enzymes that produce four-base overlap cohesive ends, homologous regions have to be available for misrepair or misrejoining. What does this mean in terms of X ray-induced aberrations? A high proportion of X ray-induced dsb result in cohesive-ends, rather than "clean" breaks, and since X ray-induced DNA damage is generally random throughout the genome, these cohesive-ends will be largely nonhomologous. On the basis of our data with restriction enzymes, such nonhomologous cohesive-ends will not be converted into aberrations by a process of misrepair. However, some small proportion of induced dsb can be predicted to interact to produce aberrations, namely those induced in repetitive DNA sequences, where homologous cohesive-ends could be produced at separate locations within and between chromosomes. The selective location of aberration breakpoints in repetitive DNA sequences could result in the formation of specific chromosome aberrations, probably representing a subset of the total aberrations induced. Clearly this hypothesis requires further testing, particularly by analyzing the breakpoints for X ray-induced chromosome aberrations at the molecular level.

THE EFFECT OF ENHANCEMENT OF MISREPAIR ON X RAY-INDUCED ABERRATIONS

It can be argued that the most likely way by which specific aberrations could be induced is by a recombination-like process between homologous DNA segments (particularly repetitive DNAs) on nonhomologous chromosomes. Such a process could take place during repair of induced DNA damage (misrepair) or during replication of a damaged template (misreplication). In the case of excision repair or recombination repair of dsb (Resnick, 1976; Szostak et al., 1983), it can be seen that misrepair is equivalent to misreplication for an error made during the resynthesis step. We have made an initial attempt to study the possible role of a recombination process in the formation of X ray-induced aberrations.

We demonstrated that the frequency of sister chromatid exchanges (SCE) was about 5 times greater when chlorodeoxyuridine (CldU) was substituted for thymidine during replication than for bromodeoxyuridine (BrdU) substitution (Heartlein et al., 1983). In addition, we demonstrated that this increase was due to errors of replication of the halogen-substituted template rather than to errors of incorporation of the halogenated base (O'Neill et al., 1983). If a chromatid interchange is regarded as an interchromosomal equivalent of an SCE, then it should be possible, if DNA synthesis is required during the formation of X ray-induced aberrations, to enhance interchange frequencies in cells containing CldU-substituted DNA compared to those in cells containing BrdU-substituted DNA. Cells were grown for two rounds of replication in BrdU and CldU, X-irradiated and then G_2 cells sampled (Hook and Preston, unpublished data). In summary, the frequency of chromatid deletions was considerably higher for BrdU-substituted chromosomes than for CldU-substituted, indicating an overall greater sensitivity of BrdU-substituted DNA to X ray-induced damage. In sharp contrast, the frequency of interchanges was 3-4 fold higher in the CldU-substituted cells, indicating that misreplication, during excision repair of X ray-induced DNA damage or recombination repair of dsb (Resnick 1976; Szostak et al., 1983), was more error-prone when the template contained CldU. This was in agreement with our observations on SCE. It was also observed, as had been previously reported by Zwanenburg et al. (1984), that the frequency of chromatid aberrations (particularly interchanges) was much higher in cells grown in CldU for two rounds of replication than in those grown in BrdU, further showing that replication errors can result in aberrations between (interchanges) as well as within (intrachanges) chromosomes. Whether a process akin to recombination is involved remains to be established.

A GENERAL MODEL FOR CHROMOSOME ABERRATION FORMATION

There is recent evidence in the literature to suggest that recombination, particularly between repetitive DNA sequences, is a plausible mechanism by which chromosome aberrations in general, and particularly specific aberrations, might be produced either "spontaneously" or following radiation or chemical treatments. For example, Hastie and Allshire (1989) review the evidence that interstitial telomere-like repetitive sequences might be hotspots for recombination, and Vernick et al (1988) provide experimental evidence to show that this is indeed the case for internal stretches of telomere-like sequences. In addition, very recently it has been demonstrated by Wahls et al. (1990) that hypervariable minisatellite DNA is a "hotspot" for homologous recombination in human cells.

Thus, it is proposed that the aberrations induced by radiations or chemical agents result from errors in replication either during S-phase synthesis, during the resynthesis step of excision repair, or during the synthesis required for recombination repair of dsb. "Spontaneous" aberrations would be formed by the same mechanism, namely errors of replication, and thus radiation-or chemically-induced DNA damages simply cause an enhanced probability of such errors occurring. In addition, the most likely regions of the genome where such a recombination process could occur is between homologous regions on homologous or nonhomologous chromosomes; a criterion met by repetitive DNA sequences.

It is also of importance to establish the possible roles of induced specific chromosome aberrations in the initiation and/or progression of tumors and in the production of particular genetic diseases. Such studies are ongoing in many laboratories, and it is already clear that, not only are aberrations in particular tumors or genetic diseases specific with regard to chromosome band location, they involve breakpoints within defined DNA sequences. Parallel studies on the mechanism of induction of such aberrations are of considerable importance.

REFERENCES

Bohr, V. A., Okumoto, D. S., and Hanawalt, P. C., 1986, Survival of UV-irradiated mammalian cells correlates with efficient DNA repair in an essential gene, Proc. Nat. Acad. Sci. USA, 83:3830-3833.
Bryant, P. E., 1984, Enzymatic restriction of mammalian cell DNA using Pvu II and Bam HI: evidence for the double-strand break origin of chromosomal aberrations, Int. J. Radiat. Biol., 46:57-65.
Bryant, P. E., 1988, Use of restriction endonucleases to study relationships between DNA double-strand breaks chromosomal aberrations and other end-points in mammalian cells, Int. J. Radiat. Biol., 54:869-890.
Hastie, N. D., and Allshire, R. C., 1989, Human telomeres: fusion and interstitial sites, TIG, 5:326-331.
Hayman, D. L., 1982, A comparative study of the relative frequency and specific pattern of chromatid interchanges induced by mono-, di- and poly-functional alkylating agents, Mutat. Res., 104:153-158.
Heartlein, M. W., O'Neill, J. P., and Preston, R. J., 1983, SCE induction is proportional to substitution in DNA for thymidine by CldU and BrdU, Mutat. Res., 107:103-109.
Heartlein, M. W., and Preston, R. J., 1985a, The effect of 3-aminobenzamide on the frequency of X-ray- or neutron-induced chromosome aberrations in cycling or noncycling human lymphocytes, Mutat. Res., 148:91-97.
Heartlein, M. W., and Preston, R. J., 1985b, An explanation of interspecific differences in sensitivity to X ray-induced chromosome aberrations and a consideration of dose-response curves, Mutat. Res., 150:299-305.
Hiss, E. A., and Preston, R. J., 1977, The effect of cytosine arabinoside on the frequency of single-strand breaks in mammalian cells following irradiation or chemical treatment, Biochim. Biophys. Acta, 478:1-8.
Holmquist, G., Gray, M., Porter, T. and Jordan, J., 1982, Characterization of Giemsa dark- and light-band DNA, Cell, 31:121-129.
Mellon, I., Bohr, V. A., Smith, C. A., and Hanawalt, P. C., 1986, Preferential DNA repair of an active gene in human cells, Proc. Nat. Acad. Sci. USA, 83:8878-8882.

Morgan, W. F., Fero, M. L., Land, M. C., and Winegar, R. A., 1988, Inducible expression and cytogenetic effects of the Eco RI restriction endonuclease in Chinese hamster ovary cells, *Mol. Cell. Biol.*, 8:3204-3211.

Natarajan, A. T., and Obe, G., 1984, Molecular mechanisms involved in the production of chromosomal aberrations, III. Restriction endonucleases, *Chromosoma*, 90:120-127.

Obe, G., Palitti, G., Tanzarella, C., Degrossi, G., and Desalvia, R., 1985, Chromosomal aberrations induced by restriction endonucleases, *Mutat. Res.*, 150:359-368.

O'Neill, J. P., Heartlein, M. W., and Preston, R. J., 1983, Sister-chromatid exchanges and gene mutations are induced by the replication of 5-bromo- and 5-chloro-deoxyuridine substituted DNA, *Mutat. Res.*, 109:259-270.

Patil, M. S., Locher, S. E., and Hariharan, P. V., 1985, Radiation-induced thymine base damage and its excision repair in active and inactive chromatin of HeLa cells, *Int. J. Radiat. Biol.*, 48:691-700.

Preston, R. J., 1980, The effect of cytosine arabinoside on the frequency of X ray-induced chromosome aberrations in normal human leukocytes, *Mutat. Res.*, 69:71-79.

Preston, R. J., 1982, DNA repair and chromosome aberrations: Interactive effects of radiation and chemicals, in: Natarajan, A. T., Obe, G., and Altmann, H. (Eds.) "DNA Repair, Chromosome Alterations and Chromatin Structure," Amsterdam: Elsevier Biomedical Press, pp. 25-35.

Preston, R. J., and Gooch, P. C., 1981, The induction of chromosome-type aberrations in G_1 by methyl methanesulfonate and 4-Nitroquinoline-N-oxide, and the non-requirement of an S-phase for their production, *Mutat. Res.*, 83:395-402.

Resnick, M. A., 1976, The repair of double-strand breaks in DNA: A model involving recombination, *J. Theor. Biol.*, 59:97-106.

Savage, J.R.K., 1977, Assignment of aberration breakpoints in banded chromosomes, *Nature*, 270:513-514.

Szostak, J. W., Orr-Weaver, T. L., and Rothstein, R. J., 1983, The double-strand-break repair model for recombination, *Cell*, 33:25-35.

Vernick, K. D., Walliker, D., and McCutchan, T. F., 1988, Genetic hypervariability of telomere-related sequences is associated with meiosis in Plasmodium falciparum, *Nucleic Acids Res.*, 16:6973-6985.

Wahls, W. P., Wallace, L. J., and Moore, P. D., 1990, Hypervariable minisatellite DNA is a hotspot for homologous recombination in human cells, *Cell*, 60:95-103.

Winegar, R. A., and Preston, R. J., 1988, The induction of chromosomal aberrations by restriction endonucleases that produce blunt-ended or cohesive-ended double-strand breaks, *Mutat. Res.*, 197:141-149.

Zwanenburg, T.S.B., Mullenders, L.H.F., Natarajan, A. T., and van Zeeland, A. A., 1984, DNA lesions, chromosomal aberrations and G_2 delay in CHO cells cultured in medium containing bromo- or chloro-deoxyuridine, *Mutat. Res.*, 127:155-168.

UNFOLDING PERSPECTIVES ON THE GENETIC EFFECTS

OF HUMAN EXPOSURES TO RADIATION

James V. Neel

Department of Human Genetics
University of Michigan
Ann Arbor, Michigan

My role in this program is to present the current status of the long-running studies on the potential genetic effects of the atomic bombs, and then indicate the direction of current thinking regarding future studies on this subject, with particular reference to studies at the DNA level. I would like to begin, however, with what will seem like a diversion, a brief review of the results of some rather recent, seemingly unrelated studies which, I believe, point to the kinds of fundamental biases which may inadvertently creep into studies of spontaneous and induced mutation rates. Such biases could be very relevant to the apparent discrepancy between the results in Japan and the experimental observations on mice, to which I will speak briefly, and should be avoided in planning for any future studies.

SPONTANEOUS AND INDUCED GENETIC VARIATION IN THE PROTEINS VISUALIZED WITH 2-D PAGE.

Some eight years ago our group began to explore the potential of two-dimensional polyacrylamide gel electrophoresis (2-D PAGE) for the study of mutation affecting protein phenotypes. Since we proposed to study human mutation rates, the cells we would examine had to be easily available. The obvious choice was the constituents of blood: lymphocytes, erythrocytes, platelets, and then of course the plasma in which they are suspended. The first step was to familiarize ourselves with the appearance of genetic variation in 2-D PAGE preparations. As our studies progressed - as well as the studies of others on brain or kidney homogenates, or on fibroblasts - less electrophoretic variation was encountered than had been characteristic of the findings with one-dimensional electrophoresis (1-D E) of, predominately, erythrocyte enzymes or plasma transport proteins.

A convenient measure of the amount of variation has been the Heterozygosity Index (HI), defined as the average frequency in percent with which heterozygotes for a given locus or group of loci are encountered in the population under study. In large scale 1-D E surveys of erythrocyte enzymes and serum proteins from representative civilized populations, the HIs were of the order of 7% (Harris, 1980, Satoh et al., 1985). By contrast the HIs encountered in these other types of preparations ranged from <1% to 5.5%. The 2-D PAGE HIs for the serum proteins were in reasonable agreement with the findings on the same proteins with 1-D E (5.5%, Rosenblum et al., 1983; Asakawa et al., 1985), but the HIs for the erythrocyte proteins scored in 2-D PAGE (3.6%, Rosenblum et al., 1984; Takahashi et al., 1986) were well below those for the erythrocyte enzymes studied by 1-D E , and the HIs for the other types of preparations - for which there was

DNA Damage and Repair in Human Tissues
Edited by B. M. Sutherland and A. D. Woodhead
Plenum Press, New York, 1990

337

no 1-D E "standard" - were even lower. For instance, three different groups of investigators reported fibroblast HIs averaging <0.4% (McConkey et al., 1979; Walton et al., 1979; Klose et al., 1983).

There are three obvious, overlapping explanations of this finding.

Technical factors. In 1-D E, proteins are usually studied one at a time, and the electrophoretic conditions can be optimized for the detection of variants of any particular protein. 2-D PAGE is a "uniform conditions" system, not optimized for the study of any particular protein, with the additional drawback that variants may sometimes migrate to areas of the gel unsuitable for scoring, or migrate to an area already occupied by a large spot, and so not be detected. We found that the 2-D PAGE technique reveals electrophoretic variants with about 80% of the efficiency of 1-D E as this is practiced in population surveys (Wanner et al., 1982). This figure of 80% applies to the fact of variant detection, rather than to the accuracy of variant subtyping. Thus, while variant under-detection may contribute to the different HIs defined with 1- and 2-DE, it appears to provide only a partial explanation of the discrepancy.

Stringent biological selection against electrophoretic variants of the proteins visualized with 2-D PAGE. McConkey et al. (1979) (see also Edwards and Hopkinson, 1980) responded to the relatively low variability of the proteins visualized in 2-D gels with the suggestion that the relatively abundant proteins scored in these studies, predominantly what it is convenient to term structural proteins, might be subject to more severe constraints with respect to tolerable variation than the transport and enzyme proteins which had been the backbone of the 1-D E studies. This suggestion implies that most electrophoretic variants of these structural proteins function as lethals either prenatally or during early childhood. There are considerations which make it unlikely this suggestion provides a satisfactory explanation. Firstly, there is now abundant evidence for genetically-determined amino acid substitutions in such structural proteins as collagen, fibrinogen and other proteins of the coagulation cascade, and receptor proteins of the cell membrane, which, while associated with disease, are not early lethals. Secondly, assuming that the loci encoding for these proteins mutate at the same average rate as the average rate now established for enzyme and transport proteins, the "genetic load" that dominant lethality would impose, in terms of pre-reproductive zygote loss, really does seem excessive.

Lower mutation rates at the loci encoding for these proteins. A much more reasonable explanation for the relative lack of genetic variation would seem to be lower average mutation rates at the loci encoding for these proteins than have been postulated from studies of enzyme and transport proteins. Locus differences in mutability are well established in experimental genetics. With respect to humans, for some years it has been apparent that the frequencies of mutation leading to a variety of dominant traits differed by a factor of ten, but it seemed unwise to generalize from the special case which dominants represent. Now it appears the same is true for nucleotide substitutions. Table 1 presents a set of mutation rates recently developed by Chakraborty and myself (in press) employing an indirect approach for a set of 19 proteins surveyed for variation in 12 Amerindian tribes. The genetic theory employed (quite reasonably) necessitates the identification of genetic variants at a locus before a mutation rate can be calculated. There were in this same survey 8 monomorphic loci, but all of these are known from other, more extensive surveys to support variants (Neel et al., 1988). If the presumably lower mutation rates at these latter loci were factored into the findings of Table 1, the range of mutation rates is, conservatively, 10-fold, and this cannot be explained by differences in the molecular weights of the protein, inasmuch as the correlation between subunit molecular weight and mutation rate is only 0.06 (P > 0.7). If, for reasons not now clear, individual locus rates can vary to this extent, then it seems reasonable to postulate locus differences in mutation rate related to the "class" of the product. In short, I suggest we must consider very seriously the possibility that the paucity of electrophoretic variants in 2-D PAGE gels reflects to some considerable extent lower mutation rates at the loci encoding for the more abundant proteins being scored in these gels. It is important in this context to emphasize that in reading 2-D gels for variation, one concentrates on the heavily-stained spots, leaving unscored hundreds - perhaps a thousand - fainter spots.

There is also some direct evidence that it is primarily mutation pressure rather than selection which determines the pattern of variation encountered in these 2-D gels. In a mutagenization experiment involving a lymphocytoid cell line treated with ethylnitrosourea, significantly more mutations were induced at loci known to be associated with variants than at the (thus far) monomorphic loci (Chu et al., 1988). Assuming a correlation between spontaneous and induced mutation rates, this result can be interpreted as indicating that the pattern of variation in these gels could as well reflect mutation pressure as the results of selection on a set of loci as mutable as the enzyme-transport protein loci. The chief weakness of this argument at present is that the identity of these proteins, the loci encoding for which are more mutable, is unknown; they might in fact be enzymes, which we have earlier suggested might as a group be more mutable. I will return to this matter of locus differences in mutability shortly.

Table 1.   Estimates of Mutation Rates Resulting in Electromorphs for a Series of 27 Loci whose Products were Examined in 12 Amerindian Tribes, after Chakraborty and Neel (in press). Individual Rates are Given for the 19 Loci at which Variants were Encountered. There were an Additional 8 Loci at which No Variants were Encountered which Must Be Assigned Rates of 0; These Rates are Included in the Average Across All Loci

Locus	Mol. Wt. ($\times 10^3$ Daltons)	Mutation rate $\pm$ s.e. $\times 10^{-5}$
ALB	66.0	1.80 ± 0.36
CRPL	53.0	1.54 ± 0.33
HP	40.0	3.18 ± 0.49
TF	90.0	1.26 ± 0.30
ACP1	15.0	4.38 ± 0.59
ADA	34.0	0.76 ± 0.23
AK1	22.0	0.24 ± 0.13
CA2	29.0	1.31 ± 0.31
ESA	28.0	0.77 ± 0.23
ESD	28.0	3.03 ± 0.49
GALT	30.0	2.98 ± 0.48
PGM1	51.0	3.48 ± 0.52
ICD	48.0	0.25 ± 0.13
LDHB	35.0	0.25 ± 0.13
MDH	35.0	0.25 ± 0.13
PEPA	46.0	0.50 ± 0.18
PEPB	55.0	0.50 ± 0.18
6PGD	52.0	1.26 ± 0.30
PHI	61.0	0.75 ± 0.23

Average:
Polymorphic loci (19)	43.1 ± 4.1	1.50 ± 0.30
All loci (27)	38.7 ± 3.5	1.06 ± 0.25

BRIEF SUMMARY OF THE FINDINGS IN THE STUDY OF THE POTENTIAL GENETIC
EFFECTS OF THE ATOMIC BOMBS

With this as background, I will now summarize as briefly as possible
the current status of the genetic follow-up studies in Japan, a preliminary
account of which is now in press (Neel et al., in press). These studies
are currently under the aegis of the Radiation Effects Research Foundation,
a joint U.S.-Japan binational foundation, on the Japanese side affiliated
with and funded through the Ministry of Welfare, on the U.S. side administered by the National Academy of Sciences, with funding from the Department
of Energy. The Genetics Program involves all the children born in Hiroshima and Nagasaki since 1946 whose parents are thought to have joint radiation exposures at the time of the bombings $\geq$ 0.001 Sv. Children _in utero_
at the time of the bombings are excluded from the study. That cohort now
numbers some 31,000 persons. Average conjoint parental gonadal exposure is
about 0.40 Sv, the amount of acute radiation commonly cited as the probable
doubling dose for man on the basis of experiments with the mouse paradigm.
Given the lapse of time between the bombings and the studies, the data per-
tain to the results of spermatogonial and dictyate-stage oocyte radiation.
A set of matched controls has also been established.

Over the years the children have been studied in many ways, new technologies being brought to bear on the problem as they appeared. At the
present time, the indicators of a potential genetic effect include still-
births, congenital defects, survival in liveborn infants, sex ratio, physical development, sex-chromosome aneuploids and balanced chromosomal rear-
raangements, and electrophoretic and activity variants of a battery of 32
polypeptides. None of these indicators has been significantly influenced
by the parental radiation exposure. The net effect is slightly positive.
On the thesis that we are not in a hypothesis-testing situation - i.e., on
the assumption that mutations were indeed produced by this exposure - we
have taken our findings at face value, as the best available evaluation of
the genetic effects of radiation on humans, and asked, what can we infer
about the human genetic doubling dose? To do this, we must estimate what
percent of those indicators with respect to which the data permit a regres-
sion-type analysis and for which the outcome is a discrete variable, can,
after the appropriate studies, be assigned to mutation occurring in the
parental generation. As Table 2 indicates, based on the estimates of
columns (a) and (b), that fraction ranges from 3 to 5% for untoward pregnancy outcomes (congenital defect and/or stillbirth and/or neonatal death)
and mortality among liveborn infants, to 100% for the sex-chromosome aneuploids and the mutant protein variants. A detailed justification for these
fractions will be supplied elsewhere (Neel et al, submitted). We have then
made two calculations, namely, the doubling dose for the phenomenon which
can be excluded at various probability levels, and the most likely doubling
dose. To calculate the former, we must estimate the regression of indicator on dose (β) and the intercept at zero dose (α). From the formula

$$DD = \frac{1}{[\beta/\alpha + Z_\alpha \sqrt{V(\beta/\alpha)}]}$$

where Z_α is the normal deviate at the desired probability level and V is
the variance of β/α, one can calculate the values for the indicators under
consideration at various confidence limits, as shown in Table 2. The α
term in this calculation is the mutational component of the intercept at
zero dose (column b, Table 2). Values presumed to be based on similar responses to radiation can be pooled. It would appear appropriate to pool
the probability level estimates for F1 mortality among liveborn infants, F1
cancer, and untoward pregnancy outcomes. The minimal estimate at the 95%
probability level which results from pooling these three estimates is 0.32
- 0.52 Sv. In the past we have been persuaded that this estimate should be
divided by 2, to convert it into a gametic estimate. We now believe this
was incorrect. Simply stated, while the estimate of the impact of sponta-

Table 2. An estsimate of the <u>zygotic</u> doubling doses that can be excluded at specific confidence levels by these data. Further explanation in text.

Trait	Observed Total Background (a)	Genetic Background (b)	Mutational Component (%, b ÷ a)	β	α	Lower confidence limit (Sv)		
						99%	95%	90%
Untoward Pregnancy Outcome	0.0502	0.0017 – 0.0027	3.4 – 5.4	0.00264 ±0.00277	0.03856 ±0.00582	0.14 – 0.23	0.18 – .29	0.21 – .33
F1 Mortality	0.0458	0.0016 – 0.0026	3.5 – 5.7	0.00076 ±0.00154	0.06346 ±0.00181	0.51 – 0.83	0.68 – 1.10	0.81 – 1.32
F1 Cancer	0.0012	0.00002 – 0.00005	2.0 – 4.0	-0.00008 ±0.00028	0.00104 ±0.00033	0.04 – 0.07	0.05 – 0.11	0.07 – 0.15
Sex-chromosome aneuploids	0.0030	0.0030	100	0.00044 ±0.00069	0.00252 ±0.00043	1.23	1.60	1.91
Protein	0.000013	0.000013	100	-0.00001 ±0.00001	0.00001 ±0.00001	0.99	2.27	7.41

* per diploid locus

neous mutation in the parental generation to the indicator reflects the contribution of two gametes, the regression term also reflects the contribution of two haploid genomes, and the factors of two cancel out. The similar estimate from pooling the data on the sex chromosome aneuploids and protein variants is 1.36 Sv. We do not believe it appropriate to attempt to combine these two estimates.

Our attempt to calculate a most probable doubling dose is summarized in Table 3. In this case we feel that because the five regression coefficients with which we are working are based on the same cohorts of children, we can combine them by simple addition. The right hand column is our estimate of the contribution each generation of spontaneous mutation to these indicators. The gametic doubling dose is simply

$$DD = \Sigma \; \alpha' / \; \Sigma \; \beta$$

where the ' indicates the use of the values presented in column b of Table 2. With this approach, we estimate the gametic doubling dose for acute radiation at between 1.69 and 2.23 Sv. In light of the discussion to come later, we note the relatively large contribution of the sex-chromosome aneuploids to this estimate.

Table 3. A Summary of the Regression of the Various Indicators on Parental Radiation Exposure and the Impact of Spontaneous Mutation on the Indicator

Trait	Regression per combined parental Sv	Contribution of spontaneous mutation
UPO	+0.00264	
F_1 Mortality	+0.00076	0.0033 -- 0.0053
Protein mutations	-0.00001	
Sex-chromosome aneuploids	+0.00044	0.0030
F_1 Cancer	-0.00008	0.00002 -- 0.00005
	0.00375	0.00632 -- 0.00835

Gametic doubling dose "Lower" = 0.00632/0.00375 = 1.69 Sv
"Upper" = 0.00835/0.00375 = 2.23 Sv

We believe we have been conservative in our assumptions and analyses. Three indicators were not folded into these doubling dose estimates, for various reasons. There was one mutation resulting in a balanced chromosomal exchange in the 8322 children of exposed who were examined and one in the 7976 controls, resulting in nearly identical mutation rates (Awa et al., 1987); these numbers were judged inadequate for a regression approach. The regression of maleness on maternal radiation - the sex-ratio regression which should much less ambiguously reveal an effect of radiation than the regression on paternal radiation - was (insignificantly) positive, rather than negative as expected in the case of a radiation-induced increase in sex-linked lethal mutations. Because, however, the loss of males implied by the change in the sex-ratio between the first trimester (115:100) and term (106:100) is so poorly understood, we saw no way to incorporate this indicator into our doubling dose estimate. Finally, there was no apparent effect of parental radiation on the child's development, at birth, at 9 months of age, or in middle school.

342

THE EXTRAPOLATION TO THE EFFECTS OF LOW-LEVEL CHRONIC RADIATION

The average gonadal dose received by the survivors of the bombings was about 0.20-0.25 Sv, with a pronounced skew to the right in the distribution of individual doses, and with some few survivors estimated to have received gonadal doses as high as 3.0 Sv. Most human concerns over the genetic effects of radiation are directed towards low-level, chronic or pulsed exposures. Our extrapolation from the observations in Japan to the latter situation must take into consideration the dose-rate factor described by Russell et al. (1958). The question of exactly how to make this extrapolation is somewhat controversial. We have accepted that the relationship between radiation and the complex of end-points we have pursued is linear-quadratic (cf. Abrahamson and Wolff, 1976), and on the basis of the distribution of gonadal doses among the survivors, applied a dose rate factor of 2. This calculation results in an estimated doubling dose for chronic radiation of 3.38 to 4.46 Sv. This range reflects only the biological uncertainty in estimating the impact of chronic radiation; allowance for the statistical uncertainty would increase that range to a considerable but indeterminate extent.

A COMPARISON WITH THE RESULTS OF EXPERIMENTS WITH MICE

Those of you who have followed the developments in mouse radiation genetics over the past 40 years will recognize that our estimate of the doubling dose is somewhat different from that usually projected on the basis of experiments with mice. We have commented on this elsewhere (Neel et al., in press); here we will be very brief. In 1972 the United Nations Scientific Committee on the Effects of Radiation, extrapolating from the experimental data on mice to humans, suggested that for chronic radiation "the use of a 100-rad doubling dose (for both sexes) will not underestimate the risk". The murine data on acute radiation effects from which that extrapolation was made have been conveniently summarized by Lüning and Searle (1971). Somewhat later, in 1977, the International Commission on Radiological Protection suggested that with respect to chronic, low-level radiation, a doubling dose of 1 Gy be used for humans (ICRP, 1977). In 1980 the Third Committee on the Biological Effects of Ionizing Radiation of the U.S. National Academy of Sciences reaffirmed that estimate of 1 Gy, somewhat arbitrarily placing upon it limits of 0.5 to 2.5 Gy. It is clear that in these extrapolations, the data from the Russell 7-locus test system (Russell, 1951), because of their excellence, volume, and exploration of dose rate factors, dominated the extrapolations, although data on mutations producing semisterility, dominant visible traits, dominant skeletal traits, and recessive lethals were also considered.

There were even at the time of the 1972 UNSCEAR report, and certainly are now, data which suggested a greater resistance of the mouse to the genetic effects of acute radiation than the data employed in the Committee extrapolations to humans. For instance, Lyon and Morris (1966, 1969) developed a six-locus test system which overlapped in only one locus with the Russell test stock. At an acute exposure of approximately 6 Gy, the spermatogonial mutation rate was some 40% of that observed with the Russell strain. Unfortunately, the control studies involved only 124,614 locus tests, in the course of which no mutations were observed; a doubling dose for this strain cannot be calculated. Bailey and Kohn (1965), in a histocompatibility system testing for mutation with respect to at least 30 loci, found no significant effect of 522 rads of X-rays, from which it was concluded that the doubling dose at the 95% probability level was >260 rad. In that same paper, Bailey and Kohn calculate from the data of Lyon et al, (1964) a doubling dose for recessive visibles (as distinct from the specific locus test) of 400 rad, and for recessive lethals, on the basis of the data of Lyon (1959), Searle (1964), and Lyon et al, (1964), a doubling dose of 80-400 rad. This latter is a higher estimate than that employed by UNSCEAR in 1982 (cf. Lüning and Searle, 1971); the difference may stem from the assumptions regarding the recessive lethal component in the mortality in controls. What can be said with assurance is that the recessive lethal induction rate in these experiments per rad appears well below the rate in the Russell system, a finding which also emerges from the later data of Roderick (1983). Finally, the dominantly-inherited cataract system developed by Kratschvilova and Ehling (1979) yielded a doubling dose estimate for acute spermatogonial radiation of approximately 1.1 Sv in early studies but 1.8 in later studies involving a different strain (cf. Favor, 1989).

Thus far I have commented on the differences between the early findings and some of the later findings with respect to specific locus tests and their variants. There have, in addition, been observations on the effect of large doses of radiation, often over repeated generations, on such less specific attributes as survival to weaning, weaning weight, litter size, and sex-ratio, well reviewed in Green (1968). These important indicators responded to a very limited extent to doses of radiation which over multiple, successive generations cumulated to as much as 20 Gy. It is an interesting commentary on the times that a number of investigators referred to these as unreliable or unsatisfactory indicators, as contrasted with specific locus systems. There was, in fact, a profound message in these indicators, namely, that the loci responsible for these traits may be less responsive to radiation mutagenesis than the loci of the specific locus tests.

The estimate derived from the Hiroshima-Nagasaki data is time and place specific and based on an approximately equal contribution to the outcome by males and females. Aneuploidy plays a larger role in the human estimate than in the mouse estimate. At this point we believe that although a reconsideration of the mouse data will result in a higher estimate of the doubling dose for mice than is currently in favor, the possibility of a real difference between mice and humans as regards the doubling dose must be taken quite seriously.

THE NEXT GENERATION OF STUDIES ON THE MUTATION RATES OF HUMANS AND MICE

We are at the end of a cycle of studies in Hiroshima and Nagasaki, and the question is: what next - if anything? This question has resulted in many discussions among the directors, the scientific councillors, the consultants, and the staff of the RERF. At the present time there are two rather obvious possible extensions of these studies. The first involves the examination of a greatly expanded battery of proteins, using two-dimensional polyacrylamide gel electrophoresis (2-D PAGE) and related technologies. The second involves studies at the DNA level. Given the orientation of this Symposium, I will not discuss the possible protein studies further, but concentrate on the emerging DNA technologies.

Before I discuss current thinking about the exact strategy, I should say a few words about the material on which any future study will be based, because this shapes the strategy. For a study of mutation, both parents of a child must be available. The majority of the children in the study cohorts were born during the first two decades after the bombings. Their parents, if still alive, are in their 60's and 70's; many are moving out of the two cities. Those who remain are not always cooperative with further studies that involve drawing a blood sample. Since any substantial new study may extend over the next decade, the non-availability of parents when necessary for a genetic study will emerge as a larger and larger issue. Accordingly, the RERF made the decision some four years ago to establish a resource of Epstein-Barr virus-transformed lymphocytoid cell lines, some 500 mother-father-one or two child constellations where one or both parents were relatively heavily exposed at the time of the bombings, and a similar and suitably matched sample where the parents were unexposed. As of January 31, 1989, 383 of the approximately 1000 family constellations projected had been established, and another 50 or so were in various stages of completion. It will be at least three more years before this resource is complete.

At this juncture I would like to refer back to my opening comments, as well as the brief discussion of the murine data. <u>If there is one lesson we have learned from the past 40 plus years of radiation genetics, it is how very careful one must be in choosing the end points.</u> Whether the new studies be based on DNA or proteins, it is necessary to take extraordinary precautions that these be representative, and the larger and more diversified the battery of indicators, the better.

Any substantial body of new data which will supplement the existing information, will be useful even if the observed difference between the children of exposed and controls does not reach statistical significance. On the other hand, I am sure we will agree that it would be intellectually satisfying at long last to achieve statistical significance with some indicator, and we now have sufficient background to estimate how much data this would require.

I presume we will agree that any future studies should involve functional genes, whether these functions are currently understood or not, so that there is ultimately a reasonable prospect of projecting to regulatory bodies and the public which is supporting these studies, the impact of an increased mutation rate on morbidity and mortality. The proteins visualized with 2-D PAGE are clearly the products of functional genes, albeit at present these proteins are largely unidentified. With respect to DNA, this strategy involves concentrating on the exons encoding for a product, rather than on the much more abundant repetitive DNA's, pseudogenes, introns, and other types of DNA of unknown or dubious function.

There is additional reason for proposing to study genes which are transcriptionally active, as suggested by their DNA structure or by the identification of a gene product. Hanawalt (1987) has summarized the evidence that the excision repair of pyrimidine dimers and certain other lesions is non-random in the mammalian genome, exhibiting a distinct preference for actively transcribed DNA sequences. Whether this finding applies to the types of lesions produced by ionizing radiation is unknown, but prudence dictates we make that assumption, and not base our studies or conclusions on DNA not known to undergo active transcription at any time.

Let us now consider the numerical requirements with respect to DNA. On the basis of studies of serum proteins and erythrocyte enzymes, we have set the rate with which mutation results in a nucleotide substitution in exons in humans at 1×10^{-8}/nucleotide/generation, or 1×10^{-5} for a gene with 1000 exon nucleotides (Neel et al., 1986). On the basis of the considerations raised earlier, I now believe this is very likely an overestimate of the mutation rate for exon nucleotides, but we will work with it. From the frequency in populations of null variants of erythrocyte enzymes (Mohrenweiser, 1981; Satoh et al., 1983) or gross insertion/ deletion/ rearrangement (I/D/R) events in DNA (Mohrenweiser et al., 1989), I will again - as before - guess that mutation yielding I/D/R's also has a frequency of 1×10^{-5}/locus/generation. Then to a first approximation, we can say the probability of a mutation of either type is roughly 2×10^{-8}/exon nucleotides scanned/generation. We will assume that the two parents of the cell line trios have received together on average 1/5 of a doubling dose. From standard power function statistics, we can calculate that on the assumption of a type I error of 0.05 and a type II error of 0.20, it would require two samples of approximately 1.8×10^9 exon nucleotides surveyed to demonstrate a statistically significant difference between the two groups. Let us assume (see below) that this study is conducted on the basis of probes derived from "active" genes, each of 500 nucleotides (1000 nucleotides per diploid child), and that there will be 500 children in each sample, then some 3.6×10^4 different probes are required to achieve these numbers. Otherwise stated, some 3.6×10^7 nucleotides should be examined for each of the children in the study if statistical significance is to be achieved. These are staggering requirements, and it may well be that in the DNA studies, as for those that have gone before, significance will not be achieved, but the data which are obtained can still be used to refine the current estimate.

I cannot emphasize too strongly how approximate these calculations are. They could easily be off by a factor of two. On the other hand, I feel reasonably confident that attaining results which will substantially advance our current understanding requires a very major effort, to the technical aspects of which we now turn. What is the most efficient way to acquire a meaningful data base? The DNA technologies are evolving so rapidly that any evaluation made today will surely be superceded within the next year or two. This rapid evolution can only accelerate as the so-called Human Genome Project gains momentum. I offer, nevertheless, some comments on the current state of the art, as recently summarized by the investigators involved in exploring in Hiroshima the feasibility of a DNA program (Satoh et al., in press).

Let us assume a suitable battery of probes can be identified. The approach among those available which seems most efficient requires as its first step the amplification of approximately 3 Kb of the cell-line genomic DNA of one of these probes by the polymerase chain reaction (PCR). This piece of DNA, which would usually be comprised of both intron and exon material, is then cleaved into 4-6 fragments. These fragments are denatured and then allowed to reanneal with an RNA standard. The fragments are then examined in the denaturing gradient gel electrophoresis (DGGE) system described by Fischer and Lerman (1983). In the presence of a mismatch in the RNA:DNA duplex, the heteroduplex will denature higher on the gel than when no mismatch is involved. Fragment position can be visualized by autoradiography or by staining with ethidium bromide. Some mismatches will be due to relatively common DNA polymorphisms, and can be disregarded. Others will be recognized as rare variants, comparable to the rare protein variants which were the basis for an earlier study of mutation rates in this population (Neel et al., 1988), and these will require family studies. As many as 4 or 5 fragments can be examined in a single gel lane. A pilot study is projected for this fall (1989). Only after this can the efficiency of the approach be evaluated. An obvious extension from this would be a two-dimensional system, completely analogous to the 2-D PAGE system for proteins, in which the first dimension would be separation based on an agarose sizing gel and the second dimension, a slab denaturing gel. First steps in this direction have recently been described by Uitterlinden et al (1989). A useful feature of both the 1-D and 2-D DNA gels is that unlike the 2-D protein gels, the expected position on the gel of the standard or type fragment can be planned, and the entire gel designed so that the fragments will be well distributed.

Our group has devoted a major effort over the past seven years to developing an algorithm for reading 2-D protein gels which an image analysis system such as marketed by Bio Image (Ann Arbor) can execute with relatively little operator intervention (Skolnick and Neel, 1986). The core of the program is a comparison of the correspondence between the spots visualized on a child's gel and the spots on the gels of his/her father and mother, or with the spots on a master, standard gel. A spot present in a child but not in either parent, or a spot in a child of half the intensity of the corresponding parental spots, is investigated as a potential mutation. It appears at present that this algorithm can be used in the analysis of isotope-labelled or ethidium bromide-stained 2-D DNA gels.

FINAL COMMENTS

In closing, I offer a few comments on parallel animal studies. Obviously, many aspects of radiation genetics can be studied to much better advantage in an experimental organism than in humans. I presume that the revision upwards in the doubling dose projections which we are suggesting will spark discussion concerning the desirability of a mouse DNA program to parallel that contemplated for the Japanese cell lines. Already difficulties in attaining true comparabiity are obvious: the human cell lines were only established 40 years after the radiation exposure. I would certainly hope that any future DNA-oriented studies on mice would involve probes comparable to those available for humans, and radiation doses more comparable to those of Hiroshima and Nagasaki than those used in past studies on the mouse - which would of course increase the magnitude of any study of mice. I am very mindful of the evidence on efficiency of DNA repair in relation to life span (Hart and Setlow, 1974; Hart et al., 1979) and for repair heterogeneity between rodent and human cells (Hanawalt, 1987), which create the basis for real differences between humans and mice. Thus, studies on the radiation genetics of murine DNA might well be more important to the clarification of aspects of DNA radiation genetics and the mouse doubling dose than to the light they would shed on the human doubling dose, the more so if we assume the DNA studies on humans will now go forward.

It is clear that any significant improvement upon our present understanding of the genetic effects of the atomic bombs, plus parallel animal studies, involves a major, major effort. The magnitude of this effort is becoming apparent at a time of decreasing relative financial resources due to national budgetary problems and (to some) increasingly attractive alternative research programs in genetics. My personal opinion is that if further studies are undertaken, they should not be token but on a scale to advance substantially our understanding of the genetic risks of radiation for human populations. We need a great deal of discussion on all aspects of these future studies. In this regard, I see such a major program on the nature and significance of radiation damage to DNA as profiting greatly from some of the developments of the Human Genome Project, providing an immediate application for some of the data issuing from that Project.

ACKNOWLEDGEMENTS

The study of the genetic effects of the atomic bombs is the work of many investigators, whose specific roles are indicated in the various pertinent citations. The author expresses his appreciation of the support of the U. S. National Cancer Institute and the Department of Energy in the personal investigations cited in this report.

REFERENCES

Abrahamson, S., and Wolff, S., 1976, Reanalysis of radiation-induced specific locus mutations in the mouse, Nature, 264:715.

Awa, A. A., Honda, T., Neriishi, S., Sotuni, T., Shimba, H., Ohtaki, K., Nakano, M., Kodama, Y., Itoh, M., and Hamilton, H. B., 1987, Cytogenetic studies of the offspring of atomic bomb survivors, in: "Cytogenetics: Basic and Applied Aspects," G. Obe and A. Basler, eds., Springer-Verlag, Berlin.

Asakawa, J., Neel, J. V., Takahashi, N., Satoh, C., Kaneoka, S., Nishikori, E., and Fujita, M., 1988, Heterozygosity and ethnic variation in Japanese platelet proteins, Hum. Genet., 78:1.

Bailey, D. W., and Kohn, H. J., 1965, Inherited histocompatibility changes in the progeny of irradiated and unirradiated inbred mice, Genet. Res., Camb. 6:330.

Chakraborty, R. and Neel, J.V., Description and validation of a method for simultaneous estimation of effective population size and mutation rate from human population data, Proc. Nat. Acad. Sci., USA, in press.

Chu, E. H. Y., Boehnke, M., Hanash, S. M., Kuick, R. D., Lamb, B. J., Neel, J. V., Niezgoda, W., Pivirotto, S., and Sundling, G., 1988, Estimation of mutation rates based on the analysis of polypeptide constituents of altered human lymphoblastoid cells, Genetics, 119:693.

Committee on the Biological Effects of Ionizing Radiations, 1980, "The Effects on Populations of Exposure to Low Levels of Ionizing Radiation," National Academy Press, Washington, D.C.

Edwards, Y. and Hopkinson, D.A., 1980, Are abundant proteins less variable?, Nature, 284:511.

Favor, J., 1989, Risk estimation based on germ cell mutations in animals, Proc. 16th Intern. Congr. Genetics. Genome, in press.

Fischer, S. G., and Lerman, L. S., 1983, DNA fragments differing by simple base-pair substitutions are separated in denaturing gradient gels: Correspondence with melting theory, Proc. Nat. Acad. Sci., USA, 80:1579.

Green, E. L., 1968, Genetic effects of radiation on mammalian populations, Ann. Rev. Genet., 2:87.

Hanawalt, P. C., 1987, Preferential DNA repair in expressed genes. Env. Health Persp., 76:9.

Harris, H., 1980, "Human Biochemical Genetics," Third, revised edition, Elsevier/North-Holland Biomedical Press, Amsterdam.

Hart, R. W., Sacher, G. A., and Hoskins, T. L., 1979, DNA repair in a short- and a long-lived rodent species, J. Gerontol., 34:808.

Hart, R., and Setlow, R. B., 1974, Correlation between deoxyribonucleic acid excision-repair and life-span in a number of mammalian species, Proc. Natl. Acad. Sci., USA, 71:2169.

International Commission on Radiation Protection, 1977, ICRP Publication 26, Pergamon Press, New York.

Klose, J., Willers, I., Singh, S., and Goedde, H. W., 1983, Two-dimensional electrophoresis of soluble and structure-bound proteins from cultured human fibroblasts and hair root cells: Qualitative and quantitative variation, Hum. Genet., 63:262.

Kratochvilova, J., and Ehling, U. H., 1979, Dominant cataract mutations induced by gamma-irradiation of male mice, Mut. Res., 63:221.

Lüning, K. G., and Searle, A. G., 1971, Estimates of the genetic risks from ionizing radiation, Mut. Res., 12:291.

Lyon, M. F., 1959, Some evidence concerning the 'mutational load' in inbred strains of mice, Heredity, Lond., 13:341.

Lyon, M. F., and Morris, T., 1966, Mutation rates at a new set of specific loci in the mouse, Genet. Res., 7:12.

Lyon, M. F., and Morris, T, 1969, Gene and chromosome mutation after large fractionated or unfractionated radiation doses to mouse spermatogonia, Mut. Res., 8:191.

Lyon, M. F., Phillips, R. J. S., and Searle, A. G., 1964, The overall rates of dominant and recessive lethal and visible mutation induced by spermatogonial x-irradiation of mice, Genet. Res., Lond., 5:448.

McConkey, E. H., Taylor, B. J., and Phan, D., 1979, Human heterozygosity: A new estimate, Proc. Natl. Acad. Sci. USA, 76:6500.

Mohrenweiser, H.W., 1981, Frequency of enzyme deficiency variants in erythrocytes of newborn infants, Proc. Natl. Acad. Sci., USA 78:5046.

Mohrenweiser, H. W., Larsen, R. D., and Neel, J. V., 1989, Development of molecular approaches to estimating germinal mutation rates. I. Detection of insertion/deletion/rearrangement variants in the human genome, Mut. Res., 212:241.

Neel, J. V., Satoh, C., Goriki, K., Asakawa, J-I., Fujita, M., Takahashi, N., Kageoka, T., and Hazama, R., 1988, Search for mutations altering protein charge and/or function in children of atomic bomb survivors: Final report, Am. J. Hum. Genet., 42:663.

Neel, J. V., Satoh, C., Goriki, K., Fujita, M., Takahashi, N., Asakawa, J., and Hazama, R., 1986, The rate with which spontaneous mutation alters the electrophoretic mobility of polypeptides, Proc. Natl. Acad. Sci. USA, 83:389.

Neel, J. V., Satoh, C., Smouse, P., Asakawa, J., Takahashi, N., Goriki, K., Fujita, M., Kageoka, T., and Hazama, R., 1988, Protein variants in Hiroshima and Nagasaki: Tales of two cities, Am. J. Hum. Genet., 43:870.

Neel, J. V., Schull, W. J., Awa, A. A., Satoh, C., Kato, H., Otake, M. and Yoshimoto, Y., The children of parents exposed to atomic bombs: Thoughts on the genetic doubling dose of radiation for humans, Am. J. Hum.. Genet., submitted.

Neel, J. V., Schull, W. J., Awa, A. A., Satoh, C., Otake, M., Kato, H., an Yoshimoto, Y., Implications of the Hiroshima-Nagasaki genetic studies for the estimation of the human "doubling dose" of radiation, Proc. 16th Intern. Congr. of Genet., Genome, in press.

Roderick, T. H., 1983, Using inversions to detect and study recessive lethals and detrimentals in mice, in: "Utilization of Mammalian Specific Locus Studies in Hazard Evaluation and Estimation of Genetic Risk," F. J. de Serres and W. Sheridan, eds., Plenum Press, New York.

Rosenblum, B. B., Neel, J. V., and Hanash, S. M., 1983, Two-dimensional electrophoresis of plasma polypeptides reveals "high" heterozygosity indices, Proc. Natl. Acad. Sci. USA, 80:5002.

Rosenblum, B. B., Neel, J. V., Hanash, S. M., Joseph, J. L., and Yew, N., 1984, Identification of genetic variants in erythrocyte lysate by two-dimensional gel electrophoresis, Am. J. Hum. Genet., 36:601.

Russell, W. L., 1951, X-ray induced mutations in mice, Cold Spring Harbor Symp. Quant. Biol., 16:327.

Russell, W. L., Russell, L. B., and Kelly, E. M., 1958, Radiation dose rate and mutation frequency, Science, 128:1546.

Satoh, C., Neel, J. V., Miura, A., Ueno, C., Arakawa, H., Omine, H., Goriki, K., and Fujita, M., 1985, Inherited thermostability variants of seven enzymes in a Japanese population, Ann. Hum. Genet., 49:11.

Satoh, C., Neel, J. V., Yamashito, A., Goriki, K., Fujita, M., and Hamilton, H. B., 1983, The frequency among Japanese of heterozygotes for deficiency variants of 11 enzymes, Amer. J. Hum. Genet., 35:656.

Satoh, C., Hiyama, K., Takahashi, N., Kodaira, M., and Neel, J. V., Approaches to DNA methods for the detection of heritable mutations in humans, Proc. Fifth Intern. Congr. on Environ. Mut.. in press.

Searle, A. G., 1964, Effects of low-level irradiation on fitness and skeletal variation in an inbred mouse strain, Genetics, 50:1159.

Skolnick, M. M., and Neel, J. V., 1986, An algorithm for comparing two-dimensional electrophoretic gels, with particular reference to the study of mutation, Adv. in Hum. Genet., 15:55.

Takahashi, N., Neel, J. V., Naguhata-Shimocichi, Y., Asakawa, J., Tanaka, Y., and Satoh, C., 1986, Inherited electrophoretic variants detected in a Japanese population with two-dimensional gels of erythrocyte lysates, Ann. Hum. Genet., 50:313.

Uitterlinden, A. G., Slagboom, P. E., Knook, D. L., and Vijg, J., 1989, Two-dimensional DNA fingerprinting of human individuals, Proc. Natl. Acad. Sci. USA, 86:2742.

United Nations Scientific Committee on the Effects of Atomic Radiation, 1972, "Ionizing radiation: Levels and effects", Vol. 2, United Nations, New York.

Walton, E., Styer, D., and Gruenstein, E.I., 1979, Genetic polymorphism in normal human fibroblasts as analyzed by two-dimensional polyacrylamide gel electrophoresis, J. Biol. Chem., 254:7951.

Wanner, L. A., Neel, J. V., Meisler, M. H., 1982, Separation of allelic variants by two-dimensional electrophoresis, Am. J. Hum. Genet., 34:209.

EFFECTS OF CALORIC RESTRICTION ON

THE MAINTENANCE OF GENETIC FIDELITY

Ronald W. Hart, Angelo Turturro, Rex A.
Pegram, and Ming W. Chou

National Center for Toxicological Research
United States Public Health Service
Jefferson, Arkansas 72079

INTRODUCTION

Comparative analysis of DNA damage and repair
determinations across different species can contribute to a
better understanding of the biological significance of these
parameters in human tissues. Previous data from such
comparative studies, used in conjunction with additional data
from a number of other areas (including life span studies) has
led to one approach which considers DNA damage and repair in
the context of longevity-assurance mechanisms (Sacher, 1977;
Hart and Turturro, 1981). The theory of longevity-assurance
mechanisms treats animal life span as the by-product of
particular processes which have evolved to protect the genomic
integrity of a species. These processes, such as DNA repair
and limiting proliferation, would also protect cells from
neoplastic transformation. Moreover, human evolution of what
appears to be the longest mammalian life span may have been
integrally dependent upon these processes, and an
understanding of these mechanisms seems critical to the
discovery of methods to improve longevity and limit toxicity
from a number of environmental exposures.

One test of the longevity-assurance theory is to utilize
a paradigm which extends life span, and evaluate different
longevity-assurance mechanisms (which have been suggested from
comparative studies) to determine how the mechanisms have been
effected. In mammals, caloric restriction (CR) is the only
paradigm which is known to consistently extend the genetically
fixed maximal life span, while concurrently reducing the
occurrence of many age-associated diseases (Sacher, 1977).
Most notable is the dramatic reduction of the incidence of
spontaneous and chemically-induced tumors in calorically
restricted rodents. Therefore, CR animals were chosen for
study as part of an integrated project to understand the
underlying protective mechanisms of caloric restriction.

DNA Damage and Repair in Human Tissues
Edited by B. M. Sutherland and A. D. Woodhead
Plenum Press, New York, 1990

Table 1.   Body Temperature and Caloric Restriction[a]

Time of Day	Diet	Body Temp.(^{o}C)
9:00 AM	AL	36.9 $\pm$ 0.04
	CR	35.8 $\pm$ 0.12
3:00 PM	AL	37.05 $\pm$ 0.05
	CR	36.1 $\pm$ 0.15
9:00 PM	AL	38.0 $\pm$ 0.01
	CR	36.7 $\pm$ 0.12
3:00 AM	AL	38.0 $\pm$ 0.05
	CR	36.8 $\pm$ 0.20

[a]Adapted from Duffy et al., 1989. Male F344 rats (18 months old) were fed NIH-31 diet ad libitum (AL) or restricted to 60% of AL (CR) starting at 14 weeks of age and continuing for the duration of the experiment. The animals were maintained on a 12/12 hr light/dark cycle with the lights on at 6:00 AM daily.

The results from our studies and other investigations indicate that caloric restriction acts at the physiological, biochemical, and molecular levels to enhance the maintenance of genetic fidelity, thereby reducing carcinogenesis and increasing life span.

PHYSIOLOGICAL ENDPOINTS

From the results of comparative studies, one of the most important longevity-assurance mechanisms appears to be the development of a large brain relative to body size (Kirkwood, 1985). An elevated brain/body weight ratio is characteristic of longer-lived species. The effects of CR are to elevate the brain/body weight ratio in rodents. Consistent with previous indications (Turturro and Hart, 1984), we found that, in the male Fischer 344 rat on NIH-31 diet, a 60% caloric restriction leads an increase (significant at the $p < 0.05$ level) of the brain weight/body weight ratio (at 12 months of age) from 0.0051 $\pm$ 0.0002 (n=11) to 0.0077 $\pm$ .0004 (n=11). There is no significant change in the liver weight/body weight ratio.

The mechanism by which an increased brain/body weight ratio may be correlated to increased longevity is unknown, however one possiblity is that increased relative brain weight indicates increased redundancy in neuronal control cells, and increased ability to withstand neuronal loss (Hart and Turturro, 1981).

Another important physiological parameter which has been correlated with life span is body temperature. Lowering body temperature is the only other mechanism found to increase longevity, and it is effective in poikilotherms (Schneider and Reed, 1985). Hibernating animals (whose body temperature is

Table 2.   Diet and Aflatoxin-DNA Binding[a]

Diet	Binding/mg DNA	Binding/Liver
AL	58 + 9	106 + 16
CR	27 + 3	42 + 3

[a]Adapted from Pegram et al., 1989. Male F344 rats were dosed with [^{3}H]aflatoxin B$_1$ (0.1 mg/kg body wt.) and sacrified at 3 hr after dosing. The animals were fed ad libitum (AL) or restricted to 60% of AL (CR) for 6 weeks prior to dosing. Binding is expressed as pmol/mg DNA, or pmol/ liver (means + SEM, n = 4).

lower than normal at times of the year) were found to live longer than non-hibernating sister species (Sacher, 1977). Caloric restriction results in a lowering of average body temperature, as shown in Table 1. This lowering is evident throughout the circadian temperature rhythm, as we have demonstrated in the mouse, rat, and in the long-lived deer mouse (Peromyscus leucopus). Presumably, spontaneous temperature-dependent DNA depurination and depyrimidination (Lindahl and Nyberg, 1972) is reduced by this alteration, leading to less spontaneous DNA damage.

The decrease in body temperature observed in the CR rats is also associated with less total oxygen consumption. In rats, average oxygen consumption was significantly reduced from an ad libitum level of 463 ml/hr to 309 ml/hr in the restricted group (Duffy et al., 1989). Similar effects occur in mice and Peromyscus. A component of this lower oxygen consumption is the smaller body size of CR rodents. The generation of oxygen free radicals during normal metabolism may be a major source of molecular damage contributing to the aging process (Harman, 1981). Reduced oxygen consumption in CR animals may result in less degenerative oxidative damage (e.g., lipid peroxidation is decreased by CR, Koizumi et al., 1987).

These changes in the CR rodents, added to the potentially lower rate of deleterious spontaneous genetic alterations attributable to decreased temperature, may culminate in less damage resulting from the normal processes of living.

DNA DAMAGE

Protection of the genome from the effects of DNA damaging agents is one of the most important mechanisms for maintaining genomic integrity. Pashko and Schwartz (1983) found decreased levels of DMBA binding to dermal DNA in food restricted mice, which they suggested may be due to modifications of metabolic activation pathways. The mycotoxin, aflatoxin B1 (AFB1), is a DNA-damaging agent which is a potent hepatocarcinogen in rats

Table 3. Diet and AFB1-DNA Adducts[a]

Diet	Picomoles Derivative/mg DNA	
	AFB1-N7-Gua	AFB1-N7-FAP
AL	44 ± 2	12 ± 2
CR	19 ± 2	3 ± 0.3

[a]Experimental conditions are described in Table 2. The [3H]AFB1-DNA adducts were hydrolyzed according to the method of Howard et al., 1983, and the separation of the AFB1-N7-guanine (AFB1-N7-Gua) and the formamido-pyrimidine (AFB1-N7-FAP) derivative was according to the method of Croy and Wogan, 1981. Values are means ± SEM, n = 4.

and has been implicated in numerous experiments as a causative agent in human liver cancer. Caloric restriction reduced by 50% the incidence of AFB1-induced hepatic tumors in male rats (Newberne and Rogers, 1986). AFB1 thus appeared to be a reasonable model compound to investigate the mechanisms of carcinogenesis which may be affected by caloric restriction.

Pegram et al. (1989) found that CR had a dramatic impact upon hepatic nuclear DNA-AFB1 binding in rats determined at three hours after administration of a single dose of AFB1 (Table 2). At this point, which approximates the peak binding time, nuclear binding (pmoles AFB1/mg DNA) in ad libitum (AL) rats was over twice that of the calorically restricted group. Moreover, total nuclear AFB1-DNA adduction per liver in the ad libitum group was 2.5 times that of the restricted rats. Analysis of the individual adducts demonstrated that much lower amounts of the major N7-guanine adduct and its stable breakdown product, the formamido-pyrimidine derivative (FAP), were present in the CR rats compared to the AL controls (Table 3).

There are many possible mechanisms which may contribute to the mitigation of damage from agents such as aflatoxin. An obvious possibility is an alteration by CR of the metabolism of an agent. For AFB1, Pegram et al. (1989) showed that the plasma concentrations of radiolabelled aflatoxin in CR rats were half the AL levels, with much more of the toxin apparently metabolized to water-soluble conjugates (Table 4). This finding is further bolstered by the determination that a higher percentage of the dose is excreted in urine in CR animals (Pegram et al., 1989). Consistent with this analysis are the results of Leakey et al., (1989), who found CR-associated elevations in certain UDP-glucuronyl-transferase activities (Table 5). UDP-gluronyl transferase is an important component of Phase 2 metabolism, which conjugates charged chemical species for excretion in the urine. Elevated activities suggest increased proficiency at excretion.

Table 4. Diet and Plasma Radioactivity After AFB1 Treatment[a]

Diet	Total Radioactivity (nCi/ml)	Protein-bound (nCi/ml)	Hydrophilic (% of non-prot.)
AL	216 ± 15	123 ± 7	11 ± 1
CR	125 ± 6	94 ± 6	25 ± 3

[a]Experimental conditions are described in Table 2. The plasma was fractionated according to the method of Wong and Hsieh, 1980. Measurements were made 3 hr after dosing. Values are means ± SEM, n = 4.

In addition to changes in conjugation activity, other mechanisms to limit DNA damage in CR animals may be more widespread. Spontaneous depurination, the mechanism by which the major adducts of aflatoxin produce mutagenic apurinic sites, is a temperature sensitive process, and the breakdown of the N7-guanine adduct to FAP is also considered a spontaneous reaction. Cooler body temperatures may result in the observed increase in ratio between the N7 adduct of AFB_1 and its derivative.

Thus, by increasing detoxification through altering xenobiotic metabolism and decreasing damage through changes in physiology and intermediary metabolism, the genome may be protected by CR from the effects of endogenous and exogenous damage.

Table 5. Diet And UDP-Glucuronyltransferase Activities[a]

Substrate	Activity (nmol/min/mg/prot.)	
	AL (n=5)	CR (n=4)
2-Aminophenol	3.3 ± 0.2	5.4 ± 0.7
Bilirubin	2.1 ± 0.2	3.5 ± 0.2
Testosterone	7.6 ± 1.2	9.4 ± 0.8
Estrone	0.7 ± 0.1	0.5 ± 0.04

[a]Adapted from Leakey et al., 1989. Experimental conditions are described in Table 1. Activities are expressed as means ± SEM.

Table 6. Diet and DNA Repair (UDS)[a]

Diet	Cell	DNA Synthesis	HU	HU+MMS	HU+UV
AL	BN	26580 ± 4325	2234 ± 373	2583 ± 257	3072 ± 259
CR	BN	18894 ± 2216	3007 ± 308	3547 ± 327*	4247 ± 408*
%change		-29%	+35%	+55%	+48%
AL	BNXF344	20954 ± 2000	4704 ± 380	6603 ± 492	9745 ± 459
CR	BNXF344	16738 ± 1428	4743 ± 425	7625 ± 420*	13044 ± 1106*
%change		-20%	+1%	+52%	+65%

[a] Adapted from Lipman et al, 1989. Repair in skin cells from male, 18 month old Brown-Norway (BN) and Brown-Norway X F344 (BNXF344) fed ad libitum (AL) or chronically restricted (60% of AL) (CR). Ultraviolet (UV) light used was at 254 nm, 20 joules/m^2. HU and MMS are methylmethanesulfonate, (0.5 mM) and hydroxyurea (2 mM), respectively. Values are cpm/million cells.
*Significantly different, p<0.01.

Table 7.   MGAP in Different Species[a]

Species	Diet	MGAP (fmols/ug DNA)
Rat (BN)	AL	0.37 + 0.04
	CR	0.64 + 0.04*
Mouse (B6C3F1)	AL	0.34 + 0.02
	CR	0.48 + 0.02*

[a]Adapted from Lipman et al., 1989.   Skin cells from male,
  18 month old Brown-Norway (BN) male and 30 month old B6C3F1
  mice, were used for the 06-methylguanine acceptor protein
  (MGAP) activity measurements. The mice were ad libitum fed
  (AL) or chronically restricted (60% of AL) (CR).
  *Significantly different, p<0.01

DNA REPAIR

     The second stage of protecting the genome is the ability
to repair DNA damage once it occurs. Lipman et al., (1989)
measured unscheduled DNA synthesis (UDS), a multi-enzyme
repair mechanism, after treatment with damaging agents in two
rat genotypes (Brown Norway (BN) and Brown Norway x Fischer
344 F1 hybrid (BNF) (Table 6).   06-Methyl-guanine-acceptor
protein activity (MGAP), a single repair enzyme, was measured
across species using the rat (BNF, 18 months) and mouse
(B6C3F1 hybrid, 30 months) (Table 7).   Table 6 shows that UDS
increased 48 and 65% in freshly isolated skin cells from 18
month old CR rats compared with their AL controls after
challenge with ultraviolet light (254 nm, 20J/m^2 UV). Also,
after treatment with methylmethane sulfonate (MMS, 0.5 mM), a
significant CR-associated increase in UDS was observed
(p<0.01, 55% for BN and 52% for BNF rats). MGAP activity
increased approximately 30% in CR mice when compared to their
AL counterparts while, in 18 month old restricted BN rats,
MGAP activity was 73% greater than in the AL group (Table 7).

     Although the mechanism of this elevation is unknown, one
key to this phenomenon may be the correlation of the changes
in body temperature to DNA repair (Table 8). MGAP levels in
phase shifted mice (i.e., CR mice were fed at 5 hr into the
dark phase of the 12 h/12 h light/dark cycle, so that the
times of maximal feeding activity for the CR and AL rats
coincided, Duffy et al., 1989) were examined at three times
during a 24 hour period. These three times represent points
where significant changes were found to occur in the
metabolism of CR rodents. The activity of MGAP exhibited a
circadian rhythm with significant increases in MGAP activity
in CR mice occurring during the period of highest metabolic
activity and body temperature.

GENE EXPRESSION

     Another longevity-assurance process involves the control
of aberrant gene expression in long-lived species. Cells from

357

Table 8. Diet, Time of Day, Temperature and MGAP[a]

Time	Diet	Body Temp.($^{\circ}$C)	MGAP (fmols/ug DNA)
4:00 AM	AL	38.0 $\pm$ 0.01	0.32 $\pm$ 0.02
	CR	36.6 $\pm$ 0.15*	0.38 $\pm$ 0.02*
7:00 AM	AL	36.5 $\pm$ 0.04	0.19 $\pm$ 0.02
	CR	35.7 $\pm$ 0.15*	0.19 $\pm$ 0.04
6:00 PM	AL	37.8 $\pm$ 0.05	0.34 $\pm$ 0.02
	CR	36.6 $\pm$ 0.15*	0.48 $\pm$ 0.02*

[a]In B6C3f1 mice, same description as in Table 7.
*Significantly different, $p < 0.01$

longer-lived species are more refractory to transformation in vitro and tumorigenesis in vivo compared to species with shorter life spans. It is possible that CR may improve this control with age. This concept has been studied experimentally by examining the expression of protooncogenes in CR animals (Nakamura et al., 1989). The evidence linking aberrant oncogene expression to carcinogenesis is substantial (Bishop, 1985). As shown in Table 9, at 2 of the 3 times of determination, hepatic c-myc protooncogene expression was significantly lower in calorically restricted B6C3F$_1$ mice than in the AL controls. These data also demonstrate that hepatic c-myc expression in these mice has a definite circadian rhythm. These circadian differences were as much as three-fold, and can affect CR or AL animals differently depending on feeding schedule.

The apparent mechanism associated with the circadian changes noted with c-myc expression seems to be body temperature-dependent. In mice (Table 9) and Peromyscus leucopus, a high correlation coefficent (>0.9) is found when c-myc expression is correlated to deep body temperature (Nakamura et al., in press).

CONCLUSIONS

Caloric restriction appears to decrease the amount of DNA damage produced endogenously by both modulating certain damage-prone pathways and by altering metabolism to more rapidly detoxify and eliminate damaging agents. The CR animals also lower their body temperature, decreasing spontaneous DNA damage. Further, any remaining damage is repaired with a more active DNA repair system. Aberrant gene expression is decreased, which is also associated with lower body temperature. Thus, CR seems to trigger in short-lived rodents many of the longevity- assurance processes used to protect the genome in longer-lived species, leading to increased life span. In this regard, the findings discussed here indicate that CR provides a good model to test the longevity- assurance theory.

Table 9.   Diet, Time, Temperature and c-myc

Protooncogene Expression[a]

Time	Diet	Body Temperature (^{o}C)	c-myc (% of Mean)
4:00 AM	AL	38.0 + 0.01	1.7 + 0.3
	CR	36.6 + 0.15*	0.4 + 0.2*
7:00 AM	AL	36.5 + 0.04	1.0 + 0.3
	CR	35.7 + 0.15*	0.4 + 0.2*
6:00 PM	AL	37.8 + 0.05	1.8 + 0.5
	CR	36.6 + 0.15*	1.3 + 0.2

[a]Adapted from Nakamura et al., 1989. Male B6C3F1 mice, 30 month old, ad libitum fed (AL) or chronically restricted (60% of AL) (CR) were used for c-myc protooncogene expression measurement.
*Significantly different, $p < 0.05$.

One theory which might explain how the triggering of the longevity- assurance genes evolved can be considered the Adaptive-Longevity Assurance Theory of CR:
1) CR mimics a situation very common in the wild, i.e. food scarity at different times of year;
2) A successful species preserves itself during these difficult times by either forming some vegetative stage (e.g., a spore) or by adapting through the development of mechanisms that extend its life span so that the organism will live to reproduce when conditions improve;
3) One of the possible mechanisms used to increase life span is to increase the effect of the same longevity-assurance genes which are responsible for the potential life span of the species.

The ability to trigger longevity-assurance processes by a simple paradigm suggests methods for enhancing these mechanisms in humans, which may ultimately lead to significant improvements in human health with decreased effects of exposures to toxic chemicals, lower cancer incidence, and increased life span.

REFERENCES

Bishop, J., 1985, Viral oncogenes, Cell, 42:23.

Croy, R.G., and Wogan, G.N., 1981, Temporal Patterns of Covalent DNA Adducts in Rat Liver after Single and Multiple Doses of Aflatoxin B_1, Cancer Res., 41:197.

Duffy, P.H., Feuers, R.J., Leakey, J.A., Turturro, A., and Hart, R.W., 1989, Effect of chronic caloric restriction on physiological variables related to energy metabolism in the male Fischer 344 rat, Mech. Ageing Dev., 48:117.

Harman, D., 1981, The aging process. Proc. Natl. Acad. Sci. 78:7124.

Hart, R.W., and Turturro, A., 1981, Evolution and longevity-assurance processes, Naturwissenschaften, 68:552.

Howard, P.C., Heflich, R.H., Evans, F.E., and Beland, F.A., 1983, Formation of DNA Adducts in vitro and in Salmonella typhimurium upon Metabolic Reduction of the Environmental Mutagen 1-Nitropyrene, Cancer Res., 43:2052.

Kirkwood, T., 1985, Comparative and evolutionary aspects of longevity. in: "Handbook of the Biology of Aging", C. Finch and E. Schneider, eds., Van Nostrand, New York.

Koizumi, A., Weindruch, R., and Walford, R.L., 1987, Influences of dietary restriction and age on liver enzyme activities and lipid peroxidation in mice, J. Nutr., 117:361.

Leakey, J., Cunny, H., Bazare, J. Jr., Webb, P., Lipscomb, J., Slikker, W. Jr., Feuers, R., Duffy, P. H., and Hart, R. W., 1989, Effects of aging and caloric restriction on hepatic drug metabolizing systems in the Fischer 344 rat. II. effects on conjugating enzymes. Mech. Ageing Dev., 48:157.

Lindahl, T. and Nyberg, B., 1972, Rate of depurination of native deoxyribonucleic acid, Biochemistry, 11:3610.

Lipman, J.M., Turturro, A., and Hart, R.W., 1989, The influence of dietary restriction on DNA repair in rodents: A preliminary study, Mech. Ageing Dev. 48:135.

Nakamura, K.D., Duffy, P.H., Turturro, A., and Hart, R.W., 1989, The effect of dietary restriction on myc protooncogene expression in mice: A preliminary study, Mech. Ageing Dev. 48:199.

Nakamura, K.D., Duffy, P.H., Lu, M., and Hart, R.W., Hepatic myc protooncogene is reduced and possibly correlated with body temperature in fasted Peromyscus leucopus mice., AGE, in press.

Newberne, P.M., and Rogers, A.E., 1986, The role of nutrients in cancer causation, in:"Diet, Nutrition, and Cancer," Y. Hsyashi, ed., Japan Soc. Press, Tokyo.

Pashko, L.L., and Schwartz, A., 1983, Effect of food restriction, dehydroepiandrosterone, or obesity on the binding of ^{3}H-7,12-dimethyl- benz(a)anthracene to mouse skin DNA. J. Gerontol. 38:8.

Pegram R.A., Allaben W.T., and Chou, M.W., 1989, Effect of caloric restriction on aflatoxin-B$_1$ DNA adduct formation and associated factors in Fischer 344 rats: Preliminary findings., Mech. Ageing Dev. 48:167.

Sacher, G., 1977, Life table modification and life prolongation, in:"Handbook of the Biology of Aging", C. Finch and L. Hayflick, eds., Van Nostrand, New York.

Schneider E.L., and Reed, J.D., 1985, Modulations of aging processes. in: "Handbook of the Biology of Aging", C. Finch and E. Schneider, eds., Van Nostrand, New York.

Turturro, A., and Hart, R.W., 1984, DNA repair mechanisms in aging, in: "Comparative Biology of Major Age-Related Diseases," D. Schiapelli and G. Migaki, eds., Liss, New York.

Wong, Z.A., and Hsieh, D.P.H., 1980, The comparative metabolism and toxicokinetics of aflatoxin B1 in the monkey, rat, and mouse, Toxicol. Appl. Pharmacol. 55:115.

ONCOGENES AND TUMOR SUPPRESSOR GENES

INVOLVED IN HUMAN LUNG CARCINOGENESIS

Curtis C. Harris[1,4], Roger Reddel[1,2], Rama Modali[1], Teresa
A. Lehman[1], Deborah Iman[1], Mary McMenamin[1], Haruhiko
Sugimura[1], Ainsley Weston[1] and Andrea Pfeifer[1,3]

[1]Laboratory of Human Carcinogenesis, Division of Cancer
Etiology, National Cancer Institute, NIH, Bldg. 37, Room
2C01, Bethesda, MD 20892

[2]Present address: Children's Medical Research Foundation,
P.O. Box 61, Camperdown N.S.W. 2050, Australia.

[3]Present address: Genetic Toxicology Section, Nestle
Research Center, Vers-Chez-Leblanc, 1026 Lausanne, CH-1800,
Vevey, Switzerland.

[4]To Whom Correspondence Should Be Addressed.

INTRODUCTION

Carcinogenesis is a multistage process involving both genetic and
epigenetic aberrations. Activation of proto-oncogenes and/or inactivation of tumor suppressor genes may occur in an early stage of carcinogenesis, i.e., tumor initiation, as well as in the later stages e.g.,
tumor conversion and progression (Fig. 1). For example, activation of
Ki-ras by base substitution mutations is an early event in human colon
carcinogenesis (Vogelstein et al., 1988), whereas amplification of N-myc
is associated with the tumor progression stage of human neuroblastoma
(Brodeur et al., 1987). In the inherited form of retinoblastoma, a
defective tumor suppressor gene, Rb-1, is found in the germline DNA and
the second Rb-1 allele is inactivated most frequently by deletion or
recombinational mechanisms during the initial stages of carcinogenesis
(Knudson, 1985; Hansen et al., 1985; Cavenee et al., 1986; Friend et
al., 1986; Fung et al., 1987). In contrast, the inactivation by somatic
mutation of both alleles of the p53 gene appears to occur during tumor
progression of human carcinomas of the colon (Baker et al., 1989),
breast and lung (Nigro et al., 1989).

One basic tenet of tumor promotion is selective clonal expansion of
the "initiated" preneoplastic cells. Possible mechanisms of tumor
promotion are listed in Table 1. Cell division and terminal differentiation of the epithelial cells are strictly balanced in the normal
bronchial epithelium. Cell-cell, cell-matrix, and cell-mediator interactions are all involved in maintaining this complex community of cells
at the tissue level of biological organization. At the cellular level,
negative and positive growth factors, signal translators, and nuclear
regulators are involved.

DNA Damage and Repair in Human Tissues
Edited by B. M. Sutherland and A. D. Woodhead
Plenum Press, New York, 1990

Table 1. Possible Selective Clonal Expansion Advantages of
          Preneoplastic and Neoplastic Cells (See Harris,
          1987)

A. Defect in control of differentiation, _e.g._, resistance
       to induction of terminal differentiation by
       endogenous and exogenous factors
B. Defect in control of growth
    1. Autocrine production of growth factors
    2. Increased sensitivity to growth factors produced by
       other cells
    3. Decreased sensitivity to inhibitors of growth
C. Differential response to cytotoxic agents
    1. Inhibition of viral cytopathological response
    2. Resistance to damage by electrophils
    3. Resistance to oxidative stress
D. Other
    1. Escape from intracellular control mediated by cell-
       cell communication
    2. Increased capacity to repair DNA damage

NEOPLASTIC TRANSFORMATION OF HUMAN BRONCHIAL EPITHELIAL CELLS

   The strategy that we have formulated for investigating the
neoplastic transformation of normal human bronchial epithelial (NHBE)
cells is shown in Table 2. Six families of activated proto-oncogenes,
ras, _raf_, _jun_, _fur_, _neu_, and _myc_ have so far been associated with human
lung cancer. Since association does not necessarily indicate causation,
human bronchial epithelial cells _in vitro_ are being used to investigate
the functional role of these genes in carcinogenesis. When transferred

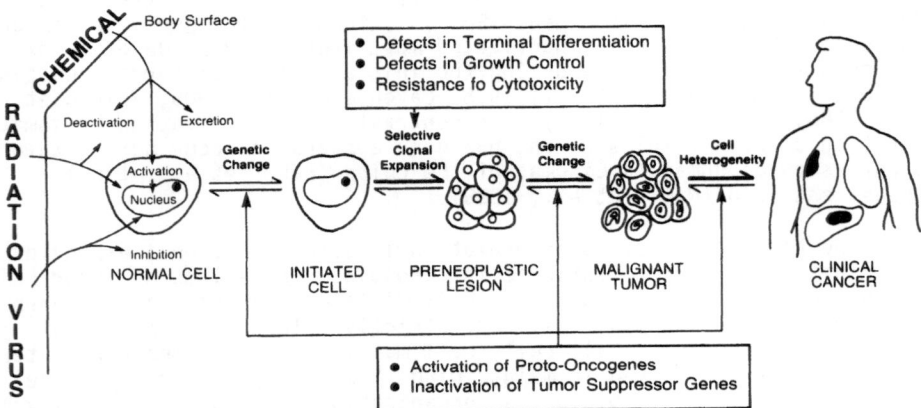

Fig. 1. Multistage carcinogenesis involving both genetic and
         epigenetic aberrations.

Table 2.   Strategy for Studying Neoplastic Transformation of
           Human Bronchial Epithelial Cells by Activated Proto-
           oncogenes

A.   Select activated proto-oncogenes associated with human
     lung cancer
B.   Transfer activated proto-oncogenes into the progenitor
     epithelial cells of bronchogenic carcinoma
C.   Select preneoplastic and neoplastic cells from
     putative suppressive normal cells
D.   Investigate dysregulation in molecular controls of
     growth and terminal differentiation
E.   Determine tumorigenic potential in athymic nude mice

---

into normal human bronchial epithelial cells by protoplast fusion, the
v-Ha-ras oncogene initiates a cascade of events leading to a decreased
responsiveness to inducers of squamous differentiation, aneuploidy,
increased lifespan, and rarely, "immortality" and tumorigenicity with
metastasis in athymic nude mice (Yoakum et al., 1985) (Table 3).
Genomic instability and apparent trans-activation of certain genes,
e.g., procollagenase IV, may be important mechanisms leading to the
phenotypic changes observed in the v-Ha-ras transformed cells.

The experiments described above and others (Rhim et al., 1981;
Namba et al., 1986; Pater and Pater, 1986; Amstad et al., 1988; Byrd et
al., 1988; Clark et al., 1988; Reddel et al., 1988a; Reznikoff et al.,
1988; Seremetis et al., 1989) indicate that "immortalization" is a rate-
limiting step in the multistage process of in vitro carcinogenesis of
human cells (Fig. 2). Therefore, we have developed human bronchial
epithelial cell lines by transfer of the SV-40 T antigen gene (Reddel et
al., 1988b). Aneuploidy is a common feature of these and other
"immortalized" human epithelial cells, and alterations in growth and
squamous differentiation pathways may also be frequently observed.

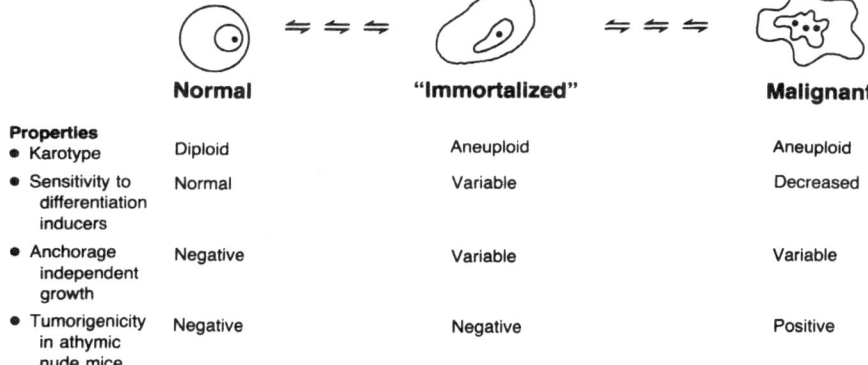

MULTISTAGE HUMAN EPITHELIAL CELL CARCINOGENESIS
IN VITRO

	Normal	"Immortalized"	Malignant
Properties			
• Karotype	Diploid	Aneuploid	Aneuploid
• Sensitivity to differentiation inducers	Normal	Variable	Decreased
• Anchorage independent growth	Negative	Variable	Variable
• Tumorigenicity in athymic nude mice	Negative	Negative	Positive

Fig. 2.   "Immortalization" appears to be a rate-limiting step in in
          vitro human cell carcinogenesis.

Table 3. Progressive Phenotypic and Genotypic Changes in
Normal Human Bronchial Epithelial Cells Transfected
with v-Ha-<u>ras</u>

---

1. Decreased response to inducers of terminal squamous
   differentiation
2. Increased response to serum mitogens
3. Increased frequency of chromosomal aberrations and
   aneuploidy
4. Increased cell population doublings
5. Cell "crisis"
6. Continuous cell line
7. Tumorigenicity
8. Increased <u>ras</u> p21 expression in tumor cells
9. Metastasis

The role of aberrant differentiation in carcinogenesis is of
considerable interest (Harris, 1982; Scott and Florine, 1982; Wille et
al., 1982; Thompson et al., 1983; Slack, 1986; Smits et al., 1987; Yuspa
et al., 1988). Our efforts in this regard have compared the growth and
squamous differentiation capabilities of NHBE cells to lung carcinoma
cells cultured under identical conditions (Lechner et al., 1983; Lechner
1984; Lechner et al., 1984). These comparative studies have indicated
that one of the differences that distinguish normal from tumorigenic
lung epithelial cells <u>in</u> <u>vitro</u> is the induction of terminal squamous
differentiation in normal cells, but not carcinoma cells, by either
serum or 12-O-tetradecanoylphorbol-13-acetate (TPA). Thus, after NHBE
cells are exposed to these agents, DNA synthesis ceases while RNA
synthesis continues for several days. In addition, the cells exhibit a
squamous morphology and eventually form cross-linked envelopes (Lechner
et al., 1984). Lung carcinoma cell lines treated with these agents do
not undergo these changes (Lechner et al., 1983; Willey et al., 1984).
Therefore, the elucidation of the mechanisms that control this differential responsiveness may be important to an understanding of carcinogenesis, especially the pathogenesis of squamous cell carcinoma which is a
common human lung cancer histology (Kraevskii, 1979).

We have recently investigated the induction of squamous differentiation in "immortalized" bronchial epithelial cells (Ke et al., 1988).
In these studies, human bronchial epithelial cells were "immortalized"
by either SV40 virus infection or transfection with the SV40 large T
antigen gene and then exposed to TPA, transforming growth factor-β_1
(TGF-β_1), or fetal bovine serum (FBS), agents that induce squamous
differentiation of normal human bronchial epithelial cells. Squamous
differentiation occurred in all ten T antigen positive cell cultures
when they were exposed to either FBS or TGF-β_1, but none differentiated
when exposed to TPA. From one cell line, designated BEAS-2B, two
subclones have been isolated. One is induced to undergo squamous
differentiation by FBS, and a second fails to undergo squamous differentiation and is mitogenically stimulated when exposed to serum. These
phenotypically different subclones provide a new <u>in</u> <u>vitro</u> cellular
system for delineating the mechanism(s) of human bronchial epithelial
cell squamous differentiation in response to FBS or TGF-β_1.

Activated <u>ras</u> oncogenes have been identified in human bronchial
carcinomas, especially adenocarcinomas (Rodenhuis et al., 1987). In
most cases the activated <u>ras</u> genes have been Ki-<u>ras</u>, but there have been
human lung cancer cell lines described with activated N-<u>ras</u> or Ha-<u>ras</u>

oncogenes (Yuasa et al., 1983; 1984). In an experimental model system, a mutated ras (activated human Ha-ras from the EJ bladder carcinoma cell line) gene linked to an immunoglobulin gene enhancer/SV40 T promoter induced multicentric adenomatous tumors (comparable to well-differentiated adenocarcinomas of the lung in man) in transgenic mice (Suda et al., 1987).

"Immortalized" human bronchial epithelial cell lines have been developed in order to define conditions under which ras and other oncogenes will reproducibly cause malignant transformation of human bronchial epithelial cells (Reddel et al., 1988b). This investigation and others have shown that human cells "immortalized" by a variety of means may be transformed by ras oncogenes (Rhim et al., 1981; Namba et al., 1986; O'Brien et al., 1986; Pater and Pater, 1986; Amstad et al., 1988; Reddel et al., 1988a). The induction of tumorigenicity in the BEAS-2B "immortalized" human bronchial epithelial cell line following infection with a recombinant retrovirus containing v-Ha-ras has been observed (Amstad et al., 1988). The anaplastic carcinomas produced in athymic nude mice by these cells have been shown to be of human epithelial origin and to have the isoenzyme phenotype and marker chromosomes characteristic of the BEAS-2B cell line. In addition, tumor cell lines from these tumors also express an abundant 21Kd protein immunoreactive with antibodies specific for the codon 12 mutation found in v-Ha-ras. This 21Kd protein is capable of being phosphorylated at threonine, position 59, in contrast to the cellular ras protooncogenes which are not. This difference indicates expression of the v-Ha-ras gene rather than activation of endogenous ras genes.

Activated ras oncogenes may have roles both in early (Guerrero et al., 1984; Zarbl et al., 1985) and late (Bondy et al., 1985; Kasid et al., 1985; Vogelstein et al., 1988) stages of the process of multistage carcinogenesis. Although exact parallels cannot be drawn between the multistep in vitro carcinogenesis described here and multistep carcinogenesis occurring in vivo, the role of ras in inducing malignancy in the already "immortalized" BEAS-2B cell line is most likely analogous to a late event.

The in vivo growth behavior and invasive potential of normal and "immortalized" human bronchial epithelial cells were studied by xeno-transplantation procedures, an in vitro assay of invasiveness, and determinations of type IV collagenase activity and mRNA expression (Bonfil et al., 1989). Immortalized BEAS-2B cells reconstituted a columnar epithelium when xenotransplanted into de-epithelialized rat tracheas transplanted sc into athymic BALB/c mice. A few adenomatous growths could be seen 16 weeks after transplantation. BZR cells, obtained by transfer of the v-Ha-ras oncogene into BEAS-2B cells, were tumorigenic in this xenotransplantation model. BZR-T33 cells, obtained from a tumor produced after injection of BZR cells, were also tumorigenic; however, they exhibited a shorter latent period. When these same cell lines were injected sc and iv into athymic BALB/c mice, BEAS-2B cells were not tumorigenic, and the BZR-T33 cells were more tumorigenic than the BZR cells. The incidence of spontaneous metastases after sc inoculation was zero for BEAS-2B cells, 33% for BZR cells, and 100% for BZR-T33 cells. Similar increasing values that correlated well with the data on in vivo growth were noted in the in vitro invasion assay, the collagenolytic ability, and the mRNA expression of type IV collagenase. Normal human bronchial epithelial cells showed the lowest values in all the assays. These progressive changes occurring in cells derived from the same parental line indicate that the presence of the v-Ha-ras oncogene in immortalized bronchial cells is associated with a full-fledged malignant phenotype, which is further enhanced by in vivo passaging.

A number of studies have demonstrated the presence of activated
c-Ki-ras oncogenes in human lung tumors (Rodenhuis et al., 1987;
Pulciani et al., 1982; Winter et al., 1985) and lung tumor cell lines
(Pulciani et al., 1982; Winter et al., 1985; Der et al., 1982; Santos et
al., 1984; Valenzuela and Groffen, 1986). The oncogene used in our
recently published study (Reddel et al., 1988a), v-Ki-ras, codes for
serine at codon 12, and this mutation has also been found in a human
bronchial adenocarcinoma cell line, A549 (Valenzuela and Groffen, 1986);
the v-Ki-ras oncogene also has a significant mutation at codon 59.
Transfer of this oncogene into an immortalized human bronchial epithelial cell line, BEAS-2B, either by infection of the cells with Ki-MSV or
by transfection of a plasmid, pHaKi, containing the v-Ki-ras coding
region resulted in neoplastic transformation.

It is of interest that the tumors induced by v-Ki-ras had adenocar-
cinomatous elements in contrast to the undifferentiated carcinomas
produced by infection of the same cells by a recombinant retrovirus
encoding v-Ha-ras (Amstad et al., 1988). This is an intriguing
observation in view of the evidence that the activated ras oncogene
found most commonly in human lung cancer is Ki-ras and that the majority
of lung carcinomas containing activated ras genes are adenocarcinomas.
However, this result should be interpreted cautiously. It is possible
that the morphologic difference is related to the experimental protocols
rather than to intrinsic differences in the effects of Ha-ras as opposed
to Ki-ras on these cells, e.g., the cells infected with the recombinant
virus encoding v-Ha-ras were G418-selected before inoculation of the
population into nude mice (Amstad et al., 1988) whereas the Ki-MSV-
infected population injected into nude mice contained a mixture of
infected and uninfected cells. At the least, this difference in
experimental protocol almost certainly accounts for the discrepancy in
tumor latency periods between v-Ha-ras-containing cells (1-3 weeks) and
v-Ki-ras-containing cells (3-6 weeks). Alternatively, it is possible
that the rapidly growing undifferentiated carcinomas induced by v-Ha-ras
may indicate a greater transforming potency either due to the
experimental protocol or due to intrinsic differences in the gene
products (including arginine and serine mutations at codon 12 in v-Ha-
ras and v-Ki-ras respectively). In support of the concept that various
mutated proteins may not be equally transforming, in vitro mutagenesis
experiments involving the c-Ha-ras gene demonstrated that replacement of
the codon 12 glycine with serine or aspartate resulted in less than 50%
of the focus-forming activity of the valine mutant (Fasano et al.,
1984).

A common feature of both Ha-ras- and Ki-ras-transformed BEAS-2B
cells was altered responsiveness to factors that induce squamous
differentiation in normal bronchial epithelial cells. As previously
reported (Ke et al., 1988), BEAS-2B cells exhibited a decreased colony
forming efficiency and clonal growth rate in response to either TGF-β_1
or FBS. In contrast, BEAS-2B cells containing either v-Ki-ras or
v-Ha-ras were unaffected by TGF-β_1 and their clonal growth rate was
increased by FBS. These fundamental changes in behavior appear to be
related to ras-induced neoplastic transformation rather than to the
experimental protocols for the following reasons. The altered
responsiveness was not due to the process of selection in nude mice
since a mitogenic response to FBS was exhibited by BEAS-2B/v-Ha-ras
cells before injection into nude mice. The G418 selection used in some
of the experimental protocols was not a major factor since tumor cell
lines established from Ki-MSV-infected BEAS-2B cells (that were not
G418-selected) also had enhanced clonal growth in the presence of serum.
The processes of gene transfer used, i.e. strontium phosphate coprecipi-

tation or retroviral infection, were not responsible for this change since BEAS-2B cells transfected with control plasmid DNA including pRSVneo or infected with ZipNeoSV(X) retrovirus and selected for G418 resistance retained an inhibitory response to serum.

Overexpression of c-raf-1 and the myc family of proto-oncogenes is primarily associated with small cell carcinoma (Gu et al., 1988; Rapp et al., 1988; Krystal et al., 1988; Graziano et al., 1987) which accounts for about 25% of human lung cancer. To determine the functional significance of the c-raf-1 and/or c-myc gene expression in lung carcinogenesis and to delineate the relation between proto-oncogene expression and tumor phenotype, we introduced both proto-oncogenes, alone or in combination, into human bronchial epithelial cells (Pfeifer et al., 1989). Two retroviral recombinants, pZip-raf and pZip-myc, containing the complete coding sequences of the human c-raf-1 and murine c-myc genes, respectively, were constructed and transfected into SV40 T antigen immortalized BEAS-2B cells. The cells were then selected for resistance to G418. BEAS-2B cells expressing both the transfected c-raf-1 and c-myc sequences formed large cell carcinomas in athymic nude mice with a latency of 4-21 weeks, whereas either pZip-raf- or pZip-myc-transfected cells were nontumorigenic after 12 months. Cell lines established from tumors revealed the presence of the co-transfected c-raf-1 and c-myc sequences and expressed morphological, chromosomal and isoenzyme markers which identified BEAS-2B cells as the progenitor cells of the tumors. Increased levels of neuron-specific enolase were detected in BEAS-2B cells containing both the c-raf-1 and c-myc genes and the derived tumor cell lines. The data demonstrate that the concomitant overexpression of the c-raf and c-myc proto-oncogenes causes neoplastic transformation of human bronchial epithelial cells resulting in large cell carcinomas with certain neuro-endocrine markers.

To determine the role of the c-raf gene in transformation in conjunction with c-myc and to study the activation of c-raf in the pathway of ras transformation in BEAS-2B cells, we examined the autophosphorylation and the serine/threonine specific kinase activity of c-raf in various BEAS-2B transfectants and in mouse 3T3 cells (Pfeifer et al., 1989). Immune-complex kinase assays were performed in which a new peptide antibody directed against the amino-terminal end of the c-raf sequence which specifically detects the 74KD c-raf protein was used. Compared to mouse 3T3 cells, autophosphorylation and serine/kinase activity were significantly higher in the immortalized BEAS-2B cells. Both activities were further increased in transfectants containing c-raf and c-myc or the v-Ha-ras oncogene. The correlation between p21 expression, c-raf kinase activity and tumorigenicity of various ras transfected BEAS-2B cell lines is under investigation. Our ongoing studies concern whether the relative efficiency with which BEAS-2B as compared to NHBE cells are transformed to tumorigenicity is associated with the level of c-raf kinase activity in these cells.

Although further characterization of the carcinomas induced by the c-raf-1 and c-myc genes is required, a correlation between the expression of these activated proto-oncogenes and the tumor phenotype is suggested. This linkage is of clinical significance with regard to therapy and prognosis, especially since the expression of c-raf-1 is associated with radiation resistance (Kasid et al., 1987; 1989). We consider that the experimental model described here should be useful to study molecular events and phenotypic markers associated with multistage lung carcinogenesis, including mechanisms involved in the cooperation of the c-raf-1 and c-myc genes in neoplastic transformation and radiation resistance.

Table 4. Strategies for Identifying and Studying Tumor
          Suppressor Genes in Lung Carcinogenesis

A. Identify chromosomal location of putative tumor
    suppressor genes
    1. Allelic deletion analysis of tumor DNA versus
        germline DNA
    2. Somatic cell genetic analysis of cellular lifespan
        and tumorigenicity
        a. Cell-cell hybrids
        b. Monochromosome-cell hybrids
B. Isolate genes by subtraction library approach
    1. Tumorigenic versus nontumorigenic hybrids
    2. Terminal squamous differentiation resistant versus
        differentiation sensitive cells
C. Isolate genes by insertion mutagenesis approach
D. Determine structure, function and tumor suppressive
    potential of isolated genes

TUMOR SUPPRESSION OF NEOPLASTIC HUMAN LUNG CELLS

Considering the large number of potential progenitor cells,
clinically evident cancer is a pathobiological event of exceedingly low
probability. Although systemic host factors, e.g. the immune system,
may largely account for its rarity, the lack of convincing reports of
"spontaneous" transformation of human cells in vitro and the difficulty
in inducing their in vitro neoplastic transformation with chemical,
physical, and viral oncogenic agents attest to the presence of inherent
suppressing factors at the biological level of the progenitor cells.
Evidence for these presumed dominant-acting "tumor suppressor" genes has
arisen primarily in epidemiological studies (Knudson, 1985); molecular
analyses of genetic loci exhibiting DNA-restriction fragment length
polymorphisms (DNA-RFLPs) show reduction to homozygosity of chromosome
13 found in retinoblastoma and osteosarcoma (Hansen et al., 1985) and of
chromosome 11 in Wilms' tumor (Koufos et al., 1984; Orkin et al., 1984;
Reeve et al., 1984; Fearon et al., 1984) and bladder cancer (Fearon et
al., 1985). Furthermore, these latter data have been corroborated by
somatic cell genetic studies with human cell hybrids (Stanbridge et al.,
1982; Sager, 1985; Kaelbling and Klinger, 1986). The tumor suppressor
gene, Rb-1, involved in retinoblastoma and a variety of other tumors
including small cell carcinoma of the lung (Harbour et al., 1988) and
breast carcinoma (T'Ang et al., 1988) has been cloned recently (Fung et
al., 1987; Friend et al., 1986; Lee et al., 1987) and was shown to
suppress the tumorigenicity of a cell line with a defective Rb-1 (Huang
et al., 1988).

Our strategy for identifying and studying additional tumor suppressor genes that are involved in human lung carcinogenesis is outlined in
Table 4. Since tumor suppressive genes may be in multiple functional
classes (Table 5) and located on several different chromosomes, a comprehensive approach is required. Our initial study has utilized allelic
sequence deletion analysis to identify the location of chromosomal
regions that may harbor putative tumor suppressor genes.

Carcinomas of the lung appear to be the result of the gross DNA and
chromosomal damage that follow exposure to mutagenic agents found
primarily in cigarette smoke and the urban environment (Doll, 1985).
Karyotype data for adenocarcinomas, large cell carcinomas and squamous

Table 5.   Examples of Functions of Putative Tumor Suppressor Genes

---

1. Induce terminal differentiation
2. Trigger senescence
3. Regulate growth
4. Inhibit proteases
5. Modulate histocompatability antigens
6. Regulate angiogenesis
7. Facilitate cell-cell communication
8. Maintain chromosomal stability

---

cell carcinomas of the lung are scarce. The available data show a considerable degree of complexity with regard to the presence of deletions, translocations, marker chromosomes and aneuploidy (Zech et al., 1985). These changes are consistent with the extensive molecular changes observed in allelic sequence deletion analysis of six chromosomes, and particularly with respect to molecular changes observed in more than 50% of informative tests for squamous cell carcinomas (Weston et al., 1989). Moreover, for each chromosome studied, with the exception of 13q, loss of heterozygosity was more extensive for squamous cell carcinomas than adenocarcinomas (Fig. 3). Interestingly, the risk of squamous cell carcinoma is greater in heavy smokers (>1 pack per day) than is the risk of adenocarcinoma (World Health Organization, 1986; Fraumeni and Blot, 1982). Additional studies are required to determine the relationship between the clastogenic effects of tobacco smoke and the widespread genetic deletions found in non-small cell carcinomas and the time of the occurrence of the deletions during the multistage process of carcinogenesis.

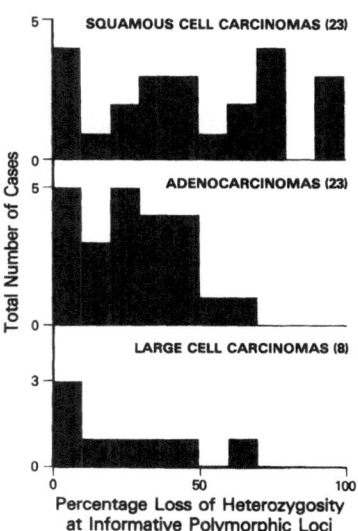

Fig. 3.   Histogram showing the extent of loss of allelic sequence heterozygosity in non-small cell carcinoma of the lung; numbers in parentheses are total number of cases analyzed at 13 polymorphic genetic loci.

Previous investigations (Brauch et al., 1987; Kok et al., 1987; Naylor et al., 1987; Yokota et al., 1987) of lung cancer have focused on small cell carcinoma and only a limited number of non-small cell carcinomas have been studied by DNA sequence deletion analysis (Brauch et al., 1987; Naylor et al., 1987; Yokota et al., 1987; Shiraishi et al., 1987). We have recently performed an extensive analysis of a sufficient number of non-small cell carcinomas, i.e., squamous cell carcinoma, large cell carcinoma and adenocarcinoma, that allow comparisons of DNA sequence deletions in different histological types (Weston et al., 1989). For example, the data consistently showed a loss of heterozygosity at 17p13 in squamous cell carcinomas but not in adenocarcinomas of the lung. Frequent loss of heterozygosity of this region of chromosome 17 has also been observed in colorectal cancer (Fearon et al., 1987) and small cell lung cancer (Yokota et al., 1987).

Loss of heterozygosity studies in human colorectal carcinomas showed frequent DNA sequence deletions in a region of chromosome 17p containing the p53 gene. Subsequently, point mutations in exon 5 of the remaining p53 allele have been shown in these tumors (Baker et al., 1989). In addition, mutations in exon 5 of the p53 gene have also been found in human osteosarcoma (Romano et al., 1989). Although the function of p53 is not known, it has been speculated that wild type p53 acts as a tumor suppressor gene, and that point mutations in the p53 gene may destroy this function. We have recently analyzed mutations in exon 5 of the p53 gene in two human non-small cell lung cancer cell lines (Modali et al., 1989). Exon 5 of p53 in these cell lines was amplified by polymerase chain reaction and the resulting product was cloned into an M13 vector for dideoxy sequencing. Sequence analysis revealed point mutations which altered the amino acid sequence of p53 in both the cell lines. We also observed co-immunoprecipitation of p53 and

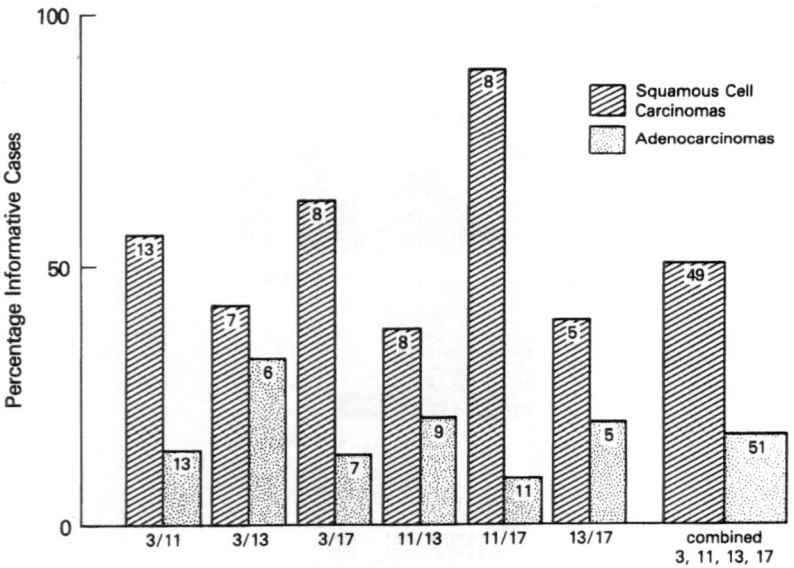

Coincident Loss of Heterozygosity for Numbered Chromosomes

Fig. 4.   For each of either 23 squamous cell or 23 adenocarcinomas of the lung coincident loss of heterozygosity is shown for different combinations of chromosomes 3, 11, 13 and 17. Numbers in bars indicate number of cases informative for the chromosomes indicated.

heat shock protein (hsp) 70/72 in these cells using both anti-hsp and anti-p53 antibodies. These results are complementary to our observations of DNA sequence deletions from chromosome 17p (D17S1) in non-small cell lung carcinomas.

Detection of loss of heterozygosity for markers on chromosome 3 (3p25-p21) was generally in agreement with other reports that use DNA-RFLPs to examine genetic loci on chromosome 3 in non-small cell lung cancer (Brauch et al., 1987; Naylor et al., 1987; Yokota et al., 1987). However, several cases remained heterozygous. Therefore, loss of heterozygosity was found to be substantially less than 100%, which is not in agreement with one previous report (Kok et al., 1987).

Among the three different histological types that were studied, it was possible to demonstrate two commonly deleted regions for chromosome 11; 11pter-p15.5 and 11p13-q13 (Weston et al., 1989). No case provided a conflict in that if both of these regions were absent then all of the polymorphic markers between them were also lost. Theoretically, it would be possible to isolate a genetic locus where loss of heterozygosity by DNA-RFLP analysis could be shown to occur both distally and proximally to that locus, e.g., the calcitonin locus would be a candidate. This could occur as the result of a translocational event or through formation of a marker chromosome. However, this was not observed. These findings are consistent with observations in pediatric tumors that describe two separate gene regions on chromosome 11 that may harbor distinctly different putative tumor suppressor genes; 11p13 in Wilms' tumor (Turleau et al., 1981; Van Heyningen et al., 1985) and 11pter-15.5 in rhabdomyosarcoma (Scrable et al., 1987).

The results for non-small cell lung cancer are very complex and suggest that some differences may occur in the spectrum of genetic deletions seen in the various histological types of lung cancer (Fig. 4). These genetic changes might also be involved in the pathogenesis of lung cancer within a 'multi-hit' framework which has been described in other cancers (Gusella, 1986; Hansen and Cavenee, 1987), and that may include loss of genes, loss of elements that affect gene expression or loss of DNA sequences that affect chromatin structure. Of the 54 tumors studied, only 20 did not show loss of heterozygosity for chromosome 11, and of those, ten showed deletions at other chromosomal loci (Weston et al., 1989). In addition, for squamous cell carcinomas, loss of DNA sequences from chromosome 17 was associated with loss of DNA sequences from chromosome 11 in 7 of 8 cases informative for both chromosomes (Fig. 4). Similarly, loss of genes on chromosome 17 was associated with loss of genes on chromosome 3 in five of seven cases. Therefore, it is argued that consistent loss of specific genes (putative tumor suppressor genes) that have been recognized in other diseases may have a role independently or in combination in non-small cell lung cancer.

Somatic cell genetic analyses of hybrids between normal and neoplastic human cells have generally shown that the normal cell has a dominant effect in suppressing the tumorigenicity of the malignant cell (Stanbridge et al., 1982; Kaelbling and Klinger, 1986; Harris, 1988). Although a rodent-human cell hybrid has been studied (Carney et al., 1979), no previous studies have examined the phenotypic properties of bronchogenic carcinomas fused with either normal or SV-40 "immortalized" (BEAS-2B) human bronchial epithelial cells. The results of these studies are summarized in Fig. 5 (Kaighn et al., 1989). The hybrids between the NHBE and the neoplastic (HuT292DM) cells had a finite lifespan, i.e., about 40 population doublings, and were nontumorigenic (5×10^6 cells, s.c., per athymic nude mouse, >6 month observation period). Although the somatic cell hybrids between BEAS-2B and HuT292DM

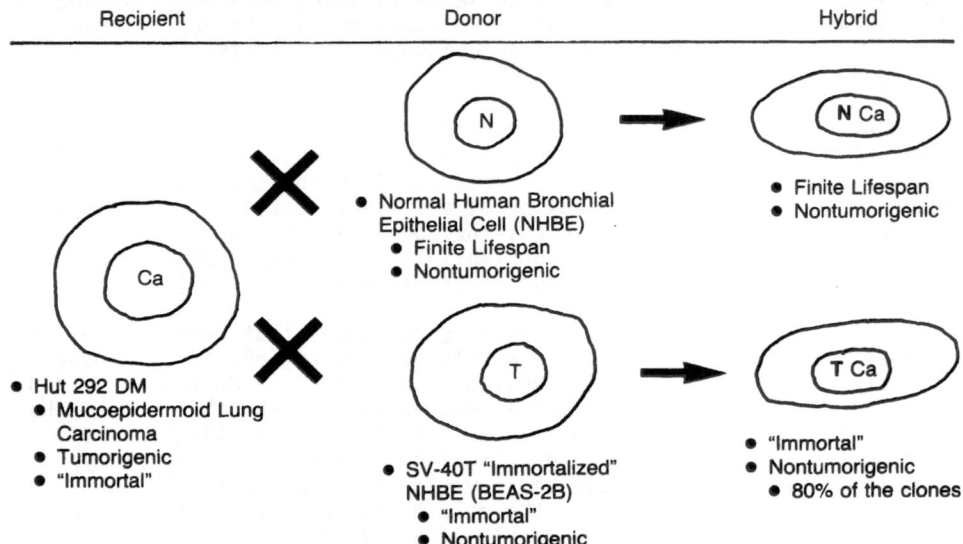

Recipient	Donor	Hybrid

Fig. 5.   Somatic cell genetic analyses of normal and neoplastic human
          lung cells.

appear to have an infinite lifespan, the majority of the cloned hybrids
were non-tumorigenic. This result indicates that genes other than those
involved in senescence can have tumor suppressive properties. In
addition, loss of DNA sequences on chromosome 11 was associated with the
emergence of tumorigenic hybrid segregants (Iman et al., unpublished
results).

      Stanbridge and coworkers (Weissman et al., 1987; Saxon et al.,
1986) have demonstrated that chromosome 11 from normal cells can be
introduced by microcell transfer into carcinomas derived from the kidney
or cervix. Guided by the results of DNA sequence deletion analysis in
non-small cell carcinomas of the lung (Weston et al., 1989), we are
systematically transferring human chromosomes 3, 11, 13 and 17 alone or
in combinations into human bronchogenic carcinoma cell lines. Our
initial findings indicate that chromosome 11-carcinoma cell hybrids have
a substantially increased tumor latency (McMenamin et al., 1989).

ACKNOWLEDGEMENTS

The editorial aid of Robert Julia is appreciated.

REFERENCES

Amstad, P., Reddel, R. R., Pfeifer, A., Malan-Shibley, L., Mark, G. E.,
      and Harris, C. C., 1988, Neoplastic transformation of a human
      bronchial epithelial cell line by a recombinant retrovirus
      encoding viral harvey ras, Mol.Carcinogenesis, 1:151.
Baker, S. J., Fearon, E. R., Nigro, J. M., Hamilton, S. R., Preisinger,
      A. C., Jessup, J. M., Van Tuinen, P., Ledbetter, D. H., Barker, D.
      F., and Nakamura, Y., 1989, Chromosome 17 deletions and p53 gene
      mutations in colorectal carcinomas, Science, 244:217.

Bondy, G. P., Wilson, S., and Chambers, A. F., 1985, Experimental metastatic ability of H-ras-transformed NIH3T3 cells, Cancer Res., 45:6005.

Bonfil, R. D., Reddel, R. R., Ura, H., Reich, R., Fridman, R., Harris, C. C., and Klein-Szanto, A. J., 1989, Invasive and metastatic potential of a v-Ha-ras-transformed human bronchial epithelial cell line, J.Natl.Cancer Inst., 81:587.

Brauch, H., Johnson, B., Hovis, J., Yano, T., Gazdar, A. F., Pettengill, O. S., Graziano, S. L., Sorenson, G. D., Poiesz, B. J., Minna, J., Linehan, M., and Zbar, B., 1987, Molecular analysis of the short arm of chromosome 3 in small-cell and non-small-cell carcinoma of the lung, N.Engl.J.Med., 317:1109.

Brodeur, G. M., Hayes, F. A., Green, A. A., Casper, J. T., Wasson, J., Wallach, S., and Seeger, R. C., 1987, Consistent N-myc copy number in simultaneous or consecutive neuroblastoma samples from sixty individual patients, Cancer Res., 47:4248.

Byrd, P. J., Grand, R. J., and Gallimore, P. H., 1988, Differential transformation of primary human embryo retinal cells by adenovirus E1 regions and combinations of E1A + ras, Oncogene, 2:477.

Carney, D. N., Edgell, C. J., Gazdar, A. F., and Minna, J. D., 1979, Suppression of malignancy in human lung cancer (A549/8) times mouse fibroblast (3P3-4E) somatic cell hybrids, J.Natl.Cancer Inst., 69:411.

Cavenee, W. K., Murphree, A. L., Shull, M. M., Benedict, W. F., Sparkes, R. S., Kock, E., and Nordenskjold, M., 1986, Prediction of familial predisposition to retinoblastoma, N.Engl.J.Med., 314:1201.

Clark, R., Stampfer, M. R., Milley, R., O'Rourke, E., Walen, K. H., Kriegler, M., Kopplin, J., and McCormick, F., 1988, Transformation of human mammary epithelial cells by oncogenic retroviruses, Cancer Res., 48:4689.

Der, C. J., Krontiris, T. G., and Cooper, G. M., 1982, Transforming genes of human bladder and lung carcinoma cell lines are homologous to the ras genes of Harvey and Kirsten sarcoma viruses, Proc.Natl.Acad.Sci.USA., 79:3637.

Doll, R., 1985, Cancer: a world wide perspective, in: "Biochemical and Molecular Epidemiology of Cancer," C. C. Harris, ed., Alan R. Liss, Inc., New York.

Fasano, O., Aldrich, T., Tamanoi, F., Taparowsky, E., Furth, M., and Wigler, M., 1984, Analysis of the transforming potential of the human H-ras gene by random mutagenesis, Proc.Natl.Acad.Sci.USA, 81:4008.

Fearon, E. R., Vogelstein, B., and Feinberg, A. P., 1984, Somatic deletion and duplication of genes on chromosome 11 in Wilms' tumours, Nature, 309:176.

Fearon, E. R., Feinberg, A. P., Hamilton, S. H., and Vogelstein, B., 1985, Loss of genes on the short arm of chromosome 11 in bladder cancer, Nature, 318:377.

Fearon, E. R., Hamilton, S. R., and Vogelstein, B., 1987, Clonal analysis of human colorectal tumors, Science, 238:193.

Fraumeni, J. F. Jr., and Blot, W. J., 1982, Lung and pleura, in: "Cancer Epidemiology and Prevention," D. Schottenfeld, and J. F. Fraumeni, eds., W.R. Saunders Co., Philadelphia.

Friend, S. H., Bernards, R., Rogelj, S., Weinberg, R. A., Rapaport, J. M., Albert, D. M., and Dryja, T. P., 1986, A human DNA segment with properties of the gene that predisposes to retinoblastoma and osteosarcoma, Nature, 323:643.

Fung, Y. K., Murphree, A. L., T'Ang, A., Qian, J., Hinrichs, S. H., and Benedict, W. F., 1987, Structural evidence for the authenticity of the human retinoblastoma gene, Science, 236:1657.

Graziano, S. L., Cowan, B. Y., Carney, D. N., Bryke, C. R., Mitter, N. S., Johnson, B. E., Mark, G. E., Planas, A. T., Catino, J. J., Comis, R. L., and Poiesz, B. J., 1987, Small cell lung cancer cell line derived from a primary tumor with a characteristic deletion of 3p, Cancer Res., 47:2148.

Gu, J., Linnoila, R. I., Seibel, N. L., Gazdar, A. F., Minna, J. D., Brooks, B. J. Jr., Hollis, G. F., and Kirsch, I. R., 1988, A study of myc-related gene expression in small cell lung cancer by in situ hybridization, Am.J.Pathol., 132:13.

Guerrero, I., Calzada, P., Mayer, A., and Pellicer, A., 1984, A molecular approach to leukemogenesis: mouse lymphomas contain an activated c-ras oncogene, Proc.Natl.Acad.Sci.USA., 81:202.

Gusella, J. F., 1986, DNA polymorphism and human disease, Annu.Rev.Biochem., 55:831.

Hansen, M. F., and Cavenee, W. K., 1987, Genetics of cancer predisposition, Cancer Res., 47:5518.

Hansen, M. F., Koufos, A., Gallie, B. L., Phillips, R. A., Fodstad, O., Brogger, A., Gedde-Dahl, T., and Cavenee, W. K., 1985, Osteosarcoma and retinoblastoma: a shared chromosomal mechanism revealing recessive predisposition, Proc.Natl.Acad.Sci.USA., 82:6216.

Harbour, J. W., Lai, S. L., Whang-Peng, J., Gazdar, A. F., Minna, J. D., and Kaye, F. J., 1988, Abnormalities in structure and expression of the human retinoblastoma gene in SCLC, Science, 241:353.

Harris, C. C., 1982, Respiratory carcinogenesis and cancer epidemiology, in: "Lung Cancer: Clinical Diagnosis and Treatment," M. Straus, ed., Grune and Stratton, New York.

Harris, C. C., 1987, Human tissues and cells in carcinogenesis research, Cancer Res., 47:1.

Harris, H., 1988, The analysis of malignancy by cell fusion: the position in 1988, Cancer Res., 48:3302.

Huang, H. J., Yee, J. K., Shew, J. Y., Chen, P. L., Bookstein, R., Friedmann, T., Lee, E. Y., and Lee, W. H., 1988, Suppression of the neoplastic phenotype by replacement of the RB gene in human cancer cells, Science, 242:1563.

Kaelbling, M., and Klinger, H. P., 1986, Suppression of tumorigenicity in somatic cell hybrids. III Cosegregation of human chromosome 11 of a normal cell and suppression of tumorigenicity in intraspecies hybrids of normal diploid x malignant cells, Cytogenet.Cell Genet., 41:65.

Kaighn, M. E., Gabrielson, E. W., Iman, D. S., Pauls, E. A., and Harris, C. C., 1989, Suppression of tumorigenicity of a human lung carcinoma line by nontumorigenic bronchial epithelial cells in somatic cell hybrids, Proc.Am.Assoc.Cancer Res., 30:445.

Kasid, A., Lippman, M. E., Papageorge, A. G., Lowy, D. R., and Gelmann, E. P., 1985, Transfection of v-rasH DNA into MCF-7 human breast cancer cells bypasses dependence on estrogen for tumorigenicity, Science, 228:725.

Kasid, U., Pfeifer, A., Weichselbaum, R. R., Dritschilo, A., and Mark, G. E., 1987, The raf oncogene is associated with a radiation-resistant human laryngeal cancer, Science, 237:1039.

Kasid, U., Pfeifer, A., Weichselbaum, R. R., Dritschilo, A., and Mark, G. E., 1989, Effect of anti-sense c-raf-1 on tumorigenicity and radiation sensitivity of human squamous carcinoma, Science, 243:1354.

Ke, Y., Reddel, R. R., Gerwin, B. I., Miyashita, M., McMenamin, M. G., Lechner, J. F., and Harris, C. C., 1988, Human bronchial epithelial cells with integrated SV40 virus T antigen genes retain the ability to undergo squamous differentiation, Differentiation, 38:60.

Knudson, A. G. Jr., 1985, Hereditary cancer, oncogenes, and antioncogenes, Cancer Res., 45:1437.

Kok, K., Osinga, J., Carritt, B., Davis, M. B., Van der Hout, A. H., Van der Veen, A. Y., Landsvater, R. M., de Leij, L. F., Berendsen, H. H., Postmus, P. E., Poppema, S., and Buys, C. H., 1987, Deletion of a DNA sequence at the chromosomal region 3p21 in all major types of lung cancer, Nature, 330:578.

Koufos, A., Hansen, M. F., Lampkin, B. C., Workman, M. L., Copeland, N. G., Jenkins, N. A., and Cavenee, W. K., 1984, Loss of alleles at loci on human chromosome 11 during genesis of Wilms' tumour, Nature, 309:170.

Kraevskii, A., 1979, Classification and pathological anatomy of lung cancer, in: "Cancer of the Lung," B. E. Peterson, ed., PSG Publishing Co., Massachusetts.

Krystal, G., Birrer, M. J., Way, J., Nau, M. M., Sausville, E., Thompson, C., Minna, J. D., and Battey, J. F., 1988, Multiple mechanisms for transcriptional regulation of the myc gene family in small-cell lung cancer, Mol.Cell Biol., 8:3373.

Lechner, J. F., McClendon, I. A., LaVeck, M. A., Shamsuddin, A. K. M., and Harris, C. C., 1983, Differential control by platelet factors of squamous differentiation in normal and malignant human bronchial epithelial cells, Cancer Res., 43:5915.

Lechner, J. F., 1984a, Inhibition of cell growth by serum, In Vitro Monograph, 5:80.

Lechner, J. F., Haugen, A., McClendon, I. A., and Shamsuddin, A. K. M., 1984b, Induction of squamous differentiation of normal human bronchial epithelial cells by small amounts of serum, Differentiation, 25:229.

Lee, W. H., Bookstein, R., Hong, F., Young, L. J., Shew, J. Y., and Lee, E. Y., 1987, Human retinoblastoma susceptibility gene: cloning, identification, and sequence, Science, 235:1394.

McMenamin, M. G., Iman, D. S., Stanbridge, E. J., Shows, T. B., and Harris, C. C., 1989, Tumor suppressor activity of microcell transferred human chromosomes in lung carcinoma cells, Proc.Am.Assoc.Cancer Res., 30:189.

Modali, R., Lehman, T. A., Weston, A., Romano, J., Appella, E., Vogelstein, B., and Harris, C. C., 1989, Mutations in the p53 gene in human lung carcinoma cell lines, Am.Soc.Hum.Genet. In press.

Namba, M., Nishitani, K., Fukushima, F., Kimoto, T., and Nose, K., 1986, Multistep process of neoplastic transformation of normal human fibroblasts by 60Co gamma rays and Harvey sarcoma viruses, Int.J.Cancer, 37:419.

Naylor, S. L., Johnson, B. E., Minna, J. D., and Sakaguchi, A. Y., 1987, Loss of heterozygosity of chromosome 3p markers in small- cell lung cancer, Nature, 329:451.

Nigro, J. M., Baker, S. J., Preisinger, A. C., Jessup, J. M., Hostetter, R., Cleary, K., Bigner, S. H., Davidson, N., Baylin, S., Devilee, P., Glover, T., Collins F. S., Weston, A., Modali, R., Harris, C. C., and Vogelstein, B., 1989, p53 gene mutations occur in diverse human tumor types, Nature, in press.

O'Brien, W., Stenman, G., and Sager, R., 1986, Suppression of tumor growth by senescence in virally transformed human fibroblasts, Proc.Natl.Acad.Sci.USA., 83:8659.

Orkin, S. H., Goldman, D. S., and Sallan, S. E., 1984, Development of homozygosity for chromosome 11p markers in Wilms' tumour, Nature, 309:172.

Pater, A., and Pater, M. M., 1986, Transformation of primary human embryonic kidney cells to anchorage independence by a combination of BK virus DNA and the Harvey-ras oncogene, J.Virol., 58:680.

Pfeifer, A., Mark, G. E., Malan-Shibley, L., Graziano, S. L., Amstad, P., and Harris, C. C., 1989, Cooperation of c-raf-1 and c-myc protooncogenes in the neoplastic transformation of SV40 T-antigen immortalized human bronchial epithelial cells, Proc.Natl.Acad.Sci.USA. In press.

Pulciani, S., Santos, E., Lauver, A. V., Long, L. K., Aaronson, S. A., and Barbacid, M., 1982, Oncogenes in solid human tumours, Nature, 300:539.

Rapp, U. R., Huleihel, M., Pawson, T., Linnoila, I., Minna, J. D., Heidecker, G., Cleveland, J. L., Beck, T., Forchhammer, J., and Storm, S. M., 1988, Role of raf oncogenes in lung carcinogenesis, Lung Cancer, 4:162.

Reddel, R. R., Ke, Y., Kaighn, M. E., Malan-Shibley, L., Lechner, J. F., Rhim, J. S., and Harris, C. C., 1988a, Human bronchial epithelial cells neoplastically transformed by v-Ki-ras: Altered response to inducers of terminal squamous differentiation, Oncogene Res., 3:401.

Reddel, R. R., Ke, Y., Gerwin, B. I., McMenamin, M. G., Lechner, J. F., Su, R. T., Brash, D. E., Park, J. B., Rhim, J. S., and Harris, C. C., 1988b, Transformation of human bronchial epithelial cells by infection with SV40 or adenovirus-12 SV40 hybrid virus, or transfection via strontium phosphate coprecipitation with a plasmid containing SV40 early region genes, Cancer Res., 48:1904.

Reeve, A. E., Housiaux, P. J., Gardner, R. J., Chewings, W. E., Grindley, R. M., and Millow, L. J., 1984, Loss of a Harvey ras allele in sporadic Wilms' tumour, Nature, 309:174.

Reznikoff, C. A., Loretz, L. J., Christian, B. J., Wu, S. Q., and Meisner, L. F., 1988, Neoplastic transformation of SV40-immortalized human urinary tract epithelial cells by in vitro exposure to 3-methylcholanthrene, Carcinogenesis, 9:1427.

Rhim, J. S., Trimmer, R., Arnstein, P., and Huebner, R. J., 1981, Neoplastic transformation of chimpanzee cells induced by adenovirus type 12--simian virus 40 hybrid virus, Proc.Natl.Acad.Sci.USA., 78:313.

Rodenhuis, S., Van de Wetering, M. L., Mooi, W. J., Evers, S. G., Van Zandwijk, N., and Bos, J. L., 1987, Mutational activation of the K-ras oncogene. A possible pathogenetic factor in adenocarcinoma of the lung, N.Engl.J.Med., 317:929.

Romano, J. W., Ehrhart, J. C., Duthu, A., Kim, C. M., Appella, E., and May, P., 1989, Identification and characterization of a p53 gene mutation in a human osteosarcoma cell line, Oncogene. In press.

Sager, R., 1985, Genetic suppression of tumor formation, Adv.Cancer Res., 44:43.

Santos, E., Martin-Zanca, D., Reddy, E. P., Pierotti, M. A., Della Porta, G., and Barbacid, M., 1984, Malignant activation of a K-ras oncogene in lung carcinoma but not in normal tissue of the same patient, Science, 223:661.

Saxon, P. J., Srivatsan, E. S., and Stanbridge, E. J., 1986, Introduction of human chromosome 11 via microcell transfer controls tumorigenic expression of HeLa cells, EMBO J., 5:3461.

Scott, R. E., and Florine, D. L., 1982, Cell cycle models for the aberrant coupling of growth arrest and differentiation in hyperplasia, metaplasia, and neoplasia, Am.J.Pathol., 107:342.

Scrable, H. J., Witte, D. P., Lampkin, B. C., and Cavenee, W. K., 1987, Chromosomal localization of the human rhabdomyosarcoma locus by mitotic recombination mapping, Nature, 329:645.

Seremetis, S., Inghirami, G., Ferrero, D., Newcomb, E. W., Knowles, D. M., Dotto, G. P., and Dalla-Favera, R., 1989, Transformation and plasmacytoid differentiation of EBV-infected human B lymphoblasts by ras oncogenes, Science, 243:660.

Shiraishi, M., Morinaga, S., Noguchi, M., Shimosato, Y., and Sekiya, T., 1987, Loss of genes on the short arm of chromosome 11 in human lung carcinomas, Jpn.J.Cancer Res., 78:1302.

Slack, J. M., 1986, Epithelial metaplasia and the second anatomy, Lancet, 2:268.

Smits, H. L., Floyd, E. E., and Jetten, A. M., 1987, Molecular cloning of gene sequences regulated during squamous differentiation of tracheal epithelial cells and controlled by retinoic acid, Mol.Cell Biol., 7:4017.

Stanbridge, E. J., Der, C. J., Doersen, C. J., Nishimi, R. Y., Peehl, D. M., Weissman, B. E., and Wilkinson, J. E., 1982, Human cell hybrids: analysis of transformation and tumorigenicity, Science, 215:252.

Suda, Y., Aizawa, S., Hirai, S., Inoue, T., Furuta, Y., Suzuki, M., Hirohashi, S., and Ikawa, Y., 1987, Driven by the same Ig enhancer and SV40 T promoter ras induced lung adenomatous tumors, myc induced pre-B cell lymphomas and SV40 large T gene a variety of tumors in transgenic mice, EMBO J., 6:4055.

T'Ang, A., Varley, J. M., Chakraborty, S., Murphree, A. L., and Fung, Y. K., 1988, Structural rearrangement of the retinoblastoma gene in human breast carcinoma, Science, 242:263.

Thompson, J. J., Zinsser, K. R., and Enterline, H. T., 1983, Barrett's metaplasia and adenocarcinoma of the esophagus and gastroesophageal junction, Hum.Pathol., 14:42.

Turleau, C., de Grouchy, J., Dufier, J. L., Phuc, L. H., Schmelck, P. H., Rappaport, R., Nihoul-Fekete, C., and Diebold, N., 1981, Aniridia, male pseudohermaphroditism, gonadoblastoma, mental retardation, and del 11p13, Hum.Genet., 57:300.

Valenzuela, D. M., and Groffen, J., 1986, Four human carcinoma cell lines with novel mutations in position 12 of c-K-ras oncogene, Nucleic Acids Res., 14:843.

Van Heyningen, V., Boyd, P. A., Seawright, A., Fletcher, J. M., Fantes, J. A., Buckton, K. E., Spowart, G., Porteous, D. J., Hill, R. E., Newton, M. S., and Hastie, N. D., 1985, Molecular analysis of chromosome 11 deletions in aniridia- Wilms tumor syndrome, Proc.Natl.Acad.Sci.USA, 82:8592.

Vogelstein, B., Fearon, E. R., Hamilton, S. R., Kern, S. E., Preisinger, A. C., Leppert, M., Nakamura, Y., White, R., Smits, A. M., and Bos, J. L., 1988, Genetic alterations during colorectal-tumor development, N.Engl.J.Med., 319:525.

Weissman, B. E., Saxon, P. J., Pasquale, S. R., Jones, G. R., Geiser, A. G., and Stanbridge, E. J., 1987, Introduction of a normal human chromosome 11 into a Wilms' tumor cell line controls its tumorigenic expression, Science, 236:175.

Weston, A., Willey, J. C., Modali, R., Sugimura, H., McDowell, E. M., Resau, J., Light, B., Haugen, A., Mann, D. L., Trump, B. F., and Harris, C. C., 1989, Differential DNA sequence deletions from chromosomes 3, 11, 13 and 17 in squamous cell carcinoma, large cell carcinoma and adenocarcinoma of the human lung, Proc.Natl.Acad.Sci.USA, 86:5099.

Wille, J. J. Jr., Maercklein, P. B., and Scott, R. E., 1982, Neoplastic transformation and defective control of cell proliferation and differentiation, Cancer Res., 42:5139.

Willey, J. C., Moser, C. E. Jr., Lechner, J. F., and Harris, C. C., 1984, Differential effects of 12-O-tetradecanoylphorbol-13-acetate on cultured normal and neoplastic human bronchial epithelial cells, Cancer Res., 44:5124.

Winter, E., Yamamoto, F., Almoguera, C., and Perucho, M., 1985, A method to detect and characterize point mutations in transcribed genes: amplification and overexpression of the mutant c-Ki-ras allele in human tumor cells, Proc.Natl.Acad.Sci.USA., 82:7575.

ACTIVATION OF CARCINOGENS BY HUMAN LIVER CYTOCHROMES P-450

F. Peter Guengerich, Tsutomu Shimada, Masahiko Iwasaki,
Mary Ann Butler, and Fred F. Kadlubar

Department of Biochemistry and Center in Molecular
Toxicology, Vanderbilt University, Nashville, Tennessee
37232 (F.P.G., T.S., M.I.) and
National Center for Toxicological Research,
Jefferson, Arkansas 72079 (M.A.B., F.F.K.)

INTRODUCTION

Over the years scientists have become aware that many chemical carcinogens are not active in themselves and that enzymatic activation to
electrophilic forms is required for tumor initiation and, perhaps, for
tumor promotion in some instances (Nebert, 1978; Weisburger, 1980; Miller
and Miller, 1981; Conney, 1982; Searle, 1984; Dipple et al., 1985). Many
of the proteins that have been recognized to have roles in the metabolism
of drugs are now implicated in both the bioactivation and detoxification
of potential mutagens and carcinogens, including enzymes involved in
oxidation and conjugation reactions (Guengerich, 1988). Most of these
enzymes are found in gene families with more or less closely related
sequences (Nebert et al., 1989), and discernment of the catalytic roles
of individual proteins in specified bioactivation and detoxication
reactions is difficult but necessary for an understanding of cancer
etiology. Levels of many of these enzymes show wide inter-individual
variation, with both genetic and environmental contributions to these
differences.

The highest concentrations of many of the enzymes involved in
carcinogen metabolism are usually found in the liver. Some of the
enzymes under consideration with regard to the influence of variation on
cancer risk include the cytochrome P-450 (P-450) enzymes, glutathione S-
transferases, epoxide hydrolases, acetyltransferases, and sulfotrans-
ferases (Guengerich, 1989b). We have focused our attention on the P-450
enzymes (Kadlubar and Hammons, 1987): more than 20 of these are found in
humans, and the levels of some can vary by two orders of magnitude among
individuals, as evidenced by both pharmacokinetic parameters (Ayesh et
al., 1984; Schellens et al., 1988) and direct measurements of protein and
mRNA (Jaiswal et al., 1985; Wrighton et al., 1987; Yoo et al., 1988;
Shimada and Guengerich, 1989a; Bork et al., 1989; Perrot et al., 1989).

IN VITRO STRATEGIES

In recent years this laboratory has been able to purify several of

DNA Damage and Repair in Human Tissues
Edited by B. M. Sutherland and A. D. Woodhead
Plenum Press, New York, 1990

381

the major P-450 enzymes from human liver samples (Distlerath et al., 1985; Shimada et al., 1986; Guengerich et al., 1986; Distlerath and Guengerich, 1987; Guengerich, 1989a). These purified enzymes have been used as antigens in the preparation of polyclonal antibodies that are capable of inhibiting catalytic activity and as probes for the isolation of cDNA clones by screening of expression libraries. A good deal of information has been accumulated, in this laboratory as well as others, on the catalytic specificities of these P-450 enzymes toward particular substrates, including both drugs and model substrates (Guengerich, 1989a).

While some information can be obtained from *in vitro* assays involving the covalent binding of radiolabeled carcinogens to DNA, the approach is insensitive in terms of the amount of enzyme required, laborious, and, most importantly, dependent upon the availability of suitable radio-labeled materials. Therefore, we sought methods that would allow us to rapidly estimate a genotoxic response without the use of radioisotopes. A number of assays are available in the area of genetic toxicology, perhaps the most common being the *Salmonella typhimurium* revertant tester strains developed by Ames and his colleagues (Ames et al., 1973; McCann et al., 1975). For our purposes we decided to use a so-called "*umu*" test (Oda et al., 1985; Shimada and Nakamura 1987; Shimada et al., 1987), which is based upon the induction of the SOS response in bacteria: a chimeric *umuC''lacZ* construct is carried in the plasmid pSK1002 in *S. typhimurium* TA1535, and activation of the recA protein activates the *umuC* gene segment to yield enhanced transcription of the *lacZ* insert and β-galactosidase production (which is measured colorimetrically—Miller, 1972). With this assay, we screened more than 70 carcinogens in the presence of NADPH-fortified liver microsomes prepared from five different individuals (organ donors). This initial screening enabled us to make decisions as to which of the compounds were most genotoxic in the assay, which compounds were "directly" genotoxic without further activation, which of the compounds were inactivated by such metabolism, and which of the particular P-450 enzymes (known to be enriched in certain of the test liver samples) might be involved in some of the reactions. Of the initial compounds tested, those selected for further study are those presented in this chapter [the other compounds examined are cited elsewhere (Shimada et al., 1989a)]. The genotoxic chemicals were then examined more extensively by using purified enzymes and, with a larger series of human liver microsomal samples, techniques of antibody inhibition, selective inhibition and stimulation with certain chemicals, and correlation of activities with known markers among the samples. More recently, some of the work has been extended to include assays with specific sequences expressed in yeast-based vectors (Beaune et al., 1986; Brian et al., 1989).

IN VITRO RESULTS: BIOACTIVATION OF PRO-MUTAGENS

Although a large number of different P-450 enzymes are found in humans, our studies have implicated only a few in the bioactivation of most of the major pro-mutagens examined. The assignment of roles for bioactivation is presented in Table 1 (Yoo et al., 1988; Shimada and Guengerich, 1989a; Shimada et al., 1989a, 1989b).

The assignment of a role for P-450j (P-450 IIE1; Nebert et al., 1989) in the activation of the short-chain nitrosamines is based upon previous work done using the detection of aldehydes that are diagnostic for oxidation of the nitrosamines to carcinogenic products (Wrighton et al., 1987; Yoo et al., 1988). We have examined a large number of nitrosamines and found that none are particularly effective at inducing

Table 1.   Pro-carcinogens Activated by Human P-450 Enzymes

$P-450_j$ (P-450 IIE1)

      N-Nitroso-N-benzyl-N-methylamine
      N-Nitroso-N-butyl-N-methylamine
      N-Nitroso-N,N-diethylamine
      N-Nitroso-N,N-dimethylamine

$P-450_{PA}$ (P-450 IA2)

      2-Acetylaminofluorene
      2-Aminoanthracene
      4-Aminobiphenyl
      2-Amino-3,5-dimethylimidazo[4,5-f]quinoline (MeIQ)
      2-Amino-3,8-dimethylimidazo[4,5-f]quinoxaline (MeIQx)
      2-Aminodipyrido[1,2-a:3',2'-d]imidazole (Glu P-2)
      2-Aminofluorene
      2-Amino-6-methyldipyrido[1,2-a:3',2'd]imidazole (Glu P-1)
      2-Amino-3-methylimidazo[4,5-f]quinoline (IQ)
      3-Amino-1-methyl-5H-pyrido[4,3-b]indole (Trp P-2)

$P-450_{NF}$ (P-450 IIIA4)

      Aflatoxin B_1
      Aflatoxin G_1
      6-Aminochrysene
      Benzo(b)fluoranthene-9,10-diol
      Benzo(a)pyrene-7,8-diol (+ and -)
      tris-(2,3-Dibromopropyl)phosphate
      7,12-Dimethylbenz(a)anthracene-3,4-diol
      Sterigmatocystin

---

the umu response (Shimada et al., 1989a). Further, nitrosamines are relatively inefficient in causing either base-pair or frameshift mutations in S. typhimurium strains. The information obtained to date is probably reliable in gauging the role of the enzyme in nitrosamine activation, although studies on the covalent binding of radiolabel to DNA would also be useful. In addition, a system with a more sensitive biological endpoint would be very helpful in the examination of more compounds.

P-450$_{PA}$ (P-450 IA2) was implicated in the activation of a variety of primary arylamines and the arylamide, 2-acetylaminofluorene. While the activation of 2-acetylaminofluorene is of little etiological consequence in the sense that it is strictly a model compound, its activation by P-450$_{PA}$ points out the fact that the chemical mechanism of P-450$_{PA}$ oxidation does not rely on the low oxidation potentials of the amines. This point is further dramatized by the observation that the enzyme was originally isolated on the basis of its ability to catalyze the O-deethylation of phenacetin (Distlerath et al., 1985). Rates of activation (measured with the umu assay) were well correlated with phenacetin O-deethylase activity and the immunochemically-determined amounts of P-450$_{PA}$ in individual human liver samples (Shimada et al., 1989a). Purified P-450$_{PA}$ was also highly active in activating all of the compounds designated in Table 1 (Shimada et al. 1989a). Microsomal activation of these compounds was strongly inhibited by either 7,8-benzoflavone (α-naphthoflavone) or antibodies that are highly specific for P-450$_{PA}$. Previously, inhibition studies had been done with polyclonal antibodies raised against the rat ortholog P-450$_{ISF-G}$ (rat P-450 IA2) (Butler et al., 1989a; Shimada et al., 1989a). Antibodies prepared against human P-450$_{PA}$ inhibited the reactions more strongly (Fig. 1) (Butler et al., 1989b), and in more recent experiments we have found that even stronger inhibition can be obtained with antisera obtained from humans who have acquired an autoimmune syndrome associated with dihydralazine-induced hepatitis.

Many of the compounds that are activated by P-450$_{PA}$ are arylamines derived from pyrolysis of foods during cooking and are extremely potent compounds in bacterial mutagenesis assays and in the *umu* assay (Kadlubar and Hammons, 1987). While the potent mutagenicity of these compounds may be rationalized in terms of the rapid rates at which bacterial enzymes can O-acetylate their N-hydroxy metabolites to DNA-binding species, several of these amines have been shown to be moderately carcinogenic, producing tumors at several sites, including the liver and intestine. Moreover, the ingestion of some of these compounds by humans consuming cooked meats has now been documented.

P-450$_{NF}$ has been implicated in the activation of a wide variety of compounds (Table 1, Shimada and Guengerich, 1989a; Shimada et al., 1989a; Shimada et al., 1989b). P-450$_{NF}$ was originally isolated on the basis of its ability to oxidize dihydropyridine drugs (i.e., nifedipine) and subsequently found to catalyze the oxidation of a number of steroids and other drugs (Guengerich et al., 1986; Guengerich, 1989a). P-450$_{PA}$ is not exclusively activating all arylamines, for P-450$_{NF}$ was implicated in the bioactivation of 6-aminochrysene (Shimada et al., 1989a). The exact mechanism of the reaction is unknown, and pathways involving N-hydroxylation or diol epoxide formation are possible (Kadlubar and Hammons, 1987).

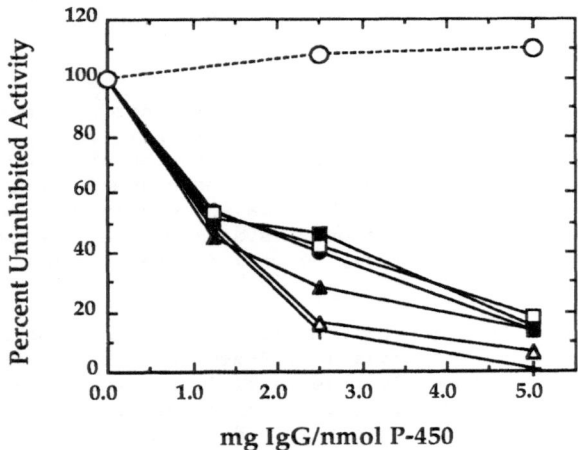

Fig. 1. Inhibition of human liver microsomal oxidation activities by rabbit anti-human P-450$_{PA}$. The indicated degrees of catalytic activity were measured in the presence of anti-P-450$_{PA}$ [mg immunoglobulin G fraction (IgG), solid lines] for 4-aminobiphenyl N-hydroxylation (●), phenacetin O-deethylation (■), caffeine 3-demethylation (▲), Glu P-1 N-hydroxylation (+), IQ N-hydroxylation (△), and 2-naphthylamine N-hydroxylation (□). The stippled line (O) shows the lack of effect of a pre-immune antibody on 4-aminobiphenyl N-hydroxylation in the same system.

A surprising result was the clear role of P-450$_{NF}$ in the activation of the aflatoxins (Shimada and Guengerich, 1989a). This finding is drama-tized by the immunoinhibition of the microsomal *umu* response to aflatoxin B$_1$ (Fig. 2), by the high degree of correlation of levels of immuno-chemically-detectable P-450$_{NF}$ and nifedipine oxidase activity with the *umu* response to aflatoxin B$_1$, and by the formation of 2,3-dihydro-2-(N^7-guanyl)-3-hydroxyaflatoxin B$_1$ adducts recovered after the incubation of calf thymus DNA with microsomes, each done with a group of different human liver samples (Fig. 3) (Shimada and Guengerich, 1989a).

Similar results were obtained in studies with aflatoxin G$_1$ and sterigmatocystin (Shimada and Guengerich, 1989a). The *umu* response (of P-450$_{NF}$) to the compounds listed in Table 1 was enhanced in the presence of 7,8-benzoflavone (Shimada and Guengerich, 1989a; Shimada et al., 1989a). These results confirm the original observations of others regarding the ability of such flavones to stimulate the bioactivation of certain compounds in human liver microsomes (Buening et al., 1981) and point to the selectivity of P-450$_{NF}$ (and related orthologs in other species—Schwab et al., 1988) in this response. The mechanism is still unclear, but it is apparent that an allosteric site of some sort must be involved and both enhanced interaction of the P-450 with its reductase and increased substrate affinity (Schwab et al., 1988) have been suggested to underlie the phenomenon. The stimulatory effect of 7,8-benzoflavone is in stark contrast to the strong inhibition observed in the case of P-450$_{PA}$ and provides a ready tool for the discernment of enzymes involved in particular P-450-mediated oxidation reactions.

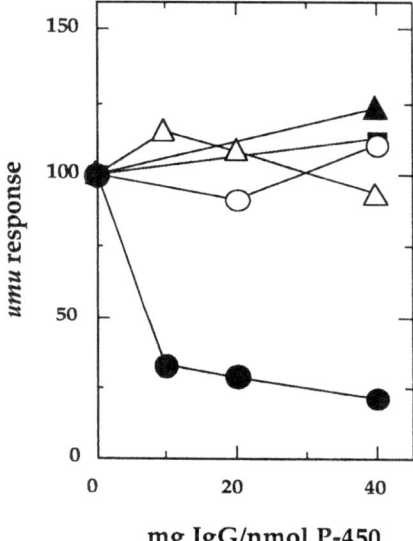

mg IgG/nmol P-450

Fig. 2. Immunoinhibition of the *umu* response to aflatoxin B$_1$ in human liver microsomes. The relative *umu* response (100 = 240 units/min/nmol P-450, liver sample number HL 110) was measured in the presence of the indicated amount of immunoglobulin G (IgG) fraction of anti-human P-450$_{NF}$ (●), anti-human P-450$_{MP}$ (○), anti-rat P-450$_{ISF-G}$ (reacts with human P-450$_{PA}$) (■), anti-rat P-450$_j$ (reacts with human P-450$_j$) (△), or anti-rat P-450$_{UT-H}$ (reacts with human P-450$_{DB}$) (▲).

The fire retardant *tris*-(2,3-dibromopropyl)phosphate is also activated by P-450$_{NF}$, and a postulated mechanism involves the formation of a bromoacrolein (Soderland et al., 1984).

A surprising outcome of these studies was that P-450$_{NF}$ plays a predominant role in the activation of dihydrodiol derivatives of carcinogenic polycyclic hydrocarbons (Shimada et al., 1989b). The assignment of such epoxidation reactions to this enzyme contrasts with the major role played by P-450 IA1 in systems involving rodents treated with polycyclic hydrocarbons (Conney, 1982; Dipple et al., 1985; Kadlubar and Hammons, 1987). However, the findings are quite consistent with the observation that the mutagenicity of 7,8-dihydroxy-7,8-dihydrobenzo(a)pyrene is enhanced by 7,8-benzoflavone (Buening et al., 1981; Conney, 1982). The microsomal *umu* response to both enantiomers of *(trans)* 7,8-dihydroxy-7,8-dihydrobenzo(a)pyrene is enhanced by 7,8-benzoflavone, the reaction is inhibited by anti-P-450$_{NF}$, and the *umu* response seen in different

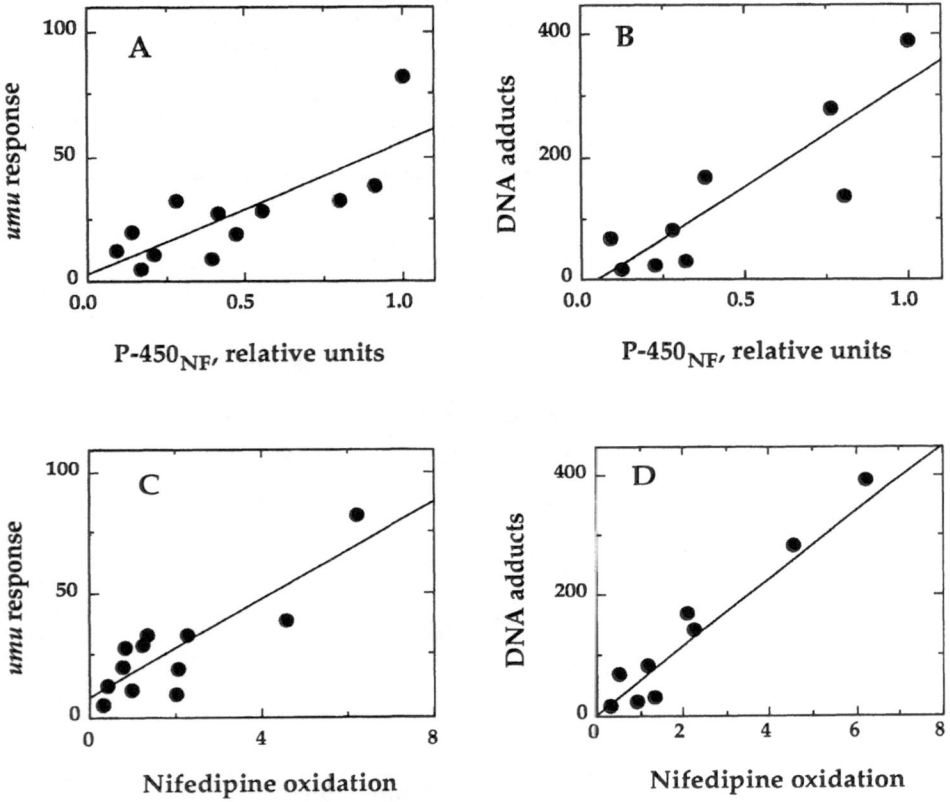

Fig. 3. Correlation of activation of aflatoxin B$_1$ with P-450$_{NF}$ and nifedipine oxidation in human liver microsomal samples. The horizontal axis shows the immunochemically estimated level of P-450$_{NF}$ (per mg microsomal protein) in Parts A and B and the nifedipine oxidase activity (nmol product formed/min/mg microsomal protein) in Parts C and D. Parts A and C show the correlation of the *umu* response (in units/min/mg microsomal protein) and Parts B and D show the amounts of 2,3-dihydro-2-(N^7-guanyl)-3-hydroxyaflatoxin B$_1$ formed in calf thymus DNA (pmol/60 min/mg microsomal protein) on the vertical axis.

microsomal samples is highly correlated with the amounts of nifedipine oxidase activity and immunochemically-determined P-450$_{NF}$ in different liver samples (Shimada et al., 1989b). The major product of the reaction appears to be the 9,10-epoxide, and the stereochemistry of the tetraols arising from the (+) dihydrodiol has been determined and is similar to that found in the oxidation catalyzed by rat P-450 IA1 (Shimada et al., 1989b). The activation of 9,10-dihydroxy-9,10-dihydrobenzo(b)fluoranthene and 3,4-dihydroxy-3,4-dihydro-7,12-dimethylbenza(a)anthracene also appears to be catalyzed by P-450$_{NF}$ in human liver, and the bay region diol epoxides derived from these diols are known to be highly tumorigenic in several assays. On the other hand, P-450$_{NF}$ does not appear to play a major role in the activation of 3,4-dihydroxy-3,4-dihydrobenz(a)- anthracene, which is capable of being epoxidized to a bay region diol epoxide, or of several dihydrodiols that are not capable of forming bay region diol epoxides (Shimada et al., 1989b).

In humans, P$_1$-450 (P-450 IA1) does not appear to be expressed to a high degree in the liver except in unusual situations, as shown by studies with specific probes for mRNA that distinguish between P-450$_{PA}$ (P-450 IA2) and P$_1$-450 (P-450 IA1) (Cresteil et al., 1988). These results are consonant with others in the immunochemical inhibition of catalytic activity (Fujino et al., 1982; Pelkonen et al., 1986). Several lines of investigation suggest that P-450$_{PA}$ does not catalyze the epoxi- dation of benzo(a)pyrene at the 7,8-position and that the enzyme most likely to be responsible for this reaction in human liver is P$_1$-450 (Shimada et al., 1989b). The amount of this enzyme present in human liver must be very low, but the rate of benzo(a)pyrene-7,8-oxide (diol) formation is also very low compared to that found in polycyclic hydrocarbon-induced rats and mice.

The activation of several of the compounds examined could not be definitively assigned to one of the P-450s under consideration in this work. In this category are 6-nitrochrysene and 3-amino-1,4-dimethyl-5H- pyrido[4,3-b]indole (Trp P-1). The activation of both was enhanced by 7,8-benzoflavone but other studies indicated lack of immuno-inhibition with anti-P-450$_{NF}$ and lack of correlation with activities known to be catalyzed by P-450$_{NF}$ (Shimada et al., 1989a). Another activity that was not assigned to a particular P-450 enzyme is benzo(a)pyrene 3-hydroxyla- tion (Shimada et al., 1989b)—this activity is of particular interest, since 3-hydroxybenzo(a)pyrene is the major phenol formed from benzo(a)- pyrene and its formation constitutes the basis of the widely used aryl hydrocarbon hydroxylase assay. The catalytic activity in human liver microsomes is slightly stimulated by 7,8-benzoflavone and is not inhib- ited by anti-P-450$_{ISF-G}$; thus, it appears that neither P-450 IA1 nor P-450 IA2 is involved in the reaction. Measurement of rates of hepatic benzo(a)pyrene 3-hydroxylation provide no information concerning the levels of these two enzymes or the capability for benzo(a)pyrene 7,8- hydroxylation.

INACTIVATION OF MUTAGENS BY P-450s

While many carcinogens require bioactivation to exert their effects, a number of compounds are directly mutagenic and their genotoxic activity is decreased by P-450 oxidation. We examined a number of compounds with the use of the umu test with similar approaches to those used to study the bioactivation of pro-carcinogens. We demonstrated that P-450$_{PA}$ plays the major role in the deactivation of furylfuramide (AF-2) and 1,3- dinitropyrene (Shimada et al., 1989c). 1,6-Dinitropyrene and 1,8- dinitropyrene are also deactivated by human liver P-450s: in the case of 1,6-dinitropyrene, P-450$_{NF}$ or a closely-related form appears to be the enzyme involved in deactivation; in the case of 1,8-dinitropyrene the principal enzyme could not be identified (Shimada and Guengerich, 1989b). Thus we see that P-450s can be important in the detoxication of carcinogens as well as their bioactivation and that apparently similar compounds (dinitropyrenes) can differ radically in terms of which P-450 enzymes are involved in detoxication. A number of other direct-acting mutagens were also examined in human liver microsomes—no NADPH-dependent inactivation was demonstrated for bleomycin, 2-nitrofluorene, 2,4,7-trinitrofluorene, N-methyl-N'-nitro-N-nitrosoguanidine, N-ethyl-N'-nitro-N-nitrosoguanidine, or daunomycin (Shimada et al., 1989c).

CONTRASTS WITH ANIMAL MODELS

Many studies have been done on the bioactivation of pro-carcinogens in experimental animals, particularly rodents. Thus, it is of interest to make comparisons between the enzymes involved in bioactivation in the different species, since many of the primary sequences are known (Nebert et al., 1989). The catalytic specificities of rat P-450j and human P-450j appear to be similar (Wrighton et al., 1987; Yoo et al., 1988) and no major differences have been found, as of yet. The specificity of the P-450 IA2 enzymes (human P-450$_{PA}$, rat P-450$_{ISF-G}$, and rabbit P-450 4 (LM4)) have been considered at length. The most notable difference observed is the lack of activity of the human enzyme towards Trp P-1(3-amino-1,4-dimethyl-5H-pyrido[4,3-b]indole). The rat enzyme readily N-hydroxylates this compound. This difference is surprising, since the compound only differs in the presence of one methyl group from Trp P-2, which is activated by both the human and rat enzymes. P-450$_{NF}$ provides many contrasts concerning species comparisons regarding bioactivation. In rats a number of different P-450 enzymes contribute to the activation of aflatoxin B$_1$ and related compounds (Ishii et al., 1986; Shimada et al., 1987), but in human liver P-450$_{NF}$ clearly predominates (Shimada and Guengerich, 1989a). This point is of interest in that some of the most active enzymes in the rat are those closely related to P-450 IIC11 (P-450$_{UT-A}$) (Shimada et al., 1987), and sequences with > 80% sequence identity are found in humans (Ged et al., 1988), but these apparently are not involved. The activation of dihydrodiol derivatives of polycyclic hydrocarbons by P-450$_{NF}$ in human liver has been discussed above, but no reports of similar activities of the rodent and rabbit orthologs have appeared. Other comparisons have been made between humans and rats in terms of the particular P-450 enzymes involved in the bioactivation of carcinogens (Shimada et al., 1989a) and point out the pitfalls in extrapolation of results from experimental animals to humans.

INDUCIBILITY, PHENOTYPING, AND FUTURE DIRECTIONS

All of the human P-450 enzymes discussed in the context of bio-activation (Table 1) are inducible and the levels of these enzymes vary widely among individuals. On the basis of information available on the *in vitro* and *in vivo* catalytic specificities of the P-450s towards drugs, we may conclude that: (1) hepatic P-450$_{PA}$ is inducible by cigarette smoking and ingestion of charbroiled foods (Pantuck et al., 1974, 1976); (2) P450$_{NF}$ is induced by barbiturates, antibiotics such as rifampicin, and some steroids (e.g., dexamethasone) (Bolt et al., 1975; Molowa et al., 1986); and (3) P-450j is induced by consumption of alcohol (Perrot et al., 1989). Levels of these enzymes can vary 50-fold among individuals and, in consideration of the abilities of these enzymes to bioactivate so many pro-carcinogens, it is of interest to know the extent to which such variations in the population affect the risk of developing tumors (Guengerich, 1988).

In some cases, direct measurements of immunoreactive protein and mRNA have been made on biopsy samples but for major phenotyping studies designed to evaluate cancer risk such approaches are probably not feasible and non-invasive procedures are needed. One possibility involves the use of peripheral blood cells. A difficulty inherent in this approach is that in none of the cases examined has the presence of a particular P-450 been correlated with hepatic levels—indeed, the only P-450 detected to date in peripheral blood cells has been the P_1-450 and the levels are extremely low (Kouri et al., 1982; Jaiswal et al., 1985). Moreover, even if one of the P-450s can be demonstrated to be present in lymphocytes or monocytes, the question of whether or not its regulation parallels that in the liver must be addressed. In principle, it would seem that peripheral blood cells might offer an advantage in that levels of DNA-carcinogen adducts could also be concurrently assessed, but whether lymphocyte DNA adducts reflect those found in target tissues is another matter of contention.

In vitro studies coupled with clinical pharmacology have led to the development of what promises to be useful techniques for non-invasive phenotyping of individuals. People have been phenotyped for P-450$_{PA}$ by measurement of phenacetin clearance (Pantuck et al., 1974, 1976), but phenacetin is not currently used, as it has now been shown to produce tumors of the renal pelvis. Recently, we have found that P-450$_{PA}$ is the major enzyme involved in the 3-demethylation of caffeine (Fig. 4).

Antibodies prepared against human P-450$_{PA}$ were shown to inhibit caffeine 3-demethylation and the N-oxidation of the human carcinogen 4-aminobiphenyl, as well as phenacetin O-deethylation (Fig. 1). Furthermore, there was an excellent correlation between caffeine 3-demethylation and the N-oxidation of 4-aminobiphenyl in liver microsomes prepared from 22 different individuals (Fig. 5).

Since hepatic caffeine 3-demethylation to 1,7-dimethylxanthine, the initial rate-limiting step in caffeine biotransformation in humans, is selectively catalyzed by P-450$_{PA}$, the level of this P-450 in humans may be characterized by determining caffeine 3-demethylation activity *in vivo*. For this purpose, we have recently modified previously established procedures for the determination of the acetylator phenotype using caffeine (Butler et al., 1989b). The molar ratio of 1,7-dimethylxanthine/ caffeine in a urine sample taken 4-5 h after an individual has consumed a cup of coffee was found to closely approximate caffeine 3-demethylation activity. Probit analysis of data from 62 individuals indicated that caffeine 3-demethylation was not normally distributed in the population (Fig. 6) and that phenotypically slow (ratio < 2.5) and rapid (ratio > 2.5) metabolizers exist, representing 77 and 23% of the population, respectively. Thus, caffeine 3-demethylation activity, a reflection of the level of P-450$_{PA}$, may be used as an indirect measure to describe the carcinogenic arylamine N-oxidation phenotype in humans.

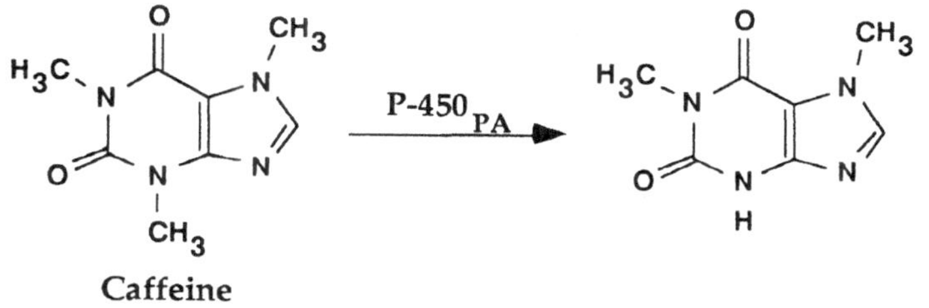

Caffeine

Fig. 4. 3-Demethylation of caffeine.

Non-invasive asays can also be used to estimate levels of P-450$_{NF}$. One approach involves measurement of pharmacokinetic parameters associated with the metabolism of the hypotensive agent nifedipine or related compounds (Schellens et al., 1988) (Fig. 7). However, it should be pointed out that secondary metabolism of the oxidation product can occur and cause difficulties in interpretation. Another approach that can be used is the measurement of urinary 6β-hydroxycortisol (Fig. 8). This measurement was originally developed to provide an estimate of total mixed-function oxidase capability (Ohnhaus and Park, 1979), but more

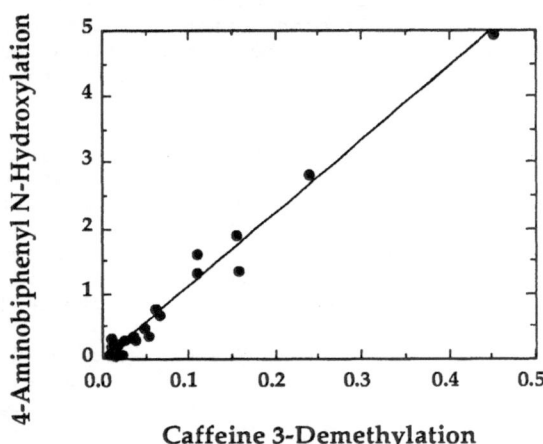

Fig. 5. Correlation of 4-aminobiphenyl N-hydroxylation and caffeine 3-demethylation in human liver microsomal samples. Both axes indicate nmol product formed/min/mg microsomal protein.

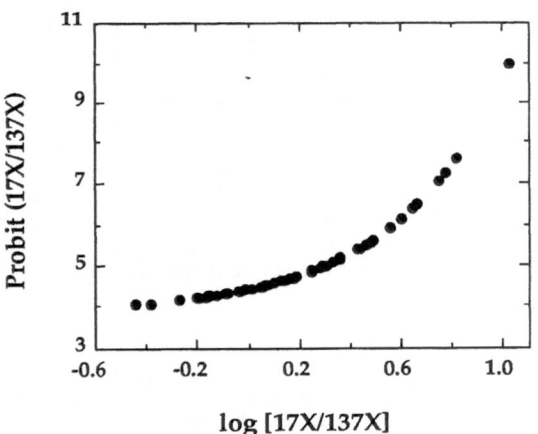

Fig. 6. Probit analysis of the urinary molar ratio of 1,7-dimethylxanthine (17X):caffeine (137X). The abscissa denotes the logarithm of the urinary molar ratio of 17X/137X, which reflects caffeine 3-demethylation activity. The ordinate represents the cumulative frequency distribution in probit units.

recently the 6β-hydroxylation of cortisol has been shown to be catalyzed by P-450$_{NF}$ or a closely related enzyme (Ged et al., 1989). This approach has the advantage that no compounds need to be administered to individuals and urine samples collected for other purposes can be used directly.

At this time, non-invasive assays for measuring P-450$_j$ are not as well-developed because of the lack of information concerning drugs as substrates for the enzyme. Of the known substrates, ethanol is of little use in phenotyping because the preponderance of metabolism occurs via the alcohol dehydrogenase pathway. One possibility might be acetaminophen, for P-450$_j$ has been demonstrated to play a major role in its oxidation to the iminoquinone (Raucy et al., 1989). However, P-450$_{PA}$ also appears to catalyze this reaction and would interfere.

With regard to overall strategy, there are two types of parameters to which variations in levels of P-450s can be linked to individuals within a specific population. The preferred situation is that in which a distinct population has been exposed to a known carcinogen and an independent means of assessing exposure is possible. One parameter is cancer itself. The other type of parameter is some measure thought to be associated with cancer, such as DNA or protein adducts. For instance, a considerable literature on the measurement of hemoglobin adducts derived from arylamines is available and the technology is in hand (Turesky et al. 1987). Levels of specific arylamine adducts (e.g., derived from food pyrolysate amines) could be measured and compared to levels of P-450$_{PA}$, measured using caffeine 3-demethylation. An opportunity is available to compare levels of urinary 2,3-dihydro-2-(N^7-guanyl)-3-hydroxyaflatoxin B$_1$, derived from DNA, with levels of urinary 6β-hydroxycortisol in

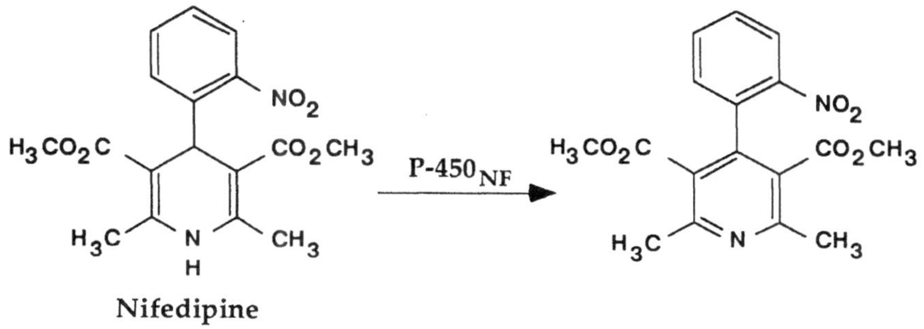

Fig. 7. Dehydrogenation of nifedipine.

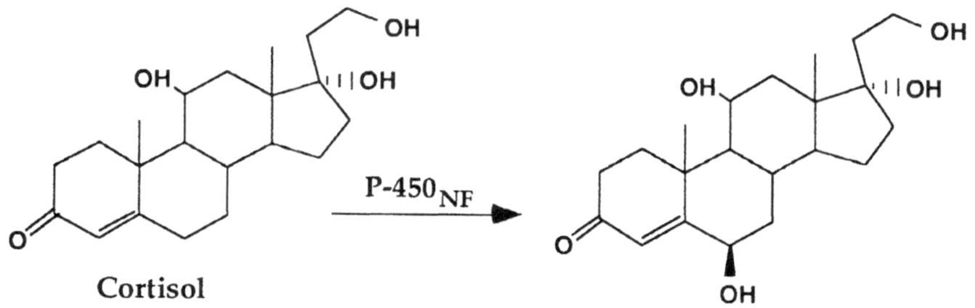

Fig. 8. 6β-Hydroxylation of cortisol.

samples derived from individuals in China and Africa who are known to consume large quantities of aflatoxins in their diets (Groopman et al., 1985, 1988). The technology for the measurement of both parameters is available (Autrup et al., 1987; Groopman and Kensler, 1987) and the high incidence of liver cancer in these areas should provide useful comparisons.

The relationship of P-450s to cancer incidence is intriguing and several instances exist where postulates have been made about the contribution of metabolism to carcinogenesis, particularly lung cancer. Kellerman et al. (1973a, 1973b) found that cigarette smokers with lung cancer showed greater inducibility of aryl hydrocarbon hydroxylase in their lymphocytes. Unfortunately many factors affect the assay, and it has been difficult to establish whether or not the previously reported trimodal variation in inducible activity really exists, and conclusions concerning genetic regulation must be considered controversial. Several groups have reported that phenotypic poor metabolizers of debrisoquine (about 10% of the people in Caucasian populations) are at decreased risk from several cancers, including those of the lung (Ayesh et al., 1984), bladder (Kaisary et al., 1987), liver (Idle et al., 1981), and head and neck (Roots et al., 1988). In the case of the lung cancers, cigarette smoking has been identified as a contributing factor; that is, the relationship appears to be demonstrable only in the smokers (Ayesh et al., 1984). Unfortunately the nature of the chemicals in cigarette smoke that cause cancer is relatively unknown and the etiology is difficult to understand. Although the concept that altered cancer risk in these situations is due to metabolic influences is attractive, the idea should still be regarded as a hypothesis. Nevertheless, opportunities to address this hypothesis in people are now available.

REFERENCES

Ames, B. N., Durston, W. E., Yamasaki, E., and Lee, F. D., 1973, Carcinogens are mutagens: a simple test system combining liver homogenates for activation and bacteria for detection, Proc. Natl. Acad. Sci. USA, 70:2281.
Autrup, H., Seremet, T., Wakhasi, J., and Wasunna, A., 1987, Aflatoxin exposure measured by urinary excretion of aflatoxin B_1-guanine adduct and hepatitis B virus infection in areas with different liver cancer incidence in Kenya, Cancer Res., 47:3430.
Ayesh, R., Idle, J. R., Ritchie, J. C., Crothers, M. J., and Hetzel, M. R., 1984, Metabolic oxidation phenotypes as markers for susceptibility to lung cancer, Nature (London), 312:169.
Beaune, P. H., Umbenhauer, D. R., Bork, R. W., Lloyd, R. S., and Guengerich, F. P., 1986, Isolation and sequence determination of a cDNA clone related to human cytochrome P-450 nifedipine oxidase, Proc. Natl. Acad. Sci. USA, 83:8064.
Bolt, H. M., Kappas, H., and Bolt, M., 1975, Effect of rifampicin treatment on the metabolism of oestradiol and 17α-oestradiol by human liver microsomes, Eur. J. Clin. Pharmacol., 8:301.
Bork, R. W., Muto, T., Beaune, P. H., Srivastava, P. K., Lloyd, R. S., and Guengerich, F. P., 1989, Characterization of mRNA species related to human liver cytochrome P-450 nifedipine oxidase and the regulation of catalytic activity, J. Biol. Chem., 264:910.
Brian, W. R., Srivastava, P. K., Umbenhauer, D. R., Lloyd, R. S., and Guengerich, F. P., 1989, Expression of a human liver cytochrome P-450 protein with tolbutamide hydroxylase activity in Saccharomyces cerevesiae, Biochemistry, 28:4993.
Buening, M. K., Chang, R. L., Huang, M-T., Fortner, J. G., Wood, A. W., and Conney, A. H., 1981, Activation and inhibition of benzo(a)-

pyrene and aflatoxin B_1 metabolism in human liver microsomes by naturally occurring flavanoids, Cancer Res., 41:67.

Butler, M. A., Guengerich, F. P., and Kadlubar, F. F., 1989a, Metabolic oxidation of the carcinogens 4-aminobiphenyl and 4,4'-methylene-bis(2-chloroaniline) by human hepatic microsomes and by purified rat hepatic cytochrome P-450 monooxygenases, Cancer Res., 49:25.

Butler, M. A., Iwasaki, M., Guengerich, F. P., and Kadlubar, F. F., 1989b, Cytochrome P-450$_{PA}$ (P-450 IA2), the phenacetin O-deethylase, is primarily responsible for the 3-demethylation of caffeine and the N-oxidation of carcinogenic arylamines, Proc. Natl. Acad. Sci. USA, in press.

Conney, A. H., 1982, Induction of microsomal enzymes by foreign chemicals and carcinogenesis by polycyclic aromatic hydrocarbons. G. H. A. Clowes Memorial Lecture, Cancer Res., 42:4875.

Cresteil, T., Jaiswal, A. K., and Eisen, H. C., 1988, Regulation of human P_1-450 gene, in: "Liver Cells and Drugs," A. Guillouzo, ed., Colloque INSERM Vol. 164, p. 51, John Libbey Eurotext, London.

Dipple, A., Michejda, C. J., and Weisburger, E. K., 1985, Metabolism of chemical carcinogens, Pharmacol. Ther., 27:265.

Distlerath, L. M., and Guengerich, F. P., 1987, Enzymology of human liver cytochromes P-450, in: "Mammalian Cytochromes P-450," F.P. Guengerich, ed., Vol. 1, p. 133, CRC Press, Boca Raton, FL.

Distlerath, L. M., Reilly, P. E. B., Martin, M. V., Davis, G. G., Wilkinson, G. R., and Guengerich, F. P., 1985, Purification and characterization of the human liver cytochromes P-450 involved in debrisoquine 4-hydroxylation and phenacetin O-deethylation, two prototypes for genetic polymorphism in oxidative drug metabolism, J. Biol. Chem., 260:9057.

Fujino, T., Park, S. S., West, D., and Gelboin, H. V., 1982, Phenotyping of cytochromes P-450 in human tissues with monoclonal antibodies, Proc. Natl. Acad. Sci. USA, 79:3682.

Ged, C., Beaune, P. H., Dalet, I., Maurel, P., and Leroux, J-P., 1989, Cortisol 6β-hydroxylase in human liver microsomes, Brit. J. Clin. Pharmacol., in press.

Ged, C., Umbenhauer, D. R., Bellew, T. W., Bork, R. W., Srivastava, P. K., Shinriki, N., Lloyd, R. S., and Guengerich, F. P., 1988, Characterization of cDNAs, mRNAs, and proteins related to human liver microsomal cytochrome P-450 S-mephenytoin 4'-hydroxylase, Biochemistry, 27:6929.

Groopman, J. D., and Kensler, T. W., 1987, The use of monoclonal antibody affinity columns for assessing DNA damage and repair following exposure to aflatoxin B_1, Pharmacol. Ther., 34:321.

Groopman, J. D., Cain, L. G., and Kensler, T. W., 1988, Aflatoxin exposure in human populations: measurements and relationship to cancer, CRC Crit. Rev. Toxicol., 19:113.

Groopman, J. D., Donahue, P. R., Zhu, J., Chen, J., and Wogan, G. N., 1985, Aflatoxin metabolism in humans: detection of metabolites and nucleic acid adducts in urine by affinity chromatography, Proc. Natl. Acad. Sci. USA, 82:6492.

Guengerich, F. P., 1988, Roles of cytochrome P-450 enzymes in chemical carcinogenesis and cancer chemotherapy, Cancer Res., 48:2946.

Guengerich, F. P., 1989a, Characterization of human microsomal cytochrome P-450 enzymes, Annu. Rev. Pharmacol. Toxicol., 29:241.

Guengerich, F. P., 1989b, Inter-individual variation in biotransformation of carcinogens: basis and relevance, in: "Monitoring People Exposed to Carcinogens: Analytical, Epidemiological, and Ethical Issues," F. Koschier, P. Skipper, and J. D. Groopman, eds., Telford Press, Caldwell, New Jersey, in press.

Guengerich, F. P., Martin, M. V., Beaune, P. H., Kremers, P., Wolff, T., and Waxman, D. J., 1986, Characterization of rat and human liver

microsomal cytochrome P-450 forms involved in nifedipine oxidation, a prototype for genetic polymorphism in oxidative drug
metabolism, J. Biol. Chem., 261:5051.

Idle, J. R., Mahgoub, A., Sloan, T. P., Smith, R. L., Mbanefo, C. O., and
Bababunmi, E. A., 1981, Some observations on the oxidation
phenotype status of Nigerian patients presenting with cancer,
Cancer Lett., 11:331.

Ishii, K., Maeda, K., Kamataki, T., and Kato, R., 1986, Mutagenic activation of aflatoxin be several forms of purified cytochrome P-450,
Mutation Res., 174:85.

Jaiswal, A. K., Gonzalez, F. J., and Nebert, D. W., 1985, Human P_1-450
gene sequence and correlation of mRNA with genetic differences in
benzo(a)pyrene metabolism, Nucl. Acids Res., 13:4503.

Kadlubar, F. F., and Hammons, G. J., 1987, Role of cytochrome P-450 in
metabolism of chemical carcinogens, in: "Mammalian Cytochromes
P-450," F. P. Guengerich, ed., Vol. 2, p. 81, CRC Press, Boca
Raton, FL.

Kaisary, A., Smith, P., Jaczq, E., McAllister, C. B., Wilkinson, G. R.,
Ray, W. A., and Branch, R. A., 1987, Genetic predisposition to
bladder cancer: ability to hydroxylate debrisoquine and mephenytoin as risk factors, Cancer Res., 47:5488.

Kellermann, G., Luyten-Kellermann, M., and Shaw, C. R., 1973a, Genetic
variation of aryl hydrocarbon hydroxylase in human lymphocytes,
Amer. J. Hum. Genetics, 25:327.

Kellermann, G., Shaw, C. R., and Luyten-Kellermann, M., 1973b, Aryl
hydrocarbon hydroxylase inducibility and bronchogenic carcinoma,
New Engl. J. Med., 298:934.

Kouri, R. E., McKinney, C. E., Slomiany, D. J., Snodgrass, D. R., Wray,
N. P., and McLemore, T. L., 1982, Positive correlation between
aryl hydrocarbon hydroxylase activity and primary lung cancer as
analyzed in cryo-preserved lymphocytes, Cancer Res., 42:5030.

McCann, J., Choi, E, Yamasaki, E., and Ames, B. N., 1975, Detection of
carcinogens as mutagens in the Salmonella/microsome test: assay
of 300 chemicals, Proc. Natl. Acad. Sci. USA, 72:5135.

Miller, E. C., and Miller, J. A., 1981, Searches for ultimate chemical
carcinogens and their reactions with cellular macromolecules,
Cancer (Phila.), 47:2327.

Miller, J. H., 1972, "Experiments in Molecular Genetics," p. 352, Cold
Spring Harbor Laboratory, Cold Spring Harbor, New York.

Molowa, D. T., Schuetz, E. G., Wrighton, S. A., Watkins, P. B., Kremers,
P., Mendez-Picon, G., Parker, G. A., and Guzelian, P. S., 1986,
Complete cDNA sequence of a cytochrome P-450 inducible by gluco-
corticoids in human liver, Proc. Natl. Acad. Sci. USA, 83:5311.

Nebert, D. W., 1978, Genetic control of carcinogen metabolism leading to
individual differences in cancer risk, Biochimie (Paris),
40:1019.

Nebert, D. W., Nelson, D. R., Adesnik, M., Coon, M. J., Estabrook, R. W.,
Gonzalez, F. J., Guengerich, F. P., Gunsalus, I. C., Johnson,
E. F., Kemper, B., Levin, W., Phillips, I. R., Sato, R., and
Waterman, M. R., 1989, The P450 superfamily: update on listing
of all genes and recommended nomenclature of the chromosomal
loci, DNA, 8:1.

Oda, Y., Nakamura, S., Oki, I., Kato, T., and Shinagawa, H., 1985,
Evaluation of the new test system (umu-test) for the detection of
environmental mutagens and carcinogens, Mutation Res., 147:219.

Ohnhaus, E. E., and Park, B. K., 1979, Measurement of urinary 6-β-
hydroxycortisol excretion as an in vivo parameter in the clinical
assessment of the microsomal enzyme-inducing capacity of anti-
pyrine, phenobarbitone, and rifampicin, Eur. J. Clin. Pharmacol.,
15:139.

Pantuck, E. J., Hsiao, K-C., Conney, A. H., Garland, W. A., Kappas, A.,

Anderson, K. E., and Alvares, A. P., 1976, Effect of charcoal-broiled beef on phenacetin metabolism in man, Science, 194:1055.

Pantuck, E. J., Hsiao, K-C., Maggiog, A., Nakamura, K., Kuntzman, R., and Conney, A. H., 1974, Effect of cigarette smoking on phenacetin metabolism, Clin. Pharmacol. Ther., 15:9.

Pelkonen, O., Pasanen, M., Kuha, H., Gachalyi, B., Kairaluoma, M., Sotaniemi, E. A., Park, S. S., Friedman, F. K., and Gelboin, H. V., 1986, The effect of cigarette smoking on 7-ethoxyresorufin O-deethylase and other monooxygenase activities in human liver: analyses with monoclonal antibodies, Brit. J. Clin. Pharmacol., 22:125.

Perrot, N., Nalpa, B., Yang, C. S., and Beaune, P., 1989, Modulation of cytochrome P-450 isozymes in human liver, by ethanol and drug intake, Eur. J. Clin. Invest., in press.

Raucy, J. L., Lasker, J. M., Lieber, C. S., and Black, M., 1989, Acetaminophen activation by human liver cytochrmes P450IIEa and P450IA2, Arch. Biochem. Biophys., 271:270.

Roots, I., Drakoulis, N., Brockmöller, J., Ritter, J., Heinemeyer, G., and Janik, T., 1988, Prevalence of poor metabolizers of debrisoquine among patients with cancer of stomach, pharynx, larynx, lung, or bladder, in: "Abstracts, Second International Meeting, International Society for the Study of Xenobiotics," p. 110, Kobe, 16-20 May, 1988.

Schellens, J. H. M., Soons, P. A., and Breimer, D. D., 1988, Lack of biomodality in nifedipine plasma kinetics in a large population of healthy subjects, Biochem. Pharmacol., 37:2507.

Schwab, G. E., Raucy, J. L., and Johnson, E. F., 1988, Modulation of rabbit and human hepatic cytochrome P-450-catalyzed steroid hydroxylations by modulation of rabbit and human hepatic cyto-chrome P-450-catalyzed steroid hydroxylations by α-naphthoflavone, Mol. Pharmacol., 33:493.

Searle, C. E., Editor, 1984, "Chemical Carcinogens," 2nd Ed., ACS Monograph 182, Vols. 1 and 2, American Chemical Society, Washington, DC.

Shimada, T., and Guengerich, F. P., 1989a, Evidence for P-450$_{NF}$, the nifedipine oxidase, being the principal enzyme involved in the bioactivation of aflatoxins in human liver, Proc. Natl. Acad. Sci. USA, 86:462.

Shimada, T., and Guengerich, F. P., 1989b, Inactivation of 1,3-, 1,6-, and 1,8-dinitropyrenes by human and rat microsomes, Cancer Res., in press.

Shimada, T., and Nakamura, S., 1987, Cytochrome P-450-mediated activation of procarcinogens and promutagens to DNA-damaging products by measuring expression of umu gene in Salmonella typhimurium TA1535/pSK1002, Biochem. Pharmacol., 36:1979.

Shimada, T., Iwasaki, M., Martin, M. V., and Guengerich, F. P., 1989a, Human liver microsomal cytochrome P-450 enzymes involved in the bioactivation of pro-carcinogens detected by umu gene response in Salmonella typhimurium TA1535/pSK1002, Cancer Res., 49:3218.

Shimada, T., Martin, M. V., Pruess-Schwartz, D., Marnett, L. J., and Guengerich, F. P., 1989b, Roles of individual forms of human cytochrome P-450 enzymes in the bioactivation of benzo(a)pyrene, 7,8-dihydroxy-7,8-dihydrobenzo(a)pyrene, and other dihydrodiol derivatives of polycyclic aromatic hydrocarbons, Cancer Res., in press.

Shimada, T., Yamazaki, H., Shimura, H., Tanaka, R., and Guengerich, F P., 1989c, Metabolic deactivation of furylfuramide by cytochrome P-450 in human and rat liver microsomes, Carcinogenesis, in press.

Shimada, T., Nakamura, S-I., Imaoka, S., and Funae, Y., 1987, Genotoxic and mutagenic activation of aflatoxin B$_1$ by constitutive forms of cytochrome P-450 in rat liver microsomes, <u>Toxicol. Appl. Pharmacol.</u>, 91:13.

Shimada, T. S., Misono, K. S., and Guengerich, F. P., 1986, Human liver microsomal cytochrome P-450 mephenytoin 4-hydroxylase, a prototype of genetic polymorphism in oxidative drug metabolism: purification and characterization of two similar forms involved in the reaction, <u>J. Biol. Chem.</u>, 261:909.

Soderland, E. J., Gordon, W. P., Nelson, S. D., Omichinski, J. G., and Dybing, E., 1984, Metabolism *in vitro* of tris(2,3-dibromopropyl)phosphate: oxidative debromination and bis(2,3-dibromopropyl)phosphate formation as correlates of mutagenicity and covalent protein binding, <u>Biochem. Pharmacol.</u>, 33:4017.

Turesky, R. J., Skipper, P. L., and Tannenbaum, S. R., 1987, Binding of 2-amino-3-methylimidazo[4,5-*f*]quinoline to hemoglobin and albumin *in vivo* in the rat. Identification of an adduct stable for dosimetry, <u>Carcinogenesis</u>, 8:1537.

Weisburger, E. K., 1980. Metabolism and activation of chemical carcinogens, <u>Mol. Cell. Biochem.</u>, 32:95.

Wrighton, S. A., Thomas, P. E., Ryan, D. E., and Levin, W., 1987, Purification and characterization of ethanol-inducible human hepatic cytochrome P-450HLj, <u>Arch. Biochem. Biophys.</u>, 258:292.

Yoo, J-S. H., Guengerich, F. P., and Yang, C-S, 1988, Metabolism of N-nitrosodialkylamines in human liver microsomes, <u>Cancer Res.</u>, 48:1499.

REPAIR OF O^6-METHYLGUANINE DAMAGE

IN NORMAL HUMAN TISSUES

Steven M. D'Ambrosio, Gulzar Wani, Mervyn Samuel,
Ruth Gibson-D'Ambrosio, and Altaf A. Wani

The Department of Radiology
Division of Radiobiology
The Department of Obstetrics and Gynecology
The Ohio State University
Columbus, Ohio 43210

INTRODUCTION

Humans are exposed to a variety of natural and man-made environmental agents. It has been estimated by Hemminiki and Vainio (1984) that humans ingest approximately 1 μg dimethylnitrosamine (DMNA) per day. Lawley (1989) estimates that the fraction of DNA guanine methylated at the O^6 position by DMNA is about 3 x 10^{-9} or 10 O^6-methylguanine (MeGua) molecules per genome containing 1.2 x 10^{10} DNA nucleotides. A study by Umbenhauer et al., (1985) directly measured the amounts of O^6-MeGua in the DNA of a non-exposed population and one exposed to DMNA in their diet. The level of O^6-MeGua in the tissue samples obtained from half of the non-exposed and the majority of exposed individuals assayed were below the detection limit (100 O^6-MeGua molecules per genome) of the assay. The remaining non-exposed individuals exhibited 116 to 176 molecules per genome, while the exposed population exhibited significantly higher values between 236 and 664 O^6-MeGua molecules per genome. Although it is very difficult to relate the actual daily ingestion of the DMNA with daily adduct formation, these and other (Poirier, 1984; Perera et al., 1987; Manchester et al., 1988) data demonstrate that human exposure to chemical agents can cause the formation of detectable levels of DNA damage. One characteristic of all of these studies is the large inter-individual variation in the levels of DNA adduct detected. This suggests that variable endogenous factors, i.e. metabolism, inactivation, and/or DNA repair, modified the reactivity of the chemical or the persistence of the adduct in the genome. In this paper we will consider the role of DNA repair as a modifying factor in alkylation induced DNA damage. Emphasis will be placed on the fate of the promutagenic and precarcinogenic O^6-alkylGua in various internal human organs and parenchymal cell types within these organs.

DNA Damage and Repair in Human Tissues
Edited by B. M. Sutherland and A. D. Woodhead
Plenum Press, New York, 1990

FORMATION OF O^6-ALKYLGUANINE

The chemistry of DNA alkylation has been thoroughly investigated by Lawley (1966) and Singer (1979). The reactivity of various types of alkylation and the adducts formed have been thoroughly characterized (Loveless, 1969; Lawley and Thatcher, 1970; Osterman-Golker et al., 1970; Lawley, 1973; Osterman-Golker, 1974; Sun and Singer, 1975; Singer, 1976, 1979). The susceptibility and the degree of modification of the nucleophilic sites in the DNA molecule to alkylation depends in large part upon the agent. Alkylsulfonates which are weakly carcinogenic and mutagenic primarily alkylate ring N-atoms (Osterman-Golker et al., 1970; Lawley, 1973). The highly mutagenic and carcinogenic N-nitroso alkylating agents, N-methyl-N-nitrosourea (MNU), N-ethyl-N-nitrosourea (ENU) and N-methyl-N-nitro-N-nitrosoguandine (MNNG), have a higher affinity for alkylating the oxygen atoms of nucleic acids (Osterman-Golker, 1974; Singer, 1976). These sites include the O^6 of Gua, O^4 and O^2 of thymine (Thy), O^2 of cytosine (Cyt) and phosphodiesters (Lawley and Thatcher, 1970; Sun and Singer, 1975). The relative abundance of alkylation at the O^6 position of Gua compared to the O positions of Thy and Cyt has facilitated its measurement and has thus allowed a detailed investigation of the O^6-alkylGua lesion in DNA (Saffhill et al., 1985).

CONSEQUENCES OF EXPOSURE

The implication of O^6-alkylGua as an important lesion in experimental carcinogenesis is based mainly on in vivo animal repair studies (Goth and Rajewsky, 1974; Osterman-Golker, 1974; Nicoll et al., 1975). Due to a spectrum of modifications, evidence relating the observed biological effects to the O^6-alkylGua adduct has been mainly circumstantial, based upon differential organ (Goth and Rajewsky, 1972; Goth and Rajewsky, 1974; Gullino et al., 1975; Sukumar et al., 1983) and cell type (Bedell et al., 1982; Swenberg et al., 1982; Lewis and Swenberg, 1983; Swenberg et al., 1985; Belinsky et al., 1987) sensitivity to transformation by the chemical and the co-incidental persistence of the O^6-alkylGua adduct. To overcome this problem, approaches involving selective incorporation of one specific adduct in DNA followed by evaluation of the changes associated with that particular lesion have been undertaken. Initial studies have focused on miscoding properties of modified bases that lead to abnormal Watson-Crick hydrogen bonding of A:T and G:C base pairs (Singer and Kroger, 1979; Saffhill, 1984, 1986). Abbott and Saffhill (1979) using *E. coli* DNA polymerase I, showed the incorporation of Thy against MNU-treated poly(dG-dC). This provided experimental evidence for the miscoding properties of O^6-MeGua. The proficiency and the nature of repairing O-alkylated adducts in vivo (Singer et al., 1978; Dolan et al., 1984; McCarthy et al., 1984; Nehls et al., 1984; Swenberg et al., 1984; Becker and Montesano, 1985; Dolan and Pegg, 1985; Richardson et al., 1985; Saffhill et al., 1985; Wani et al., 1985) plays an important role in modulating these sequence changes.

As with any type of DNA base alteration, the specific role of an individual modification contributing to eventual biological consequence needs to be evaluated. Since alkylating agents induce a spectrum of lesions in cellular DNA, it is difficult to segregate the biological consequence of one particular adduct such as O^6-alkylGua. Nevertheless, studies in vivo in bacteria, rodent, and human cells have attempted to correlate the persistence of specific O-alkylation adducts and/or levels of O^6-MT with the cell survival, mutation, and transformation by alkylating agents.

Mutagenic Properties of O^6-AlkylGua

O^6-alkylGua is miscoding and pro-mutagenic in various in vitro assays. Using the bacteriophage T7, (Dodson et al., 1982) showed that mutations in vitro increase 10- to 70-fold when O^6-alkylGua is incorporated opposite thymine in the template. O^6-MeGua positioned at a unique site in a plasmid DNA has shown the production of mutations at the selected site (Green et al., 1984). When the methyl group from the O^6-MeGua is repaired, the site again becomes sensitive to restriction endonuclease (Green et al., 1984). Similarly, when the repair activity of the host is inactivated, the mutation frequency increases several-fold (Loechler et al., 1984). Like those mutations observed with the *E. coli* polymerase I (Abbott and Saffhill, 1979), the mutations in the bacteriophage were shown to be exclusively Gua to Ade transitions induced at the preselected site (Loechler et al., 1984). As would be predicted from these experiments, this is the type of mutation that appears in MNU-induced rat mammary carcinoma (Sukumar et al., 1983).

The correlation of mammalian and human mutagenicity to specific adducts has depended upon the differential formation of adducts by the various classes of alkylating agents. ENU inducing an O^6/N7 ratio of 0.6 is a more potent mutagen than diethylsulfate (DES) having a ratio of 0.028 (Singer and Kroger, 1979; Singer and Kusmierek, 1982). EMS induces a 10- to 1000-fold higher frequency of G:C to A:T transitions than A:T to G:C transitions (Krieg, 1963; Coulondre and Miller, 1977; Ashworth et al., 1985), supporting the view that O^6-alkylGua could well be the predominant premutational lesion. A study by Newbold et al., (1980) using three methylating agents of contrasting carcinogenic potencies on mammalian (V79, Chinese hamster) cells in culture showed that the mutagenicity and not the cytotoxicity of each agent is closely paralleled by differences in the levels of O^6-MeGua. Other studies in CHO cells correlated the formation of O^6-alkylGua adducts with mutation frequency at the *hgprt* gene locus (Heflich et al., 1982; Bignami et al., 1988) but not the Na+K-ATPase (Heflich et al., 1982). In human bronchial fibroblasts, mutation at the 6-thioguanine locus showed an excellent correlation to the formation of O^6-MeGua in cellular DNA (Grafstrom et al., 1985). The role of DNA repair in modulating the mutational activity of MNNG-induced DNA damage in normal human skin fibroblasts was shown by the increase in the mutation frequency when the repair of O^6-MeGua was inhibited (Domoradzki et al., 1984, 1985).

Tumorigenicity of O^6-AlkylGua

Unlike the data available for assessing the mutational activity of the O^6-alkylGua adduct, extensive studies relating this and other specific DNA base alterations to mammalian and human cell transformation have not been performed. A study by Doniger et al., (1985) using Syrian hamster embryo cells in culture suggests that O^6-MeGua is a critical lesion for the initiation of cellular transformation. Most of the evidence for the O^6-MeGua having a role in vitro transformation is circumstantial, and is based on some very early studies (Goth and Rajewsky, 1974) in rat showing the sensitivity to ENU-induced tumors and the persistence of the O^6-MeGua in the brain, but not in the liver. Subsequent studies (Bedell et al., 1982) using distinct cells types isolated from the rat liver indicated that persistence of O^6-alkylGua in nonparenchymal cells correlated with the induction of angiosarcomas. The most recent studies to implicate O^6-alkylGua damage as being responsible for transformation via mutation comes from the studies with the *ras* oncogene. The induction of rat mammary carcinoma by a single MNU injection has consistently been shown to involve a single G:C to A:T transition at position G^{+35} of the H-*ras*-1 locus (Sukumar et al., 1983; Topal, 1988). This finding is in agreement with one of the primary mutagenic lesions of alkylating agents, like nitrosourea at the O-atom of Gua (Singer and Kroger, 1979), producing large excesses of G:C to A:T transitions (Coulondre and Miller, 1977). Thus, this mutational mechanism for the activation of *ras* oncogene fits very well with our present understanding of chemical carcinogen-induced lesions having a definite mutagenic and transforming potential in vivo (Laval and Strauss, 1985).

REPAIR OF O^6-ALKYLGUA IN HUMAN ORGANS

The repair of the O^6-alkylGua adduct in cellular DNA occurs by an O^6-MeGua-DNA alkyltransferase (O^6-MT) in bacterial (Lindahl et al., 1988) and mammalian (Pegg and Dolan, 1987) cells, including human. Unlike other repair proteins which exhibit steady-state kinetics, the O^6-MT undergoes inactivation upon stoichiometrically accepting the alkyl group from the substrate, O^6-alkylGua of the alkylated DNA (Olsson and Lindahl, 1980; Pegg et al., 1983). The protein has the highest affinity for methyl, followed by ethyl and bulkier substitutes (Pegg et al., 1983, 1984; Morimoto et al., 1985). Although these functional similarities are shared by both the bacterial, mammalian, and human O^6-MT proteins, their physical characteristics and substrate recognition differ greatly. In *E. coli* the repair protein has been isolated and the gene coding for the *E. coli* O^6-MT has been cloned and sequenced (Demple et al., 1985; Bhattacharyya et al., 1988a; Lindahl et al., 1988; Moody and Demple, 1988; Nakamura et al., 1988). The product of the *ada* gene in *E. coli* is a 39-kD precursor protein, which is processed to a heat-stable 19-20 kD active acceptor molecule (Teo, 1987; Sedgwick et al., 1988). On the other hand, the partially purified O^6-MT protein isolated from rat liver, mouse cells, human placenta, and various human cell lines is a heat-labile 18.5 to 24 kD protein (Pegg et al., 1983; Yarosh et al., 1983; Brent, 1985, 1986; Hall and Karran, 1986; Boulden et al., 1987; Bhattacharyya et al., 1988b; Myrnes and Wittwer, 1988). Unlike the *E. coli* protein, the active O^6-MT protein is not generated by the cleavage of a precursor protein. Furthermore, the human protein is not recognized by antisera recognizing the *E. coli* O^6-MT protein indicating distinct structural features (Ceccoli et al., 1988; Yarosh et al., 1988). While the *E. coli* O^6-MT recognizes O^4-methylThy and phosphotriester, the human O^6-MT is highly specific and limited to the removal of O^6-alkylGua (McCarthy et al., 1983; Brennand and Margison, 1986; Brent et al., 1988). However, due to the lability of the mammalian and human O^6-MT protein, purification of this protein and cloning of the corresponding gene(s) has been difficult. Thus, most of the studies on characterizing the repair of the O^6-alkylGua in humans have used cell-free extracts derived from adult and fetal tissues (O^6-MT activity), and cells in culture (O^6-MT activity and removal of adduct from cellular DNA).

The activity of O^6-MT is determined after incubation of the cell free protein extracts with radiolabeled alkylated DNA (Pegg and Dolan, 1987) by either: (1) measuring the amount of radiolabeled O^6-alkylGua transferred to protein, after proteolysis; or (2) directly measuring the amount of O^6-alkylGua remaining on the DNA substrate. Using these methods, Table 1 summarizes the O^6-MT activity in extracts obtained from bladder, brain, bronchial, esophageal, intestine, kidney, liver, lung, pancreas, placenta, and stomach tissue samples obtained from normal human adults and fetuses, exposed populations, tumors, tumor xenografts,

Table 1. Human O⁶-AlkylGua-DNA Alkyltransferase

Organ	Mean±S.D. (range) pmole/mg protein	Comments	Reference
Bladder	0.18 0.08	normal, adult	(Souliotis et al., 1989)
	0.32 0.06	neoplastic	(Souliotis et al., 1989)
Brain	0.07 0.04	fetal	(D'Ambrosio et al., 1987)
	0.10 0.03	fetal	(Krokan et al., 1983)
	0.08 0.04	adult	(Wiestler et al., 1984)
	0.07 0.04	adult	(Gerson et al., 1986)
	0.07 0.03	adult, astrocytoma	(Wiestler et al., 1984)
	0.03 0.01	adult, oligodendroglioma	(Wiestler et al., 1984)
	0.21 0.12	adult, meningioma	(Wiestler et al., 1984)
	0.72 0.04	adult, metastasis	(Wiestler et al., 1984)
	0.14 0.07	adult, neurinoma	(Wiestler et al., 1984)
	0.08 0.04	adult, tumors	(Wiestler et al., 1984)
	(0-2.33)	tumor xenografts	(Schold et al., 1989)
Bronchial	0.28	cultured epithelial	(Krokan et al., 1985)
	0.19 0.05	cultured fibroblast	(Grafstrom et al., 1984)
	0.14 0.03	cultured epithelial	(Grafstrom et al., 1984)
Esophageal	0.22 0.06	adult	(Grafstrom et al., 1984)
	0.19 (0.08-0.25)	exposed population	(Umbenhauer et al., 1985)
	0.33 (0.12-0.45)	tumor, exposed	(Umbenhauer et al., 1985)
Intestine	0.17 0.07	small, fetal	(D'Ambrosio et al., 1987)
	0.22 0.10	small, fetal	(Krokan et al., 1983)
	0.21 0.22	small, adult	(Myrnes et al., 1983)
	0.24 0.17	small, adult	(Gerson et al., 1986)
	0.14 0.10	large, fetal	(D'Ambrosio et al., 1987)
	0.26 (0.14-0.41)	colon, adult	(Grafstrom et al., 1984)
	0.14 0.08	colon, adult	(Myrnes et al., 1983)
	0.99 0.10	colon, adult, neoplastic	(Myrnes et al., 1983)
	0.14 0.08	colon, adult	(Gerson et al., 1986)
Kidney	0.35 0.21	fetal	Fig.1 (D'Ambrosio et al., 1987)
	0.22 0.03	fetal	(Richardson et al., 1985)
	0.19 0.01	culture epithelial	(Wani et al., 1989)
Liver	0.52 0.33	fetal	Fig.1 (Wani et al., 1985; D'Ambrosio et al., 1987)
	0.15 0.03	fetal	(Krokan et al., 1983)
	1.07 0.62	adult	(Myrnes et al., 1983)
	0.70 0.04	adult	(Pegg et al., 1982)
	0.34 0.02	adult	(Hall et al., 1984)
	0.49 0.13	adult	(Gerson et al., 1986)
	0.20 0.01	cultured epithelial	(Wani et al., 1989)

Table 1 (cont). Human O^6-AlkylGua-DNA Alkyltransferase

Organ	Mean±S.D. (range) pmole/mg protein	Comments	Reference
Lung	0.18 0.08	fetal	(D'Ambrosio et al., 1987)
	0.29 0.11	fetal	(Krokan et al., 1983)
	0.12 (0.04-0.19)	adult	(Grafstrom et al., 1984)
	0.09	adult	(Gerson et al., 1986)
Pancreas	0.27 (0.25-0.28)	fetal	(Krokan et al., 1983)
Placenta	0.12 0.06	nonsmokers	(Foiles et al., 1988)
	0.08 0.04	smokers	(Foiles et al., 1988)
Stomach	0.20 0.04	adult	(Myrnes et al., 1983)
	0.13 0.08	adult, neoplastic	(Myrnes et al., 1983)
	0.32 0.08	fetal	(Krokan et al., 1983)
	0.20 (0.08-0.26)	mucosa, exposed population	(Umbenhauer et al., 1985)

and cell cultures derived from normal bronchial, liver, and kidney tissues. These studies indicate that the highest level O^6-MT is observed in adult human liver, exhibiting 0.34 to 1.0 pmole per mg protein, while the lowest is in adult and fetal brain exhibiting 0.07 to 0.10 pmole per mg protein. This organ specific relationship is also found in the other mammalian species tested including monkey (Hall et al., 1984; Becker and Montesano, 1985) and rat (Pegg et al., 1983; Hall et al., 1984). Although one laboratory (Wani et al., 1985; D'Ambrosio et al., 1987) has shown human fetal liver to exhibit the highest level of O^6-MT among the 7 fetal tissues tested, its activity of 0.52±0.33 pmole per mg protein was 50% to 30% less than that observed in the adult liver tissue assayed by Pegg et al., (1982) and Myrnes et al., (1983). The activity in fetal stomach is much greater than the activity in adult stomach. O^6-MT activity in fetal intestinal tissues (0.17 to 0.22 pmole per mg protein) is similar to that found in the adult. One characteristic of all these studies in humans is the degree of variation within the population studied and between laboratories. For example, the values for O^6-MT in fetal liver tissue vary by 3-fold between two laboratories (Table 1). Our laboratory obtained the tissues from elected abortions while another laboratory utilized tissues from spontaneous abortuses. This same type of variation also appears in the values obtained with adult liver tissue, but is much less obvious in the other tissues assayed. These inter-laboratory variations could reflect the source and quality of the tissue, as well as the use of different methods (Pegg and Dolan, 1987) to quantify O^6-MT, or radiopurity of the substrate.

Alternatively, the variation may be due to the genetic diversity of the population, or the inducibility of the repair enzymes in individuals exposed to environmental agents prior to assay. When the data are compared within a laboratory, one observes a large range (5 to 100% of the mean) of the individual O^6-MT levels (Table 1). Our own studies (D'Ambrosio et al., 1987) with 7 fetal organs showed as much as 53% variation from the mean in 17 individual liver samples. (Values ranged 0.20 to 1.54 pmole O^6-MT per mg protein.) A second set of 12 liver and 10 kidney tissues showed similar variation in the distribution of O^6-MT of human fetal liver and kidney (Fig. 1). The range in this study was 0.34 to 1.2 and 0.38 to 0.78 pmole O^6-MT per mg protein in the liver and kidney tissues, respectively. In both of these studies we determined whether fetal factors, such as age of gestation, and maternal factors, such as smoking, drug use, and health, played a role in this variation. Only the fetal specimens obtained from one individual on phenobarbital exhibited a significant ($P<0.005$), 4-fold higher, increase in O^6-MT activity, suggesting that phenobarbital might induce O^6-MT in humans in vivo (D'Ambrosio et al., 1987). Interestingly, studies in rats fed phenobarbital also showed significantly higher levels of liver O^6-MT (Den Engelse et al., 1984). The tissues obtained from one mother with renal failure and undergoing kidney dialysis were also increased 2- to 3-fold (D'Ambrosio et al., 1987). This could suggest an environmental component in modulating the in vivo levels of O^6-MT. However, there was no significant correlation with the levels of O^6-MT in fetal (D'Ambrosio et al., 1987) or placental (Foiles et al., 1988) tissue samples obtained from maternal smokers. Similarly, individuals exposed to N-nitrosoamine in their diet and having detectable levels of O^6-MeGua in their oesophageal and stomach mucosa exhibited (Umbenhauer et al., 1985) levels O^6-MT comparable to tissue obtained from apparently normal individuals (Table 1, Myrnes et al., 1983; Grafstrom et al., 1984). These data would suggest that environmental agents do not play a major role in modulating human O^6-MT.

In samples obtained from tumors, the level of O^6-MT varies to even a greater extent, suggesting gene regulation of O^6-MT or endogenous controlling factors (Table 1). For example, tissue obtained from brain tumors exhibits O^6-MT values between 0.07 and 0.72 pmole per mg protein (Wiestler et al., 1984). Neoplastic bladder shows a 2-fold increase in the level of O^6-MT (Souliotis et al., 1989), while tumor tissue obtained from non-involved esophageal and stomach tissues of the nitrosoamine-exposed population are similar (Umbenhauer et al., 1985). If genetic factors are responsible for the individual variation in the levels of O^6-MT, then these characteristics should be preserved when the cells are established in culture. On the other hand, if the O^6-MT is controlled by endogenous factors or regulated by the expression of distinct genes, O^6-MT should be able to be modulated in culture. To help answer these questions, we have established in culture epithelial cells from human fetal liver and kidney. These cells were assayed for O^6-MT activity during isolation, upon establishment in primary culture, and at various subpassages (cumulative population doubling (CPDL) 1 through 50) (Wani et al., 1989; Table 2). Unlike that observed with the tissue, the human liver epithelial cell cultures established from 10 different tissues exhibited relatively small inter-individual variations in the O^6-MT. Values ranged between 0.17 and 0.23 pmole per mg protein during the 50 CPDL, with an overall mean of 0.196 ± 0.013 pmole per mg protein. Similarly, the level of O^6-MT varied only slightly in the kidney epithelial cell cultures with an overall mean of 0.19 ± 0.01 pmole O^6-MT per mg protein. Other studies using fibroblasts and epithelial cells derived from human bronchial tissue also showed small levels of individual variation with O^6-MT values of 0.19 ± 0.05 and 0.14 ± 0.03 pmole per mg protein, respectively (Grafstrom et al., 1984). These in vivo and in vitro data taken together may suggest that the in vivo levels of O^6-MT are modulated to a greater extent by endogenous factors regulating the expression of the O^6-MT gene. When the cells are cultured these signals are no longer present to modulate O^6-MT. If these signals could be identified and introduced into the cells in culture, then O^6-MT levels should reflect the in vivo state. This

Table 2. Stability of Human Epithelial Cellular O^6-MT in Culture

CPDL[a]	Molecules of O^6-MT per cell (x10^3) (pmole O^6-MT per mg protein)	
	Liver cells	Kidney cells
1-6	15.73 ± 4.63 (0.17)	22.20 ± 2.78 (0.29)
8-15	17.58 ± 5.55 (0.19)	16.65 ± 1.85 (0.18)
17-25	17.58 ± 5.55 (0.19)	12.95 ± 1.85 (0.14)
28-35	19.43 ± 1.85 (0.21)	13.88 ± 2.78 (0.15)
40-50	21.28 ± 1.85 (0.23)	19.43 ± 0.93 (0.21)
All[b]	18.13 ± 1.20 (0.20)	17.58 ± 1.20 (0.19)

[a]CPDL = sum[3.32log (final number of cells harvested/initial number of cells seed)]. Cells were seeded, allowed to grow to confluency and then collected for O^6-MT determination.
[b]Data is expressed at the mean±SE from 10 different cell lines, assayed in quadruplicate. Specific activity of O^6-MT was calculated from the linear portion of the protein concentration vs activity plots.
Reprinted from Wani et al., (1989) with permission.

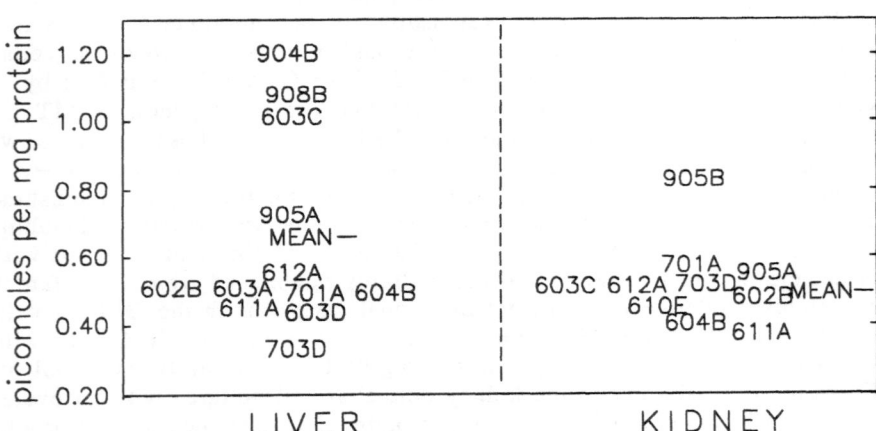

Fig. 1. The distribution of O^6-MT in human fetal liver and kidney tissue. The alphanumeric code designates individual tissue. The specific activity, in pmole O^6-MT per mg protein, for liver was 0.65±0.51, n=12; and for kidney, 0.51±0.11, n=10.

possibility is being explored, using liver and epithelial cells in chemically defined media. This data may also tell us whether the levels expressed in culture represent the actual basal or constitutive levels in the human organ. The exact mechanism, however, will have to wait for isolation and cloning of the human O^6-MT.

O^6-MT IN HUMAN CELLS

One of the greatest difficulties in predicting the human health effects of exposure to environmental agents is in extrapolating the biological responses and mechanisms from many different model systems. Due to ethical limitations of human testing, these extrapolations are based upon experimental animals, transformed animal and human cell lines, human skin fibroblasts, and human epidemiological data. Since there are many species differences in metabolism, distribution, DNA repair, chromatid organization, and life span, it is difficult to extrapolate the data directly to humans. Other systems utilizing human cells derived from tumors or normal skin may also fail to accurately predict the responses in target parenchymal cells derived from target organs. As an alternative approach, we (D'Ambrosio et al., 1983, 1988; Gibson-D'Ambrosio et al., 1986, 1987; Wani et al., 1989) and a few other laboratories (Harris and Autrup, 1983; Krokan et al., 1985; Harris, 1987) have developed conditions for establishing and maintaining epithelial cell types derived from human bronchial, kidney, lung, liver and esophageal tissues. Since over 90% of human tumors are epithelial in origin, it is important to understand the relationship between DNA base modification and disease processes in the epithelial cells derived from target internal organs. The development and utilization of in vitro systems derived from organ epithelia, which maintain in vivo specific functions, can allow for risk assessment and mechanistic studies not possible in vivo in humans. One of the problems with the use of normal epithelial cells in culture is that often they can not be maintained past the primary culture, due to the highly differentiated state of the cell. Another problem has been that many of the biochemical and metabolic functions characteristic of the cell type in vivo are lost upon culturing. Our laboratory has concentrated on cells derived from human fetal kidney and liver. We have developed procedures that allow establishment of these cells in culture, cell division for approximately 60 CPDL, and maintenance of many organ specific in vivo functions in culture (Gibson-D'Ambrosio et al., 1986, 1987; Wani et al., 1989). The cells derived from kidney exhibit ultrastructural and biochemical functions characteristic of proximate tubular epithelia of the kidney (Gibson-D'Ambrosio et al., 1987). The hepatic cells cultured from human fetal liver actively synthesize albumin and α-fetoprotein characteristic of replicatively active liver hepatocytes (Gibson-D'Ambrosio et al., 1986; Wani et al., 1989). Thus, these cells maintaining in vivo functions in culture may provide more relevant extrapolations of mechanisms of action and biological responses of environmental agents to humans. These cells allow investigation under controlled experimental conditions for studying many of the biochemical and cellular responses that may occur following human exposure to environmental agents. Using these epithelial cells we were able to (i) study the kinetics of in vivo repair, (ii) determine the mechanism of repair, and (iii) answer the question as to whether O^6-MT was inducible in human epithelial cell types.

The kinetics of repairing the O^6-MeGua adduct in liver and kidney epithelial DNA has been described (Wani et al., 1989). The loss of O^6-MeGua by both the human liver and kidney epithelial cells was biphasic, with 50% of the loss occurring within 2 hr and 1.5 hr, respectively. At the end of 4 hr, only 40% and 33% of this methylated Gua remained in the DNA of the liver and kidney cells, respectively. From these data, the liver and kidney epithelial cells would be expected to have relatively high levels of O^6-MT. Table 2 describes the levels of O^6-MT measured in cell-free protein extracts obtained from cells in CPDL 1 through 50. The cells lines tested exhibited 0.17 to 0.23 pmole O^6-MT per mg protein or approximately 15,725 to 21,275 O^6-MT molecules per cell. In comparison to in vivo tissue levels, as discussed above, these values are somewhat lower. They are similar to the values (26,000 O^6-MT molecules per cell) obtained with fibroblastic and epithelial cells cultured from bronchial tissue (Krokan et al., 1985). In contrast, other studies using normal human cell fibroblasts and lymphocytes exhibited a wide range of values between 10,000 and 140,000 O^6-MT molecules per cell (Medcalf and Lawley, 1981; Waldstein et al., 1982a; Foote and Mitra, 1984; Day et al., 1987).

When DNA damage enters the S phase of the cell cycle, the probability of a base mispairing, cell death, mutation, and transformation greatly increases (Grisham et al., 1988). DNA repair, by removing the damage before the cell enters S, can greatly reduce the biological effectiveness of exposure to the chemical agent. Thus, the biological effectiveness of any DNA damaging agent to a particular organ or cell type is the sum of the capacity of the cell to repair the damage, the rate of repair, and the time before the cell enters DNA replication. Modulation of repair, either by saturation or induction, could greatly alter the fidelity of cellular DNA replication and the biological result of exposure. Since the O^6-MT protein is stoichiometrically inactivated upon removing the alkyl group from the O^6-Gua molecule, exposure of human epithelial cells to alkylating agents like MNU and MNNG deplete intracellular levels of O^6-MT in a dose-dependent manner (Krokan et al., 1985; Wani et al., 1989). As shown in Fig. 2, a 1-hr exposure of liver and kidney epithelial cells in culture to 2, 4, and 8 µM MNNG causes a marked decrease in the amount of intracellular O^6-MT. The level of O^6-MT was almost completely restored, 48 hr following the initial treatment, in the cells treated with the 2 µM dose and not in the 4 or 8 µM dose of MNNG.

A manner in which cells can deal with chronic exposure to DNA damaging agents is by increasing the levels of O^6-MT (Day et al., 1987). E. coli are able to accomplish this by adapting to challenging dose of alkylating agents (Lindahl et al., 1988). Whether mammalian systems display a similar type of response has been somewhat contradictory with most studies performed in rodents in vivo (Swenberg et al., 1982; Pegg, 1983; Margison et al., 1985) or various mammalian cell lines (Frosina and Abbondandolo, 1985). Experiments using the rat hepatoma cell line, H4, have consistently demonstrated an enhancement of the O^6-MT by a diversity of challenging agents (Laval and Laval, 1984; Lefebvre and Laval, 1986; Frosina and Laval, 1987). These studies and others (Kaina, 1982) in V79 Chinese hamster cells showed a corresponding enhancement in cell survival and reduced mutation and chromosomal aberrations by the challenge doses of methylating agents. Induction of O^6-MT has also been observed in rat liver (Chu et al., 1981; Den Engelse et al., 1984, 1986; Schmerold and Spath, 1986), C3H/10T1/2 cells (von Hofe and Kennedy, 1988) and human lymphocytes (Waldstein et al., 1982b, 1982a). However, other studies in normal human skin fibroblasts (Karran et al., 1982; Foote and Mitra, 1984), bronchial epithelial (Krokan et al., 1985), liver hepatocytes, and kidney epithelial cells (Wani et al., 1989) have failed to exhibit an induction of O^6-MT following single or chronic exposure to low doses of alkylators. Our data using normal human fetal kidney and liver epithelial cells in culture indicate that the cells do not enhance O^6-MT activity in response to treatment by physical and chemical agents. It is possible that this discrepancy could be due to differences in cell lines, cell doubling times, and experimental protocol. Another possibility is that the enhancement may require a threshold constitutive level of O^6-MT. The rat hepatoma cell line used by Laval and coworkers (Laval and Laval, 1984; Lefebvre and Laval, 1986; Frosina and Laval, 1987) and the cell lines used by Waldstein et al., (1982a; 1982b) exhibited constitutive levels of O^6-MT in excess of 50,000 molecules per cell. The cell lines which did not show enhancement had constitutive levels of O^6-MT between 10 and 30,000 molecules per cell. Our data supports this relationship, since the unadaptable normal human fetal kidney and liver epithelial cells possess 18,500 O^6-MT molecules per cell.

Despite the fact that the normal human epithelial cells are not capable of inducing O^6-MT following the exposure to alkylating agents, the constitutive level of O^6-MT should be sufficient to repair low chronic levels of environmental or endogenous exposure to alkylating agents. Our human fetal kidney and liver epithelial cells would be able to process at least 400 O^6-MeGua adducts per cell per hr (based on 18,500 O^6-MT molecules per cell, 48 hr recovery time). This threshold may even be higher in the organ due to higher levels of in vivo O^6-MT. These levels of O^6-MT should be sufficient to repair the estimated 10 O^6-MeGua molecules formed every day in our genome by the ingestion of DMNA in our diet (Lawley, 1989). However, in the absence of an inducible activity, higher amounts of O^6-MeGua produced acutely or persistently due to chronic exposures could render the cell susceptible to the biological consequences of alkylating agents. It is interesting that in the non-exposed

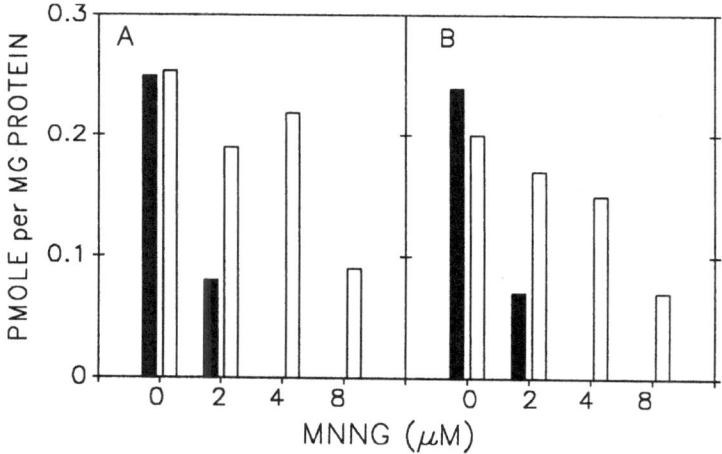

Fig. 2. Histograms comparing O^6-MT in untreated and MNNG treated cells. Normal human kidney (A) and liver epithelial cells (B) were treated in CPDL 1 through 6 with 0, 2, 4 and 8 μM MNNG for 1 hr at 37°C. Immediately following treatment (solid bar) or 48 hr post treatment (open bar) O^6-MT was assayed. Reprinted from Wani et al., (1989) with permission.

Table 3. Effect of Multiple MNNG Treatments on O^6-MT Activity

Agent	Number of Treatments[a]	Cumulative Dose	Kidney cell[b]	Liver cell[b]
		μM	molecules O^6-MT per cell $(x10^3)$[c]	
Buffer	4	0	17.58	16.65
MNNG	4	1.2	16.65	10.18
Buffer	6	0	20.35	23.13
MNNG	6	1.8	18.50	22.20
Buffer	8	0	21.28	22.20
MNNG	8	2.4	21.28	22.20

[a]Cells were treated every 6 hr with 0.3 μM MNNG. They were assayed for O^6-MT 6 hr following the last treatment.
[b]Kidney and liver cells were in CPDL 1 through 6. Treatment was begun when cells obtained 60% confluency.
[c]O^6-MT is the mean of 4 determinations from 2 experiments.
Reprinted from Wani et al., (1989) with permission.

European and exposed Chinese population detectable levels (100 to 644 molecules of O^6-MeGua per genome) of O^6-MeGua and O^6-MT (0.08 to 0.45 pmole per mg protein) were observed (Umbenhauer et al., 1985). Given that O^6-MT is inactivated upon the repair of O^6-MeGua, it is surprising that there were detectable levels of O^6-MeGua in the tissues of the population that had high levels of O^6-MT. It is possible that the damage on the chromatin was inaccessible to the repair protein, as is the case with other types of DNA damage (Bohr et al., 1987; Thomas et al., 1988). Whether the O^6-MeGua is preferentially repaired in human cells will have to wait for new technical approaches which will allow quantification of the lesion in isolated gene fragments.

ACKNOWLEDGEMENTS

Support from the NIH-NIEHS (grant ES03101) and USEPA Office of Exploratory Research (grant R812165) is gratefully acknowledged.

REFERENCES

Abbott, P.J., and Saffhill, R., 1979, DNA synthesis with methylated poly(dC-dG) templates: Evidence for a competitive nature to miscoding by O^6-methylguanine, Biochim. Biophys. Acta, 562:51.
Ashworth, D.J., Baird, W.M., Chang, C.J., Ciupek, J.D., Busch, K.L., and Cooks, R.G., 1985, Chemical modification of nucleic acids. Methylation of calf thymus DNA investigated by mass spectrometry and liquid chromatography, Biomed. Mass. Spectrom., 12:309.

Becker, R.A., and Montesano, R., 1985, Repair of O^4-methyldeoxy-thymidine residues in DNA by mammalian liver extracts, <u>Carcinogenesis</u>, 6:313.

Bedell, M.A., Lewis, J.G., Billings, K.C., and Swenberg, J.A., 1982, Cell specificity in hepatocarcinogenesis: Preferential accumulation of O^6-methylguanine in target cell DNA during continuous exposure of rats to 1,2-dimethylhydrazine, <u>Cancer Res.</u>, 42:3079.

Belinsky, S.A., White, C.M., Devereux, T.R., Swenberg, J.A., and Anderson, M.W., 1987, Cell selective alkylation of DNA in rat lung following low dose exposure to the tobacco specific carcinogen 4-(N-methyl-N-nitrosamine)-1-(3-pyridyl)-1-butanone, <u>Cancer Res.</u>, 47:1143.

Bhattacharyya, D., Tano, K., Bunick, G.J., Uberbacher, E.C., Behnke, W.D., and Mitra, S., 1988a, Rapid, large-scale purification and characterization of '*Ada* protein' (O^6-methylguanine-DNA methyltransferase) of *E. coli*, <u>Nucleic Acids Res.</u>, 16 Suppl. 14:6397.

Bhattacharyya, D., Boulden, A.M., Foote, R.S., and Mitra, S., 1988b, Effect of polyvalent metal ions on the reactivity of human O^6-methylguanine-DNA methyltransferase, <u>Carcinogenesis</u>, 9:683.

Bignami, M., Vitelli, A., Di-Muccio, A., Terlizzese, M., Calcagnile, A., Zapponi, G.A., Lohman, P.H., Den Engelse, L., and Dogliotti, E., 1988, Relationship between specific alkylated bases and mutations at two gene loci induced by ethylnitrosourea and diethyl sulfate in CHO cells, <u>Mutat. Res.</u>, 193:43.

Bohr, V.A., Phillips, D.H., and Hanawalt, P.C., 1987, Heterogeneous DNA damage and repair in the mammalian genome, <u>Cancer Res.</u>, 47:6426.

Boulden, A.M., Foote, R.S., Fleming, G.S., and Mitra, S., 1987, Purification and some properties of human DNA-O^6-methylguanine methyl-transferase, <u>J. Biosci.</u>, 11:215.

Brennand, J., and Margison, G.P., 1986, Expression of the *E. coli* O^6-methylguanine-methylphosphotriester methyltransferase gene in mammalian cells, <u>Carcinogenesis</u>, 7:185.

Brent, T.P., 1985, Isolation and purification of O^6-alkylguanine-DNA alkyltransferase from human leukemic cells. Prevention of chloroethylnitrosourea-induced cross-links by purified enzyme, <u>Pharmacol. Ther.</u>, 31:121.

Brent, T.P., 1986, Inactivation of purified human O^6-alkylguanine-DNA alkyltransferase by alkylating agents or alkylated DNA, <u>Cancer Res.</u>, 46:2320.

Brent, T.P., Dolan, M.E., Fraenkel-Conrat, H., Hall, J., Karran, P., Laval, F., Margison, G.P., Montesano, R., Pegg, A.E., Potter, P.M., Singer, B., Swenberg, J.A., and Yarosh, D.B., 1988, Repair of O-alkylpyrimidines in mammalian cells: a present consensus, <u>Proc. Natl. Acad. Sci. USA</u>, 85:1759.

Ceccoli, J., Rosales, N., Goldstein, M., and Yarosh, D.B., 1988, Polyclonal antibodies against O^6-methylguanine-DNA methyltransferase in adapted bacteria, <u>Mutat. Res.</u>, 194:219.

Chu, H.Y., Craig, A.W., and O'Connor, P.J., 1981, Repair of O^6-methylguanine in rat liver is enhanced by pretreatment with single or multiple doses of aflatoxin B_1, <u>Br. J. Cancer</u>, 43:850.

Coulondre, C., and Miller, J.H., 1977, Genetic studies of the *lac* repressor, IV. Mutagenic specificity in the *lac* I gene by *Escherichia coli*, J. Mol. Biol., 117:577.

D'Ambrosio, S.M., Oravec, C.T., and Gibson-D'Ambrosio, R.E., 1983, An in vitro human-organ-specific system for testing genotoxic agents, Ann. NY Acad. Sci., 407:426.

D'Ambrosio, S.M., Samuel, M.J., Dutta-Choudhury, T.A., and Wani, A.A., 1987, O^6-methylguanine-DNA methyltransferase in human fetal tissues: fetal and maternal factors, Cancer Res., 47:51.

D'Ambrosio, S.M., Lowder, E., and D'Ambrosio, R.E.G., 1988, Isolation and characteristics of human fetal liver hepatocytes in long term culture, J. Cell Biol., 107:78a.

Day, R.S., 3rd., Babich, M.A., Yarosh, D.B., and Scudiero, D.A., 1987, The role of O^6-methylguanine in human cell killing, sister chromatid exchange induction and mutagenesis: a review, J. Cell Sci. [Suppl], 6:333.

Demple, B., Sedgwick, B., Robins, P., Totty, N., Waterfield, M.D., and Lindahl, T., 1985, Active site and complete sequence of the suicidal methyltransferase that counters alkylation mutagenesis, Proc. Natl. Acad. Sci. USA, 82:2688.

Den Engelse, L., Floot, B.G.J., Menkveld, G.L., and Tates, A.D., 1984, Enhanced repair of O^6-methylguanine in livers of rats pretreated with phenobarbital or ENU, Mutat. Res., 130:197.

Den Engelse, L., Floot, B.G., Menkveld, G.J., and Tates, A.D., 1986, Enhanced repair of O^6-methylguanine in liver DNA of rats pretreated with phenobarbital, 2,3,7,8-tetrachlorodibenzo-p-dioxin, ethionine, or N-alkyl-N-nitrosoureas, Carcinogenesis, 7:1941.

Dodson, L.A., Foote, R.S., Mitra, S., and Masker, W.E., 1982, Mutagenesis of bacteriophage T7 in vitro by incorporation of O^6-methylguanine during DNA synthesis, Proc. Natl. Acad. Sci. USA, 79:7440.

Dolan, M.E., and Pegg, A.E., 1985, Extent of formation of O^4-methyl-thymidine in calf thymus DNA methylated by N-methyl-N-nitrosourea and lack of repair of this product by rat liver O^6-alkylguanine-DNA-alkyltransferase, Carcinogenesis, 6:1611.

Dolan, M.E., Scicchitano, D., Singer, B., and Pegg, A.E., 1984, Comparison of repair on methylated pyrimidines in poly(dT) by extracts of rat liver and *Escherichia coli*, Biochem. Biophys. Res. Commun., 123:324.

Domoradzki, J., Pegg, A.E., Dolan, M.E., Maher, V.M., and McCormick, J.J., 1984, Correlation between O^6-methylguanine-DNA-methyl-transferase activity and resistance of human cells to the cytotoxic and mutagenic effect of N-methyl-N'-nitro-N-nitrosoguanidine, Carcinogenesis, 5:1641.

Domoradzki, J., Pegg, A.E., Dolan, M.E., Maher, V.M., and McCormick, J.J., 1985, Depletion of O^6-methylguanine-DNA-methyltransferase in human fibroblasts increases the mutagenic response to N-methyl-N'-nitro-N-nitrosoguanidine, Carcinogenesis, 6:1823.

Doniger, J., Day, R.S., 3rd., and DiPaolo, J.A., 1985, Quantitative assessment of the role of O^6-methylguanine in the initiation of carcinogenesis by methylating agents, Proc. Natl. Acad. Sci. USA, 82:421.

Foiles, P.G., Miglietta, L.M., Akerkar, S.A., Everson, R.B., and Hecht, S.S., 1988, Detection of O^6-methyldeoxyguanosine in human placental DNA, Cancer Res., 48:4184.

Foote, R., and Mitra, S., 1984, Lack of induction of O^6-methylguanine-DNA methyltransferase in mammalian cells treated with N-methyl-N-nitro-N-nitrosoguanidine, Carcinogenesis, 5:277.

Frosina, G., and Abbondandolo, A., 1985, The current evidence for an adaptive response to alkylating agents in mammalian cells, with special reference to experiments with in vitro cell cultures, Mutat. Res., 154:85.

Frosina, G., and Laval, F., 1987, The O^6-methylguanine-DNA-methyl-transferase activity of rat hepatoma cells is increased after a single exposure to alkylating agents, Carcinogenesis, 8:91.

Gerson, S.L., Trey, J.E., Miller, K., and Berger, N.A., 1986, Comparison of O^6-alkylguanine-DNA alkyltransferase activity based on cellular DNA content in human, rat and mouse tissues, Carcinogenesis, 7:745.

Gibson-D'Ambrosio, R.E., Samuel, M., and D'Ambrosio, S.M., 1986, A method for isolating large numbers of viable disaggregated cells from various human tissues for cell culture establishment, In Vitro Cell. Dev. Biol., 22:529.

Gibson-D'Ambrosio, R.E., Samuel, M., Chang, C.C., Trosko, J.E., and D'Ambrosio, S.M., 1987, Characteristics of long-term human epithelial cell cultures derived from normal human fetal kidney, In Vitro Cell. Dev. Biol., 23:279.

Goth, R., and Rajewsky, M.F., 1972, Ethylation of nucleic acids by ethylnitrosourea-1-^{14}C in the fetal and adult rat, Cancer Res., 32:1501.

Goth, R., and Rajewsky, M.F., 1974, Persistence of O^6-ethylguanine in rat-brain DNA: Correlation with nervous system-specific carcinogenesis by ethylnitrosourea, Proc. Natl. Acad. Sci. USA, 71:639.

Grafstrom, R.C., Pegg, A.E., Trump, B.F., and Harris, C.C., 1984, O^6-alkylguanine-DNA alkyltransferase activity in normal human tissues and cells, Cancer Res., 44:2855.

Grafstrom, R.C., Curren, R.D., Yang, L.L., and Harris, C.C., 1985, Genotoxicity of formaldehyde in cultured human bronchial fibroblasts, Science, 228:89.

Green, C.L., Loechler, E.L., Fowler, K.W., and Essigmann, J.M., 1984, Construction and characterization of extrachromosomal probes for mutagenesis by carcinogens: Site-specific incorporation of O^6-methylguanine into viral and plasmid genomes, Proc. Natl. Acad. Sci. USA, 81:13.

Grisham, J.W., Greenberg, D.S., Kaufman, D.G., and Smith, G.J., 1988, Cycle-related toxicity and transformation in $10T_{1/2}$ cells treated with N-methyl-N'nitro-N-nitrosoguanidine, Proc. Natl. Acad. Sci. USA, 77:4813.

Gullino, P.M., Pettigrew, H.M., and Grantham, F.H., 1975, N-Nitrosomethylurea as mammary gland carcinogen in rats, J. Natl. Cancer Inst., 54:401.

Hall, J., and Karran, P. 1986, Repair of DNA lesions introduced by N-nitroso compounds, In: "Repair of DNA Lesions Introduced by N-Nitroso Compounds," B. Myrnes and H. Krokan, eds., Norwegian University Press, Oslo. pp. 73.

Hall, J.H., Bresil, H., and Montesano, R., 1984, O^6-Alkylguanine DNA alkyltransferase activity in monkey, human and rat liver, Carcinogenesis, 6:209.

Harris, C.C., 1987, Human tissues and cells in carcinogenesis research, Cancer Res., 47:1.

Harris, C.C., and Autrup, H., 1983, "Human Carcinogenesis," Academic Press, New York.

Heflich, R.H., Beranek, D.T., Kodell, R.L., and Morris, S.M., 1982, Induction of mutations and sister-chromatid exchanges in Chinese hamster ovary cells by ethylating agents, Mutat. Res., 106:147.

Hemminiki, K., and Vainio, H. 1984, Human exposure to carcinogenic components, In: "Monitoring Human Exposure to Carcinogenic and Mutagenic Agents," International Agency for Research on Cancer, Lyon. pp. 37.

Kaina, B., 1982, Enhanced survival and reduced mutation and aberration frequencies induced in V79 Chinese hamster cells pre-exposed to low levels of methylating agents, Mutat. Res., 93:195.

Karran, P., Arlett, C.F., and Broughton, B.C., 1982, An adaptive response to the cytotoxic effects of N-methyl-N-nitrosourea is apparently absent in normal human fibroblasts, Biochimie (Paris), 64:717.

Krieg, D.R., 1963, Ethyl methanesulfonate-induced reversion of bacteriophage T4rII mutants, Genetics, 48:561.

Krokan, H., Haugen, A., Myrnes, B., and Guddah, P.H., 1983, Repair of premutagenic DNA lesions in human fetal tissues: evidence for low levels of O^6-methylguanine-DNA methyltransferase and uracil-DNA glycosylase activity in some tissues, Carcinogenesis, 4:1559.

Krokan, H., Lechner, J., Krokan, R.H., and Harris, C.C., 1985, Normal human bronchial epithelial cells do not show an adaptive response after treatment with N-methyl-N'-nitro-N-nitrosoguanidine, Mutat. Res., 146:205.

Laval, F., and Laval, J., 1984, Adaptive response in mammalian cells: cross- reactivity of different pretreatments on cytotoxicity as compared to mutagenicity, Proc. Natl. Acad. Sci. USA, 81:1062.

Laval, J., and Strauss, B.S., 1985, Chemical carcinogens and proto-oncogene activation, Biochimie. (Paris), 67:391.

Lawley, P.D., 1966, Effects of some chemical mutagens and carcinogens on nucleic acids, Prog. Nucl. Acids Res. Mol. Biol., 5:89.

Lawley, P.D. 1973, Alkylation of nucleic acids and mutagenesis, In: "Molecular and Environmental Aspects of Mutagenesis," L. Prakash, F. Sherman, M.W. Miller, C.W. Lawrence, and H.W Tabor, eds., Thomas, Springfield, IL. pp. 17.

Lawley, P.D., 1989, Mutagens as carcinogens: Development of current concepts, Mutat. Res., 213:3.

Lawley, P.D., and Thatcher, C.J., 1970, Methylation of deoxyribonucleic acid cultured mammalian cells by N-methyl-N'-nitro-N-nitroso-guanidine. The influence of cellular thiol concentrations on the extent of methylation and 6-oxygen atom of guanosine as a site of methylation, Biochem. J., 116:693.

Lefebvre, P., and Laval, F., 1986, Enhancement of O^6-methylguanine-DNA-methyltransferase activity induced by various treatments in mammalian cells, Cancer Res., 46:5701.

Lewis, J.G., and Swenberg, J.A., 1983, The kinetics of DNA alkylation, repair and replication in hepatocytes, Kupffer cells, and sinusoidal endothelial cells in rat liver during continuous exposure to 1,2-dimethylhydrazine, Carcinogenesis, 4:529.

Lindahl, T., Sedgwick, B., Sekiguchi, M., and Nakabeppu, Y., 1988, Regulation and expression of the adaptive response to alkylating agents, Annu. Rev. Biochem., 57:133.

Loechler, E.L., Green, C.L., and Essigmann, J.M., 1984, In vivo mutagenesis by O^6-methylguanine built into a unique site in a viral genome, Proc. Natl. Acad. Sci. USA, 81:6271.

Loveless, A., 1969, Possible relevance of O^6-alkylation of DNA to the mutagenicity and carcinogenicity of nitrosamines and nitrosamides, Nature (Lond.), 223:206.

Manchester, D.K., Weston, A., Choi, J.-S., Trivers, G.E., Fennessey, P.V., Quintana, E., Farmer, P.B., Mann, D.L., and Harris, C.C., 1988, Detection of benzo[a]pyrene diol epoxide-DNA adducts in human placenta, Proc. Natl. Acad. Sci. USA, 85:9243.

Margison, G.P., Butler, J., and Hoey, B., 1985, O^6-Methylguanine methyltransferase activity is increased in rat tissues by ionising radiation, Carcinogenesis, 6:1699.

McCarthy, J.G., Edington, B.V., and Schendel, P.F., 1983, Inducible repair of phosphotriesters in Escherichia coli, Proc. Natl. Acad. Sci. USA, 80:7380.

McCarthy, T.V., Karran, P., and Lindahl, T., 1984, Inducible repair of O-alkylated pyrimidines in Escherichia coli, EMBO J., 3:545.

Medcalf, A.S.C., and Lawley, P.D., 1981, Time course of O^6-methylguanine removal from DNA of N-methyl-N-nitrosourea-treated human fibroblasts, Nature (Lond.), 289:796.

Moody, P.C.E., and Demple, B., 1988, Crystallization of O^6-methylguanine-DNA methyltransferase from Escherichia coli, J. Mol. Biol., 200:751.

Morimoto, K., Dolan, M.E., Scicchitano, D., and Pegg, A.E., 1985, Repair of O^6-propylguanine and O^6-butylguanine in DNA by O^6-alkylguanine-DNA alkyltransferase from rat liver and E. coli, Carcinogenesis, 6:1027.

Myrnes, B., Giercksky, K.E., and Krokan, H., 1983, Interindividual variation in the activity of O^6-methylguanine-DNA methyltransferase and uracil-DNA glycosylase in human organs, Carcinogenesis, 4:1565.

Myrnes, B., and Wittwer, C.U., 1988, Purification of the human O^6-methylguanine-DNA methyltransferase and uracil-DNA glycosylase, the latter to apparent homogeneity, Eur. J. Biochem., 173:383.

Nakamura, T., Tokumoto, Y., Sakumi, K., Koike, G., Nakabeppu, Y., and Sekiguchi, M., 1988, Expression of the ada gene of Escherichia coli in response to alkylating agents. Identification of transcriptional regulatory elements, J. Mol. Biol., 202:483.

Nehls, P., Rajewsky, M.F., Spiess, E., and Werner, D., 1984, Highly sensitive sites for guanine-O^6-ethylation in rat brain DNA exposed to N-ethyl-N-nitrosourea in vivo, EMBO J., 3:327.

Newbold, R.F., Warren, W., Medcalf, A.S.C., and Amos, J., 1980, Mutagenicity of carcinogenic methylating agents is associated with a specific DNA modification, Nature (Lond.), 283:596.

Nicoll, J.W., Swann, P.F., and Pegg, A.E., 1975, Effect of dimethylnitrosamine on persistence of methylated guanines in rat liver and kidney DNA, Nature (Lond.), 254:261.

Olsson, M., and Lindahl, T., 1980, Repair of alkylated DNA in *Escherichia coli*. Methyl group transfer from O^6-methylguanine to a protein cysteine residue, J. Biol. Chem., 255:10569.

Osterman-Golker, S., 1974, Reaction kinetics of N-methyl-N'-nitro-N-nitrosoguanidine and N-ethyl-N'-nitro-N-nitrosoguanidine, Mutat. Res., 24:219.

Osterman-Golker, S., Ehrenberg, L., and Wachtmeister, C.A., 1970, Reaction kinetics and biological action in barley of mono-functional methanesulfonic esters, Radiat. Botany, 10:303.

Pegg, A.E., 1983, Alkylation and subsequent repair of DNA after exposure to dimethylnitrosamine and related carcinogens, Rev. Biochem. Toxicol., 5:83.

Pegg, A.E., and Dolan, M.E., 1987, Properties and assay of mammalian O^6-alkylguanine-DNA alkyltransferase, Pharmacol. Ther., 34:167.

Pegg, A.E., Scicchitano, D., and Dolan, M.E., 1984, Comparison of the rates of repair of O^6-alkylguanines in DNA by rat liver and bacterial O^6-alkylguanine-DNA alkyltransferase, Cancer Res., 44:3806.

Pegg, A.E., Wiest, L., Foote, R.S., Mitra, S., and Perry, W., 1983, Purification and properties of O^6-methylguanine-DNA transmethylase from rat liver, J. Biol. Chem., 258:2327.

Pegg, A.E., Roberfroid, M., Bahr, C.V., Foote, R.S., Mitra, S., Bresil, H., Likhachev, A., and Montesano, R., 1982, Removal of O^6-methylguanine from DNA by human liver fractions, Proc. Natl. Acad. Sci. USA, 79:5162.

Perera, F.P., Santella, R.M., Brenner, D., Poirier, M.C., Munshi, A.A., Fishman, H.K., and Van Ryzin, J., 1987, DNA adducts, protein adducts, and sister chromatid exchange in cigarette smokers and nonsmokers, JNCI, 79:449.

Poirier, M.C., 1984, The use of carcinogen-DNA adduct antisera for quantitation and localization of genomic damage in animal models and the human population, Environ. Mutagen., 6:879.

Richardson, F.C., Dyroff, M.C., Boucheron, J.A., and Swenberg, J.A., 1985, Differential repair of O^4-alkylthymidine following exposure to methylating and ethylating hepatocarcinogens, Carcinogenesis, 6:625.

Saffhill, R., 1984, Differences in the promutagenic nature of 3-methylcytosine as revealed by DNA and RNA polymerizing enzymes, Carcinogenesis, 5:691.

Saffhill, R., 1986, The competitive miscoding of O^6-methylguanine and O^6-ethylguanine and the possible importance of cellular deoxynucleoside 5'-triphosphate pool sizes in mutagenesis and carcinogenesis, Biochim. Biophys. Acta, 866:53.

Saffhill, R., Margison, G.P., and O'Connor, P.J., 1985, Mechanisms of carcinogenesis induced by alkylating agents, Biochim. Biophys. Acta, 823:111.

Schmerold, I., and Spath, A., 1986, Induction of rat liver O^6-alkylguanine-DNA alkyltransferase by bleomycin, Chem. Biol. Interact., 60:297.

Schold, S.C., Brent, T.P., von Hoffe, E., Friedman, H.S., Mitra, S., Bigner, D.D., Swenberg, J.A., and Kleihues, P., 1989, O^6-Alkylguanine-DNA alkyltransferase and sensitivity to procarbazine in human brain-tumor xenografts, J. Neurosurg., 70:573.

Sedgwick, B., Robins, P., Totty, N., and Lindahl, T., 1988, Functional domains and methyl acceptor sites of the *Escherichia coli ada* protein, J. Biol. Chem., 263:4430.

Singer, B., 1976, All oxygens in nucleic acids react with carcinogenic ethylating agents, Nature (Lond.), 264:333.

Singer, B., 1979, N-Nitroso alkylating agents: formation and persistence of alkyl derivatives in mammalian nucleic acids as contributing factors in carcinogenesis, J. Natl. Cancer Inst., 62:1329.

Singer, B., and Kroger, M., 1979, Participation of modified nucleosides in translation and transcription, Prog. Nucl. Acids Res. Mol. Biol., 23:151.

Singer, B., and Kusmierek, J.T., 1982, Chemical mutagenesis, Annu. Rev. Biochem., 51:655.

Singer, B., Bodell, W.J., Cleaver, J.E., Thomas, G.H., Rajewsky, M.F., and Thon, W., 1978, Oxygens in DNA are main targets for ethylnitrosourea in normal and xeroderma pigmentosum fibroblasts and fetal rat brain cells, Nature, 276:85.

Souliotis, V.L., Giannopoulos, A., Koufakis, I., Kaila, S., Dimopoulos, C., and Kyrtopoulos, S.A., 1989, Development and validation of a new assay for O^6-alkylguanine-DNA-alkyltransferase based on the use of an oligonucleotide substrate, and its application to the measurement of DNA repair activity in extracts of biopsy samples of human urinary bladder mucosa, Carcinogenesis, 10:1203.

Sukumar, S., Notario, V., Martin-Zanca, D., and Barbacid, M., 1983, Induction of mammary carcinomas in rats by nitroso-methylurea involves malignant activation of H-*ras*-1 locus by single point mutation, Nature (Lond.), 306:658.

Sun, L., and Singer, B., 1975, The specificity of different classes of ethylating agents toward various sites of HeLa cell DNA in vitro and in vivo, Biochemistry, 14:1795.

Swenberg, J.A., Bedell, M.A., Billings, K.C., Umbenhauer, D.R., and Pegg, A.E., 1982, Cell-specific differences in O^6-alkylguanine DNA repair activity during continuous exposure to carcinogen, Proc. Natl. Acad. Sci., 79:5499.

Swenberg, J.A., Dyroff, M.C., Bedell, M.A., Popp, J.A., Huh, N., Kirstein, U., and Rajewsky, M.F., 1984, O^6-Ethyldeoxythymidine, but not O^6-ethyldeoxyguanosine, accumulates in hepatocyte DNA of rats exposed continuously to diethylnitrosamine, Proc. Natl. Acad. Sci. USA, 81:1692.

Swenberg, J.A., Richardson, F.C., Boucheron, J.A., and Dyroff, M.C., 1985, Relationships between DNA adduct formation and carcinogenesis, Environ. Health Perspect., 62:177.

Teo, I.A., 1987, Proteolytic processing of the *Ada* protein that repairs DNA O^6-methylguanine residues in *E. coli*, Mutat. Res., 183:123.

Thomas, D.C., Morton, A.G., Bohr, V.A., and Sancar, A., 1988, General method for quantifying base adducts in specific mammalian genes, Proc. Natl. Acad. Sci. USA, 85:3723.

Topal, M.D., 1988, DNA repair, oncogenes and carcinogenesis, Carcinogenesis, 9:691.

Umbenhauer, D., Wild, C.P., Montesano, R., Saffhill, R., Boyle, J.M., Huh, N., Kirstein, U., Thomale, J., Rajewsky, M.F., and Lu, S.H., 1985, O^6-Methyldeoxyguanosine in oesophageal DNA among individuals at high risk of oesophageal cancer, Int. J. Cancer, 36:661.

von Hofe, E., and Kennedy, A.R., 1988, In vitro induction of O^6-methylguanine-DNA methyltransferase in C3H/10T1/2 cells by X-rays is inhibited by nitrogen, Carcinogenesis, 9:679.

Waldstein, E.A., Cao, E.H., and Setlow, R.B., 1982a, Adaptive resynthesis of O^6-methylguanine-accepting protein can explain the differences between mammalian cells proficient and deficient in methyl excision repair, Proc. Natl. Acad. Sci. USA, 79:5117.

Waldstein, E.A., Cao, E., and Setlow, R.B., 1982b, Adaptive increase of O^6-methylguanine acceptor protein in HeLa cells following N-methyl-N'-nitro-N-nitrosoguanidine treatment, Nucleic Acids Res., 10:4595.

Wani, A.A., Wani, G., and D'Ambrosio, S.M., 1985, Repair of DNA O-alkylation damage by various human organs, Biochem. Biophys. Res. Commun., 133:589.

Wani, G., Wani, A.A., Gibson-D'Ambrosio, R.E., Samuel, M., Lowder, E., and D'Ambrosio, S.M., 1989, Absence of a DNA damage-mediated induction of human methyltransferase specific for precarcinogenic O^6-methylguanine, Teratogen. Carcinogen. Mutagen., 9:(in press).

Wiestler, O., Kleihues, P., and Pegg, A.E., 1984, O^6-Alkylguanine-DNA alkyltransferase activity in human brain and brain tumors, Carcinogenesis, 5:121.

Yarosh, D.B., Foote, R.S., Mitra, S., and Rufus, S., 1983, Repair of O^6-methylguanine in DNA by demethylation is lacking in Mer⁻ human tumor cell strains, Carcinogenesis, 4:199.

Yarosh, D.B., Rosales, N., and Ceccoli, J., 1988, Antibodies against human and E. coli O^6-methylguanine-DNA methyltransferase, J. Cell Biochem., 12A:281.

REPAIR OF O^4-ALKYLTHYMINE DAMAGE IN HUMAN CELLS

Altaf A. Wani, Gulzar Wani and Steven M. D'Ambrosio

The Department of Radiology
The Ohio State University
Columbus, Ohio 43210

INTRODUCTION

Experiments using various test systems have demonstrated that agents with carcinogenic potential are also mutagenic in both prokaryotic and eukaryotic systems (Ames, 1979; Moore et al., 1988; Yuspa et al., 1989). Model studies using experimental animals and cultured cells associate the initiation step in the process of multistage carcinogenesis, with the structural alterations of the cellular DNA (Harris and Autrup, 1983; Cairns, 1981). The modifications of DNA structure can ultimately lead to abnormal cellular function unless the induced damage is repaired prior to the commencement of the cellular DNA replication. DNA alkylating agents e.g., nitrosoureas or nitrosoguanidines are a class of chemical compounds that mediate their biological effects through interactions with nucleophilic sites in DNA and formation of alkyl adducts. The chemistry and extent of formation of these adducts as well as their subsequent fate in the living cell plays a critical role in the mutagenic and carcinogenic processes (Margison and O'Connor, 1979; O'Connor et al., 1979). Elucidation of the mechanism(s), by which a variety of different adducts elicit changes in cellular phenotype, has been an area of intense pathobiological investigation. In-depth studies have been performed on the chemistry and reactivity of different alkylation agents. It has been shown that all the oxygen sites in nucleic acids, in vitro and in vivo, are targets of alkylation particularly by ethylating mutagenic carcinogens (Singer et al., 1978; Nehls and Rajewsky, 1985). A significant proportion of total alkylation has been found to occur at the O^6 of Guanine (Gua), O^4 and O^2 of thymine (Thy), O^2 of cytosine (Cyt), and phosphodiesters, when nucleic acids are treated with agents like MNU, ENU, and MNNG (Lawley and Thatcher, 1970; Sun and Singer, 1975; Singer, 1984). Repair of the damage is perceived to play a vital part in modulating the net effects of alkylation (Saffhill, 1985). It is believed that the formation and repair of all the adducts, having a potential to initiate the errors of replication and repair, should be studied to identify their causal role in carcinogenesis (Singer, 1984, 1986; Saffhill, 1985). The adducts that are formed in relatively greater abundance, e.g., O^6-alkylguanine (O^6-alkylGua) have been thoroughly studied

DNA Damage and Repair in Human Tissues
Edited by B. M. Sutherland and A. D. Woodhead
Plenum Press, New York, 1990

over the years (Saffhill et al., 1985; D'Ambrosio et al., this volume). The data on the adducts formed in low concentrations have just begun to accumulate. This chapter will focus on various aspects of O^4-alkylthymine (O^4-alkylThy) damage particularly the repair of this minor base alkylation adduct in human cells.

BIOLOGICAL CONSEQUENCES OF O^4-ALKYLTHYMINE DAMAGE

Mutagenesis. Studies dealing with the identification of the culprit DNA alkylation lesion(s) invariably point out that, of the adducts examined, O^6-alkylGua and O^4-alkylThy are the critical modifications relevant to mutagenesis and carcinogenesis. Initial experiments attempted to elucidate the miscoding properties of modified bases that lead to abnormal Watson-Crick hydrogen bonding of A:T and G:C base pairs (Abbott and Saffhill, 1979; Singer and Kroger, 1979; Saffhill, 1984, 1986). Various characteristics attributed to O^6-alkylGua, implicating it in mutagenesis and carcinogenesis, are also displayed by O^4-alkylThy. In both in vitro and in vivo assay systems, O^4-alkylThy has been shown to be a miscoding and mutagenic lesion (Singer et al., 1983; Preston et al., 1986; Duran and Wani, 1987). In contrast to O^6-alkylGua, which directs the misincorporation of Thy, O^4-alkylThy in polynucleotide directs a large number of dGua errors (Singer et al., 1983; Duran and Wani, 1987). O^4-alkylThy triphosphate substitutes for Thy triphosphate in the polymerase I catalyzed synthesis of the alternating, poly(dA-dT) (Saffhill, 1985). In addition to G:C to A:T transitions a significant frequency of A:T to G:C transitions are induced in the *lac I* gene upon treatment of bacteria with alkylating agents (Coulondre and Miller, 1977). The mutations at A:T sites indicate the involvement of thymidine base modification by ENU. The feasibility of abnormal base pairing between O^4-alkylThy and Gua is also supported by model studies (Brennan et al., 1986). More recent mutagenesis studies of the *gpt* gene-containing bacteria suggest that the differences in the mutation spectra, by alkylating agents, may be attributed to the different ratios of O^6-alkylGua and O^4-alkylThy produced in the DNA (Richardson et al., 1987). For instance, due to its ability to form substantial amounts of O^4-alkylThy, ENU-induced mutations were shown to include A:T to G:C transition in addition to G:C to A:T transition mutations (K.K. Richardson et al., 1987).

More direct evidence on the mutagenic properties of O^4-alkylThy is provided by specific in vivo mutagenesis studies that follow the repercussions of a single adduct introduced in the test site of defined DNA sequence (Essigmann et al., 1985). In these studies a single O^4-methylthymine (O^4-MeThy) adduct was enzymatically incorporated into the amber codon of bacteriophage phiX174 *am3* duplex genome (Preston et al., 1986, 1987). A tenfold higher mutation frequency, over the control, was observed in the host that was defective for the repair of O^4-MeThy. Similarly, O^4-ethylthymine (O^4-EtThy) was targeted into a unique restriction endonuclease site before transferring the modified plasmid into the recipient bacterial cell (Duran and Wani, 1987). Mutagenicity was determined by the loss of the cognate restriction endonuclease site. The results of these gap-misrepair studies led to the conclusion that O^4-alkylThy is a highly mutagenic base modification and the initiation of the sequence alterations at the modified site depends upon several factors, including the repair capacity of the exposed host cell.

O^4-alkylThy once formed in cellular DNA acts as either dThy or dCyt (Duran and Wani, 1987; Singer et al., 1987). Sequence alteration at the O^4-alkylthy containing site, during polymerase-catalyzed DNA replication, depend upon the complementary or non-complementary base pairing as well as on the nature and timing of repair machinery attempting to reverse the damage (Duran and Wani, 1987). Based upon studies tracing the consequences of an individual lesion, the in vivo mutagenic potential of O^4-alkylThy has been demonstrated unambiguously. Moreover, the results stress that the proficiency and the nature of repair plays an essential role in modulating the sequence changes heralded by the O-alkylation damage (Singer et al., 1978; Dolan et al., 1984; McCarthy et al., 1984; Nehls et al., 1984; Swenberg et al., 1984; Becker and Montesano, 1985; Dolan and Pegg, 1985; F.C. Richardson et al., 1985; Saffhill et al., 1985; Wani et al., 1985).

Carcinogenesis. Extensive studies relating specific DNA base alteration to carcinogenesis and mammalian cell transformation have not been performed. Since exposure to alkylating carcinogens produce multiple adducts, the extent of contribution to carcinogenicity by any one lesion can be indirectly determined only by circumstantial evidence. For example, the role of O^4-alkylThy in carcinogenesis by alkylating agents can be ascertained from the work of Swenberg and coworkers using experimental animals who showed that susceptible tissues, while proficient for the removal of O^6-alkylGua, are unable to remove O^4-alkylThy (Swenberg et al., 1985). The studies using distinct cell types isolated from the rat liver indicate that persistence of O^6-alkylGua in nonparenchymal cells correlated with the induction of angiosarcomas (Swenberg et al., 1982; Bedell et al., 1982). On the other hand, hepatocytes exhibiting an efficient removal of O^6-alkylGua accumulated O^4-alkylThy in their DNA (Swenberg et al., 1984; Dyroff et al., 1986). This persistence was suggested to account for the residual heptocarcinoma induced by diethylnitrosoamine and dimethylhydrazine. The basic premise is that O^4-alkylThy accumulates in the target organ to the levels sufficient to initiate the neoplastic transformation of the affected cells.

In humans, a causal link to the formation of adducts could be evaluated from epidemiological data collated from populations with well-defined exposure histories. Although the etiology of human cancer has not been precisely established, epidemiological data attribute the major cause of cancer to the life style and exposure to environmental carcinogens (Rajewsky et al., 1977; Harris and Autrup, 1983; Yu et al., 1988). Identification of the adducts in the DNA obtained from tissues of human populations have acted as molecular dosimeters of hazardous chemical exposure (Umbenhauer et al., 1985; Lu et al., 1986; Wild et al., 1986; Manchester et al., 1988; Perera et al., 1988). O^4-alkylthymine has recently been tested as an indicator of exposure of human population to ethylating agents. Huh et al., (1989) have reported that among the individuals tested, those who died of non-cancerous disease contained O^4-EtThd at level and O^4-EtThd/Thd molar ratio of 11.7 $\pm$ 6.5 X 10^{-8} in their liver DNA. This level corresponds to approximately 340 molecules of O^4-EtThy per diploid human cell. In these studies, the patients who had died of liver and other cancers were shown to contain 4- to 5-fold higher mean levels of O^4-EtThy adducts in their liver DNA. These results clearly show the formation and accumulation of O^4-alkylThy in human cell DNA, presumably resulting from exposure to an exogenous or endogenous agent. However, the investigators did not identify the source of the agent, history of exposure, and any relationship of the accumulated adduct to the lack of its repair. On the other hand, it should be pointed out that the accumulation of elevated levels of O^6-MeGua were detected, despite a normal level of O^6-MT repair activity in the same populace (Umbenhauer et al., 1985). Although the extent of the adduct quantitated in the human liver DNA was significant, it is difficult to attribute the increased O^4-EtThy as the cause of patients' cancers. Nevertheless, it is reasonable to suggest that O^4-EtThd is continuously being formed in the human cellular DNA due to an acute or chronic exposure to some ethylating species. The adduct levels detected actually reflect a composite of both degree of formation and repair capacity of the exposed cell/organ (Montesano et al., 1985). The lack of an active repair process in susceptible individuals could predispose them to an O^4-EtThy adduct accumulation and initiate a process, conceivably resulting in death from cancer.

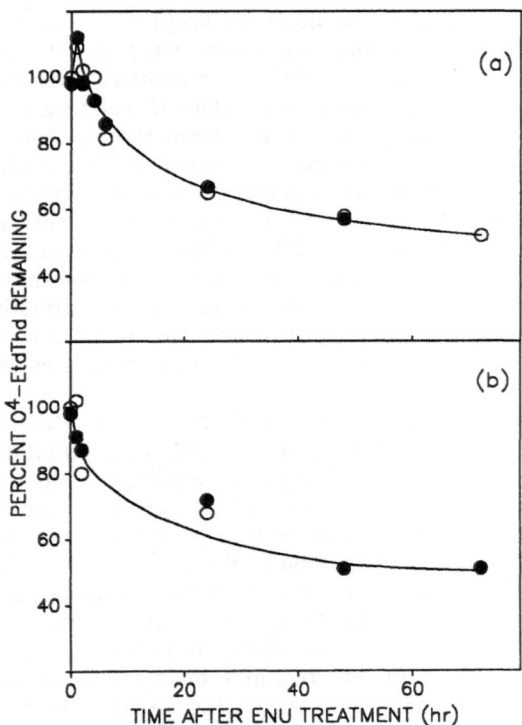

Fig. 1. The kinetics of repair of O^4-EtThd in the DNA of human cells. Normal human skin fibroblastic (a) and kidney epithelial (b) cell cultures at subpassage ~5 were treated with 1 mM ENU for 60 min. At various post-incubation times the cells were harvested and DNA extracted. O^4-EtThd was quantitated by non-competitive immunoslot blot assay using 0.4 and 0.8 ug DNA. Initial O^4-EtdThd/Thd molar ratio, calculated from the corresponding ethylated standard, was 1×10^{-6}. The results of duplicate samples of two separate experiments are presented. (From Wani and D'Ambrosio, 1987).

In vivo. The in vivo loss of O^4-alkylThy, following single dose exposure to alkylating agents, has been determined in experimental animals and cultured cells. Although few data are available, it has been determined that O^4-MeThy is lost at a relatively rapid rate compared to the loss of O^4-EtThy from the cellular alkylated DNA. The half life ($t_{1/2}$) of O^4-MeThy removal has been determined to be 20 hr for the liver DNA of rats exposed to 1,2-dimethylhydrazine (Richardson et al., 1985). Variable rates of O^4-EtThy removal have been reported for rat liver. They range from a rapid $t_{1/2}$ of 60 h (Singer et al., 1981) to 11 days (Richardson et al., 1985). In parallel studies, rat brain does not show a significant loss of O^4-EtThy from its DNA (Singer et al., 1981). Results of experiments on animal organs appear to conform with the data in cell culture. For example, rat neuronal cells proficient for the repair of O^6-EtGua did not eliminate O^4-EtThy from their DNA (Huh and Rajewsky, 1986). On the other hand, a limited number of O^4-MeThy molecules, incorporated in the DNA through the uptake of precursor nucleoside, were rapidly removed ($t_{1/2}$ = 2 to 3 hr) by cultured V79 cells (Saffhill and Fox, 1980). Repair studies using cultured human cells provide stronger evidence for the active in vivo removal of O^4-alkylThy from the modified DNA. High pressure liquid chromatography (Hplc) analysis of DNA, extracted from human fibroblastic cells treated in culture with ENU, shows O^4-EtThy repair occurring with an approximate $t_{1/2}$ of 40 to 60 h (Bodell et al., 1979). The application of sensitive immunoassays and quantitation of O^4-EtThd in ENU-treated human skin fibroblast and kidney epithelial cells indicate a gradual biphasic removal of the modified base as a function of post-treatment time in culture (Wani and D'Ambrosio, 1987a). In both cell types about 50% of the initial damage was repaired during a 72 h period (Figure 1). In these studies (Bodell et al., 1979; Wani and D'Ambrosio, 1987a), the loss of O^4-EtThy was not due to cell replication and dilution of the modified base by an increase in cellular DNA content. These kinetic data on the in vivo loss of O^4-alkylThy are consistent with an active repair process (Bodell et al., 1979; Singer et al., 1981; Richardson et al., 1985; Wani and D'Ambrosio, 1987a; Brent et al., 1988). A close review of the overall data indicates that human cells are relatively more active for the repair of the critical O^4-alkylThy adduct than the rodent cells. Enhanced repair capacity of human cells is not unique for O^4-alkylThy but is also seen for the repair of other adducts e.g., O^6-alkylGua (D'Ambrosio et al., 1987; Wani et al., 1989).

In vitro. Most of the initial understanding on the enzymology and mode of repairing O^4-alkylThy has been derived from *E. coli*, which is known to contain single or multiple forms of a transferase protein (McCarthy et al., 1983; Ahmmed and Laval, 1984; Dolan et al., 1984; McCarthy et al., 1984). Part or all of this activity in *E. coli* is due to the ability of O^6-MT protein to also recognize O^4-alkylThy. Based upon the in vivo kinetic data described above, a number of laboratories have searched for repair activity in protein extracts of mammalian tissues, including human, and cultured cells (Brent et al., 1988). These studies evaluated the ability of purified O^6-MT protein, partially purified and/or crude protein extracts to remove the O^4-alkyl group from an O^4-alkylThy containing DNA substrate (Table 1). The experiments

Table 1. Summary of the Results on Human O^4-Alkylthymine Specific Repair Activity

Source	Protein	Assay/ alkyl- substrate	Activity	Reference
Cultured cell lines				
Lymphoblast	Purified O^6-MT	Inhibition/ Me-(polydA.dT)	100-fold lower activity	(Brent, 1985)
Fibroblast	Crude extract	HPLC/ Me-(polydT)(polydA)	None	(Yarosh et al., 1985)
Fibroblast	Crude extract	HPLC/ Me-(polydT)(polydA) Me-DNA	None	(Domoradzki et al., 1984) (Dolan and Pegg, 1985)
Lymphoid	Crude extract	HPLC/ Me-(polydA.dT)	None	(Hall and Karran, 1986)
HeLa HT29	Crude extract	HPLC/ Me-dodecamer	None	(Dolan et al., 1988)
Lymphoblast	Purified O^6-MT Fractionated extract	HPLC/ Et-(polydA.dT)	None	(Brent et al., 1988)
Tissues				
Liver	Crude extract	HPLC/ Me-(polydA.dT)	50-fold lower activity	(Becker & Montesano, 1985)
Brain Intestine Liver	Crude extracts	HPLC/ Me-(polydT)(polydA)	Low or no activity	(Wani et al, 1985)
Liver	Fractionated extract	SDS-PAGE/ Me-(polydT)(polydA)	No transfer	(Yarosh et al., 1985) (Brent et al., 1988)
Kidney Liver	Crude extracts	Immunoslot blot Et-DNA	Low activity	(Wani et al. 1989, present report)

have been conducted with different types of specifically designed substrates using several approaches for the detection of O^4-alkylThy. The few studies that have analyzed the protein from human sources are discussed.

Brent (1985) has extensively purified and characterized the alkyltransferase protein from human leukemic lymphoblasts. Activity of this purified protein was tested for the recognition of the O^4-alkylThy base in DNA. The assay used was based upon the activity depletion by modified base-containing substrate. It was concluded that compared to the removal of O^6-alkylGua, human O^6-MT protein, exhibited 100-fold less activity towards O^4-alkylThy. The same purified protein preparation and also ammonium sulfate fractionated protein extract from the same cell line were tested against ENU-ethylated poly(dA.dT). An activity specific for O-alkylated pyrimidines was not observed by an assay claimed to be sensitive enough to detect 1/100th of O^6-MT activity (Brent et al., 1988). Since it is possible that the proteins involved are physically distinct and that selective removal occurs during fractionation or purification, most of the subsequent studies have been performed with cell-free protein extracts. Crude extracts from human fibroblastic cells again did not show a significant loss of O^4-MeThy from methylated poly(dT) duplexed to poly(dA) (Domoradzki et al., 1984; Yarosh et al., 1985). Protein extracts from a number of mer+ and mer- human lymphoid cell lines also showed comparable results. Recently, a model alkylated dodecamer has been successfully used as a substrate for the analysis of transferase activities (Scicchitano et al., 1986; Dolan et al., 1988). The oligomers containing a single O^4-alkylThy and radiolabeled with high specific activity ^{32}P increased the assay sensitivity at least tenfold. Nevertheless, extracts from human cell lines, HeLa and HT29, did not show a dealkylated product upon HPLC analysis (Dolan et al., 1988). In all these experiments, indicating lack of a repair activity, suitability of the substrate and protein extract was always demonstrated by running appropriate controls in parallel. For example, *E. coli* enzyme was shown to efficiently act on model duplex oligomeric or polymeric substrates while the crude extracts used contained fully active proteins specific for other alkylation adducts. Therefore, the failure to demonstrate an activity, if present, could be due to other factors, e.g., absence of a cofactor, different assay optima, and the labile nature of the repair molecule under the assay conditions provided. The latter has been suggested to be a more plausible cause by several investigators (Brent et al., 1988), using crude extracts from cultured cells and tissues.

While the data for the identification of a repair activity in human cell lines seem to be in contrast with in vivo results, the experiments with tissue extracts are more encouraging. One study has reported the presence of low levels of O^4-MeThy specific, transferase-like activity in adult human, monkey, and hepatectomized rat liver (Becker and Montesano, 1985). Activity in human liver was found to be the highest. It was suggested that the activity is either due to the same O^6-MT or a similarly regulated transferase in human liver. The affinity of the enzyme was estimated to be 30- to 50- fold less for O^4-alkylthy than O^6-alkylGua. However, the fractionated liver extracts incubated with methylated poly(dT).poly(dA) did not show a methylated protein molecule in SDS polyacrylamide gel electrophoresis (Brent et al., 1988). This supports the conclusions that the activity observed in human liver does not act by transfer of alkyl group to an acceptor molecule, as has been established for the repair of O^4-alkylThy in *E. coli*.

During our studies on DNA damage processing and consequences of specific damaged adducts in human cells, we conducted a survey of O^4-alkylThy specific activity in various human organs (Wani et al., 1985). Protein extracts from human adult liver, fetal liver, intestine, brain, kidney, lung, and skin were tested against poly(dT)methylated.poly(dA). The assay comprises the Hplc analysis of radioactive [³H]-labeled methylated bases obtained upon the enzymatic hydrolysis of the protein incubated substrate. We found a very low removal of O^4-MeThy by extracts from human liver whereas the activity in other tissues was undetectable (Wani et al., 1985). The same liver extracts were found to be proficient for the repair of other minor base-adducts like O^6-MeGua and O^2-MeThy, as reported by others (Hall and Karran, 1986; Brent et al., 1988).

In view of this data, there is no clear verdict asserting the presence or absence of a repair protein specific for O^4-alkylThy in mammalian cells. Recently some investigators in the area of O^4-alkylThy research presented a consensus, stating that the mode of O-alkylpyrimidine repair in mammalian cells differs from that of bacteria (Brent et al., 1988). They could not rule out the presence of a repair activity in mammalian cells. It is possible that a marginal enzyme activity may be present in cells which eludes detection due to inherent protein lability and the lack of sensitive assays. To obtain a clearer picture, one has to develop novel approaches for assaying a limited number of molecules responsible for repairing O^4-alkylThy in human cells. One such approach could be the development of highly sensitive assays capable of detecting subfemtomole amounts of the modified base in DNA. Furthermore, based on the rapid $t_{1/2}$ of O^4-alkylThy observed in cultured human cells, the use of extracts from human sources should be the initial candidates in these endeavors. We have recently undertaken such studies using O^4-EtThy specific antibodies to identify repair activity in human liver and kidney tissue extracts.

IMMUNOSLOT BLOT (ISB) ANALYSIS OF O^4-ALKYLTHY REPAIR ACTIVITY IN HUMAN TISSUES

Immunoglobulins have been known to possesses an exceptional ability to discern subtle alterations of biomolecular structure. Antibodies specific for a number of DNA base modifications have been developed, characterized, and applied for adduct analysis in many laboratories. The specific antibodies have been useful in quantitating DNA damage and repair in a variety of systems (Adamkiewicz et al., 1984; Wani et al., 1984, 1987b; Wani and D'Ambrosio, 1987a; Manchester et al., 1988; Mori et al., 1989). Lately, adduct specific antibodies have proven useful in tracing the exposure of humans to environmental chemicals (Umbenhauer et al., 1985; Lu et al., 1986; Wild et al., 1986; Manchester et al., 1988; Huh et al., 1989). We have developed antibodies to specific DNA base adducts, including O^4-alkylthymine (Wani et al., 1984, 1987b; Wani and D'Ambrosio, 1987a). In our studies an ISB assay was established to quantitate attomole adduct in very small amounts (ng) of alkylated DNA (Wani and D'Ambrosio, 1987a). Due to the high sensitivity of ISB assay, we have designed an in vitro repair assay for the removal of O⁴-alkylthymine in alkylated DNA incubated with cell-free extracts from different human tissues. The basic steps of this procedure are briefly described as follows.

Double-stranded calf thymus DNA (1.5 μg) ethylated with ENU (O⁴-EtThd/Thd molar ratio = 5 x 10⁻⁶) is incubated with increasing concentrations of cell-free protein extracts in a final reaction volume of 0.2 ml. Subsequently the protein is digested by treatment with proteinase-k and the DNA is denatured. The single-stranded DNA is immobilized to nitrocellulose (NC) filters and O⁴-EtThy detected by specific antibody TB3 binding. The control unmodified DNA treated under exactly same conditions is run in parallel to ensure the assay specificity for O⁴-EtThy. The amount of O⁴-EtThy present in the substrate after treatment with and without protein is calculated from comparison of the ethylated DNA standards run on the same NC filter. Specific activity is calculated from the linear portion of the activity curve.

The detection limit of the ISB repair assay is 0.1 to 0.2 fmol O⁴-EtThy or an O⁴-EtThy/Thy molar ratio of <6.3 x 10⁻⁷. Considering the specific radioactivity of alkylated substrates used in previous assays (Wani et al., 1985; Brent et al., 1988) and limitations of counting [³H] radionuclide efficiently, we estimate that the amount of O⁴-alkylThy detectable by these assays is about 25 fmoles. Reliable measurements of activity using the latter

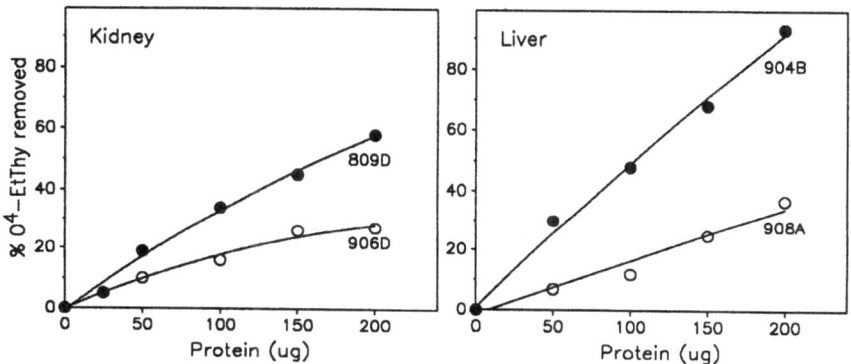

Fig. 2.   Removal of O⁴-EtThy from ethylated DNA by extracts from human kidney and liver. ENU-alkylated DNA (O⁴-EtThd/Thd molar ratio = 5 x 10⁻⁶) was reacted with indicated protein concentrations in a reaction volume of 0.2 ml under conditions essentially as described earlier (Wani et al., 1985) The protein was digested with proteinase-K and the DNA denatured by heating at 100°C for 7 min. Aliquots equivalent to ~1.2 fmol initial O⁴-EtThy concentration (corresponding to the linear portion of the parallel standard curve) were analyzed for the amount of O⁴-EtThy by antibody binding in ISB assay (Wani and D'Ambrosio, 1987a). Amount of O⁴-EtThy removed was determined from the comparison of intensities with linear standard (0.2 to 2 fmol O⁴-EtThy). Protein concentration vs activity plots are shown for individual tissue extracts exhibiting typical extremes of O⁴-EtThy removal.

assays, within or below the 25 fmole limit will be very difficult. In addition, the ISB assay can reliably detect repair activity using nanogram quantities of protein extract. Based on these considerations, the ISB repair assay affords a sensitivity at least two orders of magnitude higher than assays using radiolabeled alkylated homopolymers and HPLC analysis (Wani et al., 1985).

Results of a typical ISB repair assay are shown in Fig. 2. A protein concentration-dependent removal of O^4-EtThy from ENU ethylated substrate DNA was observed with extracts from human fetal kidney and liver. Activity in the extracts of liver tissue was relatively higher than kidney. Some extracts, for example, from liver of individual 908B and kidney of 809D, showed a higher and, in certain instances, quantitative removal of the adduct. The extremes of activity are apparent from the extent of adduct removal by the organ extracts derived from different individuals (Fig. 2). The effectiveness and specificity of the assay was established by using authentic O^4-alkylThy repair transferase from *E. coli* (McCarthy et al., 1983; Wani et al., 1985). A rapid and quantitative loss of O^4-EtThy was seen with limited units of purified enzyme (obtained from Applied Genetics, Inc). Furthermore, the tissue extracts used in these studies were found to be proficient for the removal of O^6-MeGua in O^6-MT assay (Wani et al., 1985; D'Ambrosio et al.,

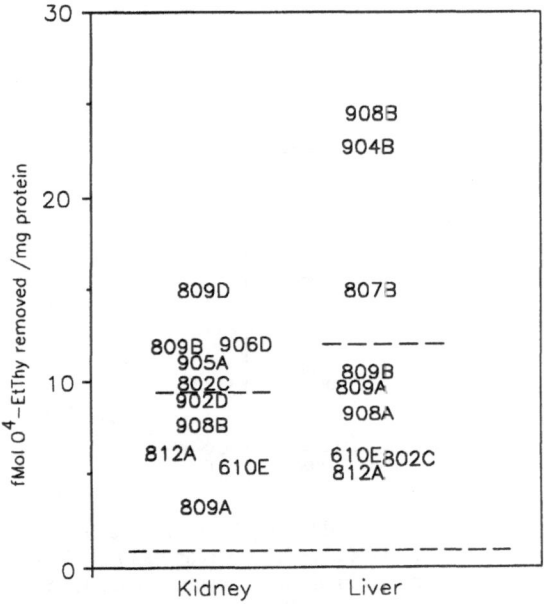

Fig. 3.   Distribution of O^4-EtThy specific activity in human kidney and liver. The activity was determined in cell-free extracts by ISB repair assay. The specific activity (fmol/mg protein) was calculated from the linear portion of the protein concentration vs activity plots. The activity values are represented by the codes for each individual specimen. The broken lines between the sample codes show the mean activity values for kidney (N=10) and liver (N=9) extracts. The dotted line at the bottom represents the limit of detection of the ISB assay.

Table 2. Effect of Free O-Alkylated Base on O^4-EtThy Specific Activity

Base added	Specific activity* (fmol/mg protein)	
	Kidney	Liver
None	12.2 (100%)	22.9 (100%)
O^6-Methylguanine (1.8 mM)	13.8 (113%)	20.4 (89%)
O^4-Methylthymine (2.3 mM)	14.0 (114%)	23.0 (101%)

*The extracts were incubated with the indicated concentration of free base at 37°C for 2 hr. Appropriate aliquots were removed and assayed for the removal of O^4-EtThy from ethylated DNA. Data are an average of two experiments.

1987; Wani et al., 1989). Direct activity comparisons of various protein extracts for the two adducts O^4-alkylThy and O^6-alkylGua, consistently shows a lower affinity for the latter. The specific activity for the removal of O^4-alkylThy is 12.04 ± 7.9 and 9.15 ± 3.5 fmol/mg protein compared to 520 ± 330 and 350 ± 210 fmoles/mg protein for O^6-alkylGua in human fetal liver and kidney tissues, respectively. In general, the level of O^4-alkylThy specific activity is 40- to 60-fold less in the human fetal tissue extracts tested.

Figure 3 shows that the activity specific for O^4-alkylThy varies widely among individuals. The observed differences in the activity between various samples appears to be due to inherent inter-individual variation. Relatively higher variation is seen in liver tissue with activity ranging from approximately 5 to 28 fmol/mg protein with a 65% deviation from the mean activity value. The corresponding deviation for the kidney was about 39%. Interestingly the samples showing higher activity for the removal of O^4-alkylThy also showed higher O^6-MT activity. The higher inter-individual variation observed in the liver and kidney extracts is frequently observed phenomena in human specimen (Myrnes et al., 1983; D'Ambrosio et al., 1987; Wani et al., 1989). Due to the small number of samples tested in these preliminary experiments (N=9), we have not made any attempts to correlate the variation to any one specific factor. However, the variation is not due to the variation in the assay used to detect the activity. Day-to-day reproducibility of the standard immunoassay allowed a reliable quantitation of the O^4-EtThy adduct in the substrate DNA. The activity for the same tissue extract, tested on different days, varied less than 10%. Thus, these data convincingly demonstrate the presence of a protein activity specific for the repair of O^4-alkylThy in DNA.

The ISB repair assay used in these studies follows the disappearance of the substrate (adduct) rather than appearance of the end product. Therefore, it is difficult to determine the exact mode of action of this putative repair activity. Several reports have, however, shown that incubation of alkyltransferase with high concentrations of modified adduct as free base results in the depletion of the activity (Brent, 1985; Dolan et al., 1985; Yarosh et al., 1986). This activity depletion is based on the ability of the transferase to utilize the alkylated free base as a weak substrate and the stoichiometric nature of the transferase reaction. Using the ISB assay we also attempted to determine if depletion of the O^4-alkylThy-specific activity would occur with methylated free bases. The human cell-free extracts were preincubated with excess of O^6-MeGua and O^4-MeThy base. Compared to the control, no significant change in activity could be seen with either base (Table 2). The lack of inhibition of the activity argues against a transferase mode of action. Such a conclusion agrees with other reports and the consensus on the subject (Brent et al., 1988).

SUMMARY

The capacity of a cell to repair damage is the first step in preventing the deleterious consequences of DNA structural alterations induced by the exposure to mutagenic carcinogens. Mammalian cells, having complex genetic organization, have evolved sophisticated mechanisms for the maintenance of integrity of their genome and normal cell function (Bohr and Hanawalt, 1988; Sancar and Sancar, 1988; Pienta et al., 1989). However, many DNA repair processes in mammalian cells are similar to those in prokaryotic cells. For example, the unique damage reversal mechanism by transferase, specific for the repair of O^6-alkylGua, results in the restoration of intact guanine base in both bacteria and mammalian cells (Olsson and Lindahl, 1980; D'Ambrosio and Wani, 1989). The proteins involved, however, are different and vary in their specificities. Mammalian transferase specific for O^6-alkylGua, more closely resembles the bacterial *ogt* gene product (Potter et al., 1987; Rebeck et al., 1988). The main O^6-alkylGua specific transferase activity in *E. coli* resides in the product of the *ada* gene (Demple et al., 1985; Nakabeppu et al., 1985). This protein possesses multiple activities including a specificity for the transfer of alkyl group from O^4-alkylthy in DNA. Such a transferase activity specific for O^4-alkylThy has not been detected in mammalian cells either as an individual activity or part of a multi-activity protein (Brent et al., 1988). Nevertheless, there is tangible evidence for the active removal of O^4-alkylthy in mammalian cells, particularly human cells. The nature, level, and mode of the O^4-alkylThy repair activity has not been fully established. Whether the repair occurs by the well known or some novel mechanism(s) has yet to be determined.

Recently Boyle et al., (1987) has provided genetic evidence for an alternate mode of repair of O^6-alkylGua in mammalian cells. The human cells, that lack O^6-MT activity were able to repair O^6-nButylGua in cellular DNA. Additional experiments, with mammalian V79 cell lines, indicated a differential specificity for various alkyl groups. It has been suggested that in these cells the repair occurs by an excision process, which is known to recognize the distortions of the DNA duplex rather than the adduct itself (Sancar and Sancar, 1988). Support for the excision mechanism is also provided by in vitro experiments, showing repair of O^6-MeGua by purified *E. coli* ABC excinuclease enzyme (Voigt et al., 1989). It is quite likely that the repair of O^4-alkylThy in mammalian cells occurs by a similar process. Whatever the mechanism, the experiments in vivo and in vitro show the activity specific for O^4-alkylThy to be very weak. To what extent it offers protection against the formation, accumulation and expression of O^4-alkylThy in human cells remains to be established.

ACKNOWLEDGEMENTS

We highly appreciate the support of our research by the NIH (grants ES02388, ES03101, CA39397) and the USEPA (grant R812165).

REFERENCES

Abbott, P.J., and Saffhill, R., 1979, DNA synthesis with methylated poly(dC-dG) templates: Evidence for a competitive nature to miscoding by O^6-methylguanine, Biochim. Biophys. Acta, 562:51.

Adamkiewicz, J., Ahrens, O., Huh, N., Nehls, P., Rajewsky, M.F., and Spiess, E., 1984, High-affinity monoclonal antibodies for the specific recognition and quantification of deoxynucleosides structurally modified by N-nitroso compounds, IARC Sci. Publ., 581.

Ahmmed, Z., and Laval, J., 1984, Enzymatic repair of O-alkylated thymidine residues in DNA: Involvement of a O^4-methylthymine-DNA methyltransferase and a O^2-methylthymine DNA glycosylase, Biochem. Biophys. Res. Commun., 120:1.

Ames, B.N., 1979, Identifying environmental chemicals causing mutations and cancer, Science, 204:587.

Becker, R.A., and Montesano, R., 1985, Repair of O^4-methyldeoxy-thymidine residues in DNA by mammalian liver extracts, Carcinogenesis, 6:313.

Bedell, M.A., Lewis, J.G., Billings, K.C., and Swenberg, J.A., 1982, Cell specificity in hepatocarcinogenesis: Preferential accumulation of O^6-methylguanine in target cell DNA during continuous exposure of rats to 1,2-dimethylhydrazine, Cancer Res., 42:3079.

Bodell, W.J., Singer, B., Thomas, G.H., and Cleaver, J.E., 1979, Evidence for removal at different rates of O-ethyl pyrimidines and ethyl phosphotriesters in two human fibroblast cell lines, Nucleic Acids Res., 6:2819.

Bohr, V.A., and Hanawalt, P.C., 1988, DNA repair in genes, Pharmacol. Ther., 38:305.

Boyle, J.M., Durrant, L.G., Wild, C.P., Saffhill, R., and Margison, G.P., 1987, Genetic evidence for nucleotide excision repair of O^6-alkylguanine in mammalian cells, J. Cell Sci. [Suppl], 6:147.

Brennan, R.G., Pyzalska, D., Blonski, W.J., Hruska, F.E., and Sundaralingam, M., 1986, Crystal structure of the promutagen O^4-methylthymidine: importance of the anti conformation of the O^4-methoxy group and possible mispairing of O^4-methylthymidine with guanine, Biochemistry., 25:1181.

Brent, T.P., 1985, Isolation and purification of O^6-alkylguanine-DNA alkyltransferase from human leukemic cells. Prevention of chloroethylnitrosourea-induced cross-links by purified enzyme, Pharmacol. Ther., 31:121.

Brent, T.P., Dolan, M.E., Fraenkel-Conrat, H., Hall, J., Karran, P., Laval, F., Margison, G.P., Montesano, R., Pegg, A.E., Potter, P.M., Singer, B., Swenberg, J.A., and Yarosh, D.B., 1988, Repair of O-alkylpyrimidines in mammalian cells: a present consensus, Proc. Natl. Acad. Sci. USA, 85:1759.

Cairns, J., 1981, The origins of human cancers, Nature, 289:353.

Coulondre, C., and Miller, J.H., 1977, Genetic studies of the lac repressor, IV. Mutagenic specificity in the lac I gene by Escherichia coli, J. Mol. Biol., 117:577.

D'Ambrosio, S.M., Samuel, M.J., Dutta-Choudhury, T.A., and Wani, A.A., 1987, O^6-methylguanine-DNA methyltransferase in human fetal tissues: fetal and maternal factors, Cancer Res., 47:51.

D'Ambrosio, S.M., and Wani, A.A. 1989, Repair of O-alkylation damage in human cells, In: "Transformation of human diploid fibroblasts," G.E. Milo, and B. Casto, eds., CRC Press, Inc., Boca Raton.

Demple, B., Sedgwick, B., Robins, P., Totty, N., Waterfield, M.D., and Lindahl, T., 1985, Active site and complete sequence of the suicidal methyltransferase that counters alkylation mutagenesis, Proc. Natl. Acad. Sci. USA, 82:2688.

Dolan, M.E., Scicchitano, D., Singer, B., and Pegg, A.E., 1984, Comparison of repair on methylated pyrimidines in poly(dT) by extracts of rat liver and Escherichia coli, Biochem. Biophys. Res. Commun., 123:324.

Dolan, M.E., Morimoto, K., and Pegg, A.E., 1985, Reduction of O^6-alkylguanine-DNA alkyltransferase activity in HeLa cells treated with O^6-alkylguanines, Cancer Res., 45:6413.

Dolan, M.E., and Pegg, A.E., 1985, Extent of formation of O^4-methylthymidine in calf thymus DNA methylated by N-methyl-N-nitrosourea and lack of repair of this product by rat liver O^6-alkylguanine-DNA-alkyltransferase, Carcinogenesis, 6:1611.

Dolan, M.E., Scicchitano, D., and Pegg, A.E., 1988, Use of oligo-deoxynucleotides containing O^6-alkylguanine for the assay of O^6-alkylguanine-DNA-alkyltransferase activity, Cancer Res., 48:1184.

Dolan, M.E., Oplinger, M., and Pegg, A.E., 1988, Use of a dodecadeoxy-
nucleotide to study repair of O^4-methylthymine lesion, <u>Mutat.</u>
<u>Res.</u>, 193:131.

Domoradzki, J., Pegg, A.E., Dolan, M.E., Maher, V.M., and McCormick,
J.J., 1984, Correlation between O^6-methylguanine-DNA-
methyltransferase activity and resistance of human cells to the
cytotoxic and mutagenic effect of N-methyl-N'-nitro-N-nitroso-
guanidine, <u>Carcinogenesis</u>, 5:1641.

Duran, H.L., and Wani, A.A., 1987, Site-specific gap-misrepair
mutagenesis by O^4-ethylthymine, <u>Biochim. Biophys. Acta</u>,
908:60.

Dyroff, M.C., Richardson, F.C., Popp, J.A., Bedell, M.A., and Swenberg,
J.A., 1986, Correlation of O^4-ethyldeoxythymidine accumulation,
hepatic initiation and hepatocellular carcinoma induction in rats
continuously administered diethylnitrosamine, <u>Carcinogenesis</u>,
7:241.

Essigmann, J.M., Fowler, K.W., Green, C.L., and Loechler, E.L., 1985,
Extrachromosomal probes for mutagenesis by carcinogens:
studies on the mutagenic activity of O^6-methylguanine built into
a unique site in a viral genome, <u>Environ. Health Perspect.</u>,
62:171.

Hall, J., and Karran, P. 1986, Repair of DNA lesions introduced by
N-nitroso compounds, In: "Repair of DNA lesions introduced by
N-Nitroso compounds," B. Myrnes, and H. Krokan, eds.,
Norwegian University Press, Oslo. pp. 73.

Harris, C.C., and Autrup, H., 1983, "Human Carcinogenesis," Academic
Press, New York.

Huh, N., and Rajewsky, M.F., 1986, Enzymatic elimination of
O^6-ethylguanine and stability of O^4-ethylthymine in the DNA of
malignant neural cell lines exposed to N-ethyl-N-nitrosourea in
culture, <u>Carcinogenesis</u>, 7:435.

Huh, N.-H., Satoh, M.S., Shiga, J., Rajewsky, M.F., and Kuroki, T., 1989,
Immunoanalytical detection of O^4-ethylthymine in liver DNA of
individuals with or without malignant tumors, <u>Cancer Res.</u>,
49:93.

Lawley, P.D., and Thatcher, C.J., 1970, Methylation of deoxyribonucleic
acid cultured mammalian cells by N-methyl-N'-nitro-N-
nitrosoguanidine. The influence of cellular thiol concentrations
on the extent of methylation and 6-oxygen atom of guanosine as
a site of methylation, <u>Biochem. J.</u>, 116:693.

Lu, S.H., Montesano, R., Zhang, M.S., Feng, L., Luo, F.J., Chui, S.X.,
Umbenhauer, D., Saffhill, R., and Rajewsky, M.F., 1986,
Relevance of N-nitrosamines to esophageal cancer in China, <u>J.</u>
<u>Cell Physiol. [Suppl]</u>, 4:51.

Manchester, D.K., Weston, A., Choi, J.-S., Trivers, G.E., Fennessey, P.V.,
Quintana, E., Farmer, P.B., Mann, D.L., and Harris, C.C., 1988,
Detection of benzo[a]pyrene diol epoxide-DNA adducts in human
placenta, <u>Proc. Natl. Acad. Sci. USA</u>, 85:9243.

Margison, G.P., and O'Connor, P.J. 1979, Nucleic acid modification by
N-nitroso compounds, In: "Chemical Carcinogenesis and DNA,"
P.L. Grover, ed., CRC Press, Boca Raton, FL. pp. 111.

McCarthy, J.G., Edington, B.V., and Schendel, P.F., 1983, Inducible repair of phosphotriesters in *Escherichia coli*, Proc. Natl. Acad. Sci. USA, 80:7380.

McCarthy, T.V., Karran, P., and Lindahl, T., 1984, Inducible repair of O-alkylated pyrimidines in *Escherichia coli*, EMBO J., 3:545.

Montesano, R., Becker, R., Hall, J., Likhachev, A., Lu, S.H., Umbenhauer, D., and Wild, C.P., 1985, Repair of DNA alkylation adducts in mammalian cells, Biochimie., 67:919.

Moore, M.M., DeMarini, D.M., deSerres, F.J., and Tindall, K.R., 1988, Mammalian cell mutagenesis, Banbury Conference, Mutat. Res., 203:69.

Mori, T., Wani, A.A., D'Ambrosio, S.M., Chang, C.C., and Trosko, J.E., 1989, In situ pyrimidine dimer determination by laser cytometry, Photochem. Photobiol., 49:523.

Myrnes, B., Giercksky, K.E., and Krokan, H., 1983, Interindividual variation in the activity of O^6-methylguanine-DNA methyltransferase and uracil-DNA glycosylase in human organs, Carcinogenesis, 4:1565.

Nakabeppu, Y., Kondo, H., Kawabata, S., Iwanaga, S., and Sekiguchi, M., 1985, Purification and structure of the intact Ada regulatory protein of Escherichia coli K12, O^6-methylguanine-DNA methyltransferase, J. Biol. Chem., 260:7281.

Nehls, P., Rajewsky, M.F., Spiess, E., and Werner, D., 1984, Highly sensitive sites for guanine-O^6-ethylation in rat brain DNA exposed to N-ethyl-N-nitrosourea in vivo, EMBO J., 3:327.

Nehls, P., and Rajewsky, M.F., 1985, Differential formation of O^6-ethylguanine in the DNA of rat brain chromatin fibers of different folding levels exposed to N-ethyl-N-nitrosourea in vitro, Cancer Res., 45:1378.

O'Connor, P.J., Saffhill, R., and Margison, G.P. 1979, N-Nitroso compounds: Biochemical mechanisms of action, In: "Environmental carcinogenesis, occurrence, risk evaluation and mechanisms," P. Emmelot, and E. Kriek, eds., Elsevier, Amsterdam, Netherlands. pp. 73.

Olsson, M., and Lindahl, T., 1980, Repair of alkylated DNA in *Escherichia coli*. Methyl group transfer from O^6-methylguanine to a protein cysteine residue, J. Biol. Chem., 255:10569.

Perera, F.P., Hemminiki, K., Young, T.L., Brenner, D., Kelly, G., and Santella, R.M., 1988, Detection of polycyclic aromatic hydrocarbon-DNA adducts in white blood cells of foundry workers, Cancer Res., 48:2288.

Pienta, K.J., Partin, A.W., and Coffey, D.S., 1989, Cancer as a disease of DNA organization and dynamic cell structure, Cancer Res., 49:2525.

Potter, P.M., Wilkinson, M.C., Fitton, J., Carr, F.J., Brennand, J., Cooper, D.P., and Margison, G.P., 1987, Characterization and nucleotide sequence of ogt, the O^6-alkylguanine-DNA- alkyltransferase gene of *E. coli*, Nucleic. Acids. Res., 15:9177.

Preston, B.D., Singer, B., and Loeb, L.A., 1986, Mutagenic potential of O^4-methylthymine in vivo determined by an enzymatic approach to site-specific mutagenesis, Proc. Natl. Acad. Sci. USA, 83:8501.

Preston, B.D., Singer, B., and Loeb, L.A., 1987, Comparison of the relative mutagenicities of O-alkylthymines site-specifically incorporated into phiX174 DNA, J. Biol. Chem., 262:13821.

Rajewsky, M.F., Augenlicht, L.H., Biessmann, H., Goth, R., Hulser, D.F., Laerum, O.D., and Lomakina, L.Y., 1977, In: "Origins of human cancer, Book B., Mechanisms of carcinogenesis," H.H. Hiah, H.H. Watson, and J.A. Winsten, eds., New York Publishing Co., New York.

Rebeck, G.W., Coons, S., Carroll, P., and Samson, L., **1988**, A second DNA methyltransferase repair enzyme in *Escherichia coli*, Proc. Natl. Acad. Sci. USA, 85:3039.

Richardson, F.C., Dyroff, M.C., Boucheron, J.A., and Swenberg, J.A., 1985, Differential repair of O^4-alkylthymidine following exposure to methylating and ethylating hepatocarcinogens, Carcinogenesis, 6:625.

Richardson, K.K., Richardson, F.C., Crosby, R.M., Swenberg, J.A., and Skopek, T.R., 1987, DNA base changes and alkylation following in vivo exposure of *Escherichia coli* to N-methyl-N-nitrosourea or N-ethyl-N-nitrosourea, Proc. Natl. Acad. Sci. USA, 84:344.

Saffhill, R., 1984, Differences in the promutagenic nature of 3-methylcytosine as revealed by DNA and RNA polymerising enzymes, Carcinogenesis, 5:691.

Saffhill, R., 1985, In vitro miscoding of alkylthymines with DNA and RNA polymerases, Chem. Biol. Interact., 53:121.

Saffhill, R., 1986, The competitive miscoding of O^6-methylguanine and O^6-ethylguanine and the possible importance of cellular deoxynucleoside 5'-triphosphate pool sizes in mutagenesis and carcinogenesis, Biochim. Biophys. Acta, 866:53.

Saffhill, R., and Fox, M., 1980, The incorporation of O^4-methylthymidine into V79 cell DNA when present in cell culture medium, Carcinogenesis, 1:487.

Saffhill, R., Margison, G.P., and O'Connor, P.J., 1985, Mechanisms of carcinogenesis induced by alkylating agents, Biochim. Biophys. Acta, 823:111.

Sancar, A., and Sancar, G.B., 1988, DNA repair enzymes, Annu. Rev. Biochem., 57:29.

Scicchitano, D., Jones, R.A., Kuzmich, S., Gaffney, B., Lasko, D.D., Essigmann, J.M., and Pegg, A.E., 1986, Repair of oligodeoxynucleotides containing O^6-methylguanine by O^6-alkylguanine-DNA-alkyltransferase, Carcinogenesis, 7:1383.

Singer, B., 1984, Alkylation of the O^6 of guanine is only one of many chemical events that may initiate carcinogenesis, Cancer Invest., 2:233.

Singer, B., 1986, O-Alkyl pyrimidines in mutagenesis and carcinogenesis: Occurrence and significance, Cancer Res., 46:4879.

Singer, B., Bodell, W.J., Cleaver, J.E., Thomas, G.H., Rajewsky, M.F., and Thon, W., 1978, Oxygens in DNA are main targets for ethylnitrosourea in normal and xeroderma pigmentosum fibroblasts and fetal rat brain cells, Nature, 276:85.

Singer, B., and Kroger, M., 1979, Participation of modified nucleosides in translation and transcription, Prog. Nucl. Acids Res. Mol. Biol., 23:151.

Singer, B., Spengler, S.J., and Bodell, W.J., 1981, Tissue-dependent enzyme-mediated repair or removal of O-ethylpyrimidines and ethylpurines in carcinogen-treated rats, Carcinogenesis, 6:1069.

Singer, B., Sagi, J., and Kusmierek, J.T., 1983, *Escherichia coli* polymerase I can use O^2-methyldeoxythymidine or O^4-methyldeoxy-thymidine in place of deoxythymidine in primed poly(dA-dT)·poly(dA-dT) synthesis, Proc. Natl. Acad. Sci. USA, 80:4884.

Singer, B., Spengler, S.J., Chavez, F., Sagi, J., Kusmierek, J.T., Preston, B.D., and Loeb, L.A., 1987, O-Alkyl deoxythymidines are recognized by DNA polymerase I as deoxythymidine or deoxycytidine, IARC Sci. Publ., 37.

Sun, L., and Singer, B., 1975, The specificity of different classes of ethylating agents toward various sites of HeLa cell DNA in vitro and in vivo, Biochemistry, 14:1795.

Swenberg, J.A., Bedell, M.A., Billings, K.C., Umbenhauer, D.R., and Pegg, A.E., 1982, Cell-specific differences in O^6-alkylguanine DNA repair activity during continuous exposure to carcinogen, Proc. Natl. Acad. Sci., 79:5499.

Swenberg, J.A., Dyroff, M.C., Bedell, M.A., Popp, J.A., Huh, N., Kirstein, U., and Rajewsky, M.F., 1984, O^6-Ethyldeoxythymidine, but not O^6-ethyldeoxyguanosine, accumulates in hepatocyte DNA of rats exposed continuously to diethylnitrosamine, Proc. Natl. Acad. Sci. USA, 81:1692.

Swenberg, J.A., Richardson, F.C., Boucheron, J.A., and Dyroff, M.C., 1985, Relationships between DNA adduct formation and carcinogenesis, Environ. Health Perspect., 62:177.

Umbenhauer, D., Wild, C.P., Montesano, R., Saffhill, R., Boyle, J.M., Huh, N., Kirstein, U., Thomale, J., Rajewsky, M.F., and Lu, S.H., 1985, O^6-Methyldeoxyguanosine in oesophageal DNA among individuals at high risk of oesophageal cancer, Int. J. Cancer, 36:661.

Voigt, J.M., Van Houten, B., Sancar, A., and Topal, M.D., 1989, Repair of O^6-methylguanine by ABC excinuclease of *Escherichia coli* in vitro, J. Biol. Chem., 264:5172.

Wani, A., Gibson-D'Ambrosio, R.E., and D'Ambrosio, S.M., 1984, Quantitation of O^6-ethylguanosine in ENU alkylated DNA by polyclonal and monoclonal antibodies, Carcinogenesis, 5:1145.

Wani, A.A., Wani, G., and D'Ambrosio, S.M., 1985, Repair of DNA O-alkylation damage by various human organs, Biochem. Biophys. Res. Commun., 133:589.

Wani, A.A., and D'Ambrosio, S.M., 1987a, Immunological quantitation of O^6-ethylthymidine in alkylated DNA: repair of minor miscoding base in human cells, Carcinogenesis, 8:1137.

Wani, A.A., D'Ambrosio, S.M., and Alvi, N.K., 1987b, Quantitation of Pyrimidine Dimers by Immunoslot Blot Following Sublethal UV-Irradiation of Human Cells, Photochem. Photobiol., 46:477.

Wani, G., Wani, A.A., Gibson-D'Ambrosio, R.E., Samuel, M., Lowder, E., and D'Ambrosio, S.M., 1989, Absence of a DNA damage-mediated induction of human methyltransferase specific for precarcinogenic O^6-methylguanine, Teratogen. Carcinogen. Mutagen., 8:(in press).

Wild, C.P., Umbenhauer, D., Chapot, B., and Montesano, R., 1986, Monitoring of individual human exposure to aflatoxins (AF) and N-nitrosamines (NNO) by immunoassays, J. Cell Biochem., 30:171.

Yarosh, D.B., Fornace, A.J., and Day, R.S., 3rd., 1985, Human O^6-alkylguanine-DNA alkyltransferase fails to repair O^4-methylthymine and methyl phosphotriesters in DNA as efficiently as does the alkyltransferase from Escherichia coli, Carcinogenesis, 6:949.

Yarosh, D.B., Hurst-Calderone, S., Babich, M.A., and Day, R.S., 3rd., 1986, Inactivation of O^6-methylguanine-DNA methyltransferase and sensitization of human tumor cells to killing by chloroethylnitrosourea by O^6-methylguanine as a free base, Cancer Res., 46:1663.

Yu, H., Harris, R.E., Kabat, G.C., and Wynder, E.L., 1988, Cigarette smoking, alcohol consumption and primary liver cancer: A case-control study in the USA, Int. J. Cancer, 42:325.

Yuspa, S.H., Kilkenny, A.E., Roop, D.R., Strickland, J.E., Tucker, R., Hennings, H., and Jaken, S., 1989, Consequences of exposure to initiating levels of carcinogens in vitro and in vivo: Altered differentiation and growth, mutations, and transformation, Prog. Clin. Biol. Res., 298:127.

ALKYLATION REPAIR IN HUMAN TISSUES

R. Montesano, J. Hall, M. Hollstein, N. Mironov and C.P. Wild

Unit of Mechanisms of Carcinogenesis, International Agency for
Research on Cancer, 150 cours Albert Thomas, 69372 Lyon Cedex
08, France

INTRODUCTION

The first evidence of alkylation of DNA by environmental chemicals was
provided by Brookes and Lawley (1960, 1961) who showed that alkylating
mustard gas formed 7-alkylguanine in nucleic acids; mustard gas was
reported in 1946 (Auerbach and Robson) to be a chemical mutagen and
respiratory tract tumours were observed among workers involved in its
manufacture (Wada et al., 1968). The carcinogenicity of the alkylating
nitrosamine dimethylnitrosamine (DMN) was first identified in the mid 1950s
(Magee and Barnes, 1956) and in the subsequent decade the importance of DNA
alkylation in the mutagenicity and carcinogenicity of such alkylating
agents became apparent. The development of the thoughts underlying
research on carcinogenic alkylating agents have been recently described in
an interesting review by Lawley (1989).

Over this time period it also became apparent that nitrosamines occur
in a variety of environmental situations and that human exposure to such
carcinogens occurs (see Bartsch and Montesano, 1984). However, it is still
not clear which human cancers can be attributed to exposure to these
carcinogens. One of the difficulties of epidemiological studies in this
context is the lack of reliable indicators of exposure to environmental
carcinogens at the individual level. The availability of markers in
humans, such as DNA adducts attributable to exposure to carcinogens, would
greatly facilitate the ascertainment of the contribution of a given
exposure in the multifactorial and multistep process of carcinogenesis, and
could also permit the examination of the relevance in humans of these DNA
modifications to the specific cellular and molecular changes leading to the
development of cancer.

The results so far obtained in our laboratory concerning: (a) the
detection of DNA alkylation adducts in human tissues; (b) the role of DNA
repair processes in determining their levels and their biological
significance; and (c) the possible link with genetic alterations observed
in oesophageal tumours are discussed.

Abbreviations: 7-medG = 7-methyldeoxyguanosine; O^6-medG = O^6-methyldeoxy-
guanosine; 3-meAde = 3-methyladenine; O^4-meThy = O^4-methylthymidine; 3-medG
= 3-methyldeoxyguanosine; O^6-meGua = O^6-methylguanine; 7-meGua = 7-methyl-
guanine

DNA Damage and Repair in Human Tissues
Edited by B. M. Sutherland and A. D. Woodhead
Plenum Press, New York, 1990

Table 1. Measurement of Exposure to Alkylating Agents

		Relative Sensitivity*
DNA Adducts in cells/tissues		
HPLC – Immunoassay	O^6–medG; 7–medG; O–^{4}meThy; 7–meGua	<10
– ^{32}P–postlabelling	O^6–medG	<10
– Fluorescence	O^6–meGua; 7–meGua	~10^2
Immunocytochemistry	O^6–medG; 7–medG	~10^2
DNA Adducts in Urine		
Immunopurification/GC–MS	3–meAde	~10^4
Protein Adducts, e.g., haemoglobin		
GC–MS	S–methylcysteine	>10^4

*Sensitivity as defined by the lowest single dose of dimethylnitrosamine in rats (μg/kg) at which alkylation is detectable above background adduct level

DNA ALKYLATION IN HUMAN TISSUES

Following metabolism, nitrosamines induce various DNA adducts by the reaction of an alkylating intermediate with the N and O atoms of DNA bases, resulting in some 12 different adducts which include 7–medG, O^6–medG, 3–meAde and O^4–meThy. These adducts, together with the methyl–phosphotriesters, account for approximately 90% of total alkylation induced by dimethyl– or diethyl–nitrosamine (see Singer and Grunberger, 1983). During the last decade, considerable methodological advances have been made to permit the measurement of low levels of DNA adducts in human tissues with a high degree of specificity and sensitivity. These methods are based on the detection and identification of the DNA adducts using high affinity antibodies, ^{32}P–post labelling techniques, fluorescence or electrochemical detection often in combination with HPLC fractionation (see Wild and Montesano, 1990a). Table 1 shows the comparative sensitivity of these various methods for the measurement of exposure to methylating agents. The approximate sensitivity is expressed relative to the capacity of the method to detect DNA– or protein–methylation adducts in rats after treatment with a single dose of DMN (see Figure 1b). Using immunoassays or ^{32}P–postlabelling techniques combined with HPLC fractionation, various DNA methylated adducts induced by a dose of 10 μg/kg or less can be detected in tissues, whereas currently fluorescence detection has an approximately 10 times lower sensitivity. Immunocytochemistry employing antibodies against O^6–medG or 7–medG has also a similar lower sensitivity. However, this method has the advantage of identifying, in a heterogenous cellular population of a given tissue, cells that are preferentially alkylated and is a method which is potentially applicable to a variety of human tissue/cell specimens. The measurement of 3–meAde in urine or of S–methyl cysteine in haemoglobin as markers of exposure to methylating agents is strongly limited by the relatively high background levels of these DNA–, protein–adducts in human body fluids.

Figure 1 shows the levels of O^6-medG in various human tissues of individuals originating from populations at different risks of certain cancers, from individuals treated with methylating chemotherapeutic drugs or exposed to toxic doses of DMN (for more details see Umbenhauer et al., 1985; Wild and Montesano, 1990a; Herron and Shank, 1980). The results for samples containing detectable levels of O^6-medG are expressed as fmole O^6-medG/mg DNA or number of adducts/parent nucleotide and ranged from approximately 1 adduct/10^8 (limit of detection) to more than 1 adduct/10^3. In oesophageal DNA, some suggestion of a higher frequency of positive samples and higher levels of O^6-medG was found in individuals from Linxian County (People's Republic of China) or Normandy (France), regions at high incidence of oesophageal cancer, compared to a low incidence area, The Rhone (France). No such differences were evident in the case of stomach tissues. These differences in the oesophageal samples, however, are based on a limited number of samples from The Rhone and Normandy and further analyses are ongoing. It is interesting that similar observations have been made by Saffhill et al. (1988) concerning the higher frequency of positive samples in high incidence areas of oesophageal cancer. Higher levels of O^6-medG were detected in some samples of placenta (Foiles et al., 1988) and oral mucosa (Wild et al., 1989). Except for the cases of acute DMN poisoning and the patients treated with chemotherapeutic agents, the nature of exposure responsible for the presence of O^6-medG in human tissues is not known, although various methylating nitrosamines have been reported in food samples from Linxian County (Singer et al., 1986).

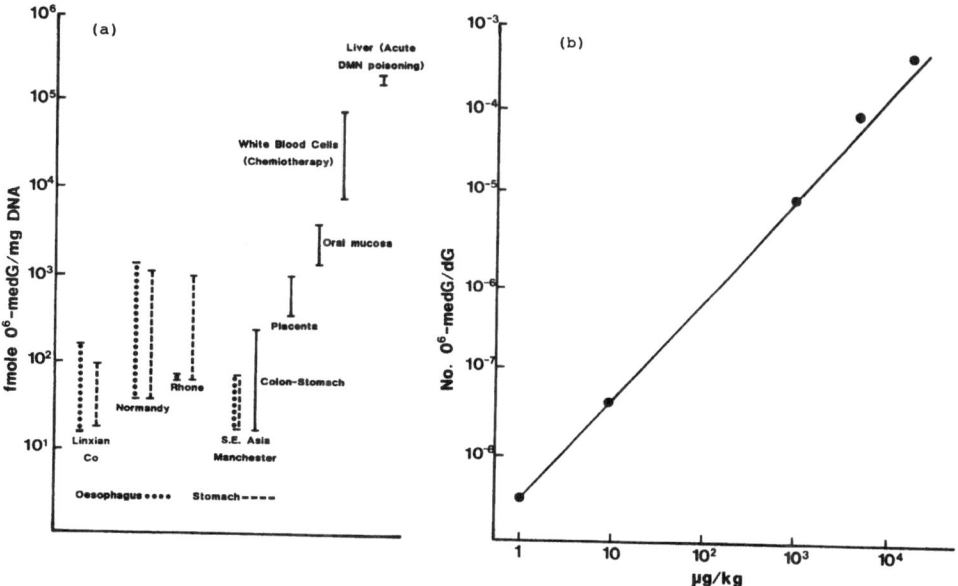

Legend to Figure 1: Levels of O^6-medG in human tissues (a) (Wild and Montesano, 1990a; Saffhill et al., 1988; Foiles et al., 1988; Herron and Shank, 1980) and in rat liver (b) exposed to single doses of DMN (Pegg and Hui, 1978).

In order to put these levels of methylation in human tissues in perspective, Figure 1b shows the levels of O^6-medG occurring in rat liver DNA after a single dose of DMN (Pegg and Hui, 1978). The level detected in most human tissues correspond to the DNA alkylation produced by a dose of approximately 10 to 100 µg/kg. Whilst it is evident that these two sets of data cannot be compared directly, it does indicate that the level of DNA alkylation observed in human tissues corresponds roughly to what one might expect from exposure to environmental methylating nitrosamines as has been discussed by Preussmann et al. (1979; see also Montesano et al., 1988).

The data collected so far have been limited by tissue availability and consequently the possibility to detect DNA alkylation adducts in peripheral blood cells (see below) would both facilitate these efforts to examine the link between a given environmental exposure and adduct formation and in addition it would permit a more valuable randomized comparison of the prevalence and level of DNA adducts among different populations. Towards this end, antibodies against the more abundant and persistent adduct 7-medG have been developed and validated (Degan et al., 1988). In experimental animals it has been shown that the level of 7-medG observed in peripheral blood cell-DNA correlates well with the level detected in liver DNA after treatment with both DMN and procarbazine (see Wild and Montesano, 1990b). Preliminary data in humans using immunoassay show that the levels in peripheral blood cell DNA range from non-detectable (<1 µmole 7-medG/mole dT) to 49 µmole/mole and higher values have been observed in some other human tissues. Studies are in progress to identify the source of exogenous or endogenous methylating agents and to exclude, using other complementary methodologies, the possible contribution in such determinations of 7-methylguanosine which is a normal constituent of t-RNA at levels of around 3.5 mmoles 7-methylguanosine per mole ribonucleosides.

REPAIR OF DNA ALKYLATION DAMAGE IN HUMAN TISSUES

The level of DNA adducts detected in humans is not only dependent upon the degree of exposure to alkylating agents but also on the capacity of a given tissue or cell to repair such adducts. In bacteria and mammalian cells each DNA alkylation adduct is repaired by specific DNA repair processes, whose activity varies from species to species and between different cell types.

The alkylated purines 7-meGua, 3-meAde and 3-meGua are removed from DNA by a direct cleavage of the glycosylic bond catalysed by a DNA glycosylase. This enzyme has been identified and characterised from a variety of mammalian cells and tissue types (reviewed Helland et al., 1987). Its preferred substrate is double stranded methylated DNA (Gallagher and Brent, 1984) and 3-meAde is more efficiently repaired than 7-meGua or 3-meGua. This glycosylase also shows activity towards the ethylated N-3 and N-7 purines but with a lower efficiency than the methylated adducts (Singer and Brent, 1981).

The O^6-alkylguanine-DNA alkyltransferase (AT) found in mammalian cells (see Yarosh, 1985) and those of E. coli (the ada+ and ogt+ gene products) (see Lindahl et al., 1988) have many properties in common, although they differ somewhat in their substrate specificity. Their mode of action involves the stoichiometric transfer of the alkyl group from the O^6-position of guanine to a cysteine receptor residue within the enzyme, resulting in the irreversible inactivation of the enzyme and restoration of the DNA structure. The AT has a greater activity on double stranded DNA than on denatured or single stranded DNA (Pegg et al., 1983; Harris et al., 1983) and exhibits a greater affinity towards short rather than long

Table 2. Repair of DNA Alkylation Adducts in Human and Rodent Tissues

Tissue		O^6-methylguanine-DNA methyltransferase[a]	Glycosylase[a]	
			3-meAde	7-meGua
Human liver	(15)[b]	1443 (710-2790)	1189 (520-2320)	22 (0-131)
Human oesophagus	(24)[c]	308 (87-481)	NT	NT
Human peripheral blood lymphocytes	(25)	370 (160-670)	NT	NT
Human placenta	(14)	73 (50-108)	NT	NT
Human stomach	(15)	199 (81-257)	NT	NT
Rat liver	(5)	130 (112-163)	536 (381-718)	37 (31-43)
Hamster liver	(8)	199 (88-298)	614 (315-946)	59 (34-111)

[a] fmol/mg protein (range of values)
[b] ( ) number of independent samples tested
[c] Tumour and non-tumour tissues
NT Not Tested

chain alkyl adducts (methyl >> ethyl, n-propyl > n-butyl > isopropyl, isobutyl > 2-hydroxyethyl), (Morimoto et al., 1985). O^6-Chloroethylguanine and O^6, N^1-ethanoguanine, the cross-link precursors formed by the clinically used bifunctional alkylating anti-cancer drugs, such as chloroethylnitrosourea are also repaired (Brent, 1986). In cells the AT level can be depleted by growth in the presence of low concentrations of MNNG, (Yarosh et al., 1984), the free base O^6-meGua or in the presence of O^6-meGua containing t-RNA (Karran, 1985).

In mammalian tissues and cells in culture treated with alkylating agents, the O-alkylpyrimidines (O^2 and O^4-alkylthymine and O^2-alkylcytosine) are lost from cellular DNA at rates higher than explicable by cell turnover and chemical instability. The exact nature of these repair processes in mammalian cells remains unclear. In E. coli, O^2-meC and O^2-meThy are repaired by the alkA$^+$ gene product, a multifunctional glycosylase and O^4-meThy by the ada$^+$ and ogt$^+$ gene products. The mammalian counterparts of these enzymes have not been clearly demonstrated to repair these lesions by the same mechanisms (reviewed Brent et al., 1988). Alternative pathways for the in vivo repair of O^6-alkylguanine and O^4-alkylthymine involving nucleotide excision repair have been demonstrated in E. coli (Samson et al., 1988) and have been implicated in the repair of O^6-butyldeoxyguanosine in human cells (Boyle et al., 1986). The involvement of such pathways in the repair of O-alkylpyrimidines in mammalian cells remains to be clarified.

Table 2 shows the activity of these two repair processes (AT and glycosylase) in various human tissues as compared to rat or hamster liver.

The AT was higher in the liver than in the other tissues and humans consistently show higher activity than other species. Liver of all three species shows a low capacity of repair 7-medG. These results, as well as the high degree of individual variation, are consistent with previous observations from different laboratories including ours (Hall et al., 1985; Gerson et al., 1986; Waldstein et al, 1982; Sagher et al. 1988).

It should be noted, however, that the data in Table 2 represent the DNA repair activity of a heterogeneous cell population, that differences in activities that could be present among the various cell population of a given tissue will have been averaged out. Belinsky et al. (1987) have shown that in rats treated with NNK, a tobacco specific nitrosamine, the level of O^6-medG in Clara cells of the lung is as much as 40 times higher than in other lung cells. In the liver of rats treated with DMN non-parenchymal cells (mainly haemangioendothelial cells) have a much lower capacity to repair O^6-medG than parenchymal liver cells and it is of interest that the great majority of tumours that develop in the liver of rats treated chronically with DMN are haemangioendothelial sarcomas (Planche-Martel et al., 1985). These two examples illustrate that the determination of the repair capacity or DNA adduct levels in the organ as a whole provide at best a limited picture. Immunohistochemical determinations of DNA adducts in frozen or fixed tissue sections would be particularly informative in this respect and would permit access to large sources of human tissue already collected and stored for other purposes. Immunohistochemical determinations of DNA adducts at the cellular level have been carried out in various experimental systems (for example, Menkveld et al., 1985; Huitfeldt et al., 1988; Nemoto et al., 1988; Wild et al., 1990) and studies are in progress in several laboratories to improve the sensitivity for their applicability to human tissue specimens.

It is of interest to determine in the same tissue sample the presence of these DNA adducts as well as the level of DNA repair enzymes responsible for their removal. However, in many instances the limited amount of tissue available undermines such determinations. Radioactively labelled methylated DNA has been used as a substrate to measure DNA repair activities. However, more recently, oligodeoxynucleotides containing single modifications such as O^6-medG and O^4-meThy have become available and shown to be substrates for AT (Scicchitano et al., 1986; Graves et al., 1987). Labelling the oligodeoxynucleotides with ^{32}P and separating the methylated and demethylated substrates by HPLC after reaction with protein extracts containing AT have provided a more sensitive approach where only small amounts of biological samples are available (Dolan et al., 1988). The availability of sensitive and highly specific antibodies recognising O^6-medG and O^4-meThy permits by immunoprecipitation the separation of the alkylated oligodeoxynucleotides from the unmodified ones. This approach is far more rapid than when the reaction products are separated by chromatography. This technique for AT measurement, requiring minute amounts of tissue, makes the assay applicable to large-scale epidemiological or clinical studies and suggests that a similar methodology could be applied for other DNA repair enzymes (Mironov et al., 1989).

ADAPTIVE RESPONSE IN MAMMALIAN CELLS AND CONTROL OF ENZYME SYNTHESIS

The repair of DNA methylation damage in E. coli involves four specific enzymes. Two are constitutively expressed (the tag⁺ and the ogt⁺ genes) and two which are inducible as part of the adaptive response to alkylating agents (the alkA⁺ and ada⁺ genes). Exposure of E. coli to non-toxic levels of MNNG induces the adaptive response which confers resistance to the killing and mutagenic effects of MNNG (Samson and Cairns, 1977). Chronic administration of DMN to rats increases the capacity of the liver to repair

O^6-medG (Montesano et al., 1979). This induction can be caused in rats by many different treatments (partial hepatectomy, nonalkylating hepatotoxins, ionising radiation) (see Saffill et al., 1985) and an induction of the uracil and 3-methyladenine DNA glycosylase has been demonstrated during cell proliferation (Gombar et al., 1981). The existence in human cells of a DNA repair response analogous to the adaptive response in E. coli is disputed (Yarosh, 1985) and with the possible exception of hepatocytes (Laval and Laval, 1984) human cells do not augment their repair capacity when exposed to methylating agents. As the AT is inactivated during the repair process and there is no apparent mechanism for the regeneration of the cysteine acceptor site, new protein must be synthesised prior to removal of additional or residual O^6-alkylG adducts. Therefore, not only the constitutive levels of the repair enzyme but the rate of resynthesis of the protein may be a critical factor in the ability of a tissue to repair the promutagenic damage prior to cell replication, and thus critically affecting the mutagenic and carcinogenic response. These phenomena of inactivation and subsequent recovery of AT following a single dose of DMN have been studied in rat and hamster liver and it can be seen that there are distinct species differences (Hall et al., unpublished).

BIOLOGICAL CONSEQUENCES OF DNA ALKYLATION/POINT MUTATION

While the relationship between alkylation adducts and the occurrence of specific mutations in DNA has been appreciated for some time (Samson and Cairns, 1977; Ellison et al., 1989), only recently has it become clear by what mechanism the induced mutations may contribute to the carcinogenic process. DNA alkylation leads to mispairing of bases, and the mutagenic activity of alkylating agents correlates with carcinogenic activity of the chemical in vivo, but this outline of a plausible pathway in carcinogenesis leaves a gap between the presence of the mutation in precancerous cells and the appearance of the transformed phenotype.

Experimental work of the last decade has identified loci in the human genome that may be the biologically relevant targets of DNA-damaging carcinogens. Oncogenes and tumour suppressor genes are transcribed regions of DNA whose protein products regulate cell growth and differentiation and can cause malignant transformation of cells when altered. It is also becoming evident that multiple genetic alterations are occurring during the development of cancer leading to fully malignant tumours (Baker et al., 1989; Harris et al., this publication). Furthermore, the transforming gene lesions found both in human cancers and in experimentally-induced animal tumours are, in some cases, DNA base substitutions such as those resulting from alkylated DNA. The most notable example of induction of transforming activity by point mutation comes from studies on the ras oncogene family. A single base change in one of three principal codons (12, 13, 61) of the H, K, or N ras gene can confer transforming properties to the p21 protein products. In the pioneering work of Barbacid and co-workers, it was shown that 90% of mammary tumours induced in rats by a single exposure to methylnitrosourea (NMU) had a transforming H-ras allele, all with an identical mutation, a G to A transition at codon 12 (61 tumours out of 61 tumours) (Zarbl et al., 1985), whereas an A to T transversion at codon 61 of the Ha-ras gene was found in mammary tumours induced by 7,12-dimethylbenz(a)anthracene (Dandekar et al., 1986), a carcinogen known to bind preferentially to adenine. These experiments provide evidence that carcinogen-specific mutations are a critical step in chemical induction of animal tumours in certain experimental models (see Barbacid, 1987). In the study of mammary tumours in NMU-exposed rats the consistent activating mutation was predictable since O^6-medG is known to give rise to G to A mutation (see Mitra et al., 1989).

Molecular biology techniques at the time of the first studies on oncogene activation in chemically-induced animal tumours did not permit empirical exclusion of the formal possibility that treatment protocols favour selective growth and malignant transformation of cells in which the specific mutation had arisen spontaneously. Current highly sensitive methods for detection of mutant cells at the single cell level now have made this a subject of intensive investigation (Kumar and Barbacid, 1988; Hollstein, personal communications).

Molecular analysis of oncogenes in human tumours supports the notion from animal experiments that ras genes are one target of chemicals that cause genetic damage and cancer. Transforming ras genes, activated by a single point mutation, have been identified in approximately 20% of human tumours, though the frequency of this lesion varies widely when the tumours are grouped according to anatomical site or cell type, from 0% (stomach carcinomas) to 50% (colon carcinomas) to 95% (pancreatic cancer) (Bos, 1988, 1989). We can imagine that the extent of ras involvement may thus depend on a variety of factors, in some instances on DNA repair capacity of the tissue or cell type, metabolic characteristics, differentiation state, the chemistry of environmmental and dietary carcinogens and their interaction with DNA and so on. It has been noted, for example, that the predominant mutation in transforming ras alleles found in human colon tumours is a G to A transition, prompting the speculation that these mutations arose as a consequence of exposure to environmental alkylating agents (Bos, 1989), reminiscent of NMU induction of mammary tumours in rats.

If environmental carcinogens that cause miscoding DNA adducts are responsible for the high incidence of specific cancers in certain geographical regions, we might expect that the prevalence of a specific activating ras mutation for that type of cancer could vary among series of samples from patients residing in different areas where different aetiological agents had been singled out by epidemiological surveys. However, data indicating a correlation in humans between a given type of exposure and the prevalence of a genetic change (point mutation, deletion, amplification, etc.) is rather limited.

Since human exposure to DNA alkylating agents has been associated with an elevated risk of oesophageal cancer in the high incidence areas of Linxian County, People's Republic of China, and Normandy, France, we tested 25 oesophageal tumours from patients, half of whom reside in Normandy, and half in the Lyon area, for presence of activating mutations in codons 12, 13 and 61 of the H, K and N-ras genes, as these are the sites where mutations can render this gene family transforming. The analysis was performed with the PCR/oligonucleotide hybridisation technique, and did not reveal any ras mutations in either group of samples tested (Hollstein et al., 1988). Other investigators reported that oesophageal carcinomas from patients residing in Linxian, People's Republic of China, have no transforming codon 12 mutations in the H or K-ras genes (Jiang et al., 1989). We have thus far no example to suggest that ras activation by point mutation can be a contributing lesion towards the development of squamous cell carcinomas of the oesophagus in humans, in which case investigations on the effects of environmental carcinogens on geographical patterns of ras gene activation may be more informative with cancers in which ras mutations have been found. Human studies to date show a conspicuous absence of ras mutations in human cancers of the breast, oesophagus, and in cervical carcinomas (Bos, 1989). It is possible that for these tumours environmental agents affect critical genes other than ras.

Cellular oncogene alterations associated with human cancers are not restricted to point mutations (Bishop, 1987) and in fact, the most

Table 3. Genetic Alterations in Oesophageal and Cervical Cancers[1]

The information contained in the boxes refers to the positive changes observed and the value in parenthesis indicates the approximate percentage of tumours with the change observed in a given set of samples.

	Allele loss	Oncogene amplification	Oncogene activation
Oesophageal carcinoma		hst-1, int-2 (45%) erbB-1 (15%) c-myc (15%) K-ras (10%)	H-, K- and N-ras
		erbB-2 H- and N-ras	
Cervical carcinoma	3p (100%)	H-, K-, N-ras hst-1, int-2 erbB-1, erbB-2 c-myc	ras

[1]Hollstein et al., 1988; unpublished data; Lu et al., 1988; Tsuda et al., 1989; Tsutsumi et al., 1988; Yokota et al., 1989; Jiang et al., 1989.

frequently observed oncogene structural alteration in human tumour DNA is gene amplification, with the caveat that: (a) amplification is one of the anomalies most easily assayed technically and, therefore, one of the most frequently tested for; and (b) an amplified gene is not necessarily contributing to the transformed phenotype; it may be a secondary event or adjacent to a second gene in the amplicon that is affecting growth behaviour, for example. In oesophageal tumours from France, we have found (Hollstein et al., unpublished data) amplification (45% of tumours positive) of the hst-1 gene coding for a protein with similarities to fibroblast growth factors, and less frequent though greater-fold amplification of the cellular homologue of the erbB oncogene, coding for the epidermal growth factor receptor (EGFR). Our results concur with results of previous studies on hst amplification in tumour samples from patients residing in Japan (Tsutsumi et al., 1988; Tsuda et al., 1988). It may be that hst 1/int2 (apparently co-amplified; Tsutsumi et al., 1988; Tsuda et al., in press) and EGFR oncogene amplification (also detected in tumours from The People's Republic of China; Lu et al., 1988) are constant features of oesophageal squamous cell carcinomas, and are related to more advanced stages of the disease. For comparison, Table 3 shows also the genetic alterations reported by other investigators for cervical carcinoma, another squamous cell tumour. Whether environmental exposures contribute to the prevalence of these lesions is unclear. Laboratory experiments have shown that many carcinogens, in addition to their properties as point mutagens via base modification and subsequent mispairing, also are recombinogenic (Schiestl, 1989), and cause gene amplification (Lavi, 1981;

Heilbronn et al., 1985; Zur Hausen et al., 1987) though the exact biochemical steps in these molecular events are less precisely understood than, e.g., G to A mutations induced by methylation at the O^6- position of guanine.

PERSPECTIVES

Biochemical-molecular epidemiology during the last decade has been mainly devoted to the development and validation of methods that could be integrated into epidemiological studies. It is now apparent that sensitive and specific methods to detect human exposures at the individual level are available and that some of these methods could be applied to field epidemiological studies. Such information on exposure now needs to be related to the occurrence of mutations and other genetic alterations that appear relevant to cancer development. Studies of this type are not yet available.

Methods are now available to detect mutations in humans that are applicable to field studies (see Albertini et al., this publication). Molecular epidemiology at the level of human oncogenes is in its infancy, but promises to offer important information on mechanisms of human carcinogenesis. It is not possible at this point to guess which oncogenes and what molecular alterations will segregate with geographical patterns of cancer incidence nor for which cancers such correlations will arise. It would be of interest to know whether or not the molecular steps leading to a particular cancer are generally the same in different regions of the world. Does the environment modulate these events, and can human exposure to specific carcinogenic compounds elicit particular molecular events in cancer genes, as animal experiments suggest?

Without detailed comprehensive studies of the type discussed in this paper, the information can be quite misleading. Mutations in the ras gene have become relatively easy to assay because the transforming biologically relevant alterations are localised. With the polymerase chain reaction/denaturing gradient gel electrophoresis (PCR/DGGE) technique (Myers et al., 1987) and other sophisticated approaches, we now have tools to learn more about transforming mutations that may be anywhere within a section of a coding sequence (e.g., as appears to be the case for the p53 tumour suppressor gene) and about events such as recombination or small deletions leading to altered function of an oncogene. These genetic alterations may occur more frequently in human cancers than we are aware of at present.

Another interesting development is that various immunological and molecular probes are becoming available that permit the determination at the cellular level of many of the alterations discussed above at the cellular level (DNA damage and subsequent induced mutations, altered oncogenic or viral proteins, regulation of DNA repair enzymes). The examination of the accumulation and interrelationships of such events in a given cell should provide valuable insight in the understanding of the carcinogenesis process.

ACKNOWLEDGEMENTS

These studies were partly supported by USA NIEHS Grant No. 5 U01 ES04281-02 and CEC Contract No EV4V 0040-F (CD).

References

Auerbach, C. and Robson, J.M., 1946, Chemical production of mutations, Nature, 157:302.

Baker, S.J., Fearon, E.R., Nigro, J.M., Hamilton, S.R., Preisinger, A.C., Jessup, J.M., VanTuinen, P., Ledbetter, D.H., Barker, D.F., Nakamura, Y., White, R. and Vogelstein, B., 1989, Chromosome 17 deletions and p53 gene mutations in colorectal carcinomas, Science, 244:217-221.

Barbacid, M., 1987, Ras genes, Ann. Rev. Biochem., 56:779-827.

Bartsch, H. and Montesano, R., 1984, Relevance of nitrosamines to human cancer, Carcinogenesis, 5:1381-1393.

Belinsky, S.A., White, C.M., Devereux, T.R., Swenberg, J.A., Anderson, M.W., 1987, Cell selective alkylation of DNA in rat lung following low dose exposure to the tobacco specific carcinogen 4-(N-methyl-N-nitrosamino)-1-(3-pyridyl)-1-butanone, Cancer Res., 47:1143-1148.

Bishop, J.M., 1987, The molecular genetics of cancer, Science, 235:305-311.

Bos, J., 1988, The ras gene family and human carcinogenesis. Mutat. Res., 195:255-271

Bos, J.L., 1989, ras oncogenes in human cancer: a review. Cancer Res., 49:4682-4689

Boyle, J.M., Margison, G.P. and Saffhill, R., 1986, Evidence for the excision repair of 0^6-n-butyldeoxyguanosine in human cells, Carcinogenesis, 7:1987-1990.

Brent, T.P., 1986, Inactivation of purified human 0^6-alkylguanine-DNA alkyltransferase by alkylating agents or alkylated DNA, Cancer Res., 46:2320-2323.

Brent, T.P., Dolan, M.E., Fraenkel-Conrat, H., Hall, J., Karran, P., Laval, F., Margison, G.P., Montesano, R., Pegg, A.E., Potter, P.M., Singer, B., Swenberg, J.A. and Yarosh, D.B., 1988, Repair of 0-alkylpyrimidines in mammalian cells: a present consensus, Proc. Natl. Acad. Sci. USA, 85:1759-1762.

Brookes, P. and Lawley, P.D., 1960, The reaction of mustard gas with nucleic acids in vitro and in vivo, Biochem J., 77:478-484.

Brookes, P. and Lawley, P.D., 1961, The reaction of mono- and di-functional alkylating agents with nucleic acids, Biochem. J., 80:496-503.

Dandekar, S., Sukumar, S., Zarbl, H., Young, L.J.T. and Cardiff, R.D., 1986, Specific activation of the cellular Harvey-ras oncogene in dimethylbenzanthracene-induced mouse mammary tumors. Molec. Cell. Biol., 6:4104-4108.

Degan, P., Montesano, R. and Wild, C.P., 1988, Antibodies against 7-methyldeoxyguanosine: its detection in peripheral blood lymphocyte DNA and potential applications to molecular epidemiology, Cancer Res., 48:5065-5071.

Dolan, M.E., Schicchitano, D. and Pegg, A.E., 1988, Use of oligodeoxynucleotides containing O^6-alkylguanine for the assay of O^6-alkylguanine-DNA-alkyltransferase activity, Cancer Res. 48:1184-1188.

Ellison, K.S., Dogliotti, E., Connors, T.d., Basu, A.K. and Essigmann, J.M., 1989, Site-specific mutagenesis by O^6-alkylguanines located in the chromosomes of mammalian cells: influence of the mammalian O^6-alkylguanine-DNA alkyltransferase, Proc. Natl. Acad. Sci. USA, 86:8620-8624.

Foiles, P.G., Miglietta, L.M., Akerkar, S.A., Everson, R.B. and Hecht, S.S., 1988, Detection of O^6-Methyldeoxyguanosine in human placental DNA, Cancer Res., 48:4184-4188.

Gallagher, P. E. and Brent, T.P., 1984, Further purification and characterisation of human 3-methyladenine DNA glycosylase. Evidence for broad specificity, Biochem. Biophys. Acta., 782:394-401.

Gerson, S.L., Trey, J.E., Miller, K. and Berger, N.A., 1986, Comparison of O^6-alkylguanine-DNA alkyltransferase activity based on cellular DNA content in human, rat and mouse tissues, Carcinogenesis, 7:745-749.

Gombar, C.T., Katz, E.J., Magee, P.N. and Sirover, M.A., 1981, Induction of the DNA repair enzymes uracil DNA glycosylase and 3-methyladenine DNA glycosylase in regenerating rat liver, Carcinogenesis, 2:595-599.

Graves, R.J., Li, B.F.L. and Swann, P.F., 1987, in: "Relevance of N-Nitroso Compounds to Human Cancer: Exposures and Mechanisms" H. Bartsch, I.K. O'Neill, and R. Shulte-Hermann, eds., IARC Scientific Publications No. 84, pp 41-43, International Agency for Research on Cancer, Lyon.

Hall, J., Brésil, H. and Montesano, R., 1985, O^6-alkylguanine DNA alkyltransferase activity in monkey, human and rat liver, Carcinogenesis, 6:209-211.

Harris, A.L., Karran, P. and Lindahl, T., 1983, O^6-Methylguanine-DNA methyltransferase of human lymphoid cells: structural and kinetic properties and absence in repair-deficient cells, Cancer Res., 43:3247-3252.

Heilbronn, R., Schlehofer, J.R., Yalkinoglu, A.O. and Zur Hausen, H., 1985, Selective DNA-amplification induced by carcinogens (initiators): evidence for a role of proteases and DNA polymerase alpha. Int. J. Cancer, 36:85-91.

Helland, D.E., Male, R., Haukanes, B.I., Olsen, L., Haugan, I. and Kleppe, K., 1987, Properties and mechanism of action of eukaryotic 3-methyladenine-DNA glycosylases, J. Cell. Sci. Suppl. 6:139-146.

Herron, D.C. and Shank, R.C., 1980, Methylated purine in human liver DNA after probable dimethylnitrosamine poisoning, Cancer Res., 40:3116-3117.

Hollstein, M.C., Smits, A.M., Galiana, C., Yamasaki, H., Bos, J.L., Mandard, A., Partensky, C. and Montesano, R., 1988, Amplification of epidermal growth factor receptor gene but no evidence of ras mutations in primary human esophageal cancers, Cancer Res., 48:5119-5123.

Huitfeldt, H.S., Sprangler, E.F., Hunt, J.M. and Poirier, M.C., 1988, Immunohistochemical localisation of DNA adducts in rat liver tissue and phenotypically altered foci during oral administration of 2-acetylaminofluorene, Carcinogenesis, 7:123-129.

Jiang, W. et al, 1989, Rapid detection of ras oncogenes in human tumors: applications to colon, esophageal and gastric cancer. Oncogene, 4:923-928.

Karran, P., 1985, Possible depletion of a DNA repair enzyme in human lymphoma cells by subversive repair, Proc. Natl. Acad. Sci. USA, 82:5285-5289.

Kumar, R. and Barbacid, M., 1988, Oncogene detection at the single cell level. Oncogene, 3: 647-651.

Laval, F. and Laval, J., 1984, Adaptive response in mammalian cells: cross reactivity of diferent pretreatments oncytotoxicity as contrasted to mutagenicity, Proc. Natl. Acad. Sci. USA, 81:1062-1066.

Lavi, S., 1981, Carcinogen-Omediated amplification of viral DNA sequences in simiabn virus 40-transformed Chinese hamster embryo cells, Proc. Natl. Acad. Sci. USA, 68:6144-6148.

Lawley, P.D., 1989, Mutagens as carcinogens: development of current concepts. Mutat. Res., 213:3-25.

Lindahl, T., Sedgwick, B., Sekiguchi, M. and Nakabeppu, Y., 1988, Regulation and expression of the adaptive response to alkylating agents, Ann. Rev. Biochem., 57: 133-157.

Lu, S.-H., Hsieh, L.-L., Luo, F.-C. and Weinstein, I.B., 1988, Amplification of the EGF receptor and c-myc genes in human esophageal cancers, Int. J. Cancer, 42:502-505.

Magee, P.H. and Barnes, J.M., 1956, The production of malignant primary hepatic tumors in the rat by feeding dimethylnitrosamine, Br. J. Cancer, 10:114-122.

Menkveld, G.J., Van der Laken, C.J., Hermsen, T., Kriek, E., Scherer, E. and Den Engelse, L., 1985, Immunohistochemical localization of O^6-ethyldeoxy-guanosine and deoxyguanosin-8-yl-(acetyl)aminofluorene in liver sections of rats treated with diethylnitrosamine, ethylnitrosourea or N-acetyl-aminofluorene, Carcinogenesis, 6:263-270.

Mironov, N.M., Wild, C.P., Martel-Planche, G., Swann, P.F. and Montesano, R., 1989, Measurement of the removal of O^6-methylguanine and O^4-methylthymine from oligodeoxynucleotides using an immunoprecipitation technique, Anal. Biochem., 183:74-79.

Mitra, G., Pauly, G.T., Kumar, R., Pei, G.K., Hughes, S.H., Moschel, R.C. and Barbacid, M., 1989, Molecular analysis of O6-substituted guanine-induced mutagenesis of ras oncogenes, Proc. Natl. Acad. Sci. USA, 86:8650-8654.

Montesano, R., Brésil, H. and Margison, G.P., 1979, Increased excision of
    O^6-methylguanine from rat liver DNA after chronic administration of
    dimethylnitrosamine, Cancer Res., 39:1789-1802.

Montesano, R., Brésil, H., Degan, P., Martel-Planche, G., Serres, M. and
    Wild, C.P., Detection in human cells of alkylated macromolecules
    attributable to exposure to nitrosamines, IARC Scientific
    Publications No. 89, Lyon, pp. 75-82.

Morimoto, K., Dolan, M.E., Scicchitano, D. and Pegg, A.E., 1985, Repair of
    O^6-propylguanine and O^6-butylguanine in DNA by O^6-alkylguanine-DNA
    alkyltransferases from rat liver and E. coli, Carcinogenesis,
    6:1027-1031.

Myers, R.M., Maniatis, T. and Lehrman, L.S., 1987, Methods in Enzymol.,
    155:501-527.

Nemoto, N., Nakatsuru, Y., Nakagawa, A. and Ishikawa, T., 1988,
    Immunohistochemical detection of anti(±)trans-7,8-dihydroxy-9,10-
    epoxy-7,8,9,10-tetrahydrobenzo(a)pyrene-bound adduct in nuclei of
    cultured HeLa cells and mouse lung tissue, J. Cancer Res., Clin.
    Oncol., 114:225-230.

Pegg, A.E. and Hui, G., 1978, Formation and subsequent removal of
    O^6-methylguanine from deoxyribonucleic acid in rat liver and kidney
    after small doses of dimethylnitrosamine, Biochem. J., 173:739-748.

Pegg, A.E., Wiest, L., Foote, R.S., Mitra, S. and Perry, W., 1983,
    Purification and propertis o O^6-methylguanine-DNA transmethylase
    from rat liver, J. Biol. Chem., 258:2327-2333.

Planche-Martel, Likhachev, A., Wild, C.P. and Montesano, R., 1985,
    Modulation of repair of O^6-methylguanine in parenchymal and
    nonparenchymal liver cells of rats treated with
    dimethylnitrosamine, Cancer Res., 45:4768-4773.

Preussmann, R., Spiegelhalder, B., Eisenbrand, G., and Janzowiski, C.,
    1979, N-Nitroso compounds in foods, in: Naturally Occurring
    Carcinogens, Mutagens and Modulators of Carcinogenesis,
    E.C. Miller, J.A. Miller, I. Hirono, T. Sugimura, and S. Takayama,
    eds., Japanese Scientific Societies Press, Tokyo, pp. 185-194.

Saffhill, R., Margison, G.P. and O'Connor, P.J., 1985, Mechanisms of
    carcinogenesis induced by alkylating agents, Biochim. Biophys.
    Acta., 823:111-145.

Saffhill, R., Badawi, A.F. and Hall, C.N., 1988, Detection of
    O^6-methylguanine in human DNA, IARC Scientific Publications No. 89,
    301-305.

Sagher, D., Karrison, T., Schwartz, L., Larson, R., Meier, P. and Strauss,
    B., 1988, Low O^6-alkylguanine DNA alkyltransferase activity in the
    peripheral blood lymphocytes of patients with therapy-related acute
    nonlymphocytic leukemia, Cancer Res., 48:3084-3089.

Samson, L. and Cairns, J., 1977, A new pathway for DNA repair in
    Escherichia choli, Nature (Lond.), 267:281-282.

Samson, L., Thomale, J. and Rajewsky, M.F., 1988, Alternative pathways for

the in vivo repair of 06-alkylguanine and 04-alkylthymine in
Escheria coli: the adaptive response and nucleotide excision
repair, EMBO J, 7:2261-2267.

Schiestl, R., 1989, Non-mutagenic carcinogens induced intrachromosomal
recombination in yeast, Nature, 337:285-288.

Scicchitano, D., Jones, R.A., Kuzmich, S., Gaffney, B., Lasko, D.D.,
Essigmann, J.M. and Pegg, A.E., 1986, Repair of oligodeoxynucleotides containing 06-methylguanine by 06-alkylguanine-DNA-
alkyltransferase, Carcinogenesis, 7:1383-1386.

Singer, B. and Brent, T.P., 1981, Human lymphoblasts contain DNA
glycosylase activity excising N-3 and N-7 methyl and ethyl purines
but not 06-alkylguanines or 1-alkyladenines, Proc. Natl. Acad. Sci.
USA, 78:856-860.

Singer, B. and Grunberger, D., 1983, "Molecular Biology of Mutagens and
Carcinogens," Plenum Press, New York & London.

Singer, G.M., Chuan, J., Roman, J., Min-Hsin Li and Lijinsky, W., 1986,
Nitrosamines and nitrosamine precursors in foods from Linxian,
China, a high incidence area for esophageal cancer, Carcinogenesis,
7:733-736.

Tsuda, T. et al, 1988, Amplification of the hst-1 gene in human esophageal
carcinomas. Jpn. J. Cancer Res., 79: 584-588.

Tsuda, T., Tahara, E., Kajiyama, G., Sakamoto, H., Terada, M. and Sugimura,
T., 1989, High incidence of coamplification of hst-1 and int-2
genes in human esophageal carcinomas, Cancer Res., 49:5505-5508.

Tsutsumi, M. et al., 1988, Coamplification of the hst-1 and int-2 genes in
human cancers. Jpn. J. Cancer Res., 79:428-432.

Umbenhauer, D., Wild, C.P., Montesano, R., Saffhill, R., Boyle, J.M., Huh,
N., Kirstein, U., Thomale, J., Rajewsky, M.F. and Lu, S.H., 1985,
06-Methyldeoxyguanosine in oesophageal DNA among individuals at
high risk of oesophageal cancer, Int. J. Cancer, 36, 661-665.

Waldstein, E.A., Cao., E.-H., Bender, M.A. and Setlow, R.B., 1982,
Abilities of extracts of human lymphocytes to remove
06-methylguanine from DNA, Mut. Res., 95:405-416.

Wada, S., Miyanashi, M., Nishimoto, Y., Kambe, S. and Miller, R.W., 1968,
Mustard gas as a cause of respiratory neoplasia in man, Lancet,
i:1161-1163.

Wild, C.P., Stich, H.F. and Montesano, R., 1989, Presence of alkylated DNA
in oral mucosal cells from cigarette smokers, Proc. Am. Assoc.
Cancer Res., 30:318.

Wild, C.P., Montesano, R., Van Benthem, J., Scherer, E. and Den Engelse,
L., 1990, Intercellular variation in aflatoxin B1 and G1 DNA adduct
levels in rat tissues: a quantitative immunocytochemical study, J.
Cancer Res. Clin. Oncol., in press.

Wild, C.P. and Montesano, R., 1990a, Detection of alkylated DNA adducts in
human tissues, in: Molecular Dosimetry of Human Cancer:
Epidemiological, Analytical and Social Considerations, P.L. Skipper
and J.D. Groopman, eds., Telford Press, in press

Wild, C.P. and Montesano, R., 1990b, Evaluation of the immunological quantitation of human exposure to aflatoxins (AF) and N-nitrosamines (NNO) in epidemiological studies, in: Immunochemical Methods for Monitoring Human Exposure to Toxic Chemicals in Foods and the Environment, Pacifichem '89, Marcel Dekker Inc., in press.

Yarosh, D.B., 1985, The role of O^6-methylguanine-DNA methyltransferase in cell survival, mutagenesis and carcinogenesis, Mutat. Res., 145:1-16.

Yarosh, D.B., Rice, M., Day, R.S., Foote, R.S. and Mitra, S., 1984, O^6-Methylguanine-DNA methyltransferase in human cells, Mutat. Res., 131:27-36.

Yokota, J., Tsukada, Y., Nakajima, T., Gotoh, M., Shimosato, Y., Mori, N., Tsunokawa, Y., Sugimura, T. and Terada, M., 1989, Loss of heterozygosity on the short arm of chromosome 3 in carcinoma of the uterine cervix, Cancer Res, 49:3598-3601.

Zarbl, H., Sukumar, S., Arthur, A.V., Martin-Zanca, D. and Barbacid, M., 1985, Direct mutagenesis of Ha-ras-1 oncogenes by N-nitroso-N-methylurea during initiation of mammary carcinogenesis in rats. Nature, 315:382.

Zur Hausen et al. (eds), 1987, The role of gene amplification in tumor initiation and promotion, Lippincott, New York.

ALBERTINI, Richard J.
 Genetics Lab.
 Dept. of Neurology
 U. of Vermont
 32 N. Prospect Street
 Burlington, VT 05401
ALVI, Nasir
 American Health Foundation
 1 Dana Road
 Valhalla, NY 10595

BAAN, Robert A.
 Dept. of Genetic Toxicol.
 Prins Maurits Lab. TNO
 MBL-TNO
 P.O. Box 46
 2280 AA Rijswijk
 The Netherlands
BEER, Janusz
 Radiation Biology Branch
 Food and Drug Administration
 12709 Twinbrook Parkway
 Rockville, MD 20857
BENNETT, Paula
 Biology Dept.
 Brookhaven Natl. Lab.
 Upton, NY 11973
BERGER, Cheryl A.
 Veterans Administration
  Med. Ctr.
 Portland Div.
 3710 SW U.S. Veterans
  Hospital Road
 P.O. Box 1034, 11C2-P
 Portland, OR 97207
BERGTOLD, David S.
 Natl. Inst. of Standards
  and Tech.
 Building 245, Room C-214
 Gaithersburg, MD 20899

BREDBERG, Anders
 Dept. of Med. Microbiol.
 U. of Lund
 Malmo General Hospital
 S-214 01 Malmo, Sweden
BREITENSTEIN, Jr., Bryce D.
 Occupational Medicine Clinic
 Brookhaven Natl. Lab.
 Upton, NY 11973

CALACE, Judith
 Biology Dept.
 Brookhaven Natl. Lab.
 Upton, NY 11973
CALHOUN, Cornelia
 SRI International
 333 Ravenwood Avenue
 Menlo Park, CA 94025
CHEN, Chun-Zhang
 Biology Dept.
 Brookhaven Natl. Lab.
 Upton, NY 11973
CHEN, Yen-Hui
 Dept. of Pharmacol.
 Health Sciences Ctr.
 State U. of New York
 Stony Brook, NY 11794
CHRISTIE, Nelwyn
 Dept. of Environmental Med.
 New York U.
 Box 817
 Tuxedo, NY 10987
CMARIK, Joan L.
 Dept. of Biochem. and Ctr.
  in Molec. Toxicol.
 Vanderbilt U.
 Nashville, TN 37215
COOGAN, Timothy P.
 N.Y. U. Med. Ctr.
 Inst. of Environmental
  Medicine
 Long Meadow Road
 Tuxedo, NY 10987

CORTESI, Roger
Office of Res. and
Development
U.S. Environmental Protection
Agency
401 M Street, S.W.
Washington, DC 20460

D'AMBROSIO, Steven M.
Div. of Radiobiol.
Dept. of Radiol.
Ohio State U.
103 Wiseman Hall
400 W. 12th Avenue
Columbus, OH 43210-1214
DE GRUIJL, Frank
Academic Hospital Utrecht
Heidelberglaan 100
P.O. Box 85500
3508 GA Utrecht
The Netherlands
DUNN, John J.
Biology Dept.
Brookhaven Natl. Lab.
Upton, NY 11973

EFTEDAL, Ingrid
Dept. of Dermatol.
Faculty of Med. in Trondheim
Unigen
prof. Brochs gt. 6
N-7030 Trondheim, Norway
EMRICK, Ann M.
Biology Dept.
Brookhaven Natl. Lab.
Upton, NY 11973
EVANS, Michele K.
Dept. of Health and Human
Services
Public Health Service
Natl. Inst. of Health
Building 37, Room 5A-19
Bethesda, MD 20892

FRANCE, Louisa L.
Biology Dept.
Brookhaven Natl. Lab.
Upton, NY 11973
FREEMAN, Steven E.
Res. Div.
Lovelace Medical Foundation
2425 Ridgecrest Drive, S.E.
Albuquerque, NM 87108

GASPARRO, Francis P.
Photobiol. Lab.
Yale U.
333 Cedar Street
New Haven, CT 06510
GORELICK, Nancy
Proctor and Gamble Company
P.O. Box 398707
Cincinnati, OH 45239-8707
GRIST, Eleanor
Biology Dept.
Brookhaven Natl. Lab.
Upton, NY 11973
GUENGERICH, F. Peter
Dept. of Biochem. and Ctr.
in Molec. Toxicol.
Vanderbilt U.
Nashville, TN 37232

HACHAM, Haim
Biology Dept.
Brookhaven Natl. Lab.
Upton, NY 11973
HALL, Janet
Intl. Agency for Res.
on Cancer
150 Cours Albert Thomas
69372 Lyon Cedex 08, France
HARRIS, Curtis C.
Lab. of Human Carcinogenesis
Natl. Cancer Inst.
Natl. Inst. of Health
Building 37, Room 2C09
9000 Rockville Pike
Bethesda, MD 20892
HELLAND, Dag
c/o W. Haseltine
Dana-Farber Cancer Inst.
44 Binney Street
Boston, MA 02142
HIRSCH, Betsy
Div. of Cytogenetics
and Genetics
U. of Minnesota
400 Church Street, S.E.
Minneapolis, MN 55455
HÖNIGSMANN, Herbert
Div. of Photobiol.
Dept. of Dermatol. I.
U. of Vienna
Alser Strasse 4
A-1090 Vienna, Austria

JORGENSEN, Timothy J.
Dept. of Radiat. Med.
Georgetown U. Sch. of Med.
3800 Reservoir Road
Washington, DC 20007

KANTOR, George J.
 Dept. of Biol. Sci.
 Wright State U.
 Dayton, OH 45435
KANJILAL, Sagarika
 Dept. of Molec. and
  Cell. Biol.
 Box 155, 108 Althouse
 Pennsylvania State U.
 State College, PA 16801
KASMAN, Krystyna
 Estee Lauder
 125 Pinelawn Road
 Melville, NY 11747
KIM, D-H.
 Dept. of Biochem. and Ctr.
  in Molec. Toxicol.
 Vanderbilt U.
 Nashville, TN 37232
KOCHEVAR, Irene
 Dept. of Dermatol.
 Wellman Lab.
 Harvard Medical School\
 Massachusetts General Hospital
 Boston, MA 02114
KRAEMER, Kenneth H.
 Natl. Cancer Inst.
 Natl. Inst. of Health
 Building 37, Room 3E-24
 9000 Rockville Pike
 Bethesda, MD 20892
KRAJCIK, Rozlyn
 Dept. of Biol. Sci.
 Wright State U.
 Dayton, OH 45435
KROKAN, Hans E.
 Unigen-Ctr. for Molec. Biol.
 Inst. of Biotech.
 U. of Trondheim
 prof. Brochs gt. 6
 N-7030 Trondheim, Norway
KYRTOPOULOS, Soterios A.
 Biol. Res. Ctr.
 Natl. Hellenic Res.
  Foundation
 48, Vas. Constantinou Avenue
 Athens, 116 35 Greece

LACKS, Sanford A.
 Biology Dept.
 Brookhaven Natl. Lab.
 Upton, NY 11973
LARCOM, Lydon L.
 Dept. of Phys. and Microbiol.
 Clemson U.
 Clemson, SC 29634-1911

LEE, Byung Mu
 Dept. of Environmental
  Health Sciences
 Johns Hopkins Sch. of Hygiene
  and Public Health
 Room 2708
 615 N. Wolfe Street
 Baltimore, MD 21205
LI, Bao Hui
 Indiana U. Sch. of Med., and
  Beijing Ctr. Hygiene and
  Epidemic Control
 Microbiology
 Indiana U. Med. Ctr.
 635 Barnhill Drive
 Indianapolis, IN 46223
LU, Xiaoqing
 Apt. 26D
 60 Haven Avenue
 New York, NY 10032
LUTZE, Louise H.
 Lab. of Radiobiol. and
  Environmental Health - LR102
 U. of California
 San Francisco, CA 94143

MADDEN, John J.
 Depts. of Psychiatry and
  Biochem.
 Emory U.
 Atlanta, GA 30322
MAMMONE, Tom
 Estee Lauder
 125 Pinelawn Road
 Melville, NY 11747
MATSUMOTO, Yoshihiro
 Basic Health Sciences
 Tower 8, Room 140
 State U. of New York
 Stony Brook, NY 11794-8651
MAYTIN, Edward V.
 Dept. of Dermatol.
 Wellman Lab. of Photomed. - 2
 Massachusetts General Hospital
 Fruit Street
 Boston, MA 02114
McGRATH, William J.
 Biology Dept.
 Brookhaven Natl. Lab.
 Upton, NY 11973
MONTELEONE, Denise C.
 Biology Dept.
 Brookhaven Natl. Lab.
 Upton, NY 11973
MONTESANO, Ruggero
 Unit of Mechanisms of
  Carcinogenesis
 Intl. Agency for Res. on Cancer
 150 Cours Albert Thomas
 69372 Lyon Cedex 08, France

455

MYHR, Brian
Dept. of Molec. and
   Cell. Toxicol.
Hazleton Lab. Amer., Inc.
Suite 400
5516 Nicholson Lane
Kensington, MD 20895

NEEL, James V.
Dept. of Human Genetics
Box 0618
U. of Michigan Med. Sch.
Ann Arbor, MI 48109-0618

OLSEN, Lisbeth Charlotte
Lab. of Biotech.
U. of Bergen
P.O. Box 3152
Arstad
N-5001 Bergen, Norway

POIRIER, Miriam C.
Natl. Cancer Inst.
Natl. Inst. of Health
Building 37, Room 3B-25
9000 Rockville Pike
Bethesda, MD 20892
PRESTON, R. Julian
Biol. Div.
P.O. Box Y
Oak Ridge Natl. Lab.
Oak Ridge, TN 37831

QUAITE, Florence E.
Biology Dept.
Brookhaven Natl. Lab.
Upton, NY 11973

RANDERATH, Kurt
Div. of Toxicol.
Dept. of Pharmacol.
Baylor Col. of Med.
One Baylor Plaza
Houston, TX 77030
RANDESI, Matthew
Biology Dept.
Brookhaven Natl. Lab.
Upton, NY 11973

REED, Eddie
Div. of Cancer Treatment
Natl. Cancer Inst.
Natl. Inst. of Health
Building 10, Room 6N-119
Bethesda, MD 20892
RIBEIRO, Eldred A.
Biology Dept.
Brookhaven Natl. Lab.
Upton, NY 11973
RITHIDECH, Kanokporn
Medical Dept.
Brookhaven Natl. Lab.
Upton, NY 11973
ROBISON, Steven H.
RCC - Genetics Lab.
U. of Vermont
32 N. Prospect Street
Burlington, VT 05401
ROTHMAN, Nathaniel
Dept. of Environmental
   Health Sciences
Johns Hopkins Sch. of Hygiene
   and Public Health
615 N. Wolfe Street
Baltimore, MD 21205

SANTELLA, Regina M.
Div. of Environmental Sci.
Columbia U.
650 W. 168th Street
New York, NY 10032
SCICCHITANO, David
American Health Foundation
1 Dana Road
Valhalla, NY 10595
SETLOW, Neva
Biology Dept.
Brookhaven Natl. Lab.
Upton, NY 11973
SETLOW, Richard B.
Biology Dept.
Brookhaven Natl. Lab.
Upton, NY 11973
SHIH, Alice
Biology Dept.
Brookhaven Natl. Lab.
Upton, NY 11973
SHIOTA, Susumu
Biology Div.
P.O. Box 2009
Oak Ridge Natl. Lab.
Oak Ridge, TN 37831
SLATKIN, Daniel N.
Medical Dept.
Brookhaven Natl. Lab.
Upton, NY 11973

STRAUSS, Bernard S.
 Depts. of Molec. Genetics
  and Cell Biol.
 U. of Chicago
 920 E. 58th Street
 Chicago, IL 60637
STRICKLAND, Paul T.
 Dept. of Environmental
  Health Sci.
 Johns Hopkins Med. Inst.
 615 N. Wolfe Street
 Baltimore, MD 21205
STUDIER, F. William
 Biology Dept.
 Brookhaven Natl. Lab.
 Upton, NY 11973
SUTHERLAND, Betsy M.
 Biology Dept.
 Brookhaven Natl. Lab.
 Upton, NY 11973
SUTHERLAND, John C.
 Biology Dept.
 Brookhaven Natl. Lab.
 Upton, NY 11973

TAICHMAN, Lorne B.
 Dept. of Oral Biol.
  and Pathol.
 Sch. of Dental Med.
 State U. of New York
 Stony Brook, NY 11794-8702
TANO, Keizo
 Biol. Div.
 P.O. Box 2009
 Oak Ridge Natl. Lab.
 Oak Ridge, TN 37831
TICE, Raymond R.
 Integrated Laboratory Systems
 P.O. Box 13501
 Research Triangle Park, NC 27709
TRUNK, John
 Biology Dept.
 Brookhaven Natl. Lab.
 Upton, NY 11973
TSIMIS, Jeannie
 Applied Genetics, Inc.
 205 Buffalo Avenue
 Freeport, NY 11520
TURTURRO, Angelo
 Dept. of Health Educ.
  and Welfare
 Public Health Service
 Food and Drug Administration
 Natl. Ctr. for Toxicol. Res.
 Jefferson, AR 72079

URBACH, Frederick
 Temple U. Sch. of Med.
 Philadelphia, PA 19140

VILPO, Juhani A.
 Dept. of Clinical Chem.
 Tampere U. Central Hospital
 SF-33520 Tampere, Finland

WANG, Gian Ping
 Dept. of Geriatrics
 Mount Sinai Med. Ctr.
 Box 1070
 One Gustave L. Levy Place
 New York, NY 10029
WANI, A. A.
 Div. of Radiobiol.
 Dept. of Radiol.
 Ohio State U.
 103 Wiseman Hall
 400 W. 12th Avenue
 Columbus, OH 43210
WANI, Maqsood
 Div. of Radiobiol.
 Dept. of Radiol.
 Ohio State U.
 103 Wiseman Hall
 400 W. 12th Avenue
 Columbus, OH 43210
WESTON, Ainsley
 Lab. of Human Carcinogenesis
 Natl. Cancer Inst.
 Natl. Inst. of Health
 Building 37, Room 2C-09
 9000 Rockville Pike
 Bethesda, MD 20892
WHITTLE, Edward J.
 Biology Dept.
 Brookhaven Natl. Lab.
 Upton, NY 11973
WOODHEAD, Avril D.
 Biology Dept.
 Brookhaven Natl. Lab.
 Upton, NY 11973

YAROSH, Daniel
 Applied Genetics, Inc.
 205 Buffalo Avenue
 Freeport, NY 11520
YOUNG, Antony R.
 Photobiology Unit
 Inst. of Dermatol.
 U. of London
 London SE 11 4th
 England

457